*Quick Reference to*
# Surgical
# Emergencies

# *Quick Reference to*
# Surgical
# Emergencies

*edited by*

## Gerald W. Shaftan, M.D.
*Professor of Surgery, State University of New York*
*Downstate Medical Center*
*Chief of the Trauma Service*
*Kings County Hospital Center*
*Brooklyn, New York*

*and*

## Bernard Gardner, M.D.
*Professor of Surgery*
*State University of New York*
*Downstate Medical Center*
*Chief of the Oncology Service*
*Kings County Hospital Center*
*Brooklyn, New York*

**with 29 Contributors**

## J. B. Lippincott Company
**Philadelphia and Toronto**

ISBN 0–397–50307–5

Library of Congress Catalog Card Number 74–1379

Printed in the United States of America

3   4   2

**Library of Congress Cataloging in Publication Data**

Shaftan, Gerald W
  Quick reference to surgical emergencies.

  1. Diagnosis, Surgical.   2. Medical emergencies.
I. Gardner, Bernard, joint author.   II. Title.
[DNLM:   1. Emergencies.   2. Surgery, Operative.
WO700 S525q 1974]
RD35.S53     617′.026     74-1379
ISBN 0–397–50307–5

# CONTRIBUTORS

**Bertram E. Bromberg, M.D.**
*Professor of Surgery*
*Division of Plastic Surgery*
*State University of New York*
*Downstate Medical Center*
*Chief, Division of Plastic Surgery*
*Kings County Hospital Center*
*Brooklyn, New York*

**Henry Burns, M.D.**
*Clinical Assistant Professor of Surgery*
*State University of New York*
*Downstate Medical Center*
*Visiting Attending*
*Kings County Hospital Center*
*Brooklyn, New York*

**Maurice L. Cohen, M.D.**
*Instructor of Surgery*
*State University of New York*
*Downstate Medical Center*
*Associate Attending Brooklyn Eye and Ear Hospital*
*Chief, Section of Otolaryngology*
*Brooklyn Cumberland Medical Center*
*Brooklyn, New York*

**Albert W. Cook, M.D.**
*Professor and Chairman*
*Department of Neurosurgery*
*State University of New York*
*Downstate Medical Center*
*Chief, Department of Neurosurgery*
*Kings County Hospital Center*
*Brooklyn, New York*

**Clarence Dennis, M.D.**
*Professor Emeritus*
*Department of Surgery*
*State University of New York*
*Downstate Medical Center*
*Brooklyn, New York*

**Bernard Gardner, M.D.**
*Professor of Surgery*
*State University of New York*
*Downstate Medical Center*
*Chief, Oncology Service*
*Kings County Hospital Center*
*Brooklyn, New York*

**Michael R. Golding, M.D.**
*Assistant Professor of Surgery*
*State University of New York*
*Downstate Medical Center*
*Active Attending*
*Kings County Hospital Center*
*Brooklyn, New York*

**David Harshaw, M.D.**
*Assistant Professor of Surgery*
*State University of New York*
*Downstate Medical Center*
*Active Attending*
*Kings County Hospital Center*
*Brooklyn, New York*

**Horace Herbsman, M.D.**
*Associate Professor of Surgery*
*State University of New York*
*Downstate Medical Center*
*Active Attending*
*Kings County Hospital Center*
*Brooklyn, New York*

**Karl E. Karlson, M.D.**
*Professor of Medical Sciences (Surgery)*
*Brown University*
*Surgeon-in-Chief, Thoracic and Cardiovascular Surgery*
*Rhode Island Hospital*
*Providence, Rhode Island*

**Donald Klotz, M.D.**
*Assistant Professor of Surgery*
*State University of New York*
*Downstate Medical Center*
*Associate Chief of Pediatric Surgery*
*Kings County Hospital Center*
*Brooklyn, New York*

**Peter K. Kottmeier, M.D.**
*Professor of Surgery*
*State University of New York*
*Downstate Medical Center*
*Chief of Pediatric Surgery*
*Kings County Hospital Center*
*Brooklyn, New York*

**Leroy S. Lavine, M.D.**
*Professor of Surgery*
*State University of New York*
*Downstate Medical Center*
*Chief, Division of Orthopedic Surgery*
*Kings County Hospital Center*
*Brooklyn, New York*

**Irving Lustrin, M.D.**
*Clinical Instructor of Surgery*
*Division of Orthopedic Surgery*
*State University of New York*
*Downstate Medical Center*
*Visiting Attending*
*Division of Orthopedic Surgery*
*Kings County Hospital Center*
*Brooklyn, New York*

**Michael J. McAlvanah, M.D.**
*Assistant Professor of Surgery*
*State University of New York*
*Downstate Medical Center*
*Active Attending*
*Kings County Hospital Center*
*Brooklyn, New York*

**Ralph Milliken, M.D.**
*Assistant Clinical Professor of*
*Anesthesiology*
*Mt. Sinai School of Medicine*
*of the City University of New York*
*Adjunct Assistant Professor*
*Health Care Administration*
*Baruch College, Graduate Division*
*City University of New York*
*New York, New York*

**Manfreds Munters, M.D.**
*Assistant Professor of Surgery*
*Division of Orthopedic Surgery*
*State University of New York*
*Downstate Medical Center*
*Active Attending*
*Kings County Hospital Center*
*Brooklyn, New York*

**Umeschandra B. Patil, M.D.**
*Assistant Professor*
*Department of Urology*
*State University of New York*
*Downstate Medical Center*
*Active Attending*
*Department of Urology*
*Kings County Hospital Center*
*Brooklyn, New York*

**Martin R. Protell, D.D.S.**
*Clinical Associate Professor*
*Department of Oral Diagnosis and*
*Radiography*
*College of Medicine and Dentistry of*
*New Jersey*
*Jersey City, New Jersey*

**Jack Rabinowitz, M.D.**
*Professor of Radiology*
*State University of New York*
*Downstate Medical Center*
*Chief, Department of Radiology*
*Kings County Hospital Center*
*Brooklyn, New York*

**J. Gordon Rubin, D.D.S.**
*Director, Dental Department*
*Hillside Hospital Division*
*Long Island Jewish Hillside Medical*
*Center*
*Glen Oaks, New York*

**Walter H. Rubins, M.D.**
*Clinical Instructor of Surgery*
*Division of Orthopedic Surgery*
*State University of New York*
*Downstate Medical Center*
*Visiting Attending*
*Division of Orthopedic Surgery*
*Kings County Hospital Center*
*Brooklyn, New York*

**Philip N. Sawyer, M.D.**
*Professor of Surgery*
*State University of New York*
*Downstate Medical Center*
*Chief, Vascular Surgery*
*Kings County Hospital Center*
*Brooklyn, New York*


**Gerald W. Shaftan, M.D.**
*Professor of Surgery*
*State University of New York*
*Downstate Medical Center*
*Chief, Trauma Service*
*Kings County Hospital Center*
*Brooklyn, New York*


**In-Chul Song, M.D.**
*Assistant Professor of Surgery*
*Division of Plastic Surgery*
*State University of New York*
*Downstate Medical Center*
*Associate Chief, Division of*
*Plastic Surgery*
*Kings County Hospital Center*
*Brooklyn, New York*


**Robert R. Sparacio, M.D.**
*Assistant Professor*
*Department of Neurosurgery*
*State University of New York*
*Downstate Medical Center*
*Active Attending*
*Kings County Hospital Center*
*Brooklyn, New York*


**S. S. Giovinda Swamy, M.D.**
*Assistant Attending*
*Brooklyn Eye and Ear Hospital*
*Brooklyn, New York*


**Bruno J. Urban, M.D.**
*Associate Professor, Department of*
*Anesthesiology*
*Duke University Medical Center*
*Durham, North Carolina*


**R. Keith Waterhouse, M.D.**
*Professor and Chairman*
*Department of Urology*
*State University of New York*
*Downstate Medical Center*
*Chief, Department of Urology*
*Kings County Hospital Center*
*Brooklyn, New York*


**Stanley W. Weitzner, M.D.**
*Professor, Department of Anesthesiology*
*State University of New York*
*Downstate Medical Center*
*Active Attending, Department of*
*Anesthesiology*
*Kings County Hospital Center*
*Brooklyn, New York*


**Donald E. Willard, M.D.**
*Assistant Professor of Surgery*
*Division of Opthalmology*
*State University of New York*
*Downstate Medical Center*
*Active Attending, Division of*
*Opthalmology*
*Kings County Hospital Center*
*Brooklyn, New York*


**Julian Zweig, M.D.**
*Assistant Professor of Surgery*
*State University of New York*
*Downstate Medical Center*
*Visiting Attending, Kings County Hospital*
*Center*
*Brooklyn, New York*

# PREFACE

A surgical emergency is an acute illness that traditionally has been treated by a surgeon. Emergency operation may or may not be part of the initial or even definitive care of such an emergency, because the scope of surgery has progressed far beyond the operating room. Emergency surgery, therefore, encompasses a wide variety of conditions for which operative treatment may be unnecessary, although the possibility that operation may be needed as part of the definitive treatment requires early involvement by a surgeon in the decisions and plan of action for a successful end result.

Recent wartime experience has pointed out the increased survival and lowered morbidity that are seen when prompt and vigorous resuscitation and treatment have been instituted for acute trauma. Improvement in the rapid transportation of acutely ill patients in civilian circumstances, as well as the increasing availability of well-equipped emergency departments manned by full-time physicians, should provide a similar decrease in civilian morbidity and mortality.

The Kings County Hospital Center is a 2,300-bed general and psychiatric hospital with 600 acute and subacute surgical beds. A large adult emergency department, which treated 187,022 patients in 1972, is manned, full-time, by attending physicians and house staff, specially trained nurses and paramedical personnel, and supplemented by a large ambulance service. There also are separate pediatric and psychiatric emergency departments with similar staffing. Of the 15,653 surgical admissions in 1972, well over 50 per cent were acute. Emergency operations represent 30 per cent of the total operative experience at our institution. A separate trauma service of 100 beds provides teaching experience to house staff under the direction of four full-time surgeons.

This book is dedicated to those physicians who may, whether in the hospital emergency department or in their offices, be faced at some time with an acute surgical emergency. It is designed to supplement their knowledge and sharpen and systemize their approach to evaluate, diagnose and give early treatment to a wide range of emergency surgical conditions.

Each of the authors has had an extensive experience in his field of expertise. The presentations are made in a format designed to allow quick reference to the condition at hand, detailing the salient features in diagnosis and treatment. In order to facilitate the understanding of both diagnosis and treatment, most chapters include a section on basic principles which provides a description of the underlying physiology, including the development of symptoms and the effects of the condition on the patient's homeostasis. The book is not intended as an encyclopedia of acute surgical conditions or as a textbook, but primarily as a quick and accurate quide to the necessary treatment of a patient often prior to the involvement of an experienced consultant. Therefore, extensive details of operative techniques are not included except as they may be needed for emergency care. However, brief descriptions of applicable operations *are* included where they may be useful to understand the direction and extent of initial emergency treatment, and postoperative management frequently is described.

Pediatric surgical emergencies have become an increasingly large portion of emergency practice. At the Kings County Hospital Center, which has, as noted, a separate pediatric emergency department, approximately 2,000 pediatric surgical emergencies are seen each month (almost one third of the total surgical emergency department visits). Since any physician may be required to face such a problem, a large section on pediatric surgical emergencies in included, which is considered to be a valuable addition to the book.

The authors and editors join in the anticipation that this book will meet an urgent need by family physicians, emergency physicians, nurses, paramedical personnel and medical students—in fact, all who deal with acutely ill patients.

Gerald W. Shaftan, M.D.
Bernard Gardner, M.D.

# CONTENTS

*Quick Reference to*
# Surgical
# Emergencies

# 1. EVALUATION OF THE ACUTELY INJURED PATIENT

*Gerald W. Shaftan,* M.D.

## Definitions

1. *The Traumatized Patient.* This is a patient injured by one or a combination of external noxious forces such as impact, deceleration, missile, thermal or chemical. The fact that these forces are external differentiates the pathology produced by them from all other disease entities (i.e., pneumonia, acute tubular necrosis), although these disease entities may subsequently be seen in a patient injury following the pathophysiologic derangements produced by the external noxious forces on the body.

2. *Management.* This term includes both the recognition and the treatment of the injury.

3 *Treatment.* This is broadly divided into:

   A. *Emergency care* of the injury to prevent increase in tissue destruction.

   B. *Definitive treatment* aimed at assisting final tissue repair and functional restoration.

## Basic Principles

1. The initial phase in the management of the injured patient is the maintenance of life-support systems. Emergency lifesaving necessarily precedes the examination of the traumatized patient. During this initial period of treatment, observation of signs with changing character, such as neurologic or abdominal findings, may be of prognostic significance and must be noted and recorded. Once immediate survival of the patient is achieved, definitive assessment of injuries and treatment may begin.

2. Priorities in management must always be salvage of:

   A. Life

   B. Limb

   C. Function

   D. Cosmesis

## Criteria for Diagnosis

1. History of injury

2. Physical evidence of trauma (*see* below)

3. Unconsciousness is considered traumatic in origin until this is disproven.

## Management

### Emergency Lifesaving

1. *Ensure Patent Airway and Ventilation.* Effective alveolar gas exchange depends on the ability of the thoracic cage to contract and expand, squeezing air out of and sucking it back into the relatively passive pulmonary parenchyma. The defects in the recently injured patient may result from:

   A. *Blockage of Upper Airway.* This is handled by an oral or nasotracheal airway or intubation, depending on the level of obstruction. Tracheostomy, except in desperate situations where intubation is impossible, is not proper at this time.

   B. *Loss of Normal Ventilatory Mechanisms.* Failure to ventilate is due in this instance to loss of lung volume because of the space-occupying pleural air or fluid or disruption of the continuity of the thoracic osseous or diaphragmatic muscular bellows. Institution of external ventilation even with severe simple pneumothorax will provide necessary life support and can be done with mouth-to-mouth, mask-and-bag or mechanical ventilators (*see* Chap. 7, Cardiopulmonary Resuscitation). Nasoric intubation will prevent gastric distention, as well as evacuating the stomach in preparation for operation.

2. *Maintain Circulation.* Circulatory assist is discussed in Chapter 7, Cardiopulmonary Resuscitation.

The control of external bleeding is most easily accomplished by clamping the bleeding vessels, direct pressure or the use of a tourniquet in distal extremity wounds. The rapid control of hemorrhage will conserve intravascular volume, which will help maintain circulation.

3. *Institute the Treatment of Shock.*

A. Shock may be recognized clinically, despite its multiple etiologies, by the presence of arterial hypotension with tachycardia resulting in a rapid, thready pulse, mental confusion or sense of impending doom, sweating, pallor and weakness.

B. Inadequate tissue perfusion is a physiologic hallmark of shock at the cellular level. An indwelling bladder catheter will provide evidence of continued renal function, a measure of tissue perfusion, as well as evidence of injury to the genitourinary system.

C. Shock may be hypovolemic—a decrease in the total volume of circulating blood; neurogenic—an increase in the venous vascular capacity; septic—similarly with an increase in the venous capacity plus comparatively obscure mechanisms permitting capillary sequestration; or cardiogenic—e.g., central pump failure as seen following myocardial infarction.

D. In most cases of trauma, the type of shock is hypovolemic, with loss of blood and colloid rather than crystalloid. However, documentation of the movement of fluid into a third space soon after injury provides a rationale for the utilization of balanced saline solution for initial resuscitation while blood is being obtained.

E. Although the maintenance of an adequate cardiac filling pressure, as evidenced by a normal or slightly elevated central venous pressure, is generally indicative of adequate vascular refilling and serially may be a satisfactory guide to the replacement of lost volume, the reversal of the clinical signs of shock is the desired end point of treatment.

F. Intravenous infusion is started with a percutaneous large bore needle or cannula. Even with peripheral venous collapse this is usually accomplished in the upper extremities, although in some instances temporary femoral vein infusion may be necessary. Surgical cutdown cannulation should be done if necessary in multiple trauma patients to provide at least two large-caliber catheters in the upper extremities, one of which is in the superior vena cava.

4. *Evaluation of the State of Consciousness.* Although not part of emergency lifesaving itself, assessment of neurologic signs at each stage of management will permit assessment of the changing character of these signs for the diagnosis of neurosurgical emergencies (*see* Chap. 20, Acute Craniocerebral Injuries).

5. *Summary of Emergency Management*

A. Ensure or institute ventilation.

B. Maintain circulation.

C. Draw blood for crossmatching and typing, baseline chemistries and hematocrit.

D. Place an intravenous line or lines—at least one intravenous line in central venous position.

E. Start a rapid infusion of 5% dextrose in lactated Ringer's solution, followed by colloid (salt-poor albumin or dextran, the latter not to exceed 1,000 ml.), as clinically indicated.

F. Transfuse with crossmatched blood if time permits; otherwise transfuse with type-specific blood, rarely with low-titer type O Rh negative blood; again clinical judgment determining type, rapidity of transfusion and volume.

G. Insert an indwelling bladder catheter.

H. Place a nasogastric sump tube attached to low suction.

## Evaluation of Injuries

Once immediate survival is assured, the patient must be completely undressed. If he is unconscious or complaining of extremity or back pain, it is always preferable to cut the clothing off. A brief history should be obtained and a systematic physical examination should be carried out and recorded.

1. *History.* This must include How? Where? and When? Not only does this information have prognostic and therapeutic importance, but it is also of medicolegal significance.

2. *Systematic Physical Examination*

A. General cutaneous examination for abrasions, contusions, lacerations and puncture wounds should be carried out. The size, character and location of each wound must be noted in the record.

Particular abrasion configurations, such as tire-tread marks, rope marks, etc., should be recorded, since these may have significant prognostic value.

B. *Head*

(1) Attention should be paid to the areas of ecchymosis, hematoma and lacerations. The latter should be palpated with a gloved finger to determine the presence of underlying fracture.

(2) Evaluation of the cranial nerves should be done (*see* Chap. 20, Acute Craniocerebral Injuries).

(3) Blood in the external auditory meatus or bleeding from the ear requires otoscopic examination. The presence of a bulging black drum or leakage of blood from the middle ear is indicative of posterior fossa skull fracture.

(4) Drainage of clear fluid from the nose (rhinorrhea) may be leakage of cerebrospinal fluid from a fracture through the cribriform plate.

(5) Extraocular motion, vision and direct and reflex pupillary reaction must be investigated for evidence of eye injury or an orbital fracture.

(6) Examination for facial fracture should be carried out by palpation of the zygoma, the nasal bones and the mandible (*see* Chap. 26, Maxillofacial Fractures).

(7) X-rays for confirmation of fractures include AP, PA and right and left laterals of the skull. Special views of the mandible, zygoma, sinuses, base of the skull and orbit are necessary for confirmation of fracture of these structures.

C. *Neck*

(1) Inspection of the neck may disclose swelling or deformity. Swelling may be due to either bleeding or air in the soft tissues of the neck. Deformity may be due to eccentric swelling or to deviation of the trachea. Note that as with the thorax, pre-existing thoracic procedures may produce deformity in both the thorax and the neck.

(2) Palpation will serve to differentiate between the extravasation of fluid or blood into the soft tissues or air. The latter has a feeling of crepitation, which is the sensation produced by moving the small bubbles of air through the planes of the tissues of the neck.

Air in the neck may come either from the pharynx, esophagus or trachea. The precise source will require more detailed evaluation. Its presence, however, is ominous.

(a) Asymmetry in the position of the trachea should also be ascertained, and the ability of the larynx to move on swallowing helps to rule out complete division of the trachea.

(b) The palpation of the common and external carotid arteries and the visualization of the filling of the superficial neck veins should be done. Marked distention of the latter presupposes mediastinal or cardiac tamponade until this is disproven.

(c) The structure of greatest importance in the neck is the cervical spinal cord. Tenderness of the cervical spine to palpation or evidence of peripheral neurologic involvement, especially in the upper extremities, should alert the examiner to stop further examination until the head has been adequately immobilized. This can be accomplished with sandbags or with a Velcro head band if the patient is on a body board.

D. *Thorax*

(1) Since equality in size, shape and motion of the two halves of the chest, together with normal resonance to percussion and breath sounds, are expected, any deviation from this equality and normality should immediately lead to the suspicion of thoracic injury.

(2) Previous thoracic operations may alter the preinjury conditions, but, in general, deformity of the thoracic wall in the absence of scars presupposes thoracic wall damage.

(3) Splinting of respiration, or "paradoxical" motion of the chest wall on breathing, as well as subjective pain on inspiration should strongly suggest that a more detailed examination for rib fracture is needed.

(4) Hyperresonance or tympany is presumptive evidence of pneumothorax, and the absence of normal mediastinal dullness or cardiac dullness with left-sided injury combined with tympany may lead to the diagnosis of tension pneumothorax without the necessity of confirmatory films.

(5) Dullness usually indicates the accumulation of fluid or blood within the pleural cavity. This can also produce mediastinal shift and embarrass circulation.

(6) In a similar manner as to the neck, if there is tenderness on palpation of the thoracic spine or evidence of distal peripheral neurologic changes, care must be exercised in the residual examination not to move the patient until x-rays rule out the possibility of dorsal vertebral fracture. If examination of the back is deemed mandatory because of subsequent findings, a "log-rolling" technique of turning the patient as a single unit should be used.

E. *Abdomen*

(1) Evaluation of the abdomen includes inspection for signs of perforation of the skin, abrasion or ecchymosis, palpa-
tion for areas of tenderness or abdominal muscular spasm, percussion for normal anatomical areas of dullness, and auscultation for the presence and quantification of the bowel sounds.

(2) The flank, buttock and back should be included in examination of the abdomen.

(3) Initial evaluation of the signs of peritoneal irritation is essential (*see* Chap. 14, Abdominal Trauma). Static findings are less important than the change in these findings.

F. *Spine*

(1) The palpation of the cervical and dorsal spine has already been discussed in relationship to the neck and thorax. This examination can be accomplished without moving the patient by passing the hand gently under the back and palpating the individual vertebral spines.

(2) Point tenderness demands consideration of this area as a site of fracture and potential cord damage, and the patient must not be moved until suitably immobilized and radiographic confirmation of normality is obtained.

G. *Pelvis*

(1) The evaluation of the integrity of the pelvis can rapidly be carried out by pressing on the pubis, compressing the iliac ala and then attempting to pull them apart.

(2) If these three maneuvers fail to produce pain, fracture is unlikely.

(3) If tenderness is elicited, an AP view of the pelvis usually will suffice for examination.

H. *Rectum*

(1) Rectal examination should be carried out even in the acutely injured patient.

(2) The presence of blood may indicate rectal or sigmoidal injury.

(3) Palpation of the level of the prostate is important. If it is high-riding, this may indicate laceration of the membranous urethra.

(4) Posterior tenderness may be due to coccygeal fracture.

I. *Extremities*

*(1)* Rapid assessment of the cutaneous, osseous, neurologic and vascular status of the extremities must be carried out.

*(2)* Disruption of the skin continuity in proximity to a clinically evident fracture is considered an open fracture until proven otherwise.

*(3)* Osseous continuity is evaluated by the presence of one or more of the possible or probable signs of fracture.

*Possible Signs of Fracture*

*(1)* Ecchymosis

*(2)* Tenderness, usually well localized

*Probable Signs of Fracture*

*(1)* Loss of normal motion and function (e.g., inability to move arms, usually because of pain, or to walk)

*(2)* False point of motion (e.g., the ability to bend the extremity or to see the extremity bent in an area where no joint exists anatomically). *This sign, like the next sign, should never be deliberately tested for, since it will produce additional soft tissue injury and may compound a closed fracture.*

*(3)* Crepitus, the audible or palpable grating of the bone ends against each other

*(4)* Axial compression tenderness. Rather than attempting to elicit tenderness by bending the extremity, both identification and even localization of probable fractures may be evaluated in the conscious patient by this technique.

*(a)* For the hand, the fingers are outstretched and the tip of each finger is percussed. Fracture in any part of the ray from the carpal bones through the phalanges will elicit pain in the respective ray. Conversely, the absence of pain is probable indication that *no* fracture exists.

*(b)* The upper extremity, including the radius and ulna, humerus, scapula and clavicle, can be rapidly assessed by percussing the outstretched upper extremity with a fist on the hyperflexed heel

of the hand. Any fracture which interrupts the osseous continuity (except avulsion fractures) will elicit localized pain.

*(c)* Evaluation of the foot is accomplished in much the same fashion as the assessment of the hand, by percussion on the tips of the toes which may have to be manually extended to accomplish end percussion.

*(d)* Assessment of the lower extremity to include calcaneus, talus, tibia and fibula, femur and the innominate bone can be done by forcibly banging with the closed fist on the heel of the outstretched extremity. Again, it must be emphasized that failure to elicit axial compression pain in the awake patient probably indicates that there is no major fracture.

*(5)* Osteophony, the transmission of sound by bone. This is a useful rapid screening evaluation for the uncooperative or obtunded patient but will elicit signs of major fractures only.

*(a)* For the upper extremity, a stethoscope is placed over the manubrium sterni, and the radial and ulnar styloid are percussed on either side.

*(b)* For the lower extremity, a stethoscope is placed over the symphysis pubis, and the medial and lateral malleoli are also percussed as one percusses a chest.

*(c)* A major fracture will produce a transmitted sound which is lower in both pitch and intensity. This is strikingly evident when the fracture is unilateral, but experience will permit such assessment even in bilateral fractures.

*Positive Signs of Fracture*

The only certain sign of fracture is x-ray confirmation of osseous discontinuity or irregularity. Specifics are discussed in Chapters 3 and 25.

*(1)*. AP, PA and right and left lateral views are necessary for skull visualization.

*(2)* AP and lateral views are necessary at a minimum for the diagnosis of fractures of the cervical thoracic and lumbar spines (note that the AP view to

visualize C-1 and C-2 is taken through the opened mouth).

*(3)* AP and lateral views are needed to diagnose fractures of the pelvis, sacrum and coccyx.

*(4)* AP and lateral views are needed for diagnosis of fractures of the upper and lower extremities down to the hands and feet.

*(5)* In the hands and feet, because of the overlapping of bones, AP and oblique projections usually will suffice.

*(6)* Examination of the ribs requires a plain film of the chest and special area study specifically for bony contrast of the region where rib fracture is clinically suspected (e.g., right lower anterior, left upper posterior, etc.).

*(7)* Special views for the facial bones, wrist, tarsus, etc. may be required.

## Determination of the Priority of Treatments

BASIC PRINCIPLES. Once the emergency lifesaving is completed and injuries are assessed, attention is directed toward the control of the most life-threatening situations. Usually initiation of treatment proceeds simultaneously with the assessment of the injuries. The following priorities are those usually followed in the ordinary civilian injury situation.

Disaster management will be discussed separately.

PRIORITY ORDER. 1. *Thoracic, cardiac and central vascular injuries,* having the greatest fatality, obviously require the highest priority. Vascular injuries, in particular, frequently require management prior to completed resuscitation or assessment.

2. *Abdominal injuries,* especially to the solid intra-abdominal viscera, can also be rapidly lethal and have the second priority.

3. *Cerebral trauma,* acute epidural or subdural hematoma, has third priority. Most other cerebral injuries are either lethal or nonlethal despite treatment and

therefore are given relatively low priority for operative treatment.

4. *Open fractures,* because of the potential for osteomyelitis, have the next highest priority.

5. *Major soft tissue injuries*

6. *Closed fractures.* The treatment priority here only involves the immobilization of the fractures to prevent compounding.

7. *Other soft tissue wounds,* especially about the face, while having a low priority in terms of life salvage, will produce better cosmetic results the earlier the repair is accomplished. The ability to do secondary reconstruction, however, places the repair of these structures at the lowest priority level.

## Definitive Treatment

1. Based upon the assessment of injuries, priority is established and treatment is planned.

2. A nasogastric tube and an indwelling catheter are placed as well as two upper extremity intravenous lines in serious injuries.

3. The management of thoracic and abdominal injuries is presented in Chapter 11, Thoracic and Cardiovascular Injuries, and Chapter 14, Abdominal Trauma.

4. Fractures are splinted (*see* Chap. 25).

5. Open wounds (*see* Chap. 10, Soft Tissue Injuries) are cleansed and dressed.

6. Replacement of circulatory volume is completed, if possible.

7. Prophylaxis against tetanus and infection is given (*see* Chap. 9).

## Management of Casualties in Mass Disaster

### Definitions

1. *Disaster.* A disaster is a volume of casualties in excess of the capabilities of the medical care facility to render effective treatment.

2. *Mass Disaster.* This is a situation in which the number of casualties are in

excess of the capability of the medical care facility to render even emergency life-saving treatment.

3. *Triage.* This is a procedure by means of which the sick and wounded are classified according to the type and urgency of the condition presented, so that they can be properly routed to appropriate medical care units.

## Basic Principles

In ordinary injury situations, the triage of casualties has already been discussed. In routine disaster situations, attention is directed toward emergency lifesaving initially, with subsequent definitive treatment of those most severely injured. In the mass disaster situation, the shortage of medical care facilities requires a reversal of the usual triage and treatment procedure so that the greatest number of casualties may be treated in the shortest period of time. Attempts at definitive mangement of the severe or potentially lethal injuries will require expenditure of considerable health-care manpower with comparatively poor salvage. The triage classification proposed by Ziperman should be used in these situations, and the classification is discussed below with comments on management.

1. *Casualties Requiring Minimal Treatment*

A. Those that only require first aid prior to discharge from the emergency department

(1) Small lacerations and contusions

(2) Second-degree burns of less than 10 per cent of the body surface not involving the face or hands

(3) Simple fractures of small bones

(4) Nonlethal asymptomatic whole body radiation

B. Those requiring hospital retention for domiciliary care only

(1) Disabling minor fracture

(2) Burns of the face or hands—patients unable to see or care for themselves

(3) Moderate neuropsychiatric disorders. This group represents the majority of those patients requiring minimal treatment who will need hospital admission.

(4) Nonlethal whole body radiation with early symptomatology (vomiting, nausea, anorexia)

2. *Casualties Requiring Immediate Care*

A. Easily accessible hemorrhage: control the bleeding.

B. Rapidly correctable mechanical respiratory defects: perform a tracheostomy.

C. Sucking chest wounds: close the wounds with occlusive dressing and insert a thoracostomy tube.

D. Severe crushing extremity wounds: amputate.

E. Incomplete amputation: complete the amputation.

F. Severe lacerations: control the bleeding and dress wounds.

G. Open fractures: control the bleeding, apply dressings and splint or amputate.

H. Severe head and neck burns requiring tracheostomy: perform a tracheostomy.

3. *Casualties Whose Surgical Treatment May Be Delayed*

A. Closed fractures of major bones

B. Moderate lacerations without extensive bleeding

C. Second-degree burns, 10-40 per cent of body surface; third-degree burns, 10-30 percent of body surface

D. Noncritical central nervous system injuries

4. *Casualties Whose Treatment Will Be Expectant Initially*

A. Critical respiratory system injuries

B. Serious cardiac or central vascular injuries

C. Penetrating or perforating abdominal wounds

D. Multiple severe injuries

E. Second- or third-degree burns over 40 per cent of the body surface

F. Lethal whole body radiation

Category 1 patients usually will not require physician time for management, so that he is freed to attend to the emergency lifesaving priority.

Patients will move to priority category 3 or 4 after emergency lifesaving is accomplished.

The objective must be restated that this triage classification is designed to treat the greatest number of patients who have the best expectancy for eventual survival.

# 2. FLUID AND ELECTROLYTE PROBLEMS

*Bernard Gardner,* M.D.

## FLUID DEPLETION

### Definitions

1. *Parenteral feeding* today is usually regarded as intravenous replacement or maintenance of the body store of water, inorganic ions and organic nutrients. Arterial infusion and hypodermoclysis are rarely used at the present time.

2. *Acute depletion* is primarily a sudden, rapid water and electrolyte change, manifested by a history of acute onset of loss, vomiting and/or diarrhea and signs of dehydration such as furrowed tongue, loss of skin turgor, dry mucous membranes, soft eyeballs, etc.

3. *Chronic depletion* is the loss of whole body mass as well as water, due to prolonged illness, starvation or chronic fluid loss. Starvation is a frequent manifestation of neoplasms because the tumor acts as a nitrogen trap, reducing available protein and fat, depleting glycogen stores and lowering serum albumin levels. Chronic loss may be seen in patients with longstanding renal disease, intestinal fistulas, etc.

4. *Dehydration* is the loss of body water. The degree of dehydration can be related to loss of body fluid by the following approximations:

    Mild dehydration—4 per cent of body weight

    Moderate dehydration—6 per cent of body weight

    Severe dehydration—8 per cent of body weight

5. *Static loss* is the fluid and electrolyte loss present on initiation of treatment.

6. *Dynamic loss* is the continuing loss of fluid and electrolytes due to metabolism and respiration, and from the skin, kidney, bowel and nasogastric suction.

### Basic Principles

1. Total body water makes up 50 to 60 per cent of the body weight and in the human is located in three compartments. The largest of these compartments is intracellular water, accounting for 60 per cent of total body water or about 30 per cent of the whole body weight (WBW); interstitial water accounts for 30 per cent of total body water (15 per cent of the WBW), and plasma or intravascular volume accounts for 10 per cent (5 per cent of the WBW). Cellular metabolism is directly related to the intracellular water volume for maintenance of cellular integrity and to the plasma volume for perfusion, which provides adequate materials for metabolism. Both of these compartments are in direct equilibrium with the interstitial fluid volume. A number of homeostatic mechanisms exist which under stress maintain the plasma volume at the expense of interstitial fluid volume so that tissue perfusion can be maintained. Slight falls in plasma volume stimulate water and salt reabsorption in the renal tubules, peripheral constriction of the arteriolar bed and shifts in blood flow designed to maintain perfusion to critical areas. When large losses of fluid occur, the major deficit will be found in the interstitial fluid compartment because it is used to refill the intravascular compartment. *Fluid replacement is therefore designed to maintain plasma volume and replace lost interstitial fluid.*

2. Fluid losses may be exogenous (i.e., vomiting, diarrhea, bleeding), or they may be endogenous into a third space. Third-space loss is defined as a loss of fluid from the effective circulating volume into a body area in which, although weighed with the patient, the fluid cannot readily be mobiliz-

ed. Examples of third-space loss would include ascites, effusions, exudation or transudation of fluid into an area of injury such as a crush or burn or for revascularization of an area after prolonged local anoxia, losses into the lumen of the intestine with obstruction, etc.

3. Urine output and central venous pressure are important adjuncts in guiding successful fluid replacement. If the central venous catheter is correctly placed, it lies in the superior vena cava and must be freely patent so that the measured level fluctuates with respiration. The absolute value of the central venous pressure is not of paramount importance, but fluid replacement is not considered adequate until a rise in CVP is demonstrated. As administered electrolytes pass into the interstitial fluid compartment from the plasma, the CVP may actually decrease. Since severe overloading of the cardiovascular system may follow persistent attempts to raise the CVP to a preset value by the use of isotonic electrolyte solutions, careful auscultation of the lungs is always necessary during fluid replacement. It must be emphasized that the CVP represents only one of several factors to be evaluated in determining successful treatment.

4. If the blood-urea nitrogen is found to be elevated and the urine output is low, it will become necessary to differentiate prerenal azotemia from chronic or acute renal failure. The treatment of the former (usually due to dehydration) is fluid replacement, whereas in the latter instance, fluid restriction after initial replacement may be desirable. Several simple tests will help to clarify this problem:

A. A BUN to creatinine ratio over 20:1 implies a prerenal azotemia.

B. Urine osmolality in excess of serum osmolality (normal, 300 mOsm./L.) implies good urinary concentrating ability rarely found with renal failure.

C. A urinary sodium concentration of under 40 mEq./L. on a spot sample implies good reabsorption capacity and prerenal azotemia.

D. An immediate increase in urinary output to a fluid or osmotic load (i.e., mannitol infusion) suggests good renal function or prerenal azotemia.

## Choice of Replacement Fluid

Table 2-1 lists the contents of some commonly used intravenous fluids. In patients with isotonic losses, or before the results of electrolyte studies are available, a balanced salt solution is the best fluid to use. An infusion of Ringer's lactate or one-half normal saline containing 44 mEq. of $NaHCO_3$ (1 ampule) can be started at once. The aim is to restore tissue perfusion and replace interstitial fluid losses. Where tissue perfusion is low due to severe dehydration, or where a more prolonged effect on plasma volume is desired (e.g., an operation is impending), the use of reconstituted albumin solutions or serum albumin is desirable. Salt solutions can be expected to affect plasma volume only for short periods of time (2 to 4 hours), whereas colloid-containing fluids have a more prolonged effect on plasma volume and CVP. With the return of electrolyte study results, it may be necessary to use specific electrolyte solutions, particularly when chloride and potassium levels may be low (e.g., in pyloric obstruction) or when sodium deficits imply a salt loss in excess of water (rare) or an underlying water intoxication syndrome (rare).

## Volume of Fluid Replacement

1. The degree of clinical dehydration gives a rough idea of the volumes to be replaced. In actual practice, the volume replacement is guided more precisely by:

A. Mental response of the patient

B. Reduction in tachycardia and restoration of blood pressure

C. Response of the CVP

D. Return of urine output to or above 40 ml./hour

E. Improvement in over-all appearance

2. The calculated approximations are valuable, however, in understanding the

## te of Replacement

1. ...rriding factor in determining ...e rate ...id replacement is whether surgery is ...ssary and how quickly it must ...e p...med. For example, in the ...resen... a gangrenous intestine, delay ...rior t...rgery is directly proportional to ...ortal... therefore, replacement of fluid ...ust b... apid enough to restore perfusion ...urinar output) so that emergency surgery ...an ... performed. In a complete mechanical simple small bowel obstruction, surgery is urgent but may be planned for 8 hours after admission; the rate of fluid administration is proportioned accordingly. Since surgery in the patient with pyloric obstruction may be delayed for several days to allow gastric decompression, fluid replacement may be more leisurely. In many instances in which no surgery is necessary, day-to-day evaluation of fluid replacement can be carried out.

This evaluation of the need for surgery necessitates a careful history and physical examination and early surgical consultation.

2. In questionable cases, all efforts should be directed to early diagnosis. Preoperative fluid replacement is essential in avoiding high surgical morbidity and difficult postoperative problems. Most anesthetic agents and surgical procedures reduce critical blood flows (to the liver and kidney), and normal perfusion should be returned and maintained intraoperatively to avoid postoperative complications. In the presence of gangrenous intestine or frank sepsis, shock may be due to release of toxic products into the blood stream rather than to fluid depletion alone and may not be correctable until the compromised intestine is resected or an abscess drained. Under such special circumstances, surgery, despite low tissue perfusion, may be lifesaving. However, these conditions represent a small percentage of acute admissions and should not alter the approach of adequate preoperative hydration.

## Chronic Depletion

1. In chronic depletion, restoration of plasma volume at the expense of interstitial fluid has already occurred, so that measured plasma volumes may be normal in spite of severe weight loss. In this instance, rapid replacement of blood or colloid may embarrass the patient's circulatory system, leading to heart failure, and slow replacement is desirable with uncomplicated chronic depletion. Use of additional calcium and magnesium replacement may be indicated in some of these patients.

2. Acute fluid loss superimposed on chronic depletion, such as intestinal obstruction due to neoplasm, requires management as in the acutely depleted patient.

### Criteria for Diagnosis

1. *Accurate History.* History of specific losses such as excessive sweating or gastric-outlet obstruction may point to specific electrolyte losses, which require replacement with solutions containing the appropriate ions. History is important not only for factors which point to these specific losses but also to determine underlying associated conditions which may alter fluid administration. A history of hypertension, chronic renal disease or heart failure may have a direct bearing on the type and rate of fluid replacement. Vomiting may not be a prominent symptom in some cases of intestinal obstruction; however, abdominal distention may indicate a large third-space loss.

2. *Physical Examination.* This is needed to estimate the degree of dehydration and the presence of third-space losses, that is, sequestrations, effusions, exudations and transudations. Physical examination should also be used to evaluate associated conditions such as pulmonary edema or liver disease which may alter the choice of replacement fluids.

**Table 2-1. The Contents of Commonly Used Repair**

| *Solution* | *mEq./L.* $Na^+$ | $K^+$ | $Cl^-$ | $HCO_3^-$ | $Ca^{++}$ | $Mg$ | |
|---|---|---|---|---|---|---|---|
| Normal saline | 154 | — | 154 | — | — | — | |
| Dextrose, 5%, in water (D5W) | — | — | — | — | — | — | |
| Dextrose, 5%, in saline (D5S) | 154 | — | 154 | — | — | — | |
| Dextrose, 5%, in ½ normal saline (D1/2 NS) | 77 | — | 77 | — | — | — | |
| Ringer's solution | 147 | 4 | 155 | — | 4 | — | |
| Ringer's lactate | 130 | 4 | 109 | (28) | 3 | — | |
| M/6 lactate | 167 | — | — | 167 | — | — | |
| Arginine HCl (1 ampule) | — | — | 100 ($^+$100 $H^+$) | — | — | — | |
| Sodium chloride, 5% | 864 | — | 864 | — | — | — | |
| Plasma | 142 | 5 | 105 | 27 | 5 | 3 | |
| Whole blood | 150 | 10 | 100 | 28 | 6 | 4 | |
| Aminosol, 5% | 10 | 17 | — | — | — | — | 200 |
| Amigen, 5% | 34 | 15 | 25 | — | 5 | 2 | 200 |
| Plasma protein fraction in 5% solution | 110 | 2 | 50 | — | — | — | 200 |

range of replacement likely to be necessary to restore the patient. It must be remembered that, in addition to static loss, dynamic loss must also be replaced. For example, a 70-kg. male with moderate dehydration will have lost roughly 4,200 ml. of fluid and will need an additional 2,000 ml./day for maintenance. Replacement may then require 6 liters of solution in the first 24 hours. The many schemas promulgated for calculation of specific electrolyte deficits are rarely used in clinical practice. It is important to remember that most acute fluid losses are isotonic and that the use of balanced salt solutions for primary replacement is desirable, rather than the use of electrolyte-free solutions such as glucose in water. When electrolyte values are available, specific deficits can then be replaced.

## Management

1. History and physical examination.
2. Draw electrolytes, blood-urea nitrogen, creatinine, hematocrit and SMA-12, if available, as a baseline.
3. Start I.V. fluids with Ringer's lactate at the rate of 1 liter/hour until evaluation for surgery is completed.
4. Gauge the rate of fluid administration by the need for surgery.
5. Monitor hourly urine output.
6. Weigh the patient.
7. Measure the central venous pressure change.
8. Note response of blood pressure, pulse and mental status.
9. Use albumin-containing solutions for prolongation of effect on perfusion volume (plasma volume).
10. Obtain necessary consultations early.
11. Give one half of the calculated fluid depletion plus maintainance fluids in 12 hours.
12. Replacement fluids should be primarily isotonic (balanced salt).
13. Use monitoring of the patient's response as a guide to remaining replacement.
14. Check the lungs frequently (by auscultation).
15. Repeat electrolyte studies as necessary.
16. Obtain an ECG to evaluate electrolyte deficit if necessary.

## HYPOKALEMIA

### Definition

Hypokalemia refers to low serum potassium levels (less than 3.5 mEq./L.).

### Basic Principles

Hypokalemia is seen in states associated with metabolic alkalosis, particularly $H^+$ loss, and potassium depletion from vomiting, excessive urine volumes or use of diuretics. In metabolic alkalosis, intracellular buffering of the bicarbonate excess occurs by the combination of bicarbonate with potassium and release of $H^+$. This accounts for the urinary excretion of $H^+$ and the paradoxical aciduria which occurs in cases of metabolic alkalosis due to primary loss of $H^+$ (i.e., pyloric stenosis). The integrity of muscular contraction and myocardial contractility are critically related to the relative concentrations of $K^+$ and $Ca^{++}$, and persisting hypokalemia may lead to death by these effects on the heart. Unreplaced urinary losses (averaging 50 to 100 mEq. of $K^+$/liter of urine) represent a common cause of hypokalemia in the postoperative patient.

### Criteria for Diagnosis

1. Serum potassium levels below 3.5 mEq./L.
2. ECG alterations: loss in amplitude of T waves, prominent U waves, S-T segment deviations.
3. The diagnosis is suspected if serum $HCO_3^-$ levels are over 34 mEq./L.

### Management

1. For states manifested by HCl loss (vomiting or significant volumes of gastric aspiration), treatment consists of replacement of HCl with normal saline. This solution produces a net acid load because the difference between the administered chloride concentration and its serum levels far exceeds the difference between the administered sodium concentration and its serum levels.
2. Where rapid correction of alkalosis is desirable, arginine HCl may be given as 1 ampule in an intravenous drip. This supplies an immediate load of 100 mEq. of $H^+$ plus 100 mEq. of $Cl^-$.
3. Administration of potassium is specific, and potassium may be added to the intravenous solutions in concentrations of 20 to 80 mEq. of KCl per liter. Levels exceeding this may be dangerous. In severe cases, we have given as much as 240 mEq. of KCl per day, but this is not recommended for routine use.

## HYPERKALEMIA

### Definition

Hyperkalemia is elevation of the serum potassium level (above 4.5 mEq./L.).

### Basic Principles

Hyperkalemia occurs most commonly in states associated with acidosis, oliguria or anuria. Hyperkalemia is the most common cause of death due to electrolyte abnormalities, and it is seen in combinations of acute and chronic renal failure due to sepsis, shock, dehydration or primary renal disease. Awareness of the possibility of hyperkalemia and its rapid diagnosis and treatment are mandatory. Sudden death due to ventricular fibrillation is a frequent concomitant of the untreated state.

### Criteria for Diagnosis

1. Serum potassium levels above 4.5 mEq./L.
2. ECG changes with mild hyperkalemia: prolonged P-R interval, low P waves, sino-atrial block
3. ECG changes with severe hyperkalemia: tenting of T waves, intraventricular block with widened QRS complexes, S-T segment shifts, ventricular fibrillation
4. Hyperkalemia should be suspected in cases of metabolic acidosis

### Management

1. Chronic treatment may be provided by use of ion-exchange resins by mouth or enema.
2. Administration of glucose and insulin (1 unit of insulin for each 2 grams of glucose) will reduce serum potassium levels.
3. Administration of hypertonic saline will reduce serum potassium.
4. For severe cases, intravenous calcium should be given to counteract the cardiac effects of potassium until the serum levels can be reduced.

## HYPONATREMIA

### Definition

Hyponatremia is a low serum sodium concentration (less than 138 mEq./L.).

### Basic Principles

Hyponatremia rather than simple reduction in serum sodium is usually secondary to excess exogenous free-water administration (glucose and water) and therefore rarely seen in acute states unless the patient has been ingesting large amounts of water or has renal failure with chronic sodium loss. Although ADH secretion responds to changes in serum osmolality, ADH secretion can be preferentially stimulated by a decrease in blood volume. Under these circumstances, we have seen inappropriate water reabsorption and dilution of serum sodium levels. Spurious low serum sodium may occur in the presence of increased serum oncotic pressure due to high glucose or keto acid levels as may occur in diabetes and other lipidemias. Osmotic transfer of water to the intravascular space is the cause.

### Management

Accurate diagnosis is necessary, and treatment may include:
1. Water restriction in dilution states due to water ingestion or inappropriate ADH secretion
2. Hypertonic saline in states due to chronic sodium loss or in patients with low serum sodium who need fluid replacement
3. Correction of high glucose levels by use of insulin

## HYPERNATREMIA

### Definition

Hypernatremia refers to high serum sodium levels (above 140 mEq./L.).

### Basic Principles

Hypernatremia is always due to either excess sodium administration or, more commonly, dehydration. Hypernatremia due to dehydration occurs frequently during the "restricted" administration of isotonic saline or lactated Ringer's solution in patients under a stimulus for maximum aldosterone secretion (e.g., cirrhosis, postoperative patients, etc.).

## Management

The management of hypernatremia basically demands the administration of sodium-free water (D5W), which will lower the serum sodium levels.

## ACID—BASE DISTURBANCES

### Definition

Acid–base disturbances refer to alterations in the blood pH and in the concentrations of the primary buffers ($HCO_3^-$ and $H_2CO_3$) in the blood.

### Basic Principles

The blood pH is governed primarily by the following formula:

$$pH = 6.1 + \log \frac{[HCO_3^-]}{[H_2CO_3]}$$

Since the concentration of $H_2CO_3 = 0.03 \times pCO_2$, the relationship can be altered to $pH \cong \frac{[HCO_3^-]}{pCO_2}$. It can be readily seen that increases in pH (alkalosis) will occur with increases in $HCO_3^-$ above 24 mEq./L. or decreases in arterial $pCO_2$ below 40 mm. Hg. Decreases in pH (acidosis) will occur when $HCO_3^-$ decreases or $pCO_2$ rises. These alterations can be brought about by metabolic or respiratory effects.

### Metabolic Alkalosis

This is associated with a rise in blood pH. The cause may be ingestion of alkalis or loss of $H^+$. The primary change is a rise in serum $HCO_3^-$ with a secondary compensatory change of a rise in $pCO_2$, (due to depression of the respiratory center).

Treatment depends on the exact cause:
1. Oral ingestion of alkali should be stopped.

2. In the vomiting patient, obstruction should be relieved if possible.
3. Administration of fluids high in chloride with respect to sodium (acid load) should be used.
4. Arginine HCl in an intravenous drip can be used.
5. Potassium supplementation may be necessary to treat associated hypokalemia.

### Metabolic Acidosis

This is associated with a fall in blood pH. The cause may be ingestion or administration of an acid load (rare) or, more commonly, the accumulation of acid products in the blood stream due to oliguria or anuria, shock or low perfusion states, ketoacidosis of starvation or uncontrolled diabetes. Metabolic acidosis can also occur with the loss of alkaline intestinal juices, such as may occur with intestinal, biliary or pancreatic fistulas. The primary change is a fall in serum $HCO_3^-$, and a secondary compensatory change is a fall in $pCO_2$ (due to stimulation of the respiratory center—hyperventilation), which is an attempt to return blood pH to normal.

Treatment depends on the underlying pathology:
1. Ion-exchange resins in renal failure
2. Aggressive treatment of associated hyperkalemia (*see* above)
3. Use of fluids such as M/6 lactate to supply bicarbonate
4. Sodium bicarbonate may be used directly I.V.
5. Dialysis may be required to treat renal failure
6. Correction of diabetes or keto-acidosis is accomplished by appropriate use of insulin and parenteral fluids

### Respiratory Alkalosis

This is reflected by a high blood pH, a primary decrease in $pCO_2$ and a compensatory decrease in serum $HCO_3^-$. This state is commonly seen in salicylate poisoning and hyperventilation due to the use of mechanical ventilators.

## Respiratory Acidosis

This is reflected by a low blood pH, a primary rise in $pCO_2$ and a secondary compensatory rise in serum $HCO_3^-$. Most commonly this is due to pulmonary disease with hypoventilation due to atelectasis, obstruction, infection or restriction of the lungs.

The critically ill surgical patient often has a combination of factors involved, with metabolic and respiratory components playing significant roles. It is vital to assess the clinical situation carefully and to make an assessment of the likely state of acid–base balance. Careful measurements of blood pH, serum $HCO_3^-$, and $pCO_2$ will then help to confirm the impression. Measurement of blood gases will delineate the respiratory components so that a total assessment can be made. Combinations of sepsis with shock (metabolic acidosis and respiratory acidosis) in patients with large nasogastric aspirations (metabolic alkalosis) receiving I.V. fluids (? effect) demand careful individual evaluation and consultation with experienced clinicians for successful treatment. The following measurements, however, are mandatory:

1. Daily weight
2. Serum $HCO_3^-$, $K^+$, $Na^+$, $Cl^-$
3. Arterial pH
4. Hourly urine output
5. Arterial $pO_2$, on room air if possible
6. Vital signs, mental status
7. Careful intake and output records
8. Frequent assessment of associated pulmonary disease by auscultation and x-ray
9. ECG monitoring to pick up electrolyte abnormalities early
10. Serum and urine osmolalities, since urine volume alone will *not* reflect renal function

# 3. ROENTGENOGRAPHIC PRINCIPLES OF EMERGENCY TRAUMA

*Jack G. Rabinowitz*, M.D.

## MULTIPLE INJURY

### Basic Principles

1. Prior to x-ray evaluation, the patient should be thoroughly examined to exclude any life-threatening condition that would require immediate treatment.

2. X-ray examinations can be performed thereafter to:

A. Confirm the clinical diagnosis

B. Determine the extent of the trauma

C. Evaluate the presence of other underlying conditions

3. Depending upon the condition of the patient, the studies can be performed either at the bedside itself, utilizing portable x-ray equipment, or by quick transport of the patient to an x-ray room.

4. Roentgenographic examination of a severely injured patient must be done carefully and promptly so as not to delay or interfere with institution of appropriate therapy.

5. Routine examinations should be avoided at this stage or at least until the patient's condition permits.

6. The initial examination should be tailored to the injury and performed with the least amount of risk and movement to the patient.

7. In the severely injured patient, bedside portable x-ray equipment may be required. These are limited and multiple views cannot be obtained. Nevertheless, they can be utilized as a preliminary guide in diagnosis and in therapy.

The following portable examinations, listed along with their diagnostic feasibility, are pertinent:

A. *Chest Examination.* At best, supine and lateral studies can be obtained. One may determine the presence of fractured ribs, pneumothorax, pulmonary contusions, pulmonary hemorrhage and mediastinal widening that may signify the presence of a ruptured esophagus or aorta or the presence of pericardial fluid.

B. *Examination of the Abdomen.* The examination can be done at the bedside, but it is best performed in an x-ray room, using high kilovoltage and a movable grid. This study may demonstrate pneumoperitoneum or hemoperitoneum.

C. *Examination of the Extremities.* In most situations, anteroposterior and lateral views can be made and obvious fractures or dislocations diagnosed.

D. *Examination of the Cervical Spine.* A lateral cross-table study to exclude fracture or dislocation should be the initial examination. Further studies can be performed thereafter.

## THORACIC INJURY

### PULMONARY CONTUSION

#### Indications

1. Chest trauma
2. Chest pain
3. Perhaps fever

#### Studies

Chest films

#### Method of Performance

Anteroposterior (AP) and lateral chest examinations should be performed in the supine or in the upright position, preferably the latter. A posteroanterior (PA) film is, however, always preferred.

#### Findings

1. Pulmonary infiltration with ill-defined borders, showing no specific segmental or lobar distribution.

2. Diffuse nodular densities either unilateral or bilateral when the trauma is more extensive.

3. All findings rapidly resolve after 48 to 72 hours.

4. There may be associated rib fractures.

## Differential Diagnosis

The association of trauma with the appearance and rapid resolution of the above findings is diagnostic for pulmonary contusion. Persistent lesions should make one consider the following diagnoses:

1. Pneumonia
2. Hematoma
3. Tumor
4. Congestive failure

### PULMONARY HEMATOMA

## Indications

1. Severe chest trauma
2. Chest pain
3. Hemoptysis
4. Fever

## Studies

1. Chest examination, PA or AP and lateral and obliques

2. Tomography (later, when necessary, to further clarify the diagnosis)

## Findings

1. Pulmonary infiltration or infiltrations with poorly defined borders, showing no segmental or lobar distribution

2. The infiltration fails to resolve within 48 to 72 hours.

3. The lesion persists for many weeks. It changes contour and, during this time, assumes a well-defined border that is now oval in shape.

4. The hematoma may contract and separate from the surrounding lung, forming, therefore, a semilunar area of lucency around the hematoma (crescent sign).

5. Complete cavitation resembling a bleb may also occur at this time.

## Differential Diagnosis

The development of the lesion as described above is characteristic and is the main differential distinguishing feature of pulmonary hematoma from the following:

1. Tumor
2. Pulmonary contusion
3. Bleb
4. Fungus ball

### PNEUMOTHORAX

## Indications

1. Chest trauma
2. Dyspnea
3. Hyperresonance on percussion

## Studies

Chest films

## Method of Performance

1. *Chest Film Exposed During Inspiration.* An anteroposterior film is usually all that is required.

2. *Chest Film Exposed During Expiration.* This film is, however, preferred when the pneumothorax is minimal and undetected on an inspiration chest film. During expiration, the lung is contracted and the surrounding pneumothorax becomes more obvious.

3. *Lateral Decubitus Film.* This examination is performed with the involved side in the uppermost position. This causes the lung to retract away from the chest wall, allowing for detection of minimal pneumothorax.

## Findings

1. A halo of air or increased lucency surrounding the lungs. The medial border of the free air is formed and outlined by the visceral pleura.

2. No parenchymal markings are noted in the area of increased lucency.

3. Minimal pleural effusion

4. Associated fractured ribs may be apparent.

5. *Tension Pneumothorax*

A. The mediastinum is shifted to the opposite side.

B. The diaphragm is depressed.

C. The intercostal spaces are bulging.

## HEMOTHORAX

### Indications

1. Trauma to the chest
2. Dyspnea
3. Dullness on auscultation and percussion.

### Studies

Chest films

### Method of Performance

1. Chest films, AP and lateral, are taken preferably in the erect position.

2. The lateral decubitus film is taken with the suspected side in the lowermost position.

### Findings

1. In the supine position, fluid collects posteriorly in the most dependent portion of the chest and causes an over-all increase in haziness to the involved side.

2. In the erect position, minimal amounts of fluid obliterate the costophrenic or cardiophrenic angles.

3. Greater amounts of fluid cast a uniform density over the lower lung, and extensive amounts of fluid will obliterate the entire hemithorax.

4. *Subpulmonary Effusion.* The fluid here is located between the inferior concave border of the lung and the convex border of the diaphragm; the fluid therefore adapts a configuration resembling the diaphragm on the upright film.

*Differential Points:*

A. The apex of the so-called diaphragmatic curve is more laterally located on the frontal film.

B. Minimal blunting in the area of the costophrenic or cardiophrenic sinus may be apparent.

C. On the left side, the distance between the gas in the fundus of the stomach and the lowermost portion of the lungs is increased.

D. A lateral film of the chest reveals the usual diaphragmatic contour to be more straight and angled. The posterior costophrenic sinus may also be obliterated.

5. Lateral decubitus films are valuable in detecting minimal amounts of pleural effusion as well as subpulmonary collections. In both, a redistribution of the fluid occurs and occupies the lateral lowermost portion of the chest.

## CHYLOTHORAX

### Indications

Chest trauma, blunt or penetrating.

### Studies

1. Chest films
2. Lymphangiogram

### Method of Performance

1. Chest films, PA or AP and lateral, and the decubitus film are taken as for hemothorax.

2. *Lymphangiogram.* A slow injection of contrast medium is made into the lymphatics located on the dorsal side of the foot. These are exposed following careful dissection. The material is drained through the lymphatic chain to the thoracic duct. Films are usually exposed at varying intervals to visualize the vessels. The nodes are best outlined 24 hours after the injection.

### Findings

1. Free pleural effusion is found as described above under Hemothorax. However, chylothorax usually is massive and occurs following a minimal delay after the onset of trauma.

2. The lymphangiogram reveals the anatomy of the lymph channels and the exact site of perforation when extravasation of the opaque material occurs outside the lymphatic chain.

## PERICARDIAL EFFUSION

### Indications

1. Chest trauma, blunt or penetrating
2. Clinical evidence of beginning cardiac tamponade, etc.

### Studies

1. Chest films
2. Fluoroscopy
3. Radioactive isotope (RISA) injection
4. $CO_2$ injection
5. Angiocardiography

### Method of Performance

1. Chest films, PA or AP and lateral, are taken in the erect position if possible.
2. Fluoroscopy is best done with image intensification.
3. *Radioactive Iodine Injection.* [131]I (RISA), 350 microcuries, is injected intravenously. This remains in the blood pool for a considerable amount of time, and large collections of blood can be detected (e.g., the cardiac chambers by direct scanning). In addition, [131]I, macro-aggregated, 300 microcuries, and Tc sulfur colloid, 600 microcuries, to outline the lung and liver respectively, are injected.
4. *Carbon Dioxide Injection.* Approximately 100 ml. of $CO_2$ are injected intravenously with the patient lying in a left lateral decubitus position (right side up). This produces a $CO_2$–fluid level in the right atrium, and films of the chest are exposed in this position.
5. *Angiocardiography.* Renografin 76, 50 ml., is injected intravenously and multiple films of the heart are exposed. The right atrium is opacified and the thickness of the right atrial wall can be outlined.

### Findings

1. On the chest PA film, an enlarging cardiac silhouette, often bilaterally symmetrical, can be seen. This feature is diagnostic if the patient's cardiac size was recently known to be normal either on x-ray or physical examination.
2. Fluoroscopy reveals decreased to absent cardiac pulsations. With image intensification, the epicardial fat pad, which is normally located on the cardiac surface, is visualized well within the apparent cardiac shadow.
3. In the isotope study, the combined scan of cardiac chambers, lungs and liver permits direct visualization of heart size, estimating the chambers and the increase in distance between the chambers and the neighboring structures.
4. In the $CO_2$ and angiocardiography studies, the thickness of the atrial wall is measured between the contrast in the atrium and the surrounding lung. This is normally approximately 2 mm. thick, and a definitive diagnosis of pericardial effusion is established when it measures greater than 5 mm. Between 2 and 5 mm., the diagnosis is questionable, particularly in the presence of pleural effusion.

## TRAUMATIC RUPTURE OF THE THORACIC AORTA

### Indications

1. Blunt or penetrating trauma
2. Dyspnea, tachycardia, hemoptysis, cyanosis, severe precordial pain and, depending upon the amount of hemorrhage and the type of rupture, *impending shock*
3. Rising blood pressure in the upper extremities associated with weakening of the femoral pulse. Dysphagia or beginning neurologic defects in the lower extremities are ominous signs.

### Studies

1. Chest films
2. Aortography

### Method of Performance

1. Chest films, PA or AP and lateral, are taken in the erect position if possible.
2. *Aortography.* A catheter is passed into the ascending aorta by way of the right axillary artery, utilizing a No. 18 thin-walled Cournand needle via percutaneous puncture. It is best not to manipulate the catheter too much within the arch of the

aorta in order not to further traumatize the perforated area. After the wire has passed into the ascending aorta, a No. 7 or 8 French thin-walled Teflon tube with multiple side holes is inserted and 50 ml. of Renografin 76 are injected under pressure at a rate of 35 ml./second. Multiple films of the aorta are obtained.

### Findings

1. *Chest Films*

A. *Widening of the upper mediastinum.* This finding may be difficult to interpret since most films are taken during expiration and in a supine position. The mediastinum in both is always slightly exaggerated. However, any *blurring of the aortic outline* should suggest the diagnosis of aortic rupture.

B. As the hematoma enlarges, the mediastinum widens, the trachea is displaced to the right and the left main stem bronchus is depressed.

C. Dissection superiorly within the mediastinal pleura obliterates the apex of the left lung.

D. An enlarging cardiac contour indicates associated hemopericardium with possible cardiac tamponade.

E. Pleural effusion suggests leakage of blood from the mediastinum into the pleural space.

2. *Aortography*

A. Opacification of the aorta demonstrates the presence of aneurysmal dilatation, usually at the immediate area and just distal to the subclavian artery. The presence of actual extravasation at this site also is possible.

B. With dissection, the false channel may also be visualized and a double channel within the aorta is obtained. The linear lucency separating both channels represents the wall of the aorta.

## RUPTURE OF THE ESOPHAGUS

### Indications

1. Previous blunt trauma or penetrating wounds by knife or missile

2. Previous history of forceful vomiting or severe coughing

3. Rapid onset of pain, prostration, dyspnea and shock; physical examination demonstrates subcutaneous emphysema in the supraclavicular area.

### Studies

1. Chest films, PA and lateral

2. Esophagogram.

### Method of Performance

1. *Chest Films*

A. PA and lateral and oblique films should be taken in the erect position if possible.

B. A lateral decubitus examination may be necessary to demonstrate the presence of pleural effusion.

2. *Esophagogram.* Water-soluble media are preferred since barium may produce undesirable effects in the mediastinum. Multiple views are necessary. The study is best performed under the image intensifier in order to observe minimal extravasation. The latter is frequently difficult to observe with routine studies.

### Findings

1. Mediastinal widening due to the presence of fluid and air. This is usually located in the lower third of the mediastinum since the most distal portion of the esophagus is most frequently involved. When the rupture occurs in other sections of the esophagus, the changes will reflect this.

2. Passage of the fluid from the mediastinum to the pleura produces an associated pleural effusion in 25 per cent of the cases. This may also be accompanied by air, and air-fluid levels will be observed in the pleura.

3. *Esophagogram.* Opaque material can be seen extravasating into, and remaining localized within, the mediastinum.

### Differential Diagnosis

In elderly persons, a fractured rib may

also account for similar clinical and x-ray features (e.g., air and fluid within the pleura). Rib fracture, however, is not associated with mediastinal widening.

## RUPTURE OF THE TRACHEA OR BRONCHUS

### Indications

Severe trauma to the chest

### Studies

1. Chest films, PA and lateral, using high-kilovoltage techniques
2. Tomography if required

### Findings

1. *Transverse Fracture of the Intrathoracic Trachea.* This usually occurs above the origin of the main bronchi. Pneumomediastinum as well as air within the neck and pleural cavity are present.
2. *Fractures of the Bronchi* (very uncommon)

    A. These are almost always associated with a fracture of the first rib. Since the latter is rare, its presence should alert one to the possibility of other underlying severe trauma (e.g., bronchial fracture).

    B. Severe and rigid angulation of the involved bronchus.

    C. Cylindrical or linear collection of radiolucency surrounding the bronchus. This is caused by air escaping from the bronchus and becoming insinuated between the bronchus and the peribronchiolar connective tissue.

    D. *Pneumomediastinum.* This occurs when the air previously described escapes outside the peribronchiolar structures into the mediastinum.

    E. All of the above findings may be best demonstrated by utilizing laminagraphy.

## TORSION OF THE LUNG

### Indications

Chest trauma

### Studies

Chest films, PA and lateral

### Findings

Reversal of the normal orientation of the pulmonary vasculature is seen. The larger and more numerous vessels are now directed upward instead of downward to the basilar lung fields.

## RIB FRACTURES

### Indications

1. Chest trauma
2. Pain on inspiration

### Studies

1. Chest films, PA or AP, lateral and oblique examinations
2. For lower rib injury, the same examinations are performed with higher kilovoltage.

### Findings

1. Pleural thickening, due to localized hematoma, is indirect evidence of costal injury.
2. Linear lucency within the shaft is due to a fracture without displacement.
3. Over-all displacement of fragments indicates obvious fracture.
4. Pleural effusion

## RUPTURE OF THE DIAPHRAGM

### Indications

Trauma to the abdomen, dyspnea, etc.

### Studies

1. Chest films, PA or AP and lateral, both in the erect position.
2. Abdominal films, supine and erect positions
3. Gastrointestinal studies if required

### Findings

1. The chest films show a soft tissue mass, suggesting elevation of the diaphragm. This may present as a fluid-

filled soft tissue mass or as an air-containing structure.

2. The mediastinum is shifted to the opposite direction.

3. On the abdominal films, the gas pattern of the abdominal viscera may be directed to the site of perforation.

4. Barium studies, particularly an upper gastrointestinal study, can be done if a diaphragmatic hernia is suspected and the diagnosis cannot be established by the previous examinations. The opaque media can be traced and will enter the abnormally located viscera.

### Differential Diagnosis

1. Eventration of the diaphragm

2. In the case of herniation, the bowel is narrowed at the site where it passes through the ruptured diaphragm. No such narrowing is encountered in eventration.

## ABDOMINAL INJURY

### Basic Principles

1. In all suspected cases of abdominal injury, when the patient's condition permits, the desired routine roentgenographic studies to be obtained should include supine and upright films of the abdomen as well as an upright study of the chest.

2. If the patient is too ill to be placed in an upright position, a lateral decubitus study of the abdomen can be substituted. This is best done with the patient lying on his left side so that the free air will collect along the right flank and will not be confused with air in the stomach. Unless otherwise stated, the above examinations will be termed *routine acute abdominal series.*

3. The need for additional studies will be determined by the nature of the trauma and by the presumptive diagnosis.

### PERFORATED INTESTINE

### Indications

1. Blunt or penetrating injury to the abdomen

2. Distended abdomen

3. Fever and possible shock

### Studies

1. Routine acute abdominal series

2. Gastrointestinal studies

### Method of Performance

1. Acute abdominal studies are performed as stated above.

2. *Gastrointestinal Studies.* An upper gastrointestinal study or enema using a water-soluble contrast agent (e.g., Gastrografin) is preferred in all cases of suspected perforation.

### Findings

1. *Pneumoperitoneum.* Free air within the abdomen is present in the supine position beneath the abdominal wall as an oval-shaped, lucent collection resembling a football. In the upright or decubitus position, the air collects, respectively, under the leaves of the diaphragm or along the lateral wall of the abdomen. Long air–fluid levels are encountered. The presence of a large pneumoperitoneum usually indicates perforation of the stomach, duodenum or colon. With small bowel perforation, little or no air may be detected.

2. *Peritonitis.* Free peritoneal fluid and an ileus pattern suggest the presence of acute peritonitis. An ileus pattern is characterized by both small and large bowel distention. The presence of fluid is recognized by an over-all increase in grayness of the film, separation of the bowel loops, loss of the hepatic angle, and decrease in size in the properitoneal fat lines.

3. *Gastrointestinal Studies.* When performed, the insertion of barium or water-soluble material into the gastrointestinal tract may demonstrate the site of perforation.

### INTRAMURAL HEMATOMA OF THE DUODENUM

### Indications

1. Blunt trauma to the abdomen

2. Pain, nausea and vomiting

## Studies

1. Routine acute abdominal studies
2. Upper gastrointestinal studies with barium

## Findings

1. *Ileus.* This is evident by the distended small and possibly large bowel.
2. Markedly distended stomach and duodenum on plain films, indicating obstruction at the duodenal level
3. Gastrointestinal studies reveal:

    A. A dilated irregular duodenum with multiple nodular defects along the wall, representing submucosal and subserous hematomas

    B. Irregularly narrowed lumen due to diffuse intramural hemorrhage

    C. Accordion pleating of the mucosa is also present and related to diffuse hemorrhage.

## RUPTURED SPLEEN

## Indications

1. Abdominal trauma
2. Left upper quadrant pain
3. Impending shock

## Studies

1. Routine acute abdominal series
2. Arteriography
3. Gastrointestinal studies

## Method of Performance

1. Acute abdominal series, routine
2. *Arteriography.* This study, when done, should be performed prior to studying the gastrointestinal tract with opaque media. The study is performed percutaneously using the Seldinger technique via either the femoral or the axillary artery. A Kifa green catheter with multiple side holes and one end hole is utilized when a flush aortogram is performed. For selective splenic arteriography, a curved-tip catheter is inserted into the celiac artery and 50 ml. of meglumine diatrizoate (Renografin 76) are injected. Serial films are obtained on the rapid film changer.

3. *Gastrointestinal Studies.* Preferably an upper gastrointestinal study is performed because of the proximity of the enlarging spleen to the stomach. This is presently rarely required.

## Findings

1. *Acute Abdominal Series*

    A. Enlarging left upper quadrant mass

    B. Displacement of the stomach shadow downward and medially

    C. Fluid within the abdominal cavity

    D. Thickened mucosal folds on the greater curvature of the stomach

    E. Pleural reaction at the base of the left pleural cavity with associated diaphragmatic elevation.

2. *Arteriography*

    A. The splenic artery and its branches are displaced and deformed

    B. Extravasation of the opaque material

    C. Irregular opacification of the splenic parenchyma with a soft tissue mass adjacent to and compressing the splenic tissue. This mass represents a subcapsular hemorrhage.

    D. Early splenic vein opacification due to rapid intraparenchymal shunting

3. *Gastrointestinal Studies*

    A. The stomach is displaced to the right and downward by the enlarged spleen.

    B. If a barium enema is performed, downward displacement of the splenic flexure is visualized.

## RUPTURE OF THE LIVER

## Indications

1. Abdominal trauma, particularly to the right side
2. Pain and impending shock conditions

## Studies

1. Routine acute abdominal series
2. Arteriography
3. Gastrointestinal studies

## Method of Performance

All studies are performed as described under Ruptured Spleen, above.

## Findings

1. *Acute Abdominal Series*
   A. Enlarging liver mass
   B. Fluid within the abdomen
   C. Elevation of the right hemidiaphragm and reactive effusion in the right pleural cavity
2. *Arteriography*
   A. Deformed and displaced hepatic artery branches
   B. Accumulation of the contrast material in the parenchyma at the site of rupture
3. *Gastrointestinal Studies.* If performed, these demonstrate the downward and medial displacement of the duodenum and the hepatic flexure.

## INJURY TO THE URINARY TRACT
### RENAL INJURY

## Indications

1. Abdominal trauma, blunt or penetrating
2. Hematuria
3. Mass in the renal area
4. Shock

Quite often, renal injury is also associated with injury to neighboring structures such as the spleen and pancreas. Renal injury should always be checked for in the presence of severe abdominal trauma.

## Studies

1. Roentgenograms of the abdomen
2. Intravenous pyelogram
3. Retrograde pyelogram
4. Renal radioisotope scan
5. Arteriography

## Method of Performance

1. *Roentgenograms of the Abdomen.* In renal trauma, usually a supine examination of the abdomen is sufficient. However, since associated intra-abdominal trauma may be present, an erect film to demonstrate the possibility of free intra-abdominal air may be required.

2. *Intravenous Pyelogram.* An intravenous pyelogram should also be done, utilizing 60 to 100 ml. of meglumine diatrizoate, 60 or 76%. The study is begun with films taken at 5 and 10 minutes after the injection. When necessary, the study is then continued at varying intervals until adequate opacification of the collecting systems is obtained. The intervals are determined by the degree of function and obstruction. If and when some opacification of the injured kidney becomes apparent, further improvement of visualization can be achieved by tomographic means.

3. *Retrograde Pyelogram.* This requires the passage of a catheter into the involved ureter, utilizing cystoscopic visualization. The value of this procedure is debatable, although it does produce greater anatomical detail. It should therefore be utilized in situations requiring a better visualized renal outline or collecting system.

4. *Renal Radioisotope Scan.* This is performed after the intravenous injection of mercury-197 and the utilization of a linear scanner to outline the function and anatomy of the kidney.

5. *Arteriography.* Selective renal arteriography is performed using 8 to 10 ml. of meglumine diatrizoate (Renografin 76) injected into the renal artery. Multiple films are obtained utilizing a serial film changer.

## Findings

1. *Roentgenograms of the Abdomen*
   A. Enlarged renal mass with poor

definition. This is due to perirenal hemorrhage.

B. Vertebral scoliosis directed away from the lesion

C. Displacement of bowel loops is also noted

D. Loss of the psoas muscle shadow due to extravasation of blood into adjacent retroperitoneal tissue

2. *Intravenous Pyelogram*

A. Decrease to nonfunction of the kidney. This can be limited to the involved area, although nonvisualization of the entire kidney can also occur.

B. The visualized collecting systems may be displaced and in some areas amputated.

C. Extravasation into the renal parenchyma or into the surrounding tissues may also be noted.

3. *Retrograde Pyelogram*

A. This will demonstrate exactly the same features as noted on the intravenous pyelogram, but with greater detail and definition.

B. Extravasation not detectable on the intravenous pyelogram will be best visualized on the retrograde study.

4. *Renal Radioisotope Scan.* Size and function of the kidney can be determined.

5. *Arteriography*

A. *Arterial Phase.* Vessel displacement, irregularity and extravasation will be noted.

B. *Nephrogram Phase.* Actual cleavage in the renal structure will be visualized as an area of lucency within the diffuse, dense renal shadow.

## URETERAL INJURY

### Indications

1. This injury occurs following penetrating injury or occasionally postoperatively due to injury to the ureter.

2. Anuria or hematuria and pain in the upper abdomen are clinically present.

### Studies

1. Roentgenograms of the abdomen
2. Intravenous pyelogram
3. Retrograde pyelogram

### Method of Performance

The studies are performed as described above under Renal Injury.

### Findings

1. *Roentgenograms of the Abdomen*

A. Enlarging renal mass

B. Extravasation with changes in the retroperitoneal structures as described above under Renal Injury

2. *Intravenous Pyelogram*

A. Nonfunction or hydro-ureter and hydronephrosis

B. Possible extravasation

3. *Retrograde Pyelogram.* This will demonstrate the actual extravasation.

## BLADDER TRAUMA

### Indications

1. Pelvic trauma
2. Pelvic fracture
3. Hematuria, pain and shock

### Studies

1. Roentgenograms of the abdomen
2. Intravenous pyelogram
3. Retrograde cystogram

### Method of Performance

1. *Roentgenograms of the Abdomen.* This study can be performed in the supine projection

2. *Intravenous Pyelogram. See* under Renal Injury, above, for method of performance.

3. *Retrograde Cystogram.* Under sterile conditions a catheter is inserted into the ureter. Approximately 150 to 200 ml. of 8 to 10% water-soluble contrast media, such as Renografin 60 or 76, are injected. Studies are performed in the frontal and both oblique positions.

## Findings

1. *Plain Film Findings*

A. Fractures or dislocations of the pelvis

B. Obliteration of the soft tissue planes due to hemorrhage and an increase in density in the pelvic area

C. Associated ileus, abnormally distended small or large bowel in the vicinity of the pelvis. This may also suggest an associated rupture into the peritoneal cavity.

2. *Intravenous Pyelogram.* This is performed only to rule out the possibility of upper urinary tract injury (*see* above).

3. *Retrograde Cystogram*

A. Extravasation into the perivesicular tissue

B. Abnormal displacement of the bladder due to the surrounding hematoma. The bladder will be either elevated, due to the extravasation or bleeding within the pelvic floor, or displaced laterally due to surrounding extravasation.

C. A soft tissue mass within the lumen of the bladder may also be present. This represents a large intravesicular hematoma.

D. Displacement and abnormal configuration of the bladder without obvious extravasation indicate a perivesicular hematoma without bladder rupture.

## INJURIES TO THE HEAD

### Basic Principles

1. The value and use of emergency x-ray studies of the skull are debatable. It is far more important to determine and treat the underlying brain injury than to diagnose the type and extent of the skull fracture. In fact, the majority of patients presenting with skull fractures demonstrate little intracranial injury, and intracranial injury occurs in 25 per cent of cases of head trauma without evidence of overt skull fracture. Many fractures are probably not diagnosed because of faulty technique, and fractures of the temporal region and base of the skull are exceedingly difficult to diagnose. The value of detailed studies of the skull in an emergency situation, therefore, remains questionable.

2. In general, four views are routinely taken: both *right and left lateral examinations of the skull,* a *frontal film* and a *Towne's projection.* The latter is an anteroposterior study with 30-degree caudal angulation of the central beam. These views will be considered as the *routine skull series.* However, under certain critical circumstances, a single lateral projection and a Towne's projection will be adequate for diagnosis.

## FRACTURE OF THE CRANIAL VAULT

### Indications

1. Injury to the skull
2. Soft tissue swelling

### Studies

Routine skull series

### Findings

1. *Linear Fracture.* The line is radiolucent, sharply edged, with no branching and no serrations.

2. *Stellate Fracture.* There are multiple linear fracture lines extending from a central area.

3. *Depressed Fracture.* There is a linear area of increased density. This represents the overlapping fragments. A zone of relative lucency usually surrounds the fragments and is caused by separation of the bone fragments.

### Differential Diagnosis

1. *Vascular Channels.* Vascular channels have a specific anatomical configuration and localization.

2. *Sutures.* These are also anatomically well outlined. In addition, they are usually irregular and serrated. Developmental variants may arise, for example, metopic suture or wormian bones.

3. *Old Fracture Line.* The fracture line is less distinct, and the margins are smoother.

## BASILAR FRACTURES

### Indications

1. Trauma
2. Bleeding from the ear, Battle's sign (subcutaneous hemorrhage around the mastoid process)

### Studies

1. Routine skull series
2. Submental-vertex projections to demonstrate the base of the skull, etc.
3. Stenver's projection to demonstrate the apex of the petrous pyramid and the internal auditory canal
4. Mayer's projection to demonstrate the petrous bone, but more specifically the attic, aditus and antrum
5. Laminagraphy

### Method of Performance

1. Routine skull series is performed as described above.
2. *Submental-vertex Projection.* The patient is supine with a pillow under the shoulders. The chin is extended and the vertex of the skull rests on the table. The x-ray tube is angled 20 degrees cephalad and directed slightly below the chin.
3. *Stenver's Projection.* The head is positioned supine on the cassette at an angle of 45 degrees. The tube is directed 12 degrees toward the top of the head. The central beam is directed below and slightly lateral to the external occipital protuberance.
4. *Mayer's Projection.* This is somewhat more complicated. The head is again positioned as above, but the tube is directed at a 45-degree angle from above caudally through the external auditory meatus.
5. *Laminagraphy.* This is performed in both the frontal and lateral projections.

### Findings

Fractures here are difficult to evaluate. Seventy-five per cent of basilar fractures involve temporal bone and arise from three directions.

1. *Squamous Fractures*
    A. *Temporal Parietal Group.* The fracture runs obliquely from upward downward.
    B. *Occipital Lateral.* The fracture line courses along the lambdoid suture toward the mastoid process.
    C. *Occipital Medial.* This is purely an occipital fracture
2. *Fractures of the Petrous Pyramid*
    A. *Longitudinal Fractures.* These fractures course along the anterior surface to one of the foramina of the middle cranial fossa. They extend posteriorly to involve portions of the middle ear.
    B. *Transverse Fractures.* These continue into the posterior cranial fossa.

## CRANIOFACIAL FRACTURES

### Indications

1. Soft tissue swelling anteriorly
2. Rhinorrhea

*Fractures of the Nasal Bones*

### Studies

1. Right and left lateral projections
2. Water's view
3. Occlusal projection (axial views)

### Method of Performance

1. Films are performed in both right and left lateral projections. In this manner, two different views of the nasal bones are taken.
2. *Water's View.* Water's view is performed with the patient's chin positioned on the table, with the forehead tilted approximately 15 degrees anteriorly. The x-ray tube is projected into the base of the skull.
3. *The Axial or Occlusal Projection.* This is performed with a dental film maintained between the teeth, and the exposure is made posteriorly behind the skull across the bridge of the nose.

### Findings

Multiple, linear lucencies are found, directed transversely or obliquely with or without depression of the fragments. The lines must be differentiated from the nasomaxillary sutures which are always present and run parallel to the dorsum of the nose in the lateral views.

### Maxillary Fractures

## Studies

1. Water's view
2. Lateral views
3. AP view

## Method of Performance

*See above.*

## Findings

1. *Transverse Maxillary Fracture* (LeFort I). This transverse fracture runs parallel to the arc of the upper teeth and may separate the teeth, alveolar processes and the hard palate.

2. *Pyramidal Fracture* (LeFort II). This type of fracture assumes a large pyramidal configuration and separates all or part of the upper jaw, the medial wall of the maxillary antrum and the nasal complex from other parts of the face.

3. *Craniofacial Separation* (LeFort III). The entire complex of facial bones here is in a fragment which separates completely from the base of the skull. These fractures may be associated with other components, fractures of the teeth, zygomatic arch, pneumocephalus, etc.

### Malar Fracture

## Indications

Malar fracture should be suspected when there has been a direct blow to the lateral aspect of the face, although this may also arise from the frontal, lateral or oblique direction.

## Studies

1. Water's view is good for evaluation of the zygomaticofrontal suture and infraorbital margin.
2. Lateral views to determine rotation of the fragments

3. Anteroposterior views
4. Basilar view to determine posterior depression of the anterior wall of the maxilla or adjacent zygomatic arch

## Findings

*Linear line or separation*
1. Zygomaticofrontal suture
2. Zygomatic arch entirely
3. Approximate junction of the zygoma with the maxilla

# FRACTURE OF THE ORBIT

## Indications

1. Facial trauma
2. Soft tissue swelling in and around the region of the orbit
3. Other fractures involving the facial bones

## Studies

1. Water's view
2. Posteroanterior views of the face
3. Lateral view
4. Oblique view of the orbit
5. Laminagraphy

## Method of Performance

1. Water's view and the posteroanterior and lateral views are performed as described above.

2. *Orbital View.* The patient's head is placed obliquely prone on the table with the orbit centered on the film. The x-ray beam is centered through the opposite side of the head, approximately 2 inches above the external auditory canal. The film demonstrates the optic foramen and the posterior wall of the orbit.

## Findings

1. *Orbital Rim*
   A. Linear lucency within the rim
   B. Displacement of the fragments with associated soft tissue
   C. Other fractures (e.g., maxillary or malar)

2. *Orbital Walls.* Water's view and oblique orbital views are most valuable for

detection. They may be difficult to interpret since the fracture extends into the base of the skull.

3. *Blowout Fractures.* These involve the thinnest portions of the bony orbit, e.g., the floor and median wall, because of sudden increase in hydrostatic pressure.

### Blowout Fracture of Orbit

#### Indications

1. Blunt trauma to the orbit
2. Enophthalmos and diplopia
3. Impaired movements of the eyeball.

#### Studies

1. Water's view
2. Laminagraphy

#### Findings

1. Soft tissue mass along the inferior orbital rim projection into the maxillary sinus
2. Depressed and displaced bony fragment projected within this mass
3. Fluid due to hemorrhage within the maxillary antrum
4. Air within the orbit

### FRACTURE OF THE MANDIBLE

#### Indications

1. Direct blow to the mandible
2. Soft tissue swelling

#### Studies

1. AP views
2. Lateral views
3. Towne's projection
4. Temporomandibular joint for dislocation

#### Findings

1. *Fracture of the Mandible.* Fractures of the body and rami of the mandible are usually obvious. The location, extent, displacement, and relationship to teeth is vital to clinical management.
2. *Dislocation of the Mandible.* The head of the mandible is anteriorly displaced. It is necessary to differentiate dislocation from fracture since therapy is quite different.

### INTRACRANIAL DAMAGE

#### Indications

1. Trauma to the head
2. Skull fractures
3. Clinical features of concussion, etc.

#### Studies

1. Routine skull series
2. Cerebral angiography
3. Aortic arch study
4. Gamma-encephalography
5. Ultrasonography

#### Method of Performance

1. Routine skull series is performed as described above.

2. *Cerebral Angiography.* This is performed by direct percutaneous puncture of the carotid artery, utilizing a Cournand or Pott's No. 16 needle. Approximately 10 ml. of meglumine diatrizoate (Renografin 76) are injected rapidly and serial films are obtained in both the AP and lateral projections. This technique adequately demonstrates the intracranial arterial systems. However, for visualization of proximal brachiocephalic vessels, an aortic arch study is recommended.

3. *Aortic Arch Study.* This is accomplished by catheterization of the brachial artery and placement of the catheter within the aortic arch. However, at this level, injection of a greater amount of contrast material is required. Simultaneous AP and lateral studies are also necessary to prevent repeat studies and reflooding of the intracranial vascular systems.

4. *Gamma-encephalography.* Radioactive mercury compounds($^{203}$Hg) and, more recently, technetium ($Tc^{99mp}$) 10 to 15 microcuries are injected intravenously. Studies are taken, utilizing the gamma camera or the rectolinear scanner. Four views are recommended.

5. *Ultrasonography.* This utilizes the echoencephalogram to detect the midline, or the M line. Any shift suggests the presence of a space-occupying mass.

## Findings

1. *Subdural Hematoma*

A. *Routine Skull Series.* Fractures may or may not be present. The pineal gland, if calcified, may be displaced. Subdural hematomas can occur in the absence of any obvious skull fractures.

B. *Cerebral Angiography.* An avascular space located between the surface of the brain and the inner wall of the skull is quite diagnostic for a hematoma. This is also associated with a shift of the anterior or middle cerebral vessels. If no shift of the midline structures occurs in the presence of a subdural hematoma, the possibility of a contralateral subdural lesion should be entertained.

C. *Gamma-encephalography.* Studies demonstrate a hot vascular area on the scan and the diagnosis is suggested by location and configuration of the activity.

D. *Ultrasonography.* This reveals a shift of the midline structures.

2. *Epidural Hematoma*

A. *Routine Skull Series.* Epidural hematoma is commonly associated with a fracture crossing the middle meningeal group, suggesting the presence of a tear of the middle meningeal artery.

B. *Cerebral Angiography.* An avascular area is presented similar to a subdural hematoma. This, however, is associated with depression of the superior sagittal sinus, meningeal vessels, or actual extravasation of the material from the meningeal artery.

C. *Gamma-encephalography* and *ultrasonography* will demonstrate the same features encountered in subdural hematoma.

3. *Intracerebral Hematoma*

A. The same skull features are encountered as for epidural hematoma.

B. *Cerebral Angiography.* An intracerebral mass is diagnosed by a combination of a shift of the anterior cerebral artery to the opposite side, with associated pressure of the middle cerebral branches to the same side.

## Differential Diagnosis

Cerebral edema

## TRAUMA TO THE VERTEBRAE

## Indications

Trauma to the spine, back pain, spasm.

## Studies

A lateral view of the spine, particularly cervical, is performed and interpreted prior to any further examination of the spine when the clinical suspicion of a vertebral fracture exists.

## Method of Performance

1. *Lateral Projection.* A translateral roentgenogram utilizing a horizontal x-ray beam is taken with the patient remaining supine. For optimum exposure of the cervical area, traction is applied to the hands to depress the shoulders. In short-necked individuals, the arm closest to the roentgen tube is raised so as to eliminate the shadow of the humeral head.

2. *Anteroposterior* and *oblique* films are added when needed.

3. *Laminagraphy.* This is performed for further detection and detail of the fracture if warranted.

## Findings

1. *Vertebral Bodies*

A. With compression fractures, there is loss of vertical height of the vertebral body, usually at the superior margin of the body.

B. With comminution, the vertebral body is shattered.

C. Fracture of the lamina at the junction with the body of the vertebrae

D. Fracture of the spinous processes at the junction with the lamina

E. A posterior element fracture may be accompanied by dislocation of the apophyseal joint

2. *Atlantoaxial Injury*

A. A fracture of the atlas at its base is slightly oblique and may extend into the body of the second cervical vertebra.

B. Rupture of the transverse ligament is difficult to demonstrate but is strongly associated with dislocation at the first and second cervical vertebral area. Laminagraphy may demonstrate this the best.

## INJURIES TO THE UPPER EXTREMITY

### SHOULDER DISLOCATION

#### Basic Principles

1. *Anterior Dislocation*

A. This may be subcoracoid, sub-glenoid or superior in position.

B. It is associated with avulsion of the capsule and fracture of the anterior rim of the glenoid.

C. It occurs following a fall on an out-stretched hand or a backward fall on the hand or elbow.

2. *Posterior Dislocation*

A. This is associated with a fracture of the posterior rim of the glenoid.

B. It occurs following a direct blow or a fall on an outstretched hand with the limb rotated inward.

#### Studies

1. Shoulder films
2. Transthoracic or axial projections

#### Method of Performance

1. Shoulder films are performed in anteroposterior and lateral projections.

2. *Transthoracic or Axial Projections*

A. The transthoracic projection is performed in an upright position, using a vertical Bucky-Potter diaphragm or grid cassette. The cassette and central ray are centered to the surgical neck of the affected humerus, with the patient standing perpen-

dicular to the film with the opposite arm raised out of the way. The ray may be angled cephalad 5 to 15 degrees.

B. An axial Bucky diaphragm will give the best results. The scapula is placed perpendicular to the film. Both shoulders are rotated as much as possible by placing the arm of the affected side on the opposite shoulder and the forearm as close to the chest as possible. The upright or the recumbent position can be used.

#### Findings

1. *Anteroposterior Projections*

A. *Anterior Dislocation.* Medial or inferior displacement of the humeral head out of the glenoid fossa suggests anterior subcoracoid or subglenoid dislocation

B. *Posterior Dislocation*

(1) Absence of the humeral head within the glenoid cavity

(2) Increased space between the glenoid fossa and the humeral head

2. *Transthoracic or Axial Projections.* There is an obvious anterior or posterior position of the humeral head in relation to the scapula.

### ACROMIOCLAVICULAR SEPARATION

#### Indications

Trauma, with pain and difficulty in moving the shoulder

#### Studies

Shoulder films

#### Method of Performance

1. Anteroposterior and lateral projections

2. An anteroposterior projection of the shoulder while holding a 15-lb. weight on the affected side is the preferred study.

#### Findings

1. There is a widening greater than several millimeters between the lateral end of the clavicle and the acromion process.

2. The clavicular end is usually higher

than the acromion, particularly when compared to the opposite side. This is best demonstrated with the patient holding the weights.

3. Calcification in the coracoclavicular ligament is a sign of previous trauma.

## FRACTURE OF THE CLAVICLE

### Basic Principles

1. Fracture of a clavicle may be caused by a direct blow to the shoulder or a fall on an outstretched hand.

2. It is common in children, with little significance.

3. In adults it is less common but more traumatic.

### Studies

1. AP projection of the shoulder
2. Oblique films if necessary

### Findings

1. *Incomplete (Greenstick) Fracture.* This is found in children, and it is difficult to evaluate.

2. *Complete Fracture with Angulation.* This may be partially obscured by overlying posterior aspects of the upper thoracic ribs.

## FRACTURE OF THE SCAPULA

### Basic Principles

Fracture of the scapula is uncommon. It is frequently associated with other injuries and factors.

### Studies

Shoulder films

### Method of Performance

1. AP and lateral projections of the shoulder
2. Tangential view

### Findings

1. *Body:* linear or comminuted; due to direct injury
2. *Neck:* frequently comminuted and impacted

3. *Coracoid process:* associated with dislocations at the coracoclavicular joint or dislocated humeral head

4. *Glenoid rim:* avulsion fracture from pull of triceps muscle. The injury is due to violent arm action.

5. *Acromion:* rare

6. *Inferior angle of the scapula:* this injury is due to violent lifting, with avulsion of the teres major or latissimus dorsi muscles.

## FRACTURE OF THE STERNUM

### Basic Principles

This type of injury is rare. It is associated with automobile injury.

### Studies

1. Lateral or oblique view of the sternum
2. Tomography when the injury is incompletely clarified by the above

### Findings

There is a transverse fracture through the body of the sternum.

### Differential Diagnosis

Anomalous development

## FRACTURE OF THE PROXIMAL HUMERUS

### Indications

1. Direct trauma or fall
2. Pain and swelling in the shoulder

### Studies

Anteroposterior and lateral or tangential projection

### Findings

1. *Neck of the Humerus*

A. *Anatomical Fracture.* Oblique fracture, complete or greenstick; the fracture is through the base of the humeral head at the junction with the upper shaft of the humerus.

B. *Surgical Neck Fracture.* This fracture is at the junction of the broad upper end of the bone and the more tubular shaft.

    *(1)* Abduction with impaction

    *(2)* Abduction with no evidence of impaction

  2. *Fracture of the Tuberosities*

    A. Fracture of the greater tuberosity is more frequent. Displacement of the fragment is obvious.

    B. Fracture of the lesser tuberosity is rare and isolated. It is caused by pull of the subscapularis muscle and is associated with posterior dislocation of the humerus.

## FRACTURE OF THE HUMERAL SHAFT

### Studies

AP and lateral projections of the humerus

### Findings

The fracture may be spiral, oblique, transverse or comminuted, with or without obvious displacement.

## FRACTURE OF THE DISTAL HUMERUS

### Indications

Pain and swelling in or about the region of the elbow

### Studies

AP and lateral projections of the elbow

### Findings

1. *Supracondylar Fracture.* This is a transverse fracture above the level of the condyles, with or without displacement.

2. *Transcondyloid Fracture.* This is a transverse fracture through the condyles, with or without displacement.

3. *Intercondylar Fracture.* This is a comminuted fracture in either a T or Y configuration, with or without complete separation of the condyles.

4. *Lateral Condylar Fracture.* The lateral condyle is rotated or displaced.

## ELBOW DISLOCATION

### Indications

Trauma, pain and swelling in the elbow

### Studies

AP and lateral projections of the elbow

### Findings

1. Posterior dislocation is the most common. The bones of the forearm are displaced backward, backward and outward, or backward and inward.

2. Anterior dislocation is rare.

    A. The bones of the forearm lie anterior and higher than the humeral condyle.

    B. There is a high association with fracture of the olecranon.

3. Lateral dislocation is very rare. It is associated with fracture of either the internal or external humeral condyle.

4. Dislocation of the radial head is frequently associated with fracture of the ulna, making either the *anterior or posterior Monteggia fracture-type.*

    A. *Anterior Monteggia Fracture.* There is an upward buckling of the fractured ulnar shaft and dislocation anteriorly of the radial head.

    B. *Posterior Monteggia Fracture.* There is dorsal buckling of the ulnar shaft and posterior displacement of the radial head.

## FRACTURE OF THE HEAD OF THE RADIUS

### Studies

AP and lateral projections of the elbow are required. Oblique films should be performed when a fracture is suspected but not identified on the original films. Occasionally an AP projection with the hand in pronation and supination is required.

### Findings

1. There is severe swelling of the elbow joint and displacement of the posterior and anterior fat pad. Radiolucent areas are noted both anterior and posterior to the distal portion of the radius. Normally the posterior fat pad is not seen and is visualized only when displaced by severe effusion

within the joint. This is a good indication for the presence of a fracture even when the fracture is not obvious. The lateral projection demonstrates this best.

2. Incomplete wedge through a portion of the radial head
3. Complete wedge with displacement
4. Transverse fracture with angulation of the head
5. Transverse fracture with impaction of the head

## FRACTURE OF THE OLECRANON PROCESS

### Studies

AP and lateral projections of the elbow

### Findings

1. Simple fracture through the base of the olecranon process, with or without displacement
2. Comminuted fracture with little or severe displacement or fragments

## FRACTURE OF THE MID FOREARM

### Studies

AP and lateral projections of the forearm with the hand in supination if possible

### Findings

1. Greenstick fracture is seen in children; it is more common at the distal end of the bone. There may be a transverse incomplete fracture, with or without buckling (torus fracture).
2. Isolated fractures of the radius and/or ulna which may be transverse or spiral, complete or incomplete, with or without displacement.
3. A fracture at the proximal portion of the ulna with dislocation (*See* Monteggia fracture dislocation under Elbow Dislocation).

## FRACTURE OF THE WRIST

### *Colles' Fracture*

### Basic Principles

Colles' fracture occurs following a fall on an outstretched hand, causing backward and outward displacement of the distal radial fragment.

### Indications

A fall, pain, swelling and wrist deformity

### Studies

1. Anteroposterior and lateral views of the wrist
2. Occasionally an oblique view when necessary

### Findings

1. Horizontal fracture through the distal part of the wrist with no displacement or minimal or gross displacement
2. The classical picture is impaction of the radial fragment, associated with avulsion of the ulnar styloid process.
3. There is disruption of the fragments with severe comminution.

### Variants

1. With Smith type (reversed Colles') fracture, angulation is ventral instead of dorsal.
2. Epiphyseal fracture is seen in children. Colles' fracture is not present at this age.

## HAND TRAUMA

### Basic Principles

1. *Routine study* for most cases of hand trauma consists of AP, lateral and oblique views of the hand.
2. In children, comparative views should be obtained.

### Method of Performance

Exposure is performed on the table top without the use of a grid. For best detail, nonscreen cassettes can be utilized.

### Findings

1. *Inferior Radial-Ulnar Dislocation*
   A. Anterior or posterior displacement of the end of the ulna
   B. Fracture of the ulnar styloid or radius is frequently presented

2. *Radiocarpal Dislocation.* This is rare and is frequently associated with fractures of the lower radius.

3. *Lunate Dislocation*

A. *Indications:* Fall on a moderately extended hand

B. *Studies:* routine; the lateral view is best for absolute diagnosis.

C. *Findings:* the lunate bone is visualized anteriorly.

4. *Perilunar Dislocation.* The carpal bones are dislocated around the lunate.

A. *Studies:* routine; the lateral view is preferred.

B. *Findings:* there is normal radial-lunate relationship, with the remaining carpal bones dislocated around the lunate.

C. *Complications:* avascular necrosis is a common sequela to lunate dislocation. It occurs only rarely with perilunar dislocation.

5. *Fracture of Navicular Bone*

A. *Studies:* routine; occasionally particular views of the navicular bone with the hand in forced ulnar deviation are required.

B. *Findings*

*(1)* Compression fracture is an early feature. There is increased *linear density* resulting from overlap of the bony margins at the fracture site.

*(2)* There is separation of the fragments, with *obvious lucency* representing the actual fracture site.

*(3)* Late features occur 2 weeks following injury: *increased radiolucency* due to absorption; *sclerosis* at the fracture margin.

C. *Complications:* avascular necrosis. Late features are fragmentation, sclerosis of bone and cyst formation.

6. *Fracture of the Triquetrum, Hamate, Greater Multangular, Lesser Multangular, Capitate and Lunate*

A. *Studies:* routine

B. *Findings: as above*

C. *Complication:* Kienböck's Disease. Osteochondritis of the lunate bone is probably secondary to trauma.

*Findings:* cystic changes, increased sclerosis and fragmentation

7. *Fracture of the Metacarpals*

A. *Indications:* trauma, crushing injury or force directly transmitted against the dorsum of the hand

B. *Studies:* routine

C. *Findings:*

*(1)* The fracture may be transverse or spiral, involving the base or body of the bone.

*(2)* Fractures at the base of the first metacarpal are frequently impacted on their medial aspect.

8. *Fracture of the Phalanges*

A. *Studies:* AP, lateral and oblique views of the finger

B. *Findings:*

*(1)* Fracture lines may be transverse, spiral or comminuted.

*(2)* In the distal phalanges, fractures are crescentic, comminuted or even longitudinal.

*(3)* Chip fractures are difficult to detect; they are usually at the base of the middle phalanx.

## INJURIES TO THE LOWER EXTREMITY

### FRACTURE OF THE HIP

**Indications**

1. Trauma to the pelvis and hip area
2. Soft tissue swelling
3. Difficulty in moving extremities, etc.

**Studies**

1. AP of the pelvis
2. Lateral projection of the femoral head

**Findings**

1. *Capsular Fracture.* The linear fracture line extends through the subcapital or the transcervical area. Abduction or impaction may be visualized. When impacted, the fracture line is represented by an area of increased density.

2. *Extracapsular Fractures*

A. *Intertrochanteric Fracture.* The

fracture line extends through the intertrochanteric line.

B. *Peritrochanteric Fracture.* There is an extension of the intertrochanteric fracture through the greater trochanter and possibly into the lesser trochanter.

C. *Subtrochanteric Fracture.* The fracture is beneath the level of the trochanters.

D. Dislocation and avulsion of the fragments can be seen in these fractures.

## DISLOCATION OF THE HIP

### Indications

As above

### Studies

As above

### Findings

1. *Anterior Dislocation*

A. The femoral head is located within the region of the obturator foramen. The head and shaft are therefore directed medially and laterally.

B. Fracture of the acetabulum may be associated with this dislocation.

2. *Posterior Dislocation.* This is the most frequent type of dislocation. It is best determined by the lateral projection. The head of the femur is seen projected superiorly and posteriorly to the acetabulum. The main shaft of the femur is directed medially.

## PELVIC TRAUMA

### Indications

1. Direct or indirect blow to the pelvis
2. Soft tissue hematoma
3. Difficulty in moving extremities
4. Hematuria, etc.

### Studies

1. AP of the pelvis
2. Lateral and oblique studies if necessary

### Method of Performance

The films can be performed in the supine position.

### Findings

1. *Avulsion Fracture.* This is due to abrupt muscular contraction of the lower extremity.

A. Avulsion of the anterior inferior iliac spine

B. Avulsion of the anterior superior iliac spine

C. Avulsion of the epiphysis of the ischium

2. *Isolated Fracture.* Fracture of the pubic rami, epiphysis pubis or sacro-iliac joint; all may demonstrate little displacement.

3. *Combined Injuries.* With severe fracture, usually more than one fracture of the pelvic ring is present, for example:

A. Pubic rami, bilateral

B. Unilateral fracture of pubic ramus, associated with separation of the symphysis pubis

C. Combined fractures with iliac and pubic segments

## FRACTURE IN THE MIDFEMORAL SHAFT

### Studies

AP and lateral projections of the thigh, including head and condyles

### Findings

Transverse, oblique or comminuted fracture, with or without displacement

## FRACTURE OF THE DISTAL FEMUR

### Studies

AP and lateral projections of the lower femur and knee

### Findings

1. *Supracondylar Fracture.* There is a transverse fracture at the level of or slightly above the condyle.

2. *Condylar or Intercondylar Fracture*

A. Intercondylar fracture is a T or Y fracture, comminuted, often displaced.

B. Single condylar fracture is uncommon with displacement

## KNEE TRAUMA

### Indications

1. Direct trauma to the knee
2. Pain and swelling
3. Ecchymosis and difficulty in moving

### Studies

1. X-ray study of the knee requires basically anteroposterior and lateral views as the routine study. When in doubt, oblique or other specific views can be requested.
2. Table-top technique without a grid is quite satisfactory.

### Findings

1. Fracture of the patella
2. Fracture of the distal femur
3. Tibial condylar fracture
4. Ligamentous injury

#### *Fracture of the Patella*

### Studies

1. Routine
2. Oblique views are important when in doubt; they will delineate the entire circumference of the bone.
3. A tangential view is taken when required. It projects the patella away from the femur.

### Findings

Fracture, transverse and occasionally vertical

### Differential Diagnosis

Bipartite or tripartite patella, congenital anomaly. The margins of the fragments are smooth and sclerotic.

#### *Tibial Condylar Fracture*

### Findings

1. Either or both condyles may be depressed. The margin is separated from the central portion of the bone.
2. The fragment may be impacted, separated or comminuted.
3. The joint is abducted when the trauma is directed from a lateral direction.

#### *Ligamentous Injury*

### Findings

1. Rupture of the lateral collateral ligament—widened lateral knee joint space
2. Rupture of the medial collateral ligament—wide medial knee joint space
3. Anterior cruciate ligament tear—fracture of the anterior portion or all of the intercondylar eminence
4. Posterior cruciate ligament tear—posterior tibial surface avulsion fracture
5. Avulsion of the tendinous insertion of the biceps femoris—the lateral surface of the tibial condyle is fractured and elevated.

## FRACTURES OF THE TIBIA AND FIBULA

### Basic Principles

The tibia is the least protected of all bones in the lower extremity and is thus commonly involved in open injuries.

### Indications

Pain, swelling and deformity in the area of the tibia and fibula

### Studies

Anteroposterior and lateral projections of the tibia and fibula

### Findings

The fractures are vertical, transverse, horizontal, torsion with or without comminution, or displacement.

## FRACTURE OF THE ANKLE

### Indications

Swelling, pain and difficulty in movement of the ankle

### Studies

AP, lateral and oblique views of the ankle

### Findings

1. *Single Malleolar Fracture.* This is an

oblique or spiral fracture through either the lateral or medial malleolus.

2. *Bimalleolar Fracture*

A. Both the lateral and medial malleoli—ankle mortise (or joint space)—may be slightly altered when displacement is present.

B. Gross displacement—Pott's fracture

3. *Trimalleolar Fracture.* The medial, lateral and posterior malleoli are involved. The articular surface is interrupted and separation is obvious.

## FOOT TRAUMA

### *Fracture of the Calcaneus*

**Indications**

Fall from a height, pain, tenderness in the region of the calcaneus.

**Studies**

Axial and lateral views of the calcaneus; tangential views if necessary.

**Findings**

1. Incomplete fracture
2. Comminuted fracture: the body of the calcaneus is completely disrupted and mutiple bony fragments are visualized.

### *Fracture of the Navicular Bone*

**Indications**

Crushing injury to the foot, pain and swelling

**Studies**

AP, lateral and oblique films of the foot

**Findings**

1. Lucency representing the fracture
2. Increased density representing compression of the bone

**Differential Diagnosis**

1. Köhler's disease—dense and compressed bone
2. Accessory ossicles

### *Fracture of the Talus, Cuboid and Cuneiform Bone*

**Indications**

As above

**Studies**

As above

**Findings**

As above

### *Fracture of the Metatarsals*

**Indications**

Pain and swelling in the region of the foot

**Studies**

AP and lateral and oblique views of the foot

**Findings**

1. *Base of the metatarsals:* linear incomplete or complete fracture with actual separation.
2. *Shaft:* the fracture may be oblique or transverse, single or multiple.

**Differential Diagnosis**

Normal epiphysis at the base of the 5th metatarsal. The epiphysis is directed vertically in contrast to the *horizontally* directed fracture.

### *Fractures of the Phalanges*

**Indications**

Trauma, ·pain and swelling in the phalanges

**Studies**

As above for the foot, with specific attention to the phalanges

**Findings**

Oblique or comminuted fracture

**Differential Diagnosis**

Sesamoid bones

# 4. RADIOLOGY OF NONTRAUMATIC SURGICAL EMERGENCIES

*Jack G. Rabinowitz*, M.D.

## ABDOMEN

### Basic Principles

X-ray examination of patients with surgical abdominal emergencies should be performed following clinical examination of the patient. The type of examination should be directed to the area suspected. In general, as in most cases pertaining to the abdomen, supine and erect films of the abdomen and a posteroanterior projection of the chest are the basic films necessary. This will be considered *routine*. Occasionally decubitus studies may and should be substituted for the erect film when the latter is too difficult to obtain. A prone view of the abdomen is also recommended to better define the outline of the rectum when this structure is in question. Special procedures, e.g., gastrointestinal studies or angiography, may then be utilized to further clarify the problem if necessary.

## LARGE BOWEL OBSTRUCTION

### Basic Principles

In elderly patients, the most frequent causes are tumor and diverticulitis. Other less common causative lesions are polyps, lipomas and adhesions.

### Indications

1. Abdominal distention
2. Vomiting
3. Minimal to no passage of gas and fecal material

### Studies

1. Routine abdominal study. Decubitus and prone position examinations are recommended when necessary.
2. Barium enema

### Method of Performance

1. Routine as indicated
   A. Lateral decubitus films are performed to further outline the distended colon. The films are exposed with the patient lying on his right or left side with the side in question in the upright position. The cassette is placed adjacent to the patient's back and an across-the-table anteroposterior film is exposed. Air rises and outlines the bowel lying superiorly.
   B. The prone film is an excellent study to outline rectal or rectosigmoid lesions. In this position, the rectum is in a superior position and air within it rises to best delineate the anatomy.
2. A barium enema is definitely indicated when colonic obstruction is suggested by routine study and the exact location of the obstruction is desired prior to surgery. Gastrografin can be substituted for barium, particularly if further definition of the colon beyond the point of obstruction is required.

### Findings

1. *Routine study.* A dilated, distended gas-filled colon is visualized and may be traced to the level of obstruction. Large air–fluid levels are demonstrated on the upright study. The colon may be recognized by:
   A. *Contour.* Haustrations differentiate the colon from the small bowel. Haustrations are short, thick and usually don't cross the entire bowel symmetrically. Valvulae conniventes characterize the small bowel.
   B. *Position.* Distended loops occupy the characteristic position of the colon: ascending and descending portions are located along the flanks; the transverse colon extends across the abdomen.

41

2. *Barium Enema.* The barium column is arrested at the level of obstruction. Specific findings are:

A. *Carcinoma.* The lumen is narrowed, irregular and scalloped. The bowel bordering the lesion both distally and proximally demonstrates shelf-like edges. This represents the margin of the mass. The sigmoid is the most frequent site—60 percent of cases.

B. *Diverticulitis.* The lumen is also narrow. The mucosa remains intact. Diverticula are usually present. An intramural abscess (or fistula) is demonstrated by the channel of barium running parallel to the narrowed elongated lumen. An inflammatory mass may produce smooth extrinsic compression.

C. *Polyp.* This is an intraluminal mass with a smooth, sharp border.

D. *Hernia.* This is an abnormal position of the involved colon. The colon tapers smoothly at the points of entry and exit through the hernial sac. The sigmoid is frequently involved.

E. *Adhesion.* This is an extrinsic linear defect upon the wall of the colon.

## SMALL BOWEL OBSTRUCTION

### Basic Principles

1. Acute small bowel obstruction may be caused by adhesions, polyps, hernias, volvulus, etc.

2. Chronic or incomplete small bowel obstruction may be caused by adhesions or a tumor. It may become acute.

### Indications

1. Distended abdomen
2. Vomiting
3. Crampy pain

### Studies

1. Routine abdominal study
2. Barium enema
3. Small bowel study

### Method of Performance

1. Routine abdominal study, as above

2. *Barium Enema.* This is performed to exclude the possibility of a proximal colonic lesion (e.g., carcinoma involving the ileocecal valve).

3. *Small Bowel Study.* This is done if and when a specific diagnosis is desired. It will locate and very frequently define the nature of the obstruction. The best studies are done with barium. Gastrografin is a poor medium for study of small bowel obstruction since it dilutes quickly because of its hyperosmolarity. Two glasses of barium are ingested and abdominal films are exposed at varying intervals, usually commencing about 15 to 20 minutes afterward. Spot films should be obtained to better outline the cause of the obstruction.

### Findings

1. *Routine Abdominal Study.* The small bowel is recognized by:

A. *Location.* Multiple distended loops are localized to the midportion of the abdomen.

B. *Contour.* Valvulae conniventes or mucosal markings are easily demonstrable when the jejunum is dilated, but they are compressed and not well defined in the distended ileum.

C. *Stepladder Appearance.* Air–fluid levels vary in height on film exposed in the erect or decubitus position, indicating hyperactive bowel. This must be distinguished from paralytic bowel or ileus. Air–fluid levels in this stage are at equal levels in the same loop.

(1) In long-standing obstruction, the stepladder appearance disappears because the bowel becomes fatigued and air–fluid levels assume similar levels.

(2) With a large amount of fluid within the bowel, air–fluid levels are minimal. Multiple soft tissue masses representing fluid-filled loops of bowel are then present.

2. *Barium Enema.* The colon is normal. With ileocecal obstruction caused by

tumor, a soft tissue mass or large filling defect will be found occupying the cecum.

3. *Small Bowel Study.* The point of obstruction is recognized by localizing discrepancy in bowel distention. The bowel distal to the point of obstruction is collapsed in contrast to the dilated proximal bowel.

*Complications: Vascular Compromise*

## Basic Principles

This occurs following long-standing simple obstruction or rapidly in complicated obstruction (e.g., closed-loop obstruction).

## Findings

*Routine Abdominal Study*

1. All the findings of small bowel obstruction

2. The bowel wall is thickened and irregular and the lumen is narrowed. This is due to the presence of edema and hemorrhage. In simple obstruction, the bowel wall remains smooth and regular.

3. Peritonitis—fluid within the peritoneum (*see* below).

## CLOSED-LOOP OBSTRUCTION

## Basic Principles

Closed-loop obstruction implies obstruction of a loop of bowel in two points. It is associated with volvulus, strangulated hernia, multiple adhesions, etc. Closed-loop obstruction is associated with early vascular compromise.

## Studies

1. Routine abdominal study
2. Barium enema
3. Small bowel study

## Method of Performance

1. Routine abdominal study, as above

2. Barium enema is to be done when plain film diagnosis suggests either cecal or sigmoid volvulus.

3. Gastrointestinal opacification studies may be performed but in most situations are unnecessary.

## Findings

*Routine Abdominal Study*

1. *Coffee-bean Sign.* The obstructed loop of bowel is twisted upon itself so that the twisted portions of bowel lie adjacent to each other. This produces the coffee-bean configuration. The two loops are distended with air and are separated by a central area of increased density composed of the two opposing thickened walls of bowel.

2. *Pseudotumor.* When the closed loop fills with fluid replacing the air, a fluid-filled soft tissue mass simulating a tumor is created.

3. *Immobility.* The closed loop is fixed and does not change configuration or position when the patient's position is altered.

## VOLVULUS

## Basic Principles

Volvulus occurs in:
1. The sigmoid
2. The cecum
3. The small bowel
4. Rarely in the stomach and in the transverse colon

## Studies

1. Routine abdominal study
2. Barium enema
3. Gastrointestinal study including small bowel series

## Findings

### Sigmoid Volvulus—Associated with Long, Mobile Mesentery

1. *Routine Abdominal Study.* A large coffee-bean or pseudotumor appearance is produced. The mass arises from the pelvis and projects to the right upper quadrant. The two limbs of the loop point downward toward the pelvis.

2. *Barium Enema.* The barium is obstructed at the rectosigmoid junction. The end of the barium column narrows gradually and has a beak-like configuration.

## Cecal Volvulus—Associated with Nonfixation of Mesentery

1. *Routine Abdominal Study.* An enlarged coffee-bean sign or a markedly enlarged loop of bowel is occupying most of the abdomen. The apex of the distended loop projects toward the left upper quadrant.

2. *Barium Enema.* A beak-like narrowing of the barium column is encountered in the ascending colon. Occasionally barium enters the twisted bowel.

## Small Bowel Volvulus

*Routine Abdominal Study.* The coffee-bean sign, pseudotumor and immobility, are all localized to the small bowel if identified.

# ILEUS

## Basic Principles

Ileus is due to partial paralysis of the bowel. It is associated with peritonitis, inflammatory or vascular disease, postoperative state, etc.

## Studies

Routine abdominal study

## Method of Performance

As indicated above

## Findings

1. *Supine Film*
    A. Sentinal loop. This is a single, distended gas-filled loop of bowel, usually the small bowel.
    B. Multiple loops of distended small bowel
    C. Combination of small and large bowel distention
2. *Upright film.* All of the above show air-fluid levels at similar levels within a single loop of bowel (no differential levels visualized).

# PERITONITIS

## Basic Principles

Peritonitis occurs following chemical, bacterial or neoplastic irritation of the peritoneum, with resulting exudate or transudate present within the peritoneal cavity.

## Studies

Routine abdominal study

## Method of Performance

As indicated above

## Findings

*Supine Film*
1. Ileus
2. Fluid in the peritoneum
    A. Over-all gray appearance to the abdomen
    B. Viscera displaced medially
    C. Distended loops are separated by fluid.

# ACUTE CHOLECYSTITIS

## Basic Principles

1. This is almost always associated with gallstones and cystic duct obstruction.
2. The causative organism may be *E. coli,* staphylococcus, etc., with secondary infection.

## Indications

1. Biliary colic
2. Fever
3. Pain, tenderness in the right upper quadrant
4. Vomiting, etc.

## Studies

1. Routine abdominal study
2. Oral cholecystogram — not indicated in the acute phase
3. Intravenous cholangiogram — usage questionable

## Method of Performance

1. Routine abdominal study, as indicated above

2. *Intravenous Cholangiogram.* Cholografin, 20 to 40 ml., is slowly injected intravenously during a minimal period of 10 minutes or with a slow-drip infusion. The latter technique is preferred. Caution must be taken regarding any ill effects or reactions. Exposures of the right upper quadrant are then taken at varying intervals beginning at approximately 20 minutes following the injection. During the acute phase, visualization of the biliary system may be markedly delayed and the study must be prolonged for many hours before being considered negative. This therefore limits the efficiency of this study. In general, opacification of the gallbladder occurs 1 to 2 hours after the common duct is visualized.

## Findings

1. *Routine Abdominal Study*
   A. Gallstones in the right upper quadrant
   B. Increased soft tissue mass in the right upper quadrant
   C. Ileus, localized or generalized; when localized, more suggestive
   D. Peritonitis
   E. Emphysematous cholecystitis — air present within the wall or lumen of the gallbladder — caused by air-producing organisms.
2. *Intravenous Cholecystogram.* Visualization of the common duct with failure to opacify the gallbladder may indicate cystic duct obstruction. The study must be adequately prolonged before true evaluation can be established.

## PANCREATITIS

### Basic Principles

1. Pancreatitis occurs in alcoholic patients or in patients with biliary tract disease.
2. Ductal and parenchymal calcifications present in chronic alcoholic pancreatitis.
3. Pseudocyst may occur rapidly following necrosis and spillage of enzymes

into adjacent tissue. The capsule is formed by surrounding tissue.

### Studies

1. Routine abdominal study
2. Upper gastrointestinal studies

### Method of Performance

Both studies are performed as indicated previously.

### Findings

1. *Routine Abdominal Study*
   A. Calcification present within the midepigastrium, simulating the configuration of the pancreas
   B. Ileus localized to the midepigastrium; sentinal loop or generalized in nature
   C. Colon cut-off sign—localized distention of the transverse colon
   D. Diffuse distention of the small and large bowel to the level of the splenic flexure
2. *Upper Gastrointestinal Study*
   A. Widening of the duodenal loop
   Б. Inverted 3 sign—caused by the displacement of the duodenum superiorly and inferiorly to the fixed ampulla of Vater
   C. Mucosal edema, predominantly in the duodenum. The stomach may be involved.
   D. Pseudocyst—displacement of bowel, particularly the stomach anteriorly

## DIVERTICULITIS

*See* above under Large Bowel Obstruction.

## APPENDICITIS

### Basic Principles

Appendicitis is associated with obstruction (e.g., fecalith).

### Studies

1. Routine abdominal study
2. Gastrointestinal studies—not recommended

## Method of Performance

Both as indicated above

## Findings

*Routine Abdominal Study*

1. Calcification—spherical and laminated stone within the right lower quadrant

2. Ileus—localized to the right lower quadrant or generalized in nature

3. Soft tissue mass in the right lower quadrant represents the entire inflammatory process; it is frequently seen with abscess.

4. Gas within the appendix, intraluminal or intramural, produced by gas-producing organism; this indicates necrosis.

## PEPTIC ULCER: PENETRATING, PERFORATED OR BLEEDING

### Indications

1. Vomiting
2. Pain
3. Shock and/or hematemesis

### Studies

1. Routine abdominal study
2. Upper gastrointestinal series
3. Arteriography

### Method of Performance

1. Routine abdominal study, as indicated above

2. Upper gastrointestinal series—the routine study is performed using barium or Gastrografin. Gastrografin is preferred since it will more easily demonstrate perforation with little or no damage to the peritoneum. For best demonstration of duodenal perforation, a glass of Gastrografin is ingested and the patient is then placed on his right side for approximately 10 minutes. Cross-table lateral exposures are then obtained using 14 × 17 films.

3. Arteriography is preferred for bleeding peptic ulcers if immediate surgery is contemplated. This should be done before or in place of the upper gastrointestinal series, utilizing a selective approach through the celiac artery.

## Findings

1. *Supine Abdominal Study.* This reveals pneumoperitoneum—football sign, air underneath the diaphragms.

2. *Upper Gastrointestinal Series.* An ulcer is revealed by:

A. A collection of barium penetrating the wall of the stomach, surrounded by an inflammatory reaction that is smooth and regular

B. Perforation is revealed by leakage of opaque material into the peritoneum.

3. *Vascular Studies Via the Celiac Artery*

A. Mucosal hyperemia—blush within the wall

B. Accumulation of opaque material within the lumen of the stomach or duodenum at the point of bleeding

## MESENTERIC OCCLUSION

### Basic Principles

1. Mesenteric occlusion can be venous or arterial.

2. Venous occlusion is associated with congestive failure, etc.

3. Arterial thrombosis is associated with arteriosclerosis. Embolus is associated with rheumatic mitral disease and atrial fibrillation.

### Studies

1. Routine abdominal study
2. Arteriography
3. Gastrointestinal series

### Method of Performance

1. Routine abdominal study, as indicated above

2. Arteriography—selective studies of superior or inferior mesenteric artery

3. Gastrointestinal series, as indicated above

## Findings

1. *Routine Abdominal Study*

A. Ileus—sentinal or multiple loops of bowel

B. Fluid in the abdomen, most likely representing hemorrhage (*see* above). A greater amount of fluid is seen in venous obstruction.

C. Distended small and large bowel terminating at the splenic flexure is a rare manifestation.

D. Thickened irregular wall of bowel is related to the secondary inflammatory changes and hemorrhage.

E. Intramural gas and portal venous gas. This ominous sign indicates mucosal necrosis. Gas in the portal system is projected peripherally within the liver.

2. *Arteriography.* A selective study will show occlusion of the vessel and possible associated collateral circulation.

3. *Gastrointestinal Series.* This is not indicated in an acute phase, but, if done, demonstrates:

A. Mucosal ulcerations, deep and irregular

B. Thumb printing—nodular defects in the wall due to intramural and serosal hematoma

C. Diffuse thickening of the wall, due to diffuse edema and hemorrhage within the bowel wall also causes coin-stacking appearance of the mucosa.

## THORAX

### PNEUMOTHORAX

*See* Chapter 3, Roentgenographic Principles of Emergency Trauma.

### PNEUMOMEDIASTINUM

*See* Chapter 3, Roentgenographic Principles of Emergency Trauma.

### ASPIRATION OF A FOREIGN BODY

## Basic Principles

This is the frequently seen in the pediatric age-group. Severity depends upon the location, size and type of foreign body (e.g., peanuts incite pneumonia after disintegration).

## Indications

1. Difficulty in breathing
2. History of foreign body ingestion

## Studies

1. Chest films, AP and lateral
2. Fluoroscopy

## Method of Performance

1. Chest films, AP and lateral, are taken in the erect position if possible
2. Fluoroscopy is best done with image intensification.

## Findings

1. *Chest films*

A. Obstructive emphysema—due to partial obstruction with ball-valve phenomenon. The segment or lobe demonstrates increased lucency due to air-trapping behind the foreign body.

B. Atelectasis—complete obstruction, collapse of the segment or lobe. This is seen as triangular density collapsing toward the hilus.

C. *Compensatory Changes*

*(1)* Compensatory emphysema within the ipsi- or contralateral lung

*(2)* Mediastinal shift toward the side of the lesion because of loss of volume

*(3)* Elevated diaphragm and narrowed intercostal spaces are not always present. These are due to the loss of pulmonary volume.

2. *Fluoroscopy.* During inspiration there is a shift of the mediastinum toward the area of involvement.

## Differential Diagnosis

*Foreign Body in the Trachea or Esophagus.* This usually lies in the path of least resistance. It assumes a sagittal direction when in the trachea and an *en face* position when in the esophagus.

## PERICARDIAL EFFUSION

*See* Chapter 3, Roentgenographic Principles of Emergency Trauma.

## DISSECTING AORTIC ANEURYSM

### Basic Principles

This occurs in patients with hypertension and in patients subject to medial necrosis (e.g., Marfan's syndrome).

### Studies

*See* Chapter 3, Roentgenographic Principles of Emergency Trauma.

## MALLORY WEISS SYNDROME

### Basic Principles

*Pathology.* There are multiple mucosal tears in the lower end of the esophagus. This occurs in patients with atrophic mucosa, following severe vomiting and retching, and is frequently seen in alcoholics.

### Studies

1. Chest film—not diagnostic (differential diagnosis is rupture of the esophagus). *See* Chapter 3, Roentgenographic Principles of Emergency Trauma.
2. Esophagogram

### Method of Performance

The esophagogram is performed with barium. Multiple views in various projections are exposed.

### Findings

1. Mucosal edema
2. Superficial tear. The barium is trapped between folds. This is very difficult to observe.

3. Possible atony of the esophagus

## BLEEDING ESOPHAGEAL VARICES

### Basic Principles

Distended and dilated esophageal veins are part of collateral circulation, following:
1. Portal vein obstruction with portal hypertension
2. Obstruction of the superior vena cava, referred to as downhill varices
3. Intrahepatic disease (cirrhosis) with sinusoidal compression.

### Studies

Esophagogram

### Method of Performance

It is preferable to do this study with thick and thin barium. Procedures are quite variable. Thick barium paste remains coated to the mucosa. Multiple spot films are then taken. In addition, thin barium may also be given following the ingestion of the thick paste. Additional procedures (e.g., the Mueller or Valsalva maneuvers) can be done to attempt better visualization of varices, but these are unnecessary. Pro-Banthine, 20 mg. I.M., has been recommended to enhance visualization.

### Findings

1. *Esophagogram*
   A. Dilated atonic esophagus
   B. Varices—irregular wormy filling defects within the lower third of the esophagus
2. *Splenoportogram.* Abnormal vessels can be demonstrated on this study, but this is truly not an emergency procedure.

# 5. RADIOGRAPHIC ASPECTS OF NEONATAL CONGENITAL PROBLEMS

*Jack G. Rabinowitz,* M.D.

## THORAX

### PNEUMOMEDIASTINUM

#### Basic Principles

1. Pneumomediastinum occurs following rapid increase of intra-alveolar pressure, with resulting rupture of the alveolar basement membrane.
2. Air escapes into the interstitial tissues and dissects along the bronchovascular structures to reach the mediastinum and occasionally the pleural cavity.
3. The condition frequently resolves spontaneously.
4. Tension pneumomediastinum may compromise the great vessels, requiring surgical intervention.

#### Indications

1. Respiratory distress
2. Crepitation on auscultation

#### Studies

Chest films

#### Method of Performance

The anteroposterior and lateral films of the chest can be taken in the supine position. They can be performed at the bedside or in the x-ray department.

#### Findings

1. Spinnaker sail sign, caused by lateral and anterior displacement of the thymus, is most often seen unilaterally but occasionally may be visualized bilaterally as an elliptical density surrounded laterally and medially by air.
2. On the lateral projection, the thymus is outlined as a tongue of tissue floating within a large air-containing retrosternal space. Normally, the latter space is oc-

cupied only by the thymus with no evidence of air.
3. Linear streaks of air may be the only sign present within the mediastinum. The air may also dissect into the soft tissues of the neck and the retroperitoneum.
4. Tension pneumomediastinum (progressive pneumomediastinum) appears as an enlarging, loculated air cyst due to the continual escape of air into the mediastinum.

## CONGENITAL LOBAR EMPHYSEMA

#### Basic Principles

Congenital lobar emphysema may be due to bronchial obstruction caused by an abnormal congenital flap of mucosal membrane or a local weakness within the bronchial wall. Both lead to a ball-valve mechanism, trapping air distal to the obstruction.

#### Indications

Increasing dyspnea and cyanosis in early infancy

#### Studies

Chest films

#### Method of Performance

Anteroposterior and lateral films can be performed in a supine position.

#### Findings

1. There is progressive overaeration of a segment or lobe.
2. Adjacent interlobar tissue is displaced so that the involved area assumes an almost spherical or cystic appearance.
3. The mediastinum is displaced to the contralateral side.

4. The intercostal spaces on the affected side are widened.

## Differential Diagnosis

1. *Pulmonary Agenesis.* Hyperlucency exists within the normal lung and contains normal bronchovascular markings.

2. *Congenital Lung Cysts, Single or Multiple.* There is little or no change in the over-all dynamics within the chest.

3. *Congenital Cystic Adenomatoid Malformation of the Lung.*

A. This is a malformation consisting of multiple cysts and hamartomas. The roentgenographic appearance is mixed, containing both solid and cystic structures.

B. It is usually asymptomatic.

C. The condition occasionally causes dyspnea and cyanosis by compressing neighboring structures.

D. Anasarca is present in 50 per cent of cases due to pressure on the great veins.

4. *Rupture or Congenital Absence of the Diaphragm.* See below.

## DIAPHRAGMATIC HERNIA

### Basic Principles

1. Diaphragmatic hernia is extension of intra-abdominal contents through a defect in the diaphragm. The hernia may be an *anterior* hernia through the foramen of Morgagni or a *posterior* hernia through the foramen of Bochdalek.

2. It may be caused by either incomplete formation of the pleuroperitoneal canal or premature return of the viscera into the peritoneum prior to closure of the pleuroperitoneal canal.

3. The nature of the hernia through the foramen of Morgagni is still undetermined since the contents are always covered with peritoneal membrane.

4. The ultimate response and prognosis following surgical repair depend upon the initial development of the ipsilateral lung tissue as well as to its capacity to expand.

### Indications

Respiratory difficulty

## Studies

1. Chest films
2. Abdominal study
3. Gastrointestinal studies

## Method of Performance

1. The chest films, AP and lateral, can be performed either in a supine or upright position. The lateral study can also be done either cross-table or in an upright position.

2. The abdominal study is best performed in a supine or upright position. If the latter cannot be obtained, a decubitus study may be performed with the involved side in the upright position.

3. The gastrointestinal series is preferably done with oral barium. The study is continued until the entire gastrointestinal tract is evaluated. Gastrografin is to be avoided in the neonatal period because of its hyperosmolarity.

## Findings

1. *Chest films*

A. Presence of cystic structures within the thoracic cavity

B. Identification of bowel wall (e.g., valvulae conniventes or haustra suggest the correct diagnosis.)

C. Associated density in the upper thoracic cavity probably represents collapse of the ipsilateral lung.

D. Displacement of the mediastinum to the opposite side

E. Right-sided hernia through the foramen of Bochdalek contains the liver in addition to the gas-filled viscera.

2. *Abdominal Study.* In the right upper quadrant in right-sided hernias the liver shadow is absent and is replaced by gas-containing viscera.

3. *Gastrointestinal Studies.* Oral studies with barium will definitely identify the position and the nature of the gastrointestinal loops.

## Differential Diagnosis

1. Congenital cystic disease of the lung
2. Staphylococcal pneumonia with

pneumatocele formation. Both congenital cystic disease of the lung and staphylococcal pneumonia are excluded by gastrointestinal studies.

3. Diaphragmatic eventration.

## ESOPHAGEAL ATRESIA

### Basic Principles

1. *Esophageal Atresia with Tracheoesophageal Fistula.* This is the most common type, occurring in approximately 85 per cent of cases. The lower esophageal segment communicates either with the trachea at the level of the bifurcation or with the proximal portion of a main bronchus.

2. *Esophageal Atresia without Tracheoesophageal Fistula.* This is found in approximately 8 per cent of cases. The lower esophageal segment remains as a small pouch at the level of the diaphragm.

3. *Esophageal Atresia with Both the Upper and Lower Esophageal Segments Communicating Separately with the Trachea*

4. *Esophageal Atresia with Only the Upper Esophageal Segment Communicating with the Trachea.* The lower pouch of the esophagus ends above the diaphragm.

5. *H-type Fistula.* The esophagus is patent, with a small fistulous communication connecting the esophagus with the trachea.

6. *Esophageal Membrane.* This is nonobstructive (may not be a true part of this entity).

### Indications

Excessive mucus regurgitation in the immediate neonatal period; fever; vomiting if and when fed.

### Studies

1. Chest films
2. Nasogastric tube insertion
3. Injection of opaque material
4. Abdominal x-ray when the abdomen is not visualized on chest films

### Method of Performance

1. Chest films, AP and lateral projections

2. *Nasogastric Tube Insertion.* A feeding tube is inserted in an effort to reach the stomach.

3. *Injection of Opaque Material.* A dose of 0.5 to 1 ml. of an opaque material, preferably Gastrografin, is injected. This is performed mainly to visualize the site of the atresia and to outline the lower margin of the upper pouch.

### Findings

1. *Chest films*

    A. Aspiration pneumonia is frequently seen in the right upper lobe.

    B. A dilated air-containing proximal esophageal pouch is best seen on the lateral projection; it is located high in the superior mediastinum. This displaces the trachea anteriorly.

2. *Nasogastric Tube Insertion.* On the chest film, the tube is coiled in the proximal pouch.

3. *Injection of Opaque Material.* The material remains collected in the upper esophageal pouch when the upper pouch is atretic.

4. *Abdominal X-ray.* This determines the presence or absence of gas within the gastrointestinal tract and therefore the presence or absence of communication of the lower esophageal pouch with the tracheobronchial tree.

## ABDOMEN

### Basic Principles

1. Under normal conditions, swallowed air reaches the stomach within minutes following birth and passes readily into the small bowel. Diffuse distribution throughout the small bowel is encountered approximately at 3 hours of age and the entire colon may be completely outlined within 5 hours.

2. In general, an abdominal film of a normal infant taken 24 hours after birth

will show gas present throughout the entire gastrointestinal tract. An upright film at this time will also demonstrate evidence of small air–fluid levels.

3. Abnormal distribution of the gas therefore aids in localizing and detecting the presence of obstructive disease in the neonatal period.

4. Radiographic evaluation of the abdomen basically requires *supine* and *upright* films of the abdomen. These studies, including a chest film, are considered the routine study.

5. Opacification studies of either the upper or lower gastrointestinal tract are necessary at times to fully clarify the underlying disease.

A barium enema is performed when a low small bowel or colonic obstruction is suspected. The barium enema outlines and locates the position of the colon, thus distinguishing the various different forms of colonic disease as well as yielding much information regarding the small bowel.

## CONGENITAL ATRESIA OF THE STOMACH

### Indications

Vomiting immediately after feeding.

### Studies

1. Routine abdominal study
2. Upper gastrointestinal study

### Method of Performance

1. Abdomen, routine
2. *Upper Gastrointestinal Series.* This is best performed using Gastrografin in small amounts to prevent vomiting and consequent aspiration.

### Findings

1. *Routine Abdominal Study*
    A. The single bubble sign is characterized by a single distended loop of gas in the epigastrium.
    B. No gas is present in the remainder of the gastrointestinal tract.
2. *Upper Gastrointestinal Series.* This

demonstrates complete obstruction of the distal end of the stomach.

### Differential Diagnosis

*Hypertrophic Pyloric Stenosis.* Atresia is detected in the immediate newborn period, whereas hypertrophic pyloric stenosis occurs slightly later. For roentgenographic differences, *see* below.

## HYPERTROPHIC PYLORIC STENOSIS

### Indications

Projectile vomiting at approximately 3 weeks of age. Hypertrophic pyloric stenosis usually occurs in the first-born male. Palpation of a hard, olive-sized muscular tumor in the right upper quadrant is diagnostic.

### Studies

1. Routine abdominal study
2. Gastrointestinal series: this is performed only when the diagnosis is not clinically apparent. Small amounts of barium are given, and the use of barium is preferred to the use of Gastrografin.

### Findings

1. *Routine Abdominal Study*
    A. Single bubble sign—dilated stomach, with some gas present distally within the small bowel
    B. The stomach demonstrates deep hyperperistaltic contractions as well as excessive fluid.
2. *Gastrointestinal Series*
    A. String sign—elongated narrow pyloric channel corresponding to the size of the muscle tumor
    B. Double-channel, or railroad sign: this is characterized by 2 elongated channels of barium. It is caused by a redundant amount of gastric mucosa within the area involved.
    C. Teat sign—projection of a portion of the lesser curvature adjacent to the pyloric muscle
    D. Shoulder sign is the actual defect

of the muscle upon the distal barium column. This and the above teat sign are caused by the peristaltic waves abutting upon the muscle tumor. Both disappear when the wave passes.

E. The tumor itself can also be visualized utilizing a *Hampton projection.* This is achieved by elevating the patient's right side to allow the air in the stomach to rise toward the antrum to outline the proximal portion of the soft tissue mass.

F. *Ancillary Findings*

(1) Gastric dilatation

(2) Hyperperistalsis

(3) Delayed emptying of the stomach

## Differential Diagnosis

1. *Antral Spasm.* This can be severe and persistent. However, the presence of a rigid narrow channel favors pyloric stenosis. Some authors believe that antral spasm associated with local inflammation and ulceration may actually be the precursor to pyloric stenosis.

2. *Atresia*—complete obstruction of the stomach (*See* above.)

## DUODENAL ATRESIA AND STENOSIS

### Basic Principles

1. *Atresia* is complete obliteration of the lumen, with or without separation of the proximal and distal segments. It is frequently associated with Down's syndrome as well as other atresias of the jejunum or ilium.

2. *Stenosis* is partial obliteration of the intestinal lumen by diffuse narrowing or by a membrane.

### Indications

1. Vomiting, most often bile-stained, within the first 24 hours of life

2. The abdomen is usually not distended in contrast to distal small bowel obstructions.

### Studies

1. Routine abdominal series
2. Gastrointestinal series

### Findings

1. *Routine Abdominal Series*

A. Double bubble sign—2 collections of gas-containing viscera in the upper abdomen. The larger collection usually represents the stomach and the smaller collection the duodenal bulb. This is best visualized in the upright position.

B. *Stenosis:* similar, although the gas may be seen distal to the dilated proximal duodenum.

2. *Gastrointestinal Series.* This demonstrates the distended stomach and duodenum and the exact site of obstruction.

## ANNULAR PANCREAS

### Basic Principles

1. *Incomplete.* There are two extensions of pancreatic tissue partially surrounding the duodenum; the ventral surface is free.

2. *Complete.* Pancreatic tissue forms a complete ring around the duodenum; this is often associated with underlying duodenal atresia.

### Indications

These depend upon the severity of the obstruction. When the obstruction is complete, bile-stained vomiting occurs within the first 24 hours of life.

### Studies and Findings

The studies and findings are similar to those in duodenal atresia and stenosis.

## MALROTATION AND MIDGUT VOLVULUS

### Basic Principles

Malrotation and midgut volvulus are alterations in the normal rotation of the midgut.

1. *Incomplete Rotation.* The small bowel is relatively normal in position. The

rotation of the cecum is incomplete and it lies anterior to the superior mesenteric artery in the left abdomen or high in the right upper quadrant. Abnormal mesenteric bands are formed that extend from the cecum across the duodenum to the right upper quadrant.

2. *Nonrotation.* The entire midgut returns to the peritoneal cavity without completing any rotation around the superior mesenteric artery. The small bowel is positioned in the right abdomen, and the colon and the cecum are positioned in the left abdomen. Fixation of the mesentery is therefore along a small and narrow area adjacent to the superior mesenteric artery. This predisposes to volvulus.

3. *Reverse Rotation.* The small bowel and colon are reversed. The duodenum lies anterior to the colon and is separated from it by the superior mesenteric artery.

### Indications

1. Occasionally intermittent bile-stained vomiting in the first week of life.

2. Shock and prostration after the first week of life

### Studies

1. Routine abdominal study
2. Barium enema
3. Upper gastrointestinal series

### Method of Performance

1. Abdomen, routine
2. *Colon Study.* This is the preferred examination, using barium.
3. *Upper Gastrointestinal Series.* This is performed with minimal amounts of barium or Gastrografin.

### Findings

1. *Routine Abdominal Study.* There is a double or triple bubble sign, due to a distended stomach and second and third portion of the duodenum.

2. *Colon Study. Barium enema* reveals a malpositioned colon.

A. The entire colon may be in the left side of the abdomen.

B. The cecum alone may point to the left side.

C. The cecum may lie in the right upper quadrant.

3. *Upper Gastrointestinal Study.* Introduction of opaque material from above demonstrates:

A. Distended loops

B. The exact level of obstruction

C. The condition of the small bowel if the barium passes the obstruction

### SMALL BOWEL ATRESIA AND STENOSIS

### Basic Principles

Atresia is the end stage of an *in utero* vascular compromise that leads to bowel infarction. If it occurs early in fetal life, the infarcted bowel is absorbed, leaving a residual atretic segment. Lesser degrees of ischemia result in stenosis or a membranous obstruction.

### Indications

Abdominal distention and vomiting within the neonatal period

### Studies

1. Routine abdominal study
2. Colon study
3. Upper gastrointestinal study

### Findings

1. *Routine Abdominal Study*

A. Distended loops of small bowel with no evidence of gas demonstrable within the large bowel

B. In the upright position, multiple air- and fluid-filled loops are seen located mainly in the left abdomen. With proximal obstruction, few loops of bowel are present. Distal small bowel occlusions may be more difficult to diagnose from colonic obstruction since the distended small bowel resembles the large bowel.

2. *Colon Study.* This is preferably performed with barium. Barium enema

demonstrates position and configuration of the colon. Microcolon is encountered in patients with distal small bowel obstructions.

3. *Upper Gastrointestinal Study.* This study is not recommended but can be done when the diagnosis is in doubt.

## Differential Diagnosis

Meconium ileus (*see* below.)

## MECONIUM ILEUS (MUCOVISCIDOSIS, CYSTIC FIBROSIS)

### Basic Principles

1. Meconium ileus is distal ileum obstruction due to markedly abnormal inspissated meconium.

2. *Classification*

A. Uncomplicated meconium ileus

B. Complicated meconium ileus (meconium ileus associated with either volvulus, atresia, perforation or meconium peritonitis)

### Indications

1. Distended abdomen

2. Loops of bowel may be seen projected through the abdomen

3. Family history of cystic fibrosis

### Studies

1. Routine abdominal study

2. Colon study

### Method of Performance

1. Abdomen, routine

2. *Colon Study.* This can be performed with barium or with Gastrografin. The latter is preferred and can be refluxed into the ileum in an attempt to relieve the obstruction. Gastrografin is hypertonic, causing increased secretion of fluid into the bowel lumen. This softens the meconium and creates a fluid medium between the meconium and the bowel wall.

### Findings

1. *Routine Abdominal Study*

A. Small bowel obstruction. Distended loops are *variable* in size; some are moderately dilated, others normal in caliber.

B. Soap-bubble appearance in the right lower quadrant due to mixing of air within the meconium

C. Delayed production of fluid levels in the upright position is caused by the viscous intestinal contents and its adherence to the bowel wall.

2. *Colon Study.* This may reveal a microcolon, usually the smallest of all obstructions.

### Complications

The following may be seen in addition to the above roentgenographic features:

1. *Volvulus* is manifested by the presence of large fluid-filled loops of bowel.

2. *Atresia* is indicated by a markedly dilated small bowel proximal to the obstruction.

3. *Meconium peritonitis* is revealed by calcifications within the peritoneum.

4. *Pseudocyst*—a huge mass of necrotic tissue containing meconium

## MECONIUM PERITONITIS

### Basic Principles

1. Meconium peritonitis is non-bacterial, chemical peritonitis resulting from intra-uterine perforation of the gastrointestinal tract.

2. Meconium undergoes calcification within 24 hours following contact with peritoneal fluid.

3. Meconium peritonitis may be associated with simple obstruction, obstruction with fibrocystic disease or with a patent gastrointestinal tract; the latter closing spontaneously *in utero.*

### Indications

Markedly distended abdomen, vomiting, etc.

## Studies

1. Routine abdominal study
2. Gastrointestinal study

## Method of Performance

1. Abdomen, routine
2. *Gastrointestinal Study.* This may be performed if a specific diagnosis is not obtained by the routine abdominal study. The entire gastrointestinal tract should then be evaluated to exclude any underlying abnormality.

## Findings

*Routine Abdominal Study* reveals calcifications. Calcium appears in clumps or in linear strands located along:

1. The lateral margin of the abdomen
2. On the surface of the liver
3. Or within the wall of the bowel

## HIRSCHSPRUNG'S DISEASE

## Basic Principles

Hirschsprung's disease is colonic obstruction due to absence of ganglion cells within the colon.

1. *Incomplete.* The absent ganglion cells are limited to the distal portion of the colon and the rectum with the latter being most commonly affected.
2. *Complete.* This is rare. It involves the entire colon and occasionally the distal small bowel. It is often misdiagnosed as small bowel obstruction.

## Indications

Obstruction, abdominal distention and vomiting commencing within the first 36 to 48 hours after birth. Passage of meconium is quite often absent or delayed.

## Studies

1. Routine abdominal study
2. Colon study

## Method of Performance

1. Abdomen, routine. Occasionally a lateral examination is performed to demonstrate the amount of air in the rectum.
2. *Colon Study.* This is preferably done with barium. False negatives may be obtained with Gastrografin.

## Findings

1. *Routine Abdominal Study*
   A. Numerous dilated gas-filled loops of intestine, with air–fluid levels present on the erect film
   B. The lateral projection, when obtained, may show a narrowed rectum.
2. *Colon Study*
   A. The distal, aganglionic segment is narrow. There is a *transition zone* at the junction of the narrow distal and dilated colon. The transition zone noted on x-ray may not represent the actual anatomical transition of ganglion cells.
   B. In the neonate, the transition zone may not be apparent. A 24-hour and even a 48-hour study of the abdomen following the barium study will reveal retention of barium.
   C. Bizarre, irregular and dysrhythmic contractions in the aganglionic segment are a suggestive feature.
   /D. In total aganglionosis the colon may be normal, small or shorter in caliber. The sigmoid is often foreshortened. No transition zone is apparent.

## Differential Diagnosis

Meconium plug syndrome (*see* below.)

## MECONIUM PLUG SYNDROME

## Indications

Abdominal distention, vomiting, no passage of meconium

## Studies

1. Routine abdominal study
2. Colon study

## Method of Performance

1. Abdomen, routine
2. *Colon study.* This is preferably per-

formed with Gastrografin to help pass the meconium plug. Barium should be given afterward to exclude the possibility of underlying Hirschsprung's disease.

## Findings

1. *Routine Abdominal Study.* The findings are similar to those in Hirschsprung's disease. Dilated loops of small and large bowel are present.

2. *Colon Study.* The meconium plug appears as a large intraluminal filling defect, occupying all or part of the lumen at the level of obstruction. The colon proximal to the plug is distended.

## ENTEROCOLITIS

### Basic Principles

1. Enterocolitis is a highly fatal, necrotizing process of the small and/or large bowel.

2. It occurs in the premature infant and in patients with underlying obstruction, particularly Hirschsprung's disease.

### Indications

Acute fulminating process with bloody diarrhea, fever, distention, vomiting and shock

### Studies

1. Routine abdominal study
2. Colon study (performed only if the diagnosis is not suspected or is in doubt).

### Findings

1. *Routine Abdominal Study.* This shows markedly distended small and large bowels.

2. *Pneumatosis Intestinales.* Air within the bowel wall may have:

A. A bubbly appearance, usually within the right lower quadrant

B. Or a diffuse linear appearance outlining the bowel wall

3. *Pneumoperitoneum.* This is free peritoneal air, resulting from perforation.

4. *Portal-venous Gas.* This is gas present within the portal-venous system, but visualized within the periphery of the liver shadow. It occurs following dissection of the gas from the bowel wall into the mesenteric vessels and the portal system.

## INTUSSUSCEPTION

### Basic Principles

1. *Definition.* Intussusception is invagination of one portion of intestine into another.

2. It is mostly functional in children below 2 years of age. Its occurrence may be related to increased fat deposition or to a change in diet.

3. It is mostly organic in patients above 2 years of age. The most common lesions are Meckel's diverticulum and polyp.

4. *Classification*

A. Entero-enteric

B. Iliocolic (most common, occurring in approximately 75% of cases)

C. Colocolic

### Indications

Young child, between 3 and 12 months of age, with abrupt, episodic crampy abdominal pains, blood in the stool, and a soft tissue mass palpable within the abdomen

### Studies

1. Routine abdominal study
2. Colon study

### Method of Performance

1. Abdomen, routine

2. *Colon Study.* This is performed with barium for diagnosis and/or for therapeutic reduction. Hydrostatic reduction is performed only when no clinical or roentgenographic evidence of peritonitis or small bowel obstruction is present. Barium is introduced under pressure, but with no palpation. The level of the barium column is maintained no higher than 3 feet above the table top. Complete reduction is considered successful only when barium flows freely into the small bowel.

If hydrostatic reduction proves unsuccessful, surgical reduction is necessary.

## Findings

1. *Routine Abdominal Study*

A. Soft tissue mass, located within the pathway of the colon

B. Failure to identify normal position of the cecum

C. Small bowel obstruction—marked dilatation of small bowel loops

D. Peritonitis—fluid within the peritoneum

2. *Barium Enema*

A. The flow of barium is arrested at the level of intussusception.

B. Concave configuration of a soft tissue mass is produced within the barium column.

C. Coil-spring appearance: barium is interspersed between the loops of intussuscepting bowel and the intussuscepted mass.

# 6. ANESTHESIA CONSIDERATIONS IN THE PATIENT FOR EMERGENCY OPERATION

*Ralph Milliken,* M.D.

Emergency surgical procedures in any age-group result in a higher operative mortality than elective operations. The amount of time that may be used to prepare the patient for operation is determined by the urgency of the surgical intervention.

## Definitions

1. *Emergency Operation.* Operations for uncontrollable massive hemorrhage, some emboli and some perforated and ruptured organs are true emergencies. In these cases delay will certainly reduce the likelihood of the patient's survival.

2. *Urgent Operation.* These are surgical procedures to correct abnormalities such as intestinal obstruction, most fractures or the drainage of the source of sepsis. Here, reasonable delay to prepare the patient is actually likely to improve the patient's chances of survival.

## Preoperative Management

1. *Major Factors to Be Corrected in Preparing the Patient for Emergency Surgery*
   A. Hydration
   B. Blood volume and/or red cell mass
   C. Electrolyte and acid–base imbalances
   D. Level of consciousness and any cause for abnormalities
   E. Impaired gastric emptying
   F. Impairment of airway patency

2. *Consideration must be given to the anesthetic agents and technique relative to the patient and the surgical problem.*
   A. Major factors in the patient's history that are of particular importance to the anesthetist

*(1)* Recent and present drug therapy

*(2)* Previous anesthetics and any complications

*(3)* Family history of anesthetic reactions

   B. Factors in physical examination that influence the choice of anesthesia

*(1)* Comatose patients require little or no anesthetic depending on the depth of coma. These patients do need high inspired oxygen, adequate ventilation and adequate muscle relaxation.

*(2)* Central venous pressure in patients with significant preoperative or intraoperative blood or fluid losses

*(3)* Pulse

*(4)* Arterial pressure

*(5)* Arterial and/or mixed venous blood gases, especially in patients with large fluid losses, abnormal acid–base or electrolyte status or disease states and operative sites that may lead to hypoxemia.

3. *Requirements for a Safe Anesthetic*
   A. In the acutely injured, the following prerequisites must be carried out before commencing the anesthetic and/or surgical procedure.

*(1)* A large bore intravenous catheter should be placed with thought given to the site of a lacerated or potentially damaged or occluded vessel. Do not place a catheter distal to such a vessel (i.e., avoid the lower extremities in abdominal trauma).

*(2)* Consider the accessibility to the I.V. during the anesthetic.

*(3)* A central venous pressure line and/or a second catheter should be used in

operations potentially involving large blood or fluid volume losses.

*(4)* The site of placement of all I.V. lines must permit protection of the puncture sites from trauma during and after surgery with the resultant displacement of the I.V. and central venous pressure catheters.

*(5)* Safety in intravenous therapy requires the following considerations at a minimum.

*(a)* Warm blood transfusions when expecting to use more than 1 unit.

*(b)* Avoid systems that would lead to air embolus.

*(c)* Avoid administration of drugs through the central venous pressure line.

B. *Monitoring That Must Be Carried Out During the Anesthetic*

*(1)* Serial central venous pressure or right atrial pressure measurements

*(2)* Continual arterial pressure recording. Consider intra-arterial monitoring in cases that may involve large blood or fluid volume losses; consider alternate sites of placement and alternate methods of noninvasive monitoring devices: Doppler ultrasonic, microphonic and oscillometric devices for providing greater accuracy.

*(3)* Periodic rechecking of blood gases and pH. Consider the necessity of administering sodium bicarbonate solutions, changing ventilation or changing inspired-oxygen concentrations based on blood gas analysis.

*(4)* Heart and breath sounds with precordial or esophageal stethoscope

*(5)* Body temperature in children and the aged

*(6)* ECG

*(7)* Ventilation monitored with ventilation meters (respirometers), blood gases, breath sounds

*(8)* Urine formation by indwelling urinary catheter if blood volume, electrolyte or sugar metabolic abnormalities exist, or if a drug with diuretic properties might be administered during or im-

mediately after surgery (e.g., head trauma)

*4. Specific Problems*

A. Airway obstruction (*See* Chap. 8, Ventilatory Support in Surgical Emergencies.)

B. Respiratory tract injury other than obstruction (burns, toxic chemicals, gastric aspiration)

C. Injury-induced airway problems

*(1)* Facial injuries so extensive that they preclude the use of a facial mask for the induction of anesthesia or awake preoxygenation in the rapid-induction intubation sequence. Alternate devices are:

*(a)* Nasal cannulae

*(b)* Nasal catheter

*(c)* Dental nasal masks

*(d)* Intermittent positive-pressure breathing mouthpiece

*(e)* Transtracheal venturi ventilation

*(2)* Glottic and lower airway injuries

D. Blood loss

*(1)* Stop hemorrhage as soon as possible in obvious bleeding.

*(2)* Provide volume replacement with:

*(a)* Balanced salt solution or saline

*(b)* Clinical dextran, limited to 1000 ml.

*(c)* Plasma derivative

*(d)* Whole blood.

*(3)* Operate *immediately* to stop internal blood loss that is of such an extent that attempted volume replacement does not improve the patient's clinical condition.

*(4)* Administer fresh-frozen plasma while investigating possible failure of clotting mechanisms.

## Anesthetic Management

### Preanesthetic Medication

1. Use the intravenous route for adequate uptake and effect.

2. Use smaller doses considering the dis-

turbed physiologic state and the use of the I.V. route for administration of drugs.

3. Consider using no medication in certain states (i.e., unconsciousness).

4. Reduce not only the dose but the variety of medication (i.e., no atropine in patients with tachycardia, no barbiturates in patients with pain).

5. Narcotics have adverse circulatory homeostatic effects especially obvious in patients with reduced blood volumes. *Use them with great care.*

## Considerations Regarding Agent and Technique

1. Use none or minimal amounts of ultra-short-acting barbiturates for induction of anesthesia in patients with reduced blood volumes.

2. Choose an anesthetic agent or technique that will reverse physiologic vasoconstriction secondary to hemorrhage *only* after the blood volume has been, or is being, aggressively replaced. Spinal and epidural blocks should not be used in a patient who may have suffered spinal cord trauma or received head trauma, and are dangerous in the circulating-volume-depleted patient. The sympathetic blockade and resultant vasodilatation over a large area of analgesia might precipitate cardiovascular collapse in these latter patients. These techniques may be used *with caution* only if analgesia need be provided for the perineum or a lower limb and if the anesthesiologist is skilled enough and has the patient's cooperation to ensure a limited spread of anesthetic solution (thus a limited vasodilatation).

3. Nerve block anesthesia should not be used proximal to a damaged nerve.

4. Regional anesthetic techniques are inherently safer and preferred in all emergency surgery, because consciousness is not lost and reflex activity and voluntary control remain intact.

5. An agent that allows a rapid awakening will enable an earlier evaluation of the level of consciousness after the anesthetic than will a longer-acting agent.

6. Elevated body temperatures indicate a higher insensible fluid loss, for which compensation should be made.

7. The $pCO_2$ should be kept at normal or lower than normal levels during all general anesthetics in order to prevent a respiratory acidosis and/or occasionally accompanying hypoxemia.

8. General anesthesia in the emergency case requires the use of an endotracheal tube to protect the tracheobronchial tree from aspiration of gastric contents that have accumulated due to the usual cessation of gastric emptying that occurs at the time of trauma and pain.

9. The use of a bite block positioned between the molars helps prevent collapsing of an oral endotracheal tube by clenched teeth.

10. Aspiration of foreign particulate matter or clear gastric secretion with a pH of 2.4 or less leads to Mendelsohn's syndrome, which is characterized by:

    A. Bronchospasm, frequently accompanied by wheezing

    B. Atelectasis

    C. Pulmonary edema

    D. Hypoxemia

    E. Bronchopneumonia

11. A high index of suspicion for gastric aspiration should be maintained in all emergency cases, but a presumptive diagnosis should be made where there is:

    A. Wheezing with no previous history of bronchoconstriction

    B. Pulmonary edema

    C. Gastric secretions recoverable on tracheobronchial or pharyngeal suctioning.

    D. Persistent hypoxemia despite lack of evidence of other causes

    E. Unexpected inequality in breath sounds

Treatment is discussed in Chapter 8, Ventilatory Support in Surgical Emergencies.

12. Be prepared to warm (or cool) any

patient who may have body temperature abnormalities.

13. In surgery that may involve the head or neck or that is performed in strange positions, the distance of the anesthesiologist from the airway markedly increases the risk of the sudden loss of a patent airway through which ventilation can be maintained. Considerations for securing the airway must be given the highest priority by surgeons and anesthesiologists. An anode (spiral reinforced) endotracheal tube is frequently best suited, since when used properly it will not collapse, and it can be used as a flexible connector.

14. Anchoring the endotracheal tube properly is of extreme importance. Both twill tape or adhesive tape may be utilized, but each has distinct advantages and disadvantages. Adhesive tape tends to decrease the usable life of all tubes, but especially anode tubes. It does not constrict the tubes and will secure them well when properly applied to all but wet or potentially wet skin. Twill tape is not affected by wet conditions but tends to collapse nonreinforced (all but anode) tubes because of the circumferential constriction that may be transmitted by the tie around the tube due to forces of displacement on the tube itself.

15. If the patient's position is changed after intubation, the breath sounds must be again checked for equality.

16. If thoracic surgery is required, controlled ventilation with inspired-oxygen concentrations high enough to maintain a good arterial oxygen tension is mandatory.

17. In any injury that may involve the chest, facilities for immediate aspiration of a tension pneumothorax must be available if a functioning chest tube is not in place. The diagnosis of tension pneumothorax should be considered with any change in compliance, blood gas tensions or breath sounds.

18. Use little or no ultra-short-acting barbiturates in patients who have:

A. Depressed level of consciousness

B. Potentially unstable cardiovascular systems

19. All patients should have individualized anesthetic doses. Patients in coma may require only oxygen, muscle relaxants and controlled ventilation. As the patient's state improves, anesthetic agents may have to be introduced cautiously.

20. In trauma involving the head, pulmonary edema may develop without fluid overload. Appropriate therapy must be instituted immediately, with consideration for adequate operative conditions regarding ventilation and brain size.

21. The endotracheal tube's external diameter must be carefully selected in children. Children should be intubated for the same reasons as adults, but a cuffed tube is not used because it would limit the internal diameter of the endotracheal tube too greatly. A snug-fitting (but not tight) endotracheal tube is the best protection against aspiration in children, considering the problems of ventilation through an endotracheal tube.

## Immediate Postanesthetic Care

1. Patients should remain on the operating table until cardiovascular hemodynamics are stabilized enough so that the patient is likely to tolerate the position changes associated with moving the patient. If this cannot be assured, consider moving the patient on the operating table to the recovery or intensive care area.

2. *Criteria to Be Evaluated Before Extubating a Patient on an Operating Table*

A. *Circulatory homeostasis* can frequently be reliably evaluated by measuring the:

(1) Peripheral perfusion, including blood pressure and central venous pressure

(2) Capillary filling by tilt testing

(3) Cardiac rhythm and ECG tracing

B. *Ventilatory adequacy* should be determined by:

*(1)* Inspiratory force. This represents a rough gauge of residual anesthetic depth, neuromuscular blockade, central respiratory drive and peripheral ventilatory mechanics. It is measured with a manometer attached directly or indirectly to the endotracheal tube.

*(2)* Tidal volume and minute volume. These are measured with the aid of respirometers when the patient is quiescent, since this will allow for a simulation of the recovery room conditions where care is less intensive than that which the anesthesiologist can render in the operating room.

*(3)* Arterial blood gases should be done in patients who are obese, who suffer from abdominal distention, extensive surgical incision (chest or abdominal) or head trauma, or who gave a history of, or suggestive of, chronic pulmonary disease or on physical examination had stigmata of pulmonary disease.

C. If spontaneous ventilation or oxygen tension while breathing room air on the operating table is inadequate, controlled ventilation with supplemental inspired oxygen through an endotracheal tube should be used to safely transport the patient.

3. Supplemental inspired oxygen should be effectively administered for:

A. All patients with abdominal or thoracic injuries and surgical incisions in those areas

B. Extensive superficial injuries

C. Moderate or severe orthopedic injuries

D. Any patient with an anesthetic lasting more than 60 minutes

E. Geriatric age-group patients

Care must be used to avoid the hazard of depressing an anoxic respiratory drive.

## ANESTHETIC TECHNIQUES

### Definitions

1. *Topical anesthesia* is the application to the mucous membranes of an anesthetic agent that will penetrate those membranes and will provide analgesia of those surfaces.

2. *Preanesthetic medication* is the use of various classes of drugs prior to the administration of an anesthetic, the primary purpose of which is to reduce anxiety. Other effects that may be desired are amnesia for the induction of the anesthetic, antisalivary effects, antiemetic effects, and vagolysis.

3. *Spinal anesthesia* is a form of extensive block anesthesia brought about by the deposition of a suitable local anesthetic solution into the spinal subarachnoid space that contains the cerebrospinal fluid, the spinal cord and spinal nerve roots.

4. *Nerve block anesthesia* is the technique of the proper application of a local anesthetic solution so that somatic nerve conduction will be interrupted. The techniques range in extent from a single nerve block to a plexus block, to a spinal or epidural anesthetic.

5. *Epidural anesthesia* is a form of extensive block anesthesia produced by injecting a suitable local anesthetic into the epidural or peridural space.

6. *Infiltration anesthesia* is the injection of a local anesthetic into tissues in order to anesthetize the nerve endings by their direct exposure to the drug.

7. *Field block anesthesia* is produced by surrounding the operative field with a continuous line of local anesthetic. Minor nerves and small sensory nerves supplying the skin over the operative field are effectively blocked by the anesthetic as they enter the field. The sensory supply to the field is the determinant of whether the block is primarily small sensory or a combination of small sensory and nerve block techniques.

8. *Regional anesthesia (analgesia)* is the abolition of pain from any region or regions of the body by reversibly interrupting sensory nerve transmission.

9. *General anesthesia* is a completely

reversible state in which the patient is safely rendered unconscious, insensitive to pain, with partial or total depression of noxious reflexes, motionless, with a varying degree of muscular relaxation and without significant depression of vital functions.

10. *Dissociative anesthesia* is a state characterized by catatonia, catalepsy, amnesia, and marked analgesia. The "dissociative" state of the central nervous system produces a condition of general anesthesia unlike that seen with any other class of agents.

## Classification

1. *Regional Anesthesia*
   A. Topical
   B. Infiltration
   C. Nerve block
      (1) Specific
      (2) Field
      (3) Intravenous
   D. Spinal or epidural
2. *General Anesthesia*
   A. Inhalation
   B. Intravenous
   C. Hypnotics
   D. Narcotic or nonnarcotic analgesics
   E. Dissociative
   F. Neuromuscular blockade

## REGIONAL ANESTHETIC TECHNIQUES AND AGENTS

### Basic Principles

1. Regional anesthetic techniques produce localized areas or regions of analgesia without depressing the sensorium, and include:
   A. Topical anesthesia
   B. Local tissue infiltration
   C. Nerve block techniques
   D. Spinal and epidural techniques
2. The class of agents used in all of these techniques is local anesthetic agents.
   A. The mechanism of action of local anesthetics is that of making the membrane

of the axon or nerve terminal incapable of depolarizing.
   (1) This membrane-stabilizing effect prevents transmission of impulses. Sympathetic nerve fibers are the most sensitive to local anesthetics.
   (2) Sympathetic paralysis is a constant accompaniment to analgesia after infiltration, nerve block or spinal or epidural anesthesia.
   B. Some agents are suited only for topical use, others for all uses (*see* Table 6-1).
   C. Vasoconstriction at the site of application of cocaine is constant.
   D. Vasodilatation enhances the removal of the agent from the site of deposition and thus shortens the duration of action.
   E. Adding a vasoconstrictor agent to the solution of an anesthetic that is associated with vasodilatation lengthens the duration of action. Agents associated with vasodilatation are lidocaine (Xylocaine) and procaine (Novocain).
   F. Relative vasoconstriction is seen with mepivacaine (Carbocaine) and prilocaine (Citanest).

### Local Anesthetic Toxicity

1. Local anesthetic toxicity is typically manifested as:
   A. *Central Nervous System Depression.* Central nervous system depression may be recognized by:
      (1) Sleepiness
      (2) Confusion
      (3) Convulsions. Seizures are a result of the paralysis of inhibiting neurons. They are treated as any other seizure except that long-term therapy is unnecessary.
   B. *Cardiovascular Collapse.* Cardiovascular collapse is due to the membrane-stabilizing action of the local anesthetic agent on the cardiac muscle, pacemaker and conduction system.
   C. *Ventilatory Insufficiency.* Ventilatory insufficiency is centrally induced.
2. Treatment of cardiovascular collapse

**Table 6-1. Regional Anesthetic Agents**

| Agent (Proprietary Name) | Potency (Procaine = 1) | Toxicity (Procaine = 1) | Recommended Concentration | | | | | | Onset of Action of Spinal Anethesia | Duration of Action of Spinal Anesthesia |
| --- | --- | --- | --- | --- | --- | --- | --- | --- | --- | --- |
| | | | Spinal | Epidural | Block of Large Nerve | Block of Small Nerve | Infiltration | Topical | | |
| Cocaine* | 4:1 | 4:1 | | | | | | 4–10% | | |
| Procaine (Novocain) | 1:1 | 1:1 | 2–5% | 2–4% | 2% | 1% | 0.5% | Does not produce topical anesthesia | 1–3 min. | ¾–1 hr. |
| Tetracaine (Pontocaine) | 10:1 | 10:1 | 0.2–0.5% | 0.2% | 0.2% | 0.1% | 0.1% | 0.5–2.0% | 5–10 min. | 2–3 hr. |
| Lidocaine (Xylocaine) | 2.0:1–2.5:1 | Varies in direct proportion to concentration (0.5%, 1:1; 1.0%, 1.4:1; 2.0%, 1.5:1) | 2–5% | 1–2% | 2% | 1% | 0.5% | 2–4% | 1–3 min. | 1–1½ hr. |
| Mepivacaine (Carbocaine) | 2.4:1 | 1.5:1 | 4% under investigation | 1.5% | 2% | 1% | 0.5% | Solution for topical anesthesia under investigation | 1–3 min. | 2–2½ hr. |

*Not recommended for use other than topical.

and/or ventilatory insufficiency consists of specific resuscitative measures until blood levels decrease and spontaneous function returns.

3. Toxic reactions are avoided by using the smallest effective volume of the smallest effective concentrations.

## TOPICAL ANESTHESIA

1. Not all local anesthetic agents are effective as topical agents. This is because some agents do not cross the mucous membrane to act on the nerve fiber terminal.

2. Endotracheal absorption of topical agents produces a blood level almost as fast as intravenous injection.

3. Topical anesthetic absorption is not delayed by a vasoconstrictor agent.

4. The blood level of a topical agent applied to mucous membranes is related to the area of application and not the concentration.

5. Topical anesthesia is inherently dangerous, and safety can only be assured by the use of meticulous technique.

## LOCAL TISSUE INFILTRATION

1. In infiltration anesthesia, ½% concentrations of all agents are effective. Greater concentrations do not increase the duration; they only increase the risk of toxic reactions.

2. Epinephrine in a concentration of 1:200,000 increases the duration of anesthesia in those agents associated with relative vasodilatation, but greater concentrations only introduce a toxicity related to the epinephrine hypertension:

    A. Cerebrovascular accidents

    B. Cardiac arrhythmias

    C. Dysphoria

3. Epinephrine should not be used:

    A. In limbs with compromised arterial circulation due to disease or trauma

    B. In such a way that it distends tissues so that sloughing and ischemia could occur

    C. When infiltrating tissues that are supplied by end arteries (i.e., digits)

4. Injected or instilled doses of local anesthetics should always be measured so that only a safe dose will be used.

## NERVE BLOCKS

### Brachial Plexus Blocks

### Anatomy

Formation of the brachial plexus is initiated in the neck when the anterior rami of C-5, C-6, C-7, C-8, T-1 and, frequently, communicating loops from C-4 and T-2 begin to merge and take positions around the subclavian artery. The plexus and artery emerge from the neck between the anterior and middle scalene muscles. They are superficial in the subclavian space at that point until the artery and nerve fibers run caudal and lateral to the first rib and emerge superficially again as the axillary artery and upper limb nerves in the axilla.

The position of the artery and nerves is maintained in the axilla and supraclavicular space, where they are relatively isolated within a tubular extension of the prevertebral fascia, thus producing a neurovascular bundle. By injecting anesthetic into the bundle, solution may reach the paravertebral fascia, where it may spread cephalad and caudad, providing block of the intercostal brachial nerve (origin, T-2) and stellate ganglion (superior cervical sympathetic ganglion).

In the area of the third part of the axillary artery, the radial nerve lies beyond the artery, the median nerve lies in front of and slightly above the artery, and the ulnar nerve lies in front of and slightly below the artery. The musculocutaneous nerve which arises from the lateral cord of the brachial plexus and innervates the lateral forearm leaves the bundle at the level of the second portion of the axillary artery. The intercostal brachial nerve arises from the second intercostal nerve and thus is not a part of the brachial plexus. It innervates the skin of the upper half of the medial and posterior part of the arm.

### Axillary (Perivascular) Brachial Plexus Block (Fig. 6-1)

1. The block is performed with the

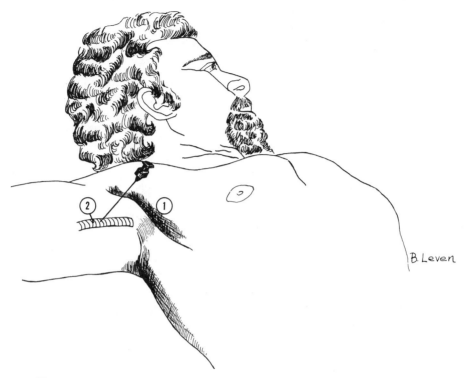

Fig. 6-1. Brachial plexus block from the axillary approach. (*1*) Anterior axillary fold. (*2*) Neurovascular bundle.

patient in the supine position with the arm abducted to 90 degrees from the body.

2. The forearm can either be extended or it can be flexed and the arm then rotated so that the head rests on the hand. The position chosen should be that which best demonstrates the axillary artery (third position) between the coracobrachial and teres major muscles.

3. A tourniquet may be placed below the axillary artery, or the physician may find it more convenient to compress and fix the artery against the humerus, using his index and middle fingers.

4. Pressure should be maintained manually or by tourniquet for 10 minutes after the solution has been injected in order to promote proximal spread of anesthetic within the neurovascular bundle and thus provide a larger and more profound anesthetic field.

5. A 22-gauge 1½-inch needle is passed through a skin wheal toward and slightly above the axillary artery. A distinct "click" may be felt as the needle pierces the fascia of the neurovascular bundle.

6. If arterial blood enters the syringe, the axillary artery has been punctured, but, since the artery lies within the neurovascular bundle, the needle should be withdrawn slightly until no blood appears on aspiration and then the physician can proceed with injection.

7. If paresthesias are obtained, the needle is withdrawn slightly, aspiration is attempted, and, if no blood is returned, injection of the anesthetic is made.

A. Eliciting paresthesias improves the likelihood of obtaining profound and extensive anesthesia.

B. If after attempting to elicit paresthesias none are obtained, the technique of puncturing the artery and then partially withdrawing the needle before injecting may be used.

8. If a tourniquet is to be used, or if the surgery involves the upper arm, a ring of subcutaneously injected anesthetic may have to be provided to anesthetize the unblocked fibers of the intercostal brachial nerve, the medial brachial cutaneous nerve or the superficial cervical plexus.

9. If these conditions can be predicted beforehand, the physician may elect to perform a supraclavicular brachial plexus block instead.

10. Onset of anesthesia takes from 10 to 40 minutes.

11. The maximum allowable dose of anesthetic should be used (50 ml. of 1% lidocaine, 30 ml. of 1½% lidocaine, or a comparable dose of another agent) in performing this block in healthy patients in order to best ensure the success of the block.

12. The larger the volume, the more likely that block of the musculocutaneous nerve will be produced.

13. *Caution:*

A. The most common serious complication of this block is intravascular injection. Since large doses of drug are being used, a toxic reaction to local anesthetic agents is likely.

B. A hematoma over the axillary artery where it may have been punctured is usually well tolerated, but when arterial puncture has occurred, pressure should be maintained over the artery for at least 5 minutes.

C. The site should be checked for further bleeding later and pressure reapplied if necessary.

## Subclavian (Perivascular) Brachial Plexus Block (Fig. 6-2)

1. The patient is supine with the head

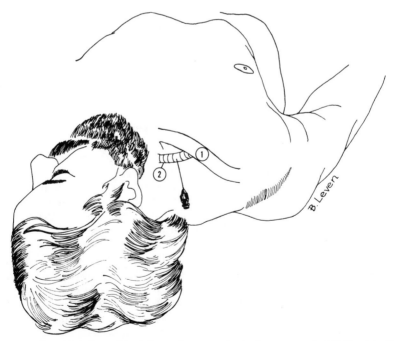

Fig. 6-2. Brachial plexus block from the supraclavicular approach. (*1*) Clavicle. (*2*) Neurovascular bundle.

gently turned away from the side to be blocked.

2. The patient should be asked to reach for his knee on the operative side in order to depress the clavicle.

3. The subclavian artery is palpated as medially as possible (where the artery emerges from between the scalene muscles).

4. With a finger still on the artery, a 22-gauge 1½-inch needle is inserted medial to the finger and directly caudad.

5. A distinct "click" may be felt as the needle pierces the fascia of the neurovascular bundle.

6. Advancing the needle further will typically elicit paresthesias, at which point the needle should be slightly withdrawn and the injections of anesthetic solution made.

7. A dose of 25 ml. of 1% lidocaine is usually sufficient if sensory block alone is desired, while 25 ml. of 1½% lidocaine will be necessary to produce muscle relaxation.

8. Eliciting paresthesias improves the likelihood of obtaining profound and extensive anesthesia.

9. Postoperatively, a chest film should be done to assess pneumothorax, although this approach rarely produces this complication.

### Block of the Radial Nerve at the Wrist

1. The radial nerve passes lateral to, and at the same depth as, the radial artery at the level of the ulnar styloid process.

2. A skin wheal is raised opposite the ulnar styloid, lateral to the radial artery, while the patient maintains his hand supinated and extended at the wrist (Fig. 6-3).

3. A 22-gauge 1½-inch needle is passed through the wheal and lateral to the artery.

4. If the patient experiences paresthesias of the thumb and back of the hand, the needle is fixed and 2 ml. of anesthetic solution (lidocaine, 1 or 1½%) should be injected.

5. Even if paresthesias are not elicited, intradermal and subcutaneous infiltration is carried out from the area lateral to the artery around the wrist and to the back of the radial half of the wrist at the level of the ulnar styloid.

6. Ten to 20 ml. of solution injected in this manner are required to provide adequate block of the dorsal branches of the radial nerve.

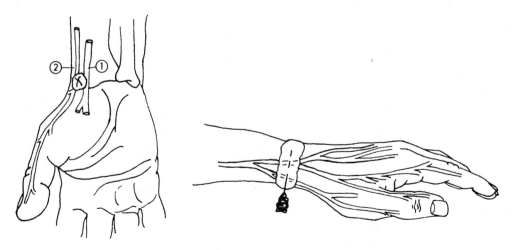

Fig. 6-3. Block of the radial nerve at the wrist. *(1)* Radial artery. *(2)* Radial nerve.

### Block of the Median
### Nerve at the Wrist

1. The median nerve lies slightly behind and to the radial side of the palmaris longus tendon at the level of the ulnar styloid process.

2. If the palmaris longus tendon is congenitally absent, the median nerve will lie between the flexor digitorum sublimis and the flexor carpi radialis tendons.

3. The patient will best demonstrate the tendons by flexing the fist at the wrist and the forearm at the elbow.

4. At the level of the ulnar styloid, a wheal is raised lateral to the palmaris longus tendon, or in case of its absence, ¼-inch lateral to the sublimis tendon (Fig. 6-4).

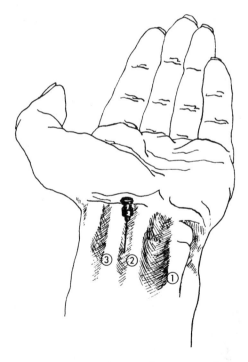

Fig. 6-4. Block of the median nerve at the wrist. (*1*) Tendon of the flexor carpi ulnaris muscle. (*2*) Tendon of the palmaris longus muscle. (*3*) Tendon of the flexor carpi radialis muscle.

5. The hand can then be relaxed and placed in a supinated position.

6. A short 25-gauge needle is then directed perpendicularly through the wheal until paresthesias of the palm, index and middle finger and radial side of the ring finger are felt.

7. The needle is then fixed and 5 to 10 ml. of solution (lidocaine, 1 or 1½%) are injected.

8. If paresthesias are not readily elicited, the needle should be redirected in a fanwise motion until paresthesias are elicited.

### Block of the Ulnar Nerve

1. The ulnar nerve divides into dorsal and volar branches about 2 inches above the wrist. The dorsal branch passes underneath the tendon of the flexor carpi ulnaris and then runs superficially to supply the dorsum of the little finger and the adjacent surface of the ring finger. The volar branch travels medial to, and slightly behind, the ulnar artery.

2. The patient lies with the hand supinated.

A. At the level of the ulnar styloid process, the ulnar artery is palpated medial to the tendon of the flexor carpi ulnaris and a skin wheal is produced (Fig. 6-5).

B. A short 25-gauge needle is passed through the wheal medial to the artery.

C. Paresthesias of the little finger should be sought, and a dose of 5 to 10 ml. of anesthetic solution (lidocaine, 1 or 1½%) is injected.

D. If paresthesias are not readily elicited, the needle should be redirected medially in a fanwise motion until they are elicited.

E. The dorsal branch is anesthetized by intradermal and subcutaneous infiltration along a line drawn from the original skin wheal to the middle of the back of the wrist.

F. Alternatively, ulnar nerve block can be carried out by infiltration of the nerve at the elbow (Fig. 6-6).

(*1*) A short 25-gauge needle is used

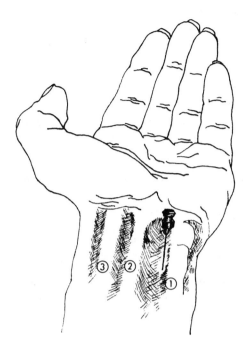

Fig. 6-5. Block of the ulnar nerve at the wrist. (*1*) Tendon of the flexor carpi ulnaris muscle. (*2*) Tendon of the palmaris longus muscle. (*3*) Tendon of the flexor carpi radialis muscle.

to raise a wheal over the palpable nerve in the groove posterior to the medial epicondyle.

(*2*) The needle is then advanced down to the nerve until paresthesias are experienced.

(*3*) A dose of 5 to 10 ml. of anesthetic solution is injected.

### Digital Nerve Block

**Anatomy**

The volar and dorsal surfaces of the upper and lower limb digits are each innervated by specific terminal nerve branches. As a result, both the dorsal and volar

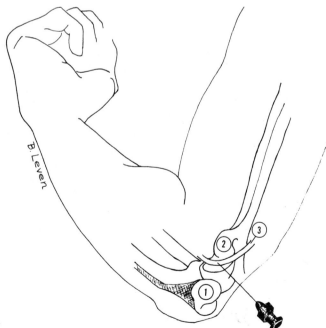

Fig. 6-6. Ulnar nerve block at the elbow. (*1*) Olecranon process. (*2*) Medial epicondyle of the humerus. (*3*) Ulnar nerve.

nerves must be blocked in order to provide adequate analgesia.

## Technique

1. A wheal is raised on the dorsolateral surfaces of the interdigital fold with a fine needle (Fig. 6-7).

2. A 1½-inch 22-gauge needle is directed through the wheal toward the bone and also passed dorsally and ventrally, so that a ring of local anesthetic solution is placed in the soft tissue of the digit between the periosteum and tendons and the skin.

3. *Caution:*

A. A vasoconstrictor agent should never be added to the local anesthetic solution because the digital arteries are end arteries and intense vasoconstriction may result in necrosis and loss of part or all of a digit.

B. Ten ml. of lidocaine, ½ to 1% solution, should not be exceeded in small digits because the digit will not absorb a greater volume without compromising its circulation.

*Femoral Nerve Block*

## Anatomy

The femoral nerve (L-2, L-3, L-4) runs down from the lumbar plexus in the groove between the psoas major and iliac muscles and enters the anterior thigh by passing lateral and slightly deeper to the femoral artery as they both pass deep to the inguinal ligament.

The anterior branch of the nerve innervates the skin covering the anterior surface of the thigh and the sartorius muscle. The posterior branches innervate the skin over the medial side of the calf to the medial malleolus of the knee joint, the medial ligament of the knees and the quadriceps muscles.

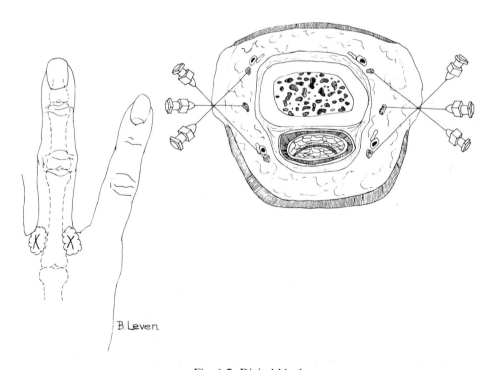

B. Leven

Fig. 6-7. Digital block.

## Technique

1. With the patient in the supine position, the femoral artery is palpated and a 1½- or 2-inch 22-gauge needle is directed lateral to it until either paresthesias (experienced as electric shocks in the knee or medial aspect of the leg) are elicited or the needle demonstrates an arterial pulsation (Fig. 6-8).

2. If paresthesias are elicited and test aspiration is negative for blood, a dose of 10 ml. of 1% lidocaine, or a comparable drug and dose, is injected; then the block should proceed as described below, except that only an additional dose of 10 ml of 1% lidocaine is injected.

3. If paresthesias are not obtained, an additional dose of 20 ml. of 1% lidocaine is injected in fanwise motion (laterally) from

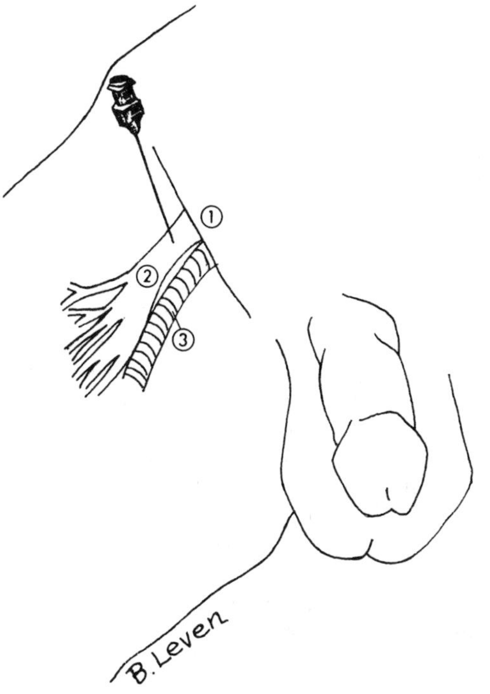

Fig. 6-8. Technique for femoral nerve block. (*1*) Inguinal ligament. (*2*) Femoral nerve. (*3*) Femoral artery.

that depth to the subcutaneous tissue. This motion should ensure blockage of both branches of the nerve since they frequently have divided above the inguinal ligament.

4. Puncture of the femoral artery requires prolonged pressure over the artery, but the block may continue.

### Sciatic Nerve Block

## Anatomy

The sciatic nerve (L-4, L-5, S-1, S-2, S-3) leaves the pelvis through the greater sciatic notch. Covered by the gluteus maximus muscle, the nerve runs down the leg, passing a point approximately equidistant from the ischial tuberosity and the greater trochanter.

## Technique

1. The patient should be placed in the lateral position with the side to be blocked up, tilted slightly forward, with the upper hip and knee joints bent.

2. A line is drawn between the greater trochanter and the posterior superior iliac spine. The long axis of the femur should underlie the continuation of this line.

3. The original line is bisected and a line at right angles is drawn caudal and mesad for 1½ to 2 inches. This point should overlie the sciatic nerve as it emerges through the greater sciatic foramen.

4. A skin wheal and deep infiltration are done (Fig. 6-9).

5. A 3-inch 22-gauge needle is then inserted perpendicular to all planes of the skin and advanced until either paresthesias (felt as a spraying electric sensation radiating down the leg to the foot) are elicited or bone is encountered.

6. The bone encountered is likely to be the rim of the greater sciatic notch. The depth of the needle at the point where it encountered bone should be noted, and the needle should be withdrawn to the subcutaneous tissue and redirected, but not to a depth greater than ¾ of an inch of the previous bone-contact depth.

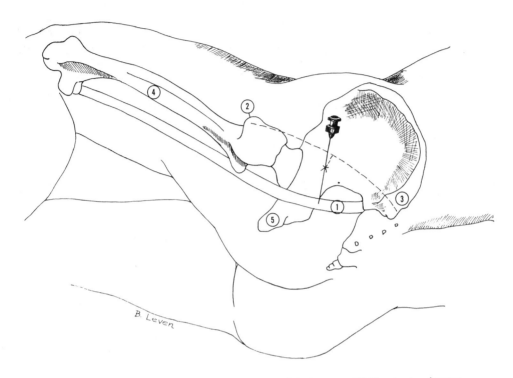

B. Leven

Fig. 6-9. Technique for sciatic nerve block. (*1*) Sciatic nerve. (*2*) Greater trochanter of the femur. (*3*) Posterior superior iliac spine. (*4*) Femur. (*5*) Ischial tuberosity.

7. The needle should be redirected perpendicular to the line connecting the trochanter and spine, since eliciting paresthesias increases the success rate of the block.

8. A dose of 25 ml. of lidocaine is needed for muscular relaxation.

9. After paresthesias are elicited, a complete block is obtained in from 5 to 30 minutes.

10. Analgesia is obtained over the skin of the back of the thigh, the back and lateral aspect of the leg and usually all of the toes, with the occasional exception of the dorsum of the great toe.

11. Muscle relaxation is obtained in the back of the thigh, the leg and the foot.

*Field Block of the Inguinal Region*

1. With the patient supine, the anterior superior iliac spine is noted. A line is drawn from the spine to the umbilicus.

2. A point 1 inch medial to the spine and along this line is the site of puncture with a 2-inch 22-gauge needle; the needle then contacts the inside shelf of the iliac bone by a slight lateral angulation.

3. A volume of 5 ml. of anesthetic is deposited in the fascial plane along the shelf. This should anesthetize the lateral femoral cutaneous nerve.

4. The needle is withdrawn to the subcutaneous tissues and redirected medially, and it may be felt to pierce the external oblique fascia, the internal oblique and the transversalis muscles.

5. When the transversalis fascia is pierced, a dose of 3 ml. of local anesthetic (lidocaine, ½%, or a comparable dose of another agent) is deposited, and the needle

is withdrawn to the subcutaneous tissue while injecting an additional 2 ml. of the anesthetic.

6. The needle is then redirected more medially and another dose of 5 ml. of solution is similarly deposited along each of 3 additional needle tracts for a total injection of 25 ml.

7. These maneuvers should provide anesthesia to the ilioinguinal and iliohypogastric nerves.

8. A 3-inch 22-gauge needle is inserted at the anterior superior iliac spine and directed medially and laterally from the initial wheal, so that the dermal, subcutaneous and muscular tissues along a line drawn from the spine to the umbilicus are infiltrated with 20 ml. of solution. This blocks branches of the lower intercostal nerves.

9. Twenty ml. of solution are used to infiltrate the skin and subcutaneous tissues parallel and caudal to the ilioinguinal ligament from the anterior superior iliac spine to the medial thigh. This injection blocks overlapping innervation of this area by the lateral femoral cutaneous and lumboinguinal nerves.

10. A femoral nerve block is then produced by passing a needle lateral to the femoral artery and infiltrating the subcutaneous tissues lateral to the artery with 20 ml. of solution injected fanwise and laterally.

11. A wheal of anesthesia is raised over the pubic tubercle. A needle is directed above and lateral to the superior ramus of the pubis and deep to the rectus muscle. Fifteen ml. of anesthetic solution are injected at this point into the space of Retzius (the space between the bladder, the rectus muscle and the pubic bone). This injection should effectively block the nerves traveling along with the spermatic cord.

12. Superficial infiltration of the skin and subcutaneous tissue over the line of incision is then performed, using minimal amounts of anesthetic.

13. The peritoneum underlying the in-

ternal inguinal ring, the spermatic sympathetic plexus and the genitofemoral nerve may require additional blocking under direct vision as they are exposed surgically.

*Intravenous Regional Anesthesia*

1. A vein in the region of the limb near the surgical field but 180 degrees from the field is best suited for placement of the needle in intravenous regional anesthesia (Fig. 6-10).

2. A deflated occlusive arterial tourniquet is placed proximal to the field.

3. If a single-dose injection is to be used, a fine-gauge scalp vein needle is well suited. If the block is to be reintroduced, a plastic catheter placed under sterile conditions is best suited. The needle or catheter is introduced into the vein with the aid of a venous tourniquet. The tourniquet is released and the needle securely taped.

4. The limb is either raised to a vertical position for 5 minutes or an Esmarch or elastic bandage is wrapped tightly over the limb up to the level of the arterial tourniquet in order to exsanguinate the limb.

5. The arterial tourniquet is inflated above arterial pressure and the limb lowered or the bandage removed.

6. A dose of 30 to 100 ml. (depending on the extent of block) of a ½% solution of anesthetic is injected slowly through the needle.

7. If the block is to be a single episode, the scalp vein needle can be removed and pressure is applied over the skin puncture.

8. The limb is gently massaged in order to increase the spread of the solution. During this time, the anesthetic molecules leave the vessels and attach themselves to nerve trunks, blocking conduction.

9. If the patient complains of tourniquet pain, a second tourniquet may be placed more distal to the original one and inflated. The proximal tourniquet may then be released.

10. This block has an effective time of about 90 minutes. When the tourniquet is

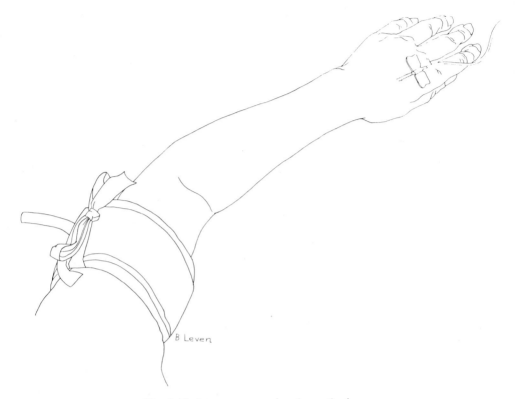

Fig. 6-10. Intravenous regional anesthesia.

released, the anesthetic will be slowly picked up, allowing approximately 5 minutes of additional analgesia.

11. If a plastic catheter has been used, the limb can be re-exsanguinated and reinjected, obtaining another period of anesthesia.

12. *Caution:* When the tourniquet is released, the anesthetic is circulated and systemic toxicity may become manifest at this time.

## SPINAL ANESTHESIA

1. Spinal anesthesia is produced by depositing the local anesthetic agent in the cerebrospinal fluid that bathes the spinal cord and nerve roots.

2. By making the anesthetic solution either heavy or light in relation to the cerebrospinal fluid, the solution can usually be directed to localize at a selected area of the spinal cord, producing analgesia, motor and sympathetic paralysis in the approximately corresponding segments.

3. Spinal anesthesia is prolonged by:

A. Using long-acting local anesthetic agents

B. Adding epinephrine to the anesthetic solution.

4. Fewer agents are approved for spinal anesthesia because of the local irritant properties of some agents.

## EPIDURAL ANESTHESIA

1. Epidural anesthesia requires that the local anesthetic agent be deposited in the epidural or peridural space either:

A. At the segments to be blocked

B. Or at a lower segment and "pushed" up by volume displacement

2. Deposition can be:

A. Directly through a needle in the epidural space

B. Through a catheter threaded through a needle already in the epidural space

3. The epidural space contains:

A. Spinal cord and meninges

B. Nerve roots and their coverings

C. Blood vessels

D. Fat

4. These structures necessitate a greater amount of local anesthetic to be deposited in the epidural space before anesthesia appears.

5. The induction time for epidural anesthesia is longer than that for spinal anesthesia since the anesthetic agent has more tissues to penetrate before becoming effective.

6. Epidural anesthesia can be prolonged by using:

A. Long-acting local anesthetics

B. Local anesthetics with epinephrine added

C. Repeated doses, most commonly accomplished with a temporarily placed epidural catheter

7. Spinal anesthesia and epidural anesthesia involve sympathetic paralysis to a large number of segments.

8. Hypotension results from a dilatation of the vascular space without a corresponding increase in blood volume.

9. Choice of agent for spinal or epidural anesthesia is based on:

A. Desired duration of anesthesia

B. Advisability of adding epinephrine to an anesthetic solution

C. A possibility of an allergy or sensitivity to an agent or class of agents

D. Individual preference for agents

## SAFETY IN REGIONAL ANESTHESIA

1. Experience indicates that anesthetic hazards increase manyfold when unconsciousness is induced by general anesthesia.

2. Regional anesthesia techniques are safer and preferable when available in the patient for emergency surgery, because consciousness is not lost and because the patient retains reflex activity.

3. Patients who do not lend themselves to regional anesthesia are:

A. Infants and children

B. Confused, demented and psychotic patients

C. Extremely apprehensive patients

## GENERAL ANESTHESIA

### Basic Principles

1. Certain procedures are best suited for general anesthesia. A suitable general anesthetic encompasses:

A. Relief of pain

B. Obtundation of some reflexes

C. Muscle relaxation adequate for surgical manipulation

D. Unconsciousness and amnesia to obviate mental trauma

2. The ideal anesthetic agent should have these properties:

A. Rapid induction and emergence

B. Nonirritating and pleasant to inhale

C. Provide excellent muscle relaxation in light planes

D. Have no adverse effects on organs or organ systems

E. Be nonflammable

3. No agent presently available has all these properties.

4. The current practice of general anesthesia frequently involves the administration of many drugs and agents, including:

A. Ultra-short-acting barbiturates for a shortened induction

B. Inhalation agent or agents for anesthesia maintenance

C. Neuromuscular blocking agents for adequate surgical conditions

D. An intravenous analgesic

E. Intravenous drugs to antagonize the effects of C and D

## AVAILABLE GENERAL ANESTHETIC AGENTS

### *Inhalation Agents*

**Ether**

1. Flammable
2. Liquid at room temperature but vaporizes readily
3. Unpleasant odor
4. Prolonged, stormy, unpleasant induction and a prolonged emergence. *The properties of flammability and prolonged induction and emergence generally make ether unsuitable for emergency surgery.*
5. Stimulates salivary and tracheobronchial secretions
6. Nausea and vomiting are stimulated on induction, emergence and into the recovery period.
7. Catecholamine output is increased during ether anesthesia. The increased blood level of catecholamines tends to stabilize the blood pressure and pulse during the anesthetic.
8. Ventilation is not depressed until deep levels because reflex activity acts as a ventilatory drive.
9. Ether provides the best muscle relaxation of any inhalation anesthetic. A synergism exists between the relaxant properties of ether and the curariform drugs.

**Cyclopropane**

1. Flammable
2. Mild, pleasant odor
3. Rapid induction and awakening
4. Induction is so rapid that it is popular as an inhalation replacement in the rapid-induction intubation sequence when it is judged that barbiturate administration is too hazardous.
5. Mild stimulation of salivary secretions; induction vomiting is rare.
6. Moderate muscle-relaxant properties in surgical depths of 15 to 25% inhaled concentrations
7. Moderate synergism with curariform drugs
8. High oxygen concentrations can be administered simultaneously because of cyclopropane's potency as an anesthetic and analgesic
9. Little accompanying cardiovascular depression
10. Recommended in patients with coronary artery disease
11. Endogenous catecholamine release accompanies cyclopropane administration, and this typically provides remarkable blood pressure stability.
12. Cardiac pacemaker irritability accompanies the elevated blood catecholamines.
13. Ventricular arrhythmias occur relatively frequently at only a mild elevation of arterial carbon dioxide tension.
14. Epinephrine or epinephrine-containing solutions should not be injected during cyclopropane anesthesia due to the extreme likelihood of precipitating serious ventricular arrhythmias due to a summation of cardiac-irritant properties.
15. Cardiovascular stability is gained at the expense of peripheral vasoconstriction and tissue perfusion. A further decrease in tissue perfusion may be undesirable in the blood-volume-depleted patient who is only marginally perfusing certain tissues.
16. Ventilatory depression worsens as the anesthetic level deepens.
17. Controlled ventilation is necessary in order to maintain a normal or approximately normal carbon dioxide tension in all but the highest depths.
18. Cyclopropane is administered typically in a closed circle to avoid the spilling of cyclopropane into the room and to reduce the flammability hazard and the cost of its administration.
19. Awakening is rapid but is frequently punctuated by a short period of emesis for which the patient is typically amnesic.

**Halothane**

1. Most popular anesthetic agent in the English-speaking world
2. Lowest over-all mortality rate of any general anesthetic

**Table 6-2. General Anesthetic Agents**

| Agent (Proprietary Name) | Physical State | Vaporization at Room Temperature | Flammability | Odor | Induction Time | Emergence | Nausea and Vomiting | Catecholamine Production | Muscle Relaxation | Potency* |
|---|---|---|---|---|---|---|---|---|---|---|
| Ether | Liquid | Rapid | Explosive | Unpleasant | Prolonged and stormy | Prolonged | Common | Increased | Good | 1.92% |
| Cyclopropane | Gas | | Explosive | Mild, pleasant | Rapid | Rapid | Moderate on emergence | Increased | Moderate | 9.2% |
| Halothane (Fluothane) | Liquid | Readily | None | Pronounced but not unpleasant | Rapid | Rapid | Rare | Decreased | Mild | 0.74% |
| Methoxyflurane (Penthrane) | Liquid | Poor | None | Pronounced unpleasant | Prolonged | Prolonged | Rare | Probably reduced | Moderate | 0.16% |
| Nitrous oxide | Gas | | Supports combustion | Sweet | Rapid | Rapid | Rare | Probably increased | Poor | 101% (greater than 1 atmosphere required) |

*Minimum alveolar concentration required to produce anesthesia.

3. Physically stable because of the three fluoride atoms and one each of chloride and bromide attached to a two-carbon chain

4. Nonflammable because of the effects of the halogen atoms

5. No stimulation of nausea, vomiting or salivary secretions

6. Pronounced odor, but not unpleasant

7. Liquid at room temperature, but readily vaporized with a variety of apparatus

8. Extremely potent; thus, overdosage is easy and so it needs careful control of its vaporization and inhaled concentration.

A. Sophisticated vaporizing equipment is utilized in order to accurately meter the concentration of halothane delivered from the anesthesia machine.

B. It is typically administered in a relatively high flow of gases in order to accurately control the inspired concentration.

9. Poor analgesic properties

10. Decreased blood catecholamines associated with halothane administration

11. Direct vasodilator and mild sympathetic ganglionic blocker effects

12. Cardiovascular depressant effects are noted as a clinically decreased blood pressure.

13. Vasodilatation probably protects perfusion even at low mean blood pressures.

14. Ventilatory depression progresses as anesthesia deepens.

15. Nitrous oxide administration lessens the required inspired concentration and thus modifies these effects.

16. Mild muscle relaxant properties and mild synergism with nondepolarizing muscle relaxants

17. Rapid induction and emergence

18. Cutaneous vasodilatation is typically present.

A. A lowered body temperature is associated due to heat loss.

B. On awakening, many of these patients initiate voluntary muscle shivering known as "halothane shakes" in order to produce body heat. This shivering causes an increased oxygen consumption.

19. Halothane undergoes biotransformation (i.e., it undergoes metabolic degradation in the human).

## Halothane-Induced Disease

Halothane hepatitis is a disease that can be fatal. It is observed clinically as jaundice, fever and chills a few days after halothane anesthesia. The clinical picture is impossible to differentiate from viral hepatitis. Histologically a varied picture is seen.

DNA production in lymphocytes taken from a patient in the post acute phase is seen when the lymphocytes are exposed to halothane. Lymphocyte stimulation and clinical history provide the best presumptive evidence that a hepatitis may be caused by halothane.

Hepatitis is probably an immunologically induced phenomenon and so a patient challenge would verify the diagnosis. A patient in the quiescent phase would be exposed to an extremely small dose of halothane for a very limited time. If acute hepatitis follows, this is the strongest evidence for the diagnosis of halothane hepatitis.

Hepatitis is rare, occurring in less than one out of 10,000 anesthetics.

## Methoxyflurane

1. Halogenated ether

2. Physically stable liquid at room temperature; poorly vaporized due to a low vapor pressure

3. Nonflammable.

4. Pronounced odor, moderately unpleasant

5. Prolonged induction and awakening. Nitrous oxide is frequently simultaneously administered as a supplement in order to achieve greater depth of anesthesia without

the administration of large doses of methoxyflurane.

6. No stimulation of nausea, vomiting or salivary secretions is commonly experienced.

7. Catecholamine secretions are reduced and myocardial depression is evident as a moderately depressed blood pressure.

8. Ventilation is progressively depressed as the anesthetic level is deepened.

9. Moderate muscle relaxation in surgical depths

10. A synergism exists with the curariform agents.

11. Most potent anesthetic in common usage

12. Extremely potent analgesic

13. It has been found extremely useful for burn dressing and cast changes in light depths.

14. Methoxyflurane undergoes biotransformation. A stimulation of DNA production occurs in the lymphocytes of a patient in the postacute hepatitis phase when the lymphocytes are exposed to methoxyflurane.

## Methoxyflurane-Induced Diseases

1. Postanesthetic hepatitis indistinguishable from that seen with halothane is reported. There seems to be a cross-sensitivity between halothane and methoxyflurane as hepatitis stimulants.

2. Fatal high-output renal failure is reported. It is associated with:

A. Prolonged anesthetics

B. Overweight patients

C. Surgical depths of methoxyflurane anesthesia

Histologically, calcium oxalate crystals are seen in the renal tubules. Abnormally elevated serum fluoride levels are associated with the oliguria.

The mechanism is presumed to be a toxic effect of fluoride that is split from the methoxyflurane molecule. Safety suggests that methoxyflurane should be administered in light depths, supplemented by nitrous oxide and muscle relaxants for a period of less than 4 hours.

## Nitrous Oxide and Balanced Anesthesia

1. Nonirritating, sweet smelling

2. Nonflammable, inorganic gas, that will support combustion with oxygen released by decomposition of the $N_2O$ molecule

3. It is considered to be the least toxic anesthetic agent.

4. It is successfully used for burn dressings and cast changes where unconsciousness is not necessary.

5. Rapid induction and emergence are available in high-flow systems, since the relatively impotent nitrous oxide must replace much of the body's nitrogen before it can have much effect.

6. Weak anesthetic, moderate analgesic and amnesic

7. It is most frequently used in combination with other agents and/or drugs.

A. Muscle relaxants can be used as adjunctive agents. A large amount of muscle relaxant is needed to provide a quiet surgical field because of the limited analgesia available. The excess muscle relaxant is needed to overcome muscular tone and reflexes present due to the inadequate pain relief afforded by the nitrous oxide.

B. Low concentrations of potent inhalation anesthetics may be added to nitrous oxide to reduce the amount of muscle relaxants needed. By using only small doses of inhalation agents, the rapid reversibility of the nitrous oxide anesthetic is not lost.

C. Intravenous agents can be used to enhance the central nervous system depressant properties of nitrous oxide. Barbiturates, tranquilizers, narcotics or any combination of these are frequently used. Unless these nonretrievable agents are rapidly removed or destroyed, they tend to compromise the rapid reversibility of the nitrous oxide.

### *Intravenous Agents*

### Basic Principles

1. Nonvolatile, thus administered intravenously
2. They are diverse pharmacologically and chemically.
3. They typically have unsatisfactory pharmacologic side effects and so are used most frequently with simultaneous nitrous oxide in order to avoid excess depression.
4. The intravenous agents can be pharmacologically deactivated by one or more methods:
   A. Dilution within tissue and/or water compartments
   B. Attachment to pharmacologically inactive receptors
   C. Metabolic inactivation by the blood, liver or kidneys
   D. Excretion of intact or metabolized molecules by the kidneys and/or other excretory route
5. Selection of intravenous agents requires an understanding of the patient's physiologic state and the pharmacology and disposition of the alternative agents.
6. Control of anesthesia with these agents is difficult because of:
   A. Nonretrievability of the drugs
   B. Patient tolerance
   C. Latency between administration and pharmacologic effect
   D. Difficult interpretation of depth of anesthesia
7. Intolerance, idiosyncratic and allergic phenomena are more common with intravenous agents than with inhalation agents
8. Nonretrievability of the drugs may be the cause of a prolonged and/or disoriented emergence.

### Classification

Commonly used nonvolatile, intravenous agents are categorized into:
1. Hypnotics used for basal narcosis (deep state of hypnosis)
2. Narcotics or narcotic–tranquilizer combinations used for basal narcosis and analgesia
3. "Dissociative" anesthetic agents
4. Adjunctive anesthetic agents

### Hypnotics or Ultra-Short-Acting Barbiturates

1. These are most commonly used for induction of anesthesia but they are occasionally used for basal anesthesia. They are:
   A. Thiopental (Pentothal)
   B. Thiamylal (Surital)
   C. Methohexital (Brevital)
2. Pharmacologically they are very much alike, although thiopental and thiamylal are sulfur-substituted barbiturates.
3. Ultra-short-acting barbiturates get their name because of their brief duration of action.
4. Induction doses of these agents cause a brief hypnosis, during which time an inhalation agent is typically introduced.
5. Ventilation is depressed with even small doses.
6. The ventilatory pattern will frequently become irregular.
7. Moderate amnesia is available from a deep dose of the ultra-short-acting barbiturates, and so they have gained popularity for use in cardioversion.
8. Cardiac contractility is so depressed that it is unsafe to use these agents alone for anesthesia without other agents that provide analgesia without a similar degree of cardiac depression.
9. Laryngospasm, coughing, sneezing, retching and vomiting can be seen after even a small dose. The cough and spasm reflexes seem to be enhanced, since bronchospasm has occurred on injection of the ultra-short-acting barbiturates.
10. Cessation of their pharmacologic effect is due to removal of the barbiturates from the brain to muscle and fat tissue.
11. Basal narcosis is produced by repeated generous doses, so that there is an accumulation of barbiturate at the

pharmacologically active site. Thus, the patient derives hypnosis and obtundation of some reflexes.

12. Nitrous oxide is typically administered during basal narcosis, so that there is a summation of analgesic effects and a reduction in the dose of barbiturate needed. Muscle relaxation during basal narcosis, nitrous oxide anesthesia is inadequate for abdominal surgery.

## Narcotic and Nonnarcotic Analgesics

1. Narcotics and some nonnarcotic analgesics are extremely effective analgesics, and it is for this property that they are used in anesthesia.

2. Ventilatory depression of some degree is a constant pharmacologic effect in anesthetic doses. By administering nitrous oxide simultaneously, less narcotic can be used due to the summation of analgesic effects. On withdrawing the nitrous oxide, the patient will typically become responsive.

3. Ventilation must be supported during narcotic, nitrous oxide anesthesia in the emergency patient in order to avoid a respiratory acidosis and frequently accompanying hypoxemia. Artificial ventilation removes the spontaneous ventilatory pattern, one of the better signs of anesthetic depth.

4. Ventilation must be carefully observed in the recovery room because the long-term ventilatory depression accompanying some narcotics may prove disastrous.

5. All narcotics and effective nonnarcotic analgesics have been used. Most commonly used are meperidine and morphine. The narcotics with retained psychotropic effects of hypnosis are most useful. Narcotics without sedative effects should be supplemented with tranquilizers in order to ensure that the patients are actually asleep and will not remember the events and conversations of surgery.

6. Muscle relaxation for abdominal surgery is inadequate with these drugs, and muscle-relaxant drugs must be used to provide adequate conditions.

7. Cardiovascular instability is common, as demonstrated by tilt testing. Blood-volume-depleted patients represent a great risk.

8. Cardiovascular stability may be adversely affected by the tranquilizers commonly used as supplements.

9. Innovar is the most commonly used narcotic tranquilizer preparation. It is a mixture of droperidol (a butyrophenone-derived tranquilizer) and fentanyl (approximately 150 times as potent as morphine) in a 50:1 mixture. Droperidol is a mild vasodilator (perhaps an adrenergic blocking agent) with a 6-hour pharmacologic half-life. Fentanyl has a half-life of approximately 30 minutes. Most frequently only the fentanyl is used for supplemental doses.

10. The use of Innovar has advantages over the use of meperidine and morphine in that overdosage is difficult due to the relatively short duration of action of fentanyl.

11. Innovar can be successfully used for preanesthetic medication and for supplemental sedation and analgesia during regional anesthesia.

## Dissociative Anesthesia—Ketamine

1. This form of anesthesia produces a state of:

    A. Catalepsy

    B. Amnesia

    C. Marked analgesia

2. Ketamine is the only drug of this nature currently marketed in the United States.

3. Route of administration may be:

    A. Intramuscular with an onset of action within a few minutes

    B. Intravenous with an onset of action almost immediately.

4. Ventilatory depression is only seen for a short time after intravenous administration.

5. Blood pressure is usually well maintained.

6. A mild tachycardia is often noted.

7. Muscle relaxation is not consistent, and so pharmacologic paralysis and supported ventilation are necessary for a relaxed field.

8. Pharyngeal and laryngeal reflexes are inconsistently retained, and so all patients with potentially full stomachs would have to be handled by intubation with a cuffed endotracheal tube.

9. Patient movements common during the anesthetic, but it is not in response to pain. This is part of the cataleptic state, and it makes judgment of depth extremely difficult.

10. Vivid hallucinations are a complaint of a large minority of patients. This can be reduced somewhat by preanesthetic medication, but the hallucinations discourage the use of ketamine in young adults, in whom hallucinations are seen most frequently.

11. Recovery after ketamine is more prolonged than after the fast-acting inhalation agents, and vomiting is occasionally seen at this time.

## Neuromuscular Blocking Agents

1. Neuromuscular blocking agents (voluntary muscle relaxants) have revolutionized anesthesiology. Previously only deep general or extensive regional anesthesia could allow for a muscularly relaxed field. The ill and traumatized patient was at great risk under these circumstances.

2. Neuromuscular blocking agents can provide for a profoundly relaxed surgical field with relatively light planes of general anesthesia. A patient can be totally paralyzed, and, as long as ventilation is artificially maintained, there will be no ill effects. Optimal operating conditions are now potentially available to the high-risk patient.

3. *Anesthetic Management of Patients Receiving Neuromuscular Blocking Agents*

A. The anesthesiologist commits himself to maintain adequate ventilation for the patient when using these drugs. Artificial ventilation eliminates the availability of one of the prime indicators of depth of anesthesia, the pattern of ventilation. The commitment to maintain satisfactory ventilation for the patient continues into the recovery room and beyond.

B. Succinylcholine has no pharmacologic antagonist.

C. The curariform agents have a mechanism of antagonism. Drugs are administered that poison the acetylcholinesterases, so that more acetylcholine becomes available and the competition between acetylcholine and the relaxant molecules is shifted to where the relaxant molecules are displaced. This displacement allows acetylcholine to depolarize the membrane.

D. Patients administered muscle relaxants need careful recovery room care, since despite their seemingly awake status they may "fatigue" and be unable to maintain a clear airway. All patients who have had muscle relaxants are at a potentially higher risk.

# 7. CARDIOPULMONARY RESUSCITATION

*Bruno J. Urban*, M.D.
*Stanley W. Weitzner*, M.D.

## Definitions

1. *Cardiac arrest* is defined as sudden and unexpected cessation of effective circulation. This may be caused by ventricular standstill or severe arrhythmias.

2. *Respiratory arrest* is defined as sudden and unexpected cessation of effective ventilation. Ventilatory efforts may be completely absent or minimal.

Clinically, cessation of either effective circulation or ventilation causes the arrest of the other in short succession, and both may have to be assisted for successful resuscitation. If treatment is not immediate, the ensuing tissue hypoxia and acidosis will result in damage to vital organs (the brain first) and finally death.

## Principles of Management

There are four distinct phases in the management of cardiopulmonary arrest:
1. Diagnosis
2. Emergency treatment
3. Definitive treatment
4. Postresuscitation care

Brain damage normally occurs 4 to 6 minutes after the arrest; therefore, prompt diagnosis and restoration of effective brain circulation is necessary for successful resuscitation. This interval may be shortened by pre-existing diseases which impair oxygen transport to the tissues. Diagnostic procedures and definitive treatment of underlying diseases are delayed in favor of immediate treatment of the arrest.

## Diagnosis

The diagnosis is entirely clinical; the following signs constitute criteria for emergency treatment:

1. Loss of pulse where previously present. A major artery, preferably the carotid, should be palpated.

2. Absent or gasping ventilatory efforts

3. Unconsciousness in a previously alert individual which does not respond to the supine position

4. Pupillary dilation. Enlargement of the pupil will start approximately 45 seconds following the cessation of cerebral circulation and will be completed 1 minute later.

5. Skin color. Cyanosis or extreme pallor may be present.

Auscultation of heart sounds, blood pressure measurements, electrocardiography and other auxiliary diagnostic techniques are unnecessary and waste time. They should be performed after the institution of emergency treatment.

## Emergency Treatment

The following steps are taken, each of which may be sufficient for the return of spontaneous, effective, cardiopulmonary action.

1. Place the patient in a supine position and deliver a sharp blow to the chest wall overlying the heart. Sometimes this will restore spontaneous heart action if performed early after an arrest due to cardiac standstill.

2. Summon help as you initiate the next step. The physical efforts of resuscitation are such that one person can rarely sustain them over any extended period of time. Additional personnel are also mandatory for the planning of definitive treatment and the mobilization of postresuscitation care facilities.

The sequence of further treatment is summarized by the ABC mnemonic:
A = Airway
B = Breathing
C = Circulation

3. Establish an airway.

A. Remove foreign material from the oral cavity. Remove dentures only if loose; often the airway can be kept patent more easily with a set of dentures in place.

B. Upper airway obstruction is most frequently produced by the tongue impinging against the posterior pharyngeal wall (Fig. 7-1). This is treated by hyperextension of the head. One hand is placed under the neck while the other is pressing

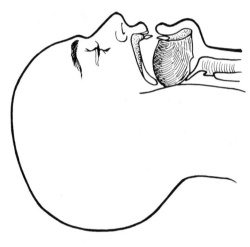

Fig. 7-1.

the forehead backward; additionally, the jaw is displaced forward (Fig. 7-2). Maintaining this position will ensure the patency of the airway in most cases. A pillow or folded sheet placed under the head will facilitate this task.

4. Begin artificial ventilation.

A. Artificial ventilation should be started either by the mouth-to-mouth or mouth-to-nose method. The resuscitator places himself beside the patient and forcefully exhales a deep breath into the patient's mouth (or nose) while the nostrils (or mouth) are occluded to prevent leakage (Fig. 7-3). This should be done rapidly for the first several breaths; later a respiratory rate of approximately 15 breaths per minute is adequate. If resuscitation is performed by one person only, 2 quick breaths should alternate with 15 chest compressions. With more people available, a satisfactory relation between artificial circulation and ventilation develops automatically.

B. As soon as possible, ventilation with a mask and breathing bag should be instituted. In this way, high inspiratory oxygen concentrations can be delivered to the patient. The last three fingers of the left

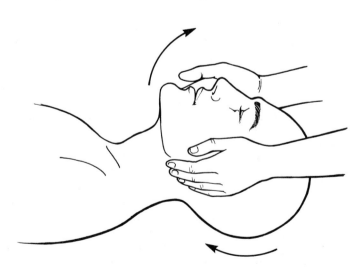

Fig. 7-2.

hand maintain the airway patent by keeping the jaw displaced forward (Fig. 7-2). The fingers should be placed on the lower mandible and not over the soft tissues of the floor of the mouth, or else additional obstruction may be produced. The mask is applied to the face and held in position between the thumb and index finger (Fig. 7-3A). A gas-tight seal is usually effected by gently pressing the mask against the face; excessive pressure will flex the neck and thereby tends to cause obstruction. The right hand squeezes the bag (Fig. 7-3B).

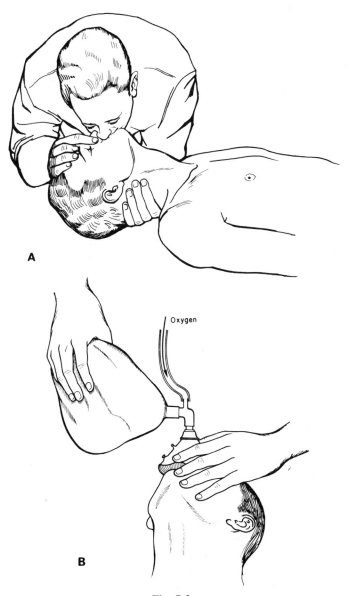

Fig. 7-3.

Commonly used mask-bag combinations are described below:

*(1) Mask, Nonrebreathing Valve, Self-inflating Bag* (Fig. 7-4). This combination has the advantage of being useable with room air only, although oxygen can be added through a side arm. Due to the stiffness of the bag, this device is more difficult to learn to use, and changes in resistance and compliance are not as easily appreciated. Inspiratory oxygen concentrations will be lower than with other combinations, even in the presence of high

flows. On exhalation, the bag will fill preferentially with room air. A slow hand release of the bag will partly compensate for this. Modification for use with high oxygen concentrations can be achieved by the addition of a T-adaptor and a piece of corrugated tubing (Fig. 7-4). During inflation, the continuously flowing oxygen is stored in the tubing and drawn into the self-inflating bag on exhalation.

*(2) Mask, Rovenstine Elbow, Rubber Bag* (Fig. 7-5). Oxygen flows through the nipple of the elbow into the

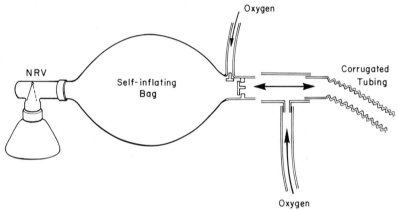

Fig. 7-4. Mask, non-rebreathing valve (NRV), and self-inflating bag. The T-adaptor and corrugated tubing, which are added to increase the inspiratory oxygen concentrations, are depicted on the right side of the schematic. In use, the T-adaptor is connected to the tail of the bag, and the upper oxygen inlet is sealed.

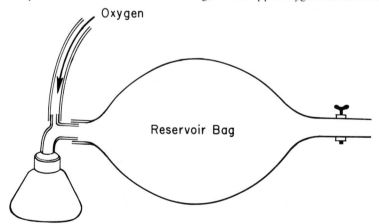

Fig. 7-5. Mask, Rovenstine Elbow, rubber bag. The Rovenstine Elbow is a curved, metal, modified T-adaptor which connects the oxygen supply, the bag, and the mask.

reservoir bag, which is kept filled by adjustment of the tail clamp. Gas is pushed into the lungs by squeezing the bag; on exhalation, it returns into the bag and finally exits through the tail. High flows of oxygen, approximately three times the minute volume (e.g., 20 to 25 L./minute for an adult), are necessary to avoid significant rebreathing of exhaled gas. Nevertheless, some rebreathing will always occur, but it is inconsequential compared to the gain in oxygenation.

*(3) Mask, Nonrebreathing valve, Bag* (Fig. 7-6). With this combination, the flow of oxygen into the bag has only to equal the minute volume. Contamination of the inspiratory gas is prevented by the nonrebreathing valve. The adjustable tail clamp will prevent both collapse and overdistention of the bag. (The latter would impair valve function.) This device will provide effective ventilation with the highest inspired oxygen concentrations.

C. Artificial ventilation of the type described above provides a continuous feedback between the patient and the resuscitator. Changes in resistance and compliance are immediately appreciated and compensated. This does not hold true for mechanical ventilators, and they should not be used with a mask for emergency resuscitation. For instance, in cases of airway obstruction, if there is a leak, the machines may continue to function, ventilating the mask dead space, the stomach or the room. Pressure-cycled ventilators are absolutely contraindicated, because they will cycle on each compression of the chest.

D. Changes in resistance to inflation are usually due to the inability to maintain a patent airway. In this case, a proper-size oro- or nasopharyngeal airway should be inserted (Figs. 7-7 and 7-8). However, these devices are not without danger. An oral airway too small for the particular patient may cause additional obstruction by pushing the base of the tongue against the posterior pharyngeal wall; one too large may bend the epiglottis against the laryngeal opening. Nasal airways may give rise to the same complications and, in addition, may enter the esophagus or produce bleeding. Intubation of the trachea has no

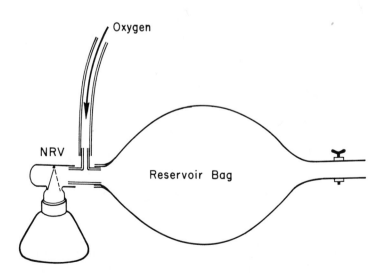

Fig. 7-6. NRV = non-rebreathing valve.

place in emergency treatment. It belongs to the phase of definitive therapy.

5. Begin artificial circulation. This is effected by closed-chest cardiac massage, which will restore 30 to 50 percent of normal cardiac output.

A. The patient is positioned on a hard surface (e.g., the floor). Any resiliency of

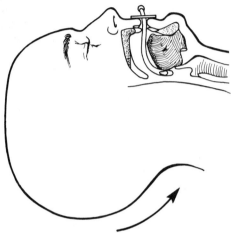

Fig. 7-7. Oropharyngeal airway in place. Compare Fig. 7-1 and note that the tongue is elevated (anteriorly) from the posterior wall of the pharynx.

the supporting surface cushions the effects of chest compression and renders it less effective. If the patient is in bed, a stiff board should be placed under his back.

B. The resuscitator kneels (or stands) at the side of the patient. The heel of one hand is placed over the lower third of the sternum, excluding the ensiform process (Fig. 7-9). The second hand is placed on top of the first. The fingers are kept straight and should barely touch the chest. The arms are held extended at the elbows. The force of compression is generated by bending at the hips moving the shoulders forward and utilizing the weight of the upper trunk. It should be sufficient to displace the sternum about 4 to 5 cm. Pushing the hands downward moves the sternum backward and compresses the heart between the posterior surface of the sternum and the anterior surface of the vertebral column (Fig. 7-10). Rapid compression is followed by rapid release; the maneuver is repeated about 60 times per minute. To facilitate venous return, the legs should be elevated if at all possible.

For infants, the resuscitator stands at the head. He slides his fingers under the

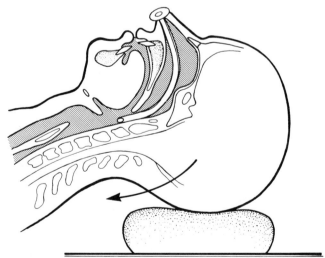

Fig. 7-8. A nasopharyngeal airway in place. (Compare Fig. 7-1.) Elevating the occiput and extending the head help lift the tongue away from the posterior pharyngeal wall.

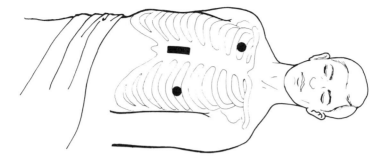

Fig. 7-9. The darkened rectangular area denotes where the heel of the hand is placed for closed-chest cardiac massage. The two darkened circular areas indicate where defibrillator electrodes should be placed.

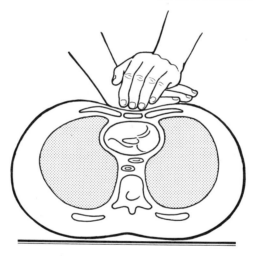

Fig. 7-10.

scapulae and superimposes his thumbs on the midsternum. The chest is compressed by pressing the ball of the lower thumb downward. In older children, the pressure is applied to the lower third as well as to the midsternum. Here, the fingertips or the heel of one hand may be used.

C. Mechanical aids (e.g., Cardiac Press) have been constructed to facilitate external cardiac massage. In principle, they consist of a plunger attached to a lever which is connected by an elbow joint to a rigid board. The board is placed under the patient. Position and height of the plunger are then adjusted so that the plunger rests on the lower third of the sternum. By pushing the lever down, the plunger displaces the sternum posteriorly. This downward excursion is limited and is adjustable for optimal compression. Because a rigid support connects the lever to the board beneath the patient, no cushioning can occur and all the force applied is used to compress the heart. In other devices, plunger and support are fixed in a frame, and the plunger is propelled pneumatically. Again, proper positioning of the plunger and adjustment of its excursion are needed for maximal efficiency.

D. Complications of closed-chest cardiac compression include rib fractures, rupture or contusion of viscera and pneumothorax. To minimize morbidity, the applied pressure should be just enough to effect adequate cerebral circulation. This requires a minimum systolic pressure of 60 mm. Hg. Clinically, this is judged by a palpable carotid pulse and observing changes in the size of the pupil. Reversal of pupillary dilatation is always a sign of adequate brain circulation. Pulsation of the major arteries is often difficult to ascertain, since chest compressions may also result in a strong venous pulse and soft tissue impulses.

E. External chest compression has replaced open-chest cardiac massage as the method of choice. *Internal cardiac massage should be performed only by trained physicians* with proper equipment in cases in which the following exist:

*(1)* The thorax is already opened or traumatically deformed (e.g., in penetrating chest wounds or flail chest).

*(2)* External chest compressions are ineffective (e.g., in severe kyphoscoliosis).

*(3)* Major intrathoracic pathology is suspected (e.g., cardiac tamponade).

*(4)* External defibrillation is expected to fail (e.g., during hypothermia).

6. Maintain a physiologic pH. Severe metabolic acidosis will occur even in the presence of effective resuscitative efforts. A lowered pH impairs cardiac muscle function and lessens the chance of spontaneous restoration of an effective heartbeat. In addition, many drugs, especially the catecholamines, exert most of their action at physiologic pH ranges.

A. Sodium bicarbonate is given intravenously to counteract acidosis. One 50-ml. ampule (3.75 gm. or 44.6 mEq.) is injected every 5 to 7 minutes. In children, the dose is 1 to 2 mEq./kg. of body weight. As soon as possible, arterial blood samples should be drawn and analyzed for acid–base changes to direct further treatment. The addition of bicarbonate buffer will drive the reaction, $H_2O + CO_2 \leftrightharpoons H^+ + HCO_3^-$, toward the left and liberate $CO_2$. Effective ventilation is therefore mandatory for the normalization of pH. In the absence of rapid $CO_2$ removal, the administration of bicarbonate will actually lower pH.

B. Instead of bicarbonate, tris buffer (THAM) may be given in dosages of 1 to 2 mEq./kg. This chemical acts by binding hydrogen$^+$ ions and shifting the equation, $H_2O + CO_2 \leftrightharpoons H^+ + HCO_3^-$, to the right. By lowering $CO_2$, it also exerts an effect inside the cell. THAM is excreted by the kidneys, which may be damaged by the impaired circulation. It also causes hypoglycemia and thus may interfere with the evaluation of the patient's status. Large doses therefore should be avoided.

C. To be effective, both drugs have to be administered intravenously. A large vessel should be selected, and a catheter or plastic cannula is inserted to avoid infiltration. Since the superficial veins are usually collapsed, percutaneous cannulation of the subclavian vein has been found useful. It offers the additional advantage of reliable monitoring of central venous pressure. A needle or cannula with syringe attached is inserted at a point one to two fingerbreadths below the clavicle in the midclavicular line. Introduction is facilitated by a small stab wound to eliminate skin resistance. The needle is directed mediad and slightly cephalad, aiming at a point just beneath the posterior surface of the head of the clavicle. Intraluminal position is determined by the aspiration of blood. Once the vessel is entered, a catheter is advanced through the needle, or the plastic cannula is pushed in a few millimeters while the stylet is withdrawn. Fixation is accomplished by taping to the skin. If percutaneous attempts fail, a cutdown has to be performed. Sterile technique is desirable but may have to yield to speed of performance.

Lactated Ringer's solution is the crystalloid solution of choice for maintaining the intravenous line. Its advantage rests in its ability to temporarily restore major fluid losses. The times at which drugs and fluids are administered must be recorded.

7. Emergency treatment can be carried out for any period of time. If not interrupted, it ensures adequate cerebral perfusion until definitive treatment can start.

### Definitive Treatment

Definitive treatment consists of treating the precipitating causes of cardiac arrest. It should be instituted as soon as possible to minimize systemic sequelae.

1. Inject epinephrine, 0.5 to 1.0 mg., intravenously. This amount should be diluted in 5 to 10 ml. of physiologic solution. Intravenous administration is preferred to intracardiac injection. The latter may damage the heart and should be used only if an intravenous line cannot be established. Intracardiac injections are performed with a 22-gauge, 10-cm. needle inserted at a point in the fourth intercostal space approximately 5 cm. to the left of the sternal border. *Avoid intramyocardial injections; inject only after easy aspiration of blood.*

The administration of epinephrine may be repeated every 5 to 7 minutes without prior electrocardiographic diagnosis. In cardiac standstill, the drug may help start cardiac action; in case of ventricular fibrillation, it may facilitate defibrillation by countershock. To be effective, prior normalization of pH is necessary.

2. *Intubation.* The trachea is intubated with a cuffed tube through the mouth or nose. The procedure must be performed in a well-oxygenated patient, and resuscitative measures should not be interrupted for more than 15 seconds in attempting to do this.

A. The mechanical problem of in-

tubation consists in aligning the three axes of larynx, pharynx and mouth. Flexing the neck by positioning a pillow under the head will straighten the angle between the axes of larynx and pharynx; hyperextending the head in the atlantooccipital joint will straighten the angle between the axes of pharynx and mouth. There remains only one obstacle to the exposure of the vocal cords, the soft tissues of the floor of the mouth. This is overcome with the laryngoscope blade, which lifts the jaw and pushes the tongue to the side (Fig. 7-11).

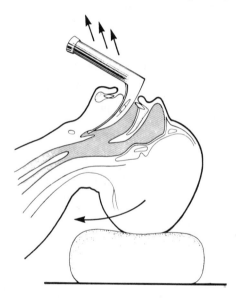

Fig. 7-11.

B. Prior to intubation, the equipment is checked for completeness and malfunction. Equipment consists of one larynogoscope handle with two blades of proper size (one curved and one straight), three endotracheal tubes each for oral or nasal use, a Magill forceps, a stylet, lubricant and a suction apparatus with several catheters. The tubes are cuffed, or of adjacent sizes, and fitted with a straight (oral) or curved (nasal) connector. For adults, the most commonly used sizes are from No. 36 to No. 42 French (No. 8 to No. 12

Magill). Laryngoscope blades are also manufactured in different sizes, and the appropriate one is selected by estimating the distance between the patient's teeth and larynx. Cuffed tubes are not used in infants or small children because a gas-tight fit is produced by the narrow cricoid ring. In selecting the proper tube, one rule of thumb states that the diameter of the tube should correspond to the diameter of the patient's fifth finger or of the nostril. Intubation in the younger age-groups is easier with a straight blade because the larynx is situated higher in the neck.

C. Intubation involves the following steps:

*(1)* The intubator is at the head of the patient. The head is hyperextended and a pillow or folded sheet is placed under it. The laryngoscope is held in the left hand, while the mouth is being opened with the right hand. The blade is inserted from the right corner of the mouth. This avoids damage to the brittle front teeth and shortens the distance to the larynx. The tongue is pushed to the left. Once the uvula is seen, the tip of the laryngoscope is directed toward the midline until the epiglottis is visible. When using a curved blade, its tip is allowed to rest in the vallecula in front of the epiglottis. A straight blade is advanced further, lifting the epiglottis up. The laryngoscope is then pulled upward in a direction perpendicular to the axis of the neck (Fig. 7-11). This compresses the soft tissue of the floor of the mouth, allowing exposure of the laryngeal opening. In more difficult cases, the whole head can be lifted up (and suspended) from the laryngoscope. The direction of the pull is important. If the laryngoscope is used as a lever with the upper teeth as the fulcrum, the larynx will be pushed out of sight, and soft tissues as well as the upper teeth might be damaged. It is not necessary to expose the larynx completely. Identification of the posterior aspect of the rima glottidis is sufficient for intubation.

*(2)* A well-lubricated tube is inserted, again proceeding from the right side of the mouth toward the midline. This ensures a clear field of view until the larynx is entered. The tube is advanced to the point where the proximal end of the cuff is just visible below the vocal cords.

*(3)* For nasal intubation, the tube is first inserted through the nose into the pharynx; then the steps outlined for oral intubation are followed. By twisting and pushing the part of the tube protruding from the nose, the tip of the tube can be directed (under direct vision) from the pharynx into the larynx. Should this maneuver prove difficult, Magill forceps are introduced from the right side of the mouth, and the tip of the tube is grasped and inserted into the larynx. If Magill forceps are not available, any long forceps may be used. It may be helpful to have an assistant advancing the tube on command, while the tip is directed by the forceps.

*(4)* Once in place, the endotracheal tube is immediately connected to the breathing bag and ventilation is resumed. The cuff is inflated just enough so that no air is felt escaping on inhalation when the larynx is palpated. In order to avoid compression of the tube, the laryngoscope is left in the oral cavity until final fixation. Both lungs are checked for aeration by auscultation.

D. Successful intubation does not guarantee unimpeded ventilation. The tube might slip into the bronchus, become dislodged, kinked or obstructed by external compression (e.g., biting). In order to prevent these complications, endotracheal tubes have to be secured. This is done by taping the tube to the skin and inserting an oral airway or bite block. Since kinking occurs most frequently in the part of the tube protruding from the mouth, fixation with a bite block is a more effective method. The simplest bite block is a roll of gauze (approximately 2 cm. in diameter) wrapped with adhesive tape. It is inserted between the right molars before the laryngoscope blade is withdrawn. The tube is taped to it and both are taped to the skin. The bite block must be long enough to stabilize the tube up to the connector; the connector should not be taped.

Nasal tubes are taped to the skin of the nose and, in addition, may be secured with umbilical tape around the neck. It is important to employ a curved connector. Since soft nasotracheal catheters are exceptionally prone to kinking, any protrusion beyond the nostrils should be avoided.

E. After intubation, a mechanical ventilator may be employed. Only volume-preset machines may be used because pressure-cycled devices (e.g., Bird Mark VII or a Bennett PR-2) will initiate a new ventilatory cycle with each compression of the chest. The resulting high respiratory rates and low tidal volumes will not produce an adequate alveolar ventilation. As soon as possible, the volume of ventilation should be adjusted according to blood gas analysis.

F. Rarely, pathologic changes may make it impossible to establish or maintain a patent airway. In these cases, one of the following procedures may be performed.

*(1) Tracheostomy.* Although this is usually an elective procedure carried out over an indwelling tracheal catheter, it may be lifesaving in otherwise intractable upper airway obstruction. *It should be performed by experienced physicians only.*

*(2) Conitomy* (cricothyreotomy). This procedure consists of stabbing a knife blade transversely through the cricothyroid membrane. A curved metal tube (or any suitable substitute) is inserted through the incision into the larynx and trachea. Since the membrane lies close to the skin without interposed major structures, little bleeding is encountered normally.

*(3) Transtracheal Ventilation.* This recently described procedure may prove to be best suited to cope with otherwise intractable airway obstruction. A 16-gauge needle (or plastic cannula) is inserted percutaneously into the trachea either through the cricothyroid membrane or any prominent and easily palpated part of the trachea. Position is ascertained by the aspiration of air. The needle is fixed with tape when lying in the middle of the tracheal lumen and pointing toward the thoracic cavity. The hub is connected by means of a closed interrupter to an oxygen supply source of approximately 50 p.s.i. pressure. The interrupter may be a mechanical or electrical timer or simply a folded rubber hose compressed with a strong clamp. Intermittent short bursts of oxygen delivered through the tracheal needle will adequately ventilate the lungs. If the airway is not completely occluded, additional air may be drawn in during the burst by a Venturi action. Exhalation is passive and usually not impeded because upper airway obstructions tend to be inspiratory only. This method of ventilation will gain the time to secure the airway permanently with a "semielective" tracheostomy.

3. *Electrocardiographic Diagnosis.* The definitive treatment of cardiac arrest requires electrocardiographic diagnosis. Mechanical compression of the chest is briefly interrupted to obtain recordings free of artifacts. The following two groups of conduction disturbances are most commonly encountered.

A. *Ventricular Fibrillation*

*(1)* The most effective way to terminate this condition is to apply an electrical countershock with either direct or alternating current. For adults the usual energy is 200 watt-seconds D.C. or 500 to 1,000 volts A.C. for 0.1 to 0.25 second. The recommended dosages are marked on the defibrillators. They vary with body resistance and have to be adjusted according to clinical response. The dosage for children is proportionally lower (e.g., 100 watt-seconds D.C.). One starts defibrillation with the lowest recommended energy for the particular apparatus and steps it up if no response occurs.

*(2)* The electrodes are generously

pasted with conductive jelly and placed at the apex of the heart and parasternally just below the right clavicle (Fig. 7-9). Firm pressure is applied. In order to prevent accidents, discharge of the countershock must be under the control of the person holding the electrodes. Resuscitation procedures continue until just before shocking. Then all personnel are told to step back and avoid any contact with the patient; the patient cable of the ECG is disconnected, and the countershock is administered.

(3) Coarse fibrillation is more easily amenable to this treatment. Fine fibrillation can be converted into the coarse type by the intravenous administration of epinephrine (0.5 to 1.0 mg. diluted in 5 to 10 ml. 5% G/W). Should weak fibrillation persist, 5 ml. of 10% calcium chloride (0.5 gm.) may be given intravenously.

(4) If ventricular fibrillation persists after countershock, the above maneuvers are repeated. Higher energy levels or a series of A.C. shocks in succession may also be of value. If fibrillation recurs, antiarrhythmic drugs such as lidocaine (2 mg./kg. intravenously) should be tried before repeating the procedure. Lidocaine levels may be maintained by infusion, the usual concentration being 1 mg. per 1 ml. of solution.

(5) Defibrillation frequently results in conversion to a regular rhythm. However, attempts must sometimes be continued for prolonged periods of time until success, or obvious signs of cerebral death, can be determined.

B. *Ventricular standstill, slow idioventricular rhythm and extreme sinus bradycardia* are less frequent causes of cardiac arrest and may also develop following defibrillation. While they persist, external cardiac compressions must continue. Myocardial depressants should be avoided (e.g., discontinue the lidocaine drip). Certain drugs are particularly effective in initiating or enhancing cardiac rhythmicity.

(1) Isoproterenol has both an inotropic and a chronotropic effect. The preferred method of administration is by an intravenous infusion of 2 mg. of isoproterenol in 500 ml. of solution. In this way the dose can be titrated according to the observed effects. Isoproterenol is the drug of choice in starting the heart after defibrillation. As a potent peripheral vasodilator, it may produce hypotension. This side effect is counteracted by the rapid infusion of lactated Ringer's solution or by small doses of a peripheral vasopressor (e.g., phenylephrine).

(2) Epinephrine. In addition to its already described use, epinephrine can be given in a dilute intravenous infusion (2 to 3 mg. dissolved in 500 ml. 5% G/W). The drug produces a combined inotropic, chronotropic and vasopressor effect. Its drawback rests in its potential to induce ventricular fibrillation.

(3) Calcium chloride. This inotropic drug is administered slowly (intravenously) in doses of 0.5 gm. (5 ml. of a 10% solution).

(4) Vasopressors are restricted to combatting hypotension in the presence of an elevated central venous pressure. Hypotension with a low central venous pressure should be treated with infusions (e.g., lactated Ringer's solution). To avoid fluid overload, a combination of infusion and vasopressor may be used, especially for the reversal of drug-induced hypotension (e.g., after isoproterenol). Phenylephrine given by intravenous infusion (10 mg. diluted in 250 ml. 5% G/W) serves well in titrating the blood pressure.

(5) Atropine sulfate in doses of 0.4 mg. intravenously is given to relieve sinus bradycardia and improve atrioventricular conduction. This dose may be repeated every minute up to a total of 2 mg. Very slow administration may initially result in further slowing of the heart rate.

(6) Electrical pacing of the heart. An external cardiac pacemaker may be tried if drugs are ineffective in restoring

spontaneous cardiac activity. The rate of pacing is set to approximately 70 to 80 per minute, and the voltage is adjusted to the value required in the particular patient. Internal cardiac pacing usually produces better results than external pacing. A bipolar catheter electrode is inserted percutaneously by cutdown or subclavian needle into the right ventricle. The position of the tip is adjusted to achieve maximum response to minimal stimulation by monitoring the electrocardiogram. *The procedure should be restricted to experienced physicians only.*

4. In spite of aggressive and continuing resuscitative efforts, cerebral damage and death may occur. In general, therapy is considered unsuccessful, and may be discontinued, if after one hour of effective resuscitation no signs of spontaneous cardiopulmonary activity can be observed and the pupils remain dilated.

## Postresuscitation Care

Intensive treatment will be necessary for at least the first three days following cardiac arrest. It is considered to be completed only if the patient's vital functions are restored, the cause for the accident is determined and measures for its permanent correction are started. A detailed outline of postresuscitation care is beyond the scope of this discussion, but, in general, the following steps are taken:

1. The patient is transferred to a special care unit equipped with continuous monitoring devices. Arrhythmias and an unstable blood pressure are commonly seen following cardiac arrest and must be treated immediately to prevent recurrence of arrest.

2. Ventilatory support is continued and adjusted with repeated arterial blood gas determinations. The current practice tries to avoid both respiratory acidosis and alkalosis. The $CO_2$ tension is kept at about 35 torr. Oxygen tensions must be adequate to ensure complete saturation of hemoglobin. An unstable thoracic cage (the result of broken ribs during chest compression) may necessitate internal fixation for longer periods of time with a volume-preset ventilator (*see* Chap. 11, Thoracic and Cardiovascular Injuries).

3. The arterial pH should be maintained close to normal. This may necessitate frequent arterial analyses and the further administration of alkalinizing agents. Blood electrolytes are followed closely and maintained within the normal range.

4. Cerebral edema will compound possible brain damage secondary to cardiac arrest. Its prevention and treatment are of importance. To this end, hydrocortisone is given, and hypothermia to about 32° C. is instituted. Large doses of barbiturates may be given to decrease cerebral oxygen consumption, and they will also help suppress convulsions. In our experience this treatment has shown promising results.

5. Cardiac glycosides and vasopressors may be needed. Infusions of lidocaine may be needed as well, to suppress arrhythmias.

6. Urinary output is closely monitored; it should be maintained above 30 ml./hour. The early administration of mannitol is helpful in this respect. Later, diuretics (furosemide is our drug of choice at this time) are indicated. If these are unsuccessful, dialysis should be considered.

7. The complications of resuscitation have to be treated. These might necessitate the use of chest tubes, antibiotics and even corrective surgery. If ventilatory support is deemed necessary for any length of time, a tracheostomy should be performed.

8. The underlying disease, having manifested itself by triggering a cardiopulmonary arrest, must be diagnosed. The diagnostic and therapeutic procedures outlined above involve the close collaboration of different specialties; therefore, consultants should be called early and frequently.

# 8. VENTILATORY SUPPORT IN SURGICAL EMERGENCIES

*Ralph Milliken*, M.D.

## Definition

Respiratory failure is the inability of the patient to provide sufficient oxygen to the tissues to maintain aerobic metabolism. This chapter will deal with primary and secondary pulmonary failure, although inadequate oxygenation may also be caused by failure of perfusion or oxygen extraction.

## Basic Principles

### Central Mechanisms for Ventilatory Depression

1. Direct injury to the brain or spinal cord associated with inadequate motor function
2. Cerebral embolization (fat, clot, etc.) and resultant deficits
3. Generalized central nervous sytem depression secondary to sedative, hypnotic or analgesic drugs.
4. Central-nervous-system-induced ventilatory dysfunction secondary to metabolic abnormality (acid–base or electrolyte disturbance, etc.)

### Deranged Physiology Seen in Peripheral Ventilatory Failure

1. Decreased compliance (chest wall, lung or total chest) with resultant increased work of breathing (e.g., pulmonary fibrosis, immobilization of chest wall, etc.)
2. Altered ventilation-perfusion function with underperfusion of nonventilated alveoli and resultant hypoxemia (e.g., atelectasis, pneumonia, etc.)
3. Increased dead space ventilation with ventilation of nonperfused alveoli secondary to shock, pulmonary emboli, etc.
4. Increased dead space/tidal volume ratio secondary to atelectasis with relative overventilation of the unaffected lung areas

### Airway Obstruction with Secondary Ventilatory Failure

1. Soft tissue obstruction of the upper airway, head or neck. This may be caused by loss of consciousness produced by natural (sleep) or unnatural (coma) events. It may be caused by airway trauma.
2. Trauma to both the soft and/or hard tissue of the upper airway, head or neck
3. The above may be complicated by aspiration of material into the lower airway, resulting in:
   A. Obstruction of the tracheobronchial tree or larynx
   B. Atelectasis of the lung
   C. Lung abscess
   D. Pneumonia
   E. Mendelsohn's syndrome (aspiration of gastric juice)
   F. Suffocation
4. Glottic trauma (lacerated or paralyzed vocal cords, fractured larynx, neck hematoma with compression), resulting in obstruction
5. Tracheobronchial trauma (lower airway), resulting in obstruction (e.g., lacerated or ruptured trachea)

### Chest Injury with Associated Ventilatory Insufficiency

1. Pain with resulting shallow, splinting respiration
2. Multiple rib fractures, sternal fractures or costochondral separations, resulting in an unstable segment and paradoxical respiration
3. Space-occupying lesion of the chest (hemothorax, pneumothorax, chylothorax or hemopneumothorax, rup-

ture of the diaphragm, etc.) with partial or total collapse of one or both lungs

4. Lung contusions with pulmonary interstitial edema, local airway and alveolar obstruction, and limited or massive hemorrhage

5. Respiratory burn and/or tissue damage

## Distant Injuries with Associated Ventilatory Insufficiency

1. Abdominal injuries with associated pain that produces shallow, splinting respirations

2. Abdominal distention that interferes with ventilation

3. Orthopedic trauma with possible concomitant fat emboli

### Criteria for Diagnosis

### Signs of Ventilatory Insufficiency

1. Hypoxia is diagnosed by blood gas analysis where the arterial oxygen tension ($pAO_2$) is less than 80 torr. Cyanosis is an unreliable sign of the state of arterial oxygenation. Tissue hypoxia is frequently first reflected by mental confusion or restlessness. Tissue hypoxia can lead to cellular death. Signs of hypoxia are:

A. *Hyperventilation.* This is initiated by the effect of the low $pAO_2$ on the chemoreceptors, which stimulate the ventilatory center.

B. *Sympathetic Stimulation.* Hypoxia is the most potent sympathetic stimulant, acting on chemoreceptors and perhaps vasomotor centers. Initially the heart rate is increased and in turn the cardiac output is increased.

2. Hypercapnia is an arterial carbon dioxide tension ($pACO_2$) greater than 45 torr. Initially hypercapnia stimulates the ventilatory center to augment ventilation. Hypercapnia is best diagnosed by blood gas analysis. Signs of hypercapnia are:

A. Hyperventilation noted as increased frequency and depth of ventilation

B. Sympathetic stimulation reflected

in an increased heart rate and an increased cardiac output

3. Hypotension can be precipitated by ventilatory insufficiency due to the presence of hypoxia or hypercapnia. Since carbon dioxide is a local vasodilator, and since compensation for both hypoxia and hypercapnia cause vasoconstriction, either vasoconstriction or vasodilatation may be present.

4. Dyspnea is the subjective appreciation of attempting to increase ventilation without being able to do so. Not all dyspnea represents ventilatory insufficiency.

## Factors Predisposing to Ventilatory Insufficiency

1. Pulmonary disease existing prior to surgery or trauma is a significant factor.

2. Cigarette smoking increases degenerative lung changes, and heavy cigarette smoking is highly correlated with postoperative respiratory complications.

3. Obesity predisposes to ventilatory insufficiency through a variety of mechanisms.

4. Increasing age increases pulmonary complications.

5. Pain increases pulmonary complications through the mechanism of:

A. Ineffective tracheal toilet and retained secretions

B. Atelectasis promoted by inadequate attempts at deep breathing

The closer a surgical incision is to the thorax, the more likely the interference with ventilatory function.

6. Abdominal distention is a frequent cause of ventilatory complications. The distention produces restriction of lung and chest movements.

7. Central depressant drugs, including anesthetics and narcotics, increase the incidence of pulmonary complications because of the loss of spontaneous deep breathing which is believed to have a pulmonary protective effect.

## Management

### Establishing an Airway

1. A patent airway is a prerequisite for ventilatory support.

2. Remove any debris in the upper and lower airway when possible. Use a head-low position to aid drainage of blood and foreign material away from the larynx.

3. Airway management in emergency situations is similar to that in elective anesthetic procedures, but it is appropriately altered when necessary.

4. Oropharyngeal and nasopharyngeal airways have only slight short-term use.

### Indications for Endotracheal Intubation

1. To establish and maintain a free airway in patients who cannot be treated satisfactorily by oro- or nasopharyngeal airways

2. To prevent aspiration of foreign material into the tracheobronchial tree by sealing off the trachea with a cuff

3. To permit effective positive-pressure ventilation that cannot be provided safely or effectively with a mask

4. To permit effective removal of tracheobronchial secretions or foreign material

The performance of endotracheal intubation is discussed in Chapter 7, Cardiopulmonary Resuscitation.

### Routes of Endotracheal Intubation

1. Transoral and transnasal routes are frequently chosen in the emergency situation in order to provide immediate ventilatory support. The transoral route is typically the easiest route.

2. The transnasal route may be chosen if the following situations exist:

A. The mouth or jaw is traumatized or anatomically abnormal so that oral intubation is difficult or impossible and/or the nasal route is easier.

B. Moderate or long-term ventilatory support is likely to be needed and the nasal route is more comfortable for the patient, and thus is preferred.

3. Tracheostomy is chosen:

A. Whenever a patient cannot tolerate an endotracheal tube

B. When the need for an artificial airway will extend beyond 48 to 72 hours (We frequently will maintain endotracheal intubation for 7 or more days.)

C. When passage of an endotracheal tube is impossible or dangerous by any other route

### Methods of Endotracheal Intubation

1. *Awake Intubation Via the Upper Airway*

A. In using an awake intubation, the anesthetist attempts to pass an endotracheal tube through the vocal cords and into the trachea, where the cuff is inflated in order to protect the trachea from soilage. Since the tube cannot be passed in the fully conscious, reflex-intact patient, the anesthetist attempts to lower the level of consciousness and/or obtund the reflexes. In doing this, the risk of vomiting and aspiration is increased since the patient's airway is less protected than in the awake, reflex-intact state. This risk is reduced since the anesthetist should be prepared to suction vigorously if vomiting does occur. The anesthetist must work quickly once he starts the awake intubation sequence. In preparing a nostril for awake nasal intubation, a topical anesthetic with vasoconstricting properties should be placed in the most patent nostril, usually the one with the freest flow of gas. An endotracheal tube is then passed through the nose, through the pharynx and past the vocal cords into the trachea.

B. Methods available to obtund the gag reflex are:

*(1)* Sedation

*(2)* Topical anesthesia

*(3)* Superior laryngeal nerve block bilaterally; transtracheal topical injection

2. *Effective, Drug-induced Un-*

*conscious Intubation* (rapid-induction intubation sequence)

A. This technique would be used in the patient who:

(1) Will be having a general anesthetic for surgery

(2) Would be so restless, uncooperative or apprehensive that general anesthesia is needed for intubation and/or tracheostomy

B. The team approach must be used for this type of intubation. A surgeon should be scrubbed and gowned and prepared to do an immediate tracheostomy if intubation attempts are unsuccessful and ventilation cannot be maintained with a mask and bag. A sterile tray with instruments and cannulae for the tracheostomy should be prepared and available before the induction. Another individual (anesthetist, surgeon or circulating nurse) should be available to assist the anesthesiologist during intubation. This person should be holding a functioning large bore suction device, preferably stiff to enable its accurate placement during use. This device would be used if vomitus appeared in the pharynx. The anesthesiologist's assistant can aid also in monitoring the patient, repositioning the operating table after intubation, and providing help in other tasks at the beginning of the anesthetic.

C. The rapid-induction intubation sequence results in a telescoping of the induction time into a very short period. An absolute loss of the excitement stage should be achieved, and the sequence should achieve a rapid intubation with the aim of protecting the airway by a cuffed endotracheal tube. Rapid induction for emergency anesthetics utilizes preoxygenation by mask, the rapid administration of a predetermined amount of ultra-short-acting barbiturate and typically a short-acting muscle relaxant, followed immediately by endotracheal intubation without attempting to ventilate the patient once the sequence is begun until endotracheal intubation has been accomplished. This technique relies heavily upon the proper preinduction evaluation of the anatomy of the upper airway and upon the physiologic condition of the patient, so that no predictable problems regarding endotracheal intubation exist and adverse drug reactions do not occur.

D. The sequence is best preceded by emptying the stomach, using induced emesis and/or a nasogastric tube. By decreasing the contents of the stomach, there should be less likelihood of vomiting or regurgitation. The use of a nasogastric or other stomach tube is no assurance that the stomach has been thoroughly emptied. During the anesthetic, a large bore stomach tube should be passed again and allowed to drain continuously.

E. The blockage of the esophagus or gastric cardia with a balloon affair is difficult to accomplish, uncomfortable to the patient, hazardous in that the balloon may be regurgitated or may produce incomplete blockage, and thus is unreliable. It is not commonly used because it is time-consuming and unreliable.

F. Cricoid cartilage pressure (Sellick maneuver) is effective because the cricoid cartilage is a complete cartilaginous ring with a broad posterior surface that can effectively occlude the esophagus against the cervical vertebral bodies.

G. Fowler's position is used to decrease the likelihood of passive regurgitation with induction of unconsciousness and muscle relaxation. By placing the patient in a head-up position, the larynx is placed above the gastric cardia, thus requiring additional pressure to be expended before gastric contents can be pushed into the pharynx. Since the fasciculations of succinylcholine-induced skeletal muscle paralysis increase intragastric pressure irregularly, this position adds to the safety of the rapid-induction intubation sequence. It also adds safety where the stomach is not fully emptied.

H. The prophylactic use of neutralizing solutions taken orally by the awake patient prior to induction will not avoid the serious sequence of regurgitation or vomiting.

I. Awakening from anesthesia is a hazardous time due to the depression of natural reflexes which may not protect the airway from gastric aspiration. These protective reflexes should be demonstrated by "bucking on the tube," checking the patient's response to verbal commands, adequate ventilation, etc.

## Hazards of Rapid-Induction Intubation

1. During controlled respiration, overdosage (relative or absolute) can result from either intravenous drugs or gaseous anesthetics delivered in too high a concentration. The protective effects of spontaneous ventilation lost by induced muscle paralysis increase the hazards of some anesthetics. Complications of overdosage can be missed if the anesthetist is too busy during rapid induction to adequately observe the patient.

2. Passive regurgitation and active vomiting are significant hazards since the possibility of a full stomach is the indication for a rapid-induction intubation sequence. The administration of atropine increases the competency of the gastric cardia, and its use should be considered prior to the rapid-induction intubation sequence.

3. Hypotension during rapid induction may be due to relative or absolute overdoses of intravenous or gaseous agents used in the sequence. The Fowler's position frequently used as an aid to reduce regurgitation predisposes to hypotension by causing blood-pooling, particularly when associated with anesthetic agents that cause vasodilation or reduced blood volume. Positive-pressure ventilation after intubation may lead to hypotension if it is too vigorous, reducing venous return to the right heart.

4. Reflex circulatory responses to intubation are common. Most frequently seen are hypertension, tachycardia and arrhythmias. Cardiac arrest may be seen.

5. Pharmacologic hazards of rapid-induction techniques are most frequently related to barbiturates. A dose of ultra-short-acting barbiturate should be individualized for each patient, but, because of the need for rapid unconsciousness to avoid regurgitation, overdosage leading to adverse effects may occur. Succinylcholine chloride is the most commonly chosen muscle relaxant used for rapid-induction techniques because its effects are induced with the shortest latency period. The pharmacology of these drugs is reviewed in Chapter 6, Anesthesia Considerations in the Patient for Emergency Operation.

## Oxygen Therapy

1. Oxygen therapy is used to combat hypoxia. Oxygen therapy in the hypoxic patient is used to achieve the following goals:

A. To ensure adequate tissue oxygenation

B. To obviate the need for compensatory hypoxic responses such as increased peripheral sympathetic activity, increased cardiac output and hyperventilation

2. Satisfactory oxygen therapy achieves an arterial oxygen tension of 90 to 150 torr, but the causes of hypoxia must be investigated since oxygen therapy alone may not be adequate treatment. Repeated $paO_2$ determinations should be made to monitor the success of therapy. Techniques of oxygen therapy include the following commonly used devices:

A. Nasal catheter

B. Nasal cannula

C. Face mask with or without a reservoir bag and with or without non-rebreathing valves

D. Face hood

E. Oxygen tent

F. Respirators

Patients receiving oxygen must be carefully observed, since administered oxygen will cause ventilatory depression in a patient whose principal ventilatory stimulus was hypoxia.

## Respirator Therapy

1. *Indications for Respirator Therapy*

A. When other forms of oxygen therapy are unsuccessful in combating hypoxia

B. When spontaneous ventilatory effort is not adequate in providing adequate alveolar ventilation and carbon dioxide homeostasis. A few patients have a constantly elevated $pACO_2$, but they are in homeostasis and do not need respirator therapy.

C. In occasional cases of acute, severe pulmonary edema

D. Chest injuries, including chest surgery and cases involving unstable chest segments

E. Head injury and neurologic deterioration where ventilatory stimuli are suppressed

F. Abdominal distention that interferes with respiration

G. Other conditions that are noted above

2. *Management of Patients Receiving Respirator Therapy*

Expert consultation should be obtained for all patients who are to receive respiratory therapy. An etiologic diagnosis should be made as soon as possible. Initial respiratory monitoring of patients started on respirator therapy should include:

A. Arterial blood gases repeated as often as necessary in order to ensure that the therapy is providing the desired results

B. Measurement of inspiratory force

C. Total chest compliance

D. Chest x-ray

E. A determination of the per cent of cardiac output shunted past nonventilating areas

F. A determination of the fraction of inspired gas and the ventilated areas not participating in gas exchange, i.e., the dead space

G. Vital signs

H. Intake and output

3. *Types of Ventilators and Their Selection and Use*

A. Tank and cuirass ventilators function by providing a negative pressure outside the chest. This produces a negative intrathoracic pressure which closely simulates normal breathing. These ventilators are typically cumbersome, bulky, noisy devices, which discourage good nursing care, are difficult to adjust finely, and as a result are infrequently utilized.

B. Intermittent positive-pressure ventilators (IPPV) function by applying positive pressure to the airway by mask, endotracheal tube or tracheostomy, thus forcing inspiration. Expiration may be assisted by a negative pressure generated by the ventilator.

*(1)* Pressure-limited ventilators will deliver a volume of gas until a preset inspiratory pressure is reached within the patient circuit. When this pressure is developed, the ventilator will automatically switch to the expiratory phase. The volume of gas delivered by the ventilator can vary with each inspiration. The length of expiration can be preset by using an apnea control as in a Bird ventilator series or by a frequency control device as in the Bennett ventilator. Both the Bird and the Bennett ventilators allow for patient initiation of inspiration.

*(2)* Volume-limited ventilators deliver at least a minimum predetermined volume of gas at a predetermined rate regardless of the pressure required (within certain limitations). The volume of gas, the inspired concentration of oxygen and the minimum ventilatory frequency can be predetermined by the operator while using the Ohio Model 560, Bennett MA-1 and Engstrom ventilators. The first two ventilators allow for patient initiation of mechanical inspiration while the Engstrom is only a "controller," i.e., it is not designed to assist the patient's inspiratory efforts,

but only provides predetermined volumes at predetermined rates.

C. Selection of a ventilator and its proper use should be made with the aid of a physician experienced in ventilator therapy. In the short term when consultative services may not be available, the following goals should be considered.

*(1)* Adequate arterial oxygen tensions of 70 to 100 torr should be maintained. A ventilator that will provide such tensions should be selected, since hypoxia can cause brain damage and hyperoxia can initiate pulmonary damage. Problems involving adequate oxygenation may be solved by hyperventilation, utilizing high inspired-oxygen concentrations or continuous positive-pressure ventilation. These techniques typically require volume-limited ventilators and sophisticated supervision. Demonstration of adequate oxygenation by blood gas analysis should be provided as soon as possible after initiation of ventilation.

*(2)* Adequate ventilation (the minute pulmonary gas exchange) is needed to maintain a normal arterial carbon dioxide tension. Ventilation requirements for patients with normal lungs are easily predicted by nomograms and are usually easily provided by pressure-limited ventilators. Patients with deranged pulmonary physiology may have ventilation requirements that can only be satisfied by the use of volume-limited ventilators. Arterial

carbon dioxide tensions of 30 to 50 torr are most desirable. Adequacy of ventilation can be confirmed by gas and tidal sampling, rebreathing technique and most accurately by blood gas analysis (*see* above).

*(3)* Humidification of inspired gases to 100 per cent water-vapor tension at body temperature is usually achieved in the upper airway. This humidification maintains a relatively low viscosity of tracheobronchial secretions, enabling them to be swept out by normal ciliary action and normal coughing. If normal humidification is not maintained, mucus becomes inspissated and pathologic changes can develop in the lungs. Efficient adjunct humidification and warming of inspired gases should be provided for patients on long-term ventilator therapy. This is usually accomplished by a heated humidifier or nebulizer connected into the patient inspiratory circuit.

D. Increase in the $pAO_2$ may be achieved by increasing the concentration of inspired oxygen, increasing the ventilatory volume or in selected patients by maintaining a positive end-expiratory pressure (PEEP).

Alteration in the $pACO_2$ is accomplished either by altering the ventilatory "dead space" or by adjusting the ventilatory rate of the respirator.

E. It cannot be overemphasized that expert consultation is invaluable in ventilator management.

# 9. SURGICAL INFECTIONS

*Horace Herbsman,* M.D.

## Definitions

Infection is an inflammatory response to the entrance and growth of micro-organisms in tissues, resulting from one type of organism or from a mixture of several types. It may take the following forms:

1. *Cellulitis.* This is a diffuse inflammatory involvement of the skin and subcutaneous tissues.

2. *Lymphangitis.* This is an inflammation of the lymphatic vessels leading from the site of infection.

3. *Abscess.* This is a localized collection of liquefied tissues and pus.

4. *Septicemia.* This is generalized circulatory bacterial invasion associated with toxemia

## Basic Principles

Infection can occur spontaneously or, more commonly, secondary to a wound. All wounds, both traumatic and surgical, provide a suitable environment for the growth of bacteria. Factors which influence the development of an infection are:

1. *Type of Bacteria.* Certain organisms, by virtue of their growth characteristics and toxin production, are more virulent than others and have the ability to produce rapidly lethal infections.

2. *Degree of Contamination.* Small amounts of bacterial contamination can often be effectively cleared by the tissues, but, when the number of bacteria introduced exceeds the critical level of resistance, infection will develop.

3. *Type of Wound.* Large wounds and wounds near unclean areas of the body are more prone to infection. Devitalized tissue

and foreign bodies in the wound will predispose the wound to infection.

4. *Duration of Wound.* The longer a wound remains untreated, the more likely it is to become infected.

5. *Host Resistance.* General good health and previously acquired immunity will enhance resistance to infection.

## Criteria for Diagnosis

1. *Clinical Diagnosis.* A detailed history and physical examination are essential to proper diagnosis, with particular emphasis on the onset and duration of symptoms and the physical characteristics of the infected area. Chills, fever and malaise indicate systemic involvement.

2. *Laboratory Diagnosis*

  A. *Local Tests*

    *(1)* Any exudate obtained from the infected area should be examined microscopically.

    *(2)* Culture and sensitivity determinations under both aerobic and anaerobic conditions are essential.

    *(3)* In certain instances, such as chronic granulomatous infections, biopsy may be performed, utilizing the tissue for histologic and bacteriological examination.

  B. *Systemic Tests*

    *(1)* Complete blood counts, including a leukocyte count, differential count and hematocrit, may yield important information. A leukocytosis with a shift to the left is usual in bacterial infection and may be an important baseline for assessing recovery.

    *(2)* Blood cultures are essential where septicemia is suspected.

    *(3)* Occasionally, skin and ag-

glutination tests may prove helpful, such as in brucellosis and tuberculosis.

## Management

### Local Management

1. Areas of cellulitis and lymphangitis are treated by rest and elevation to promote venous and lymphatic drainage.

2. Moist heat is applied to the inflamed area to produce local hyperemia and aid drainage of exudate.

3. Appropriate surgical drainage is performed where indicated.

A. Fluctuation, indicating the presence of fluid within an abscess cavity, is an indication for incision and drainage. Occasionally, an aneurysm may be mistaken for an abscess. The careful observer will remember to check for pulsation and bruit before incising the area.

B. If doubt exists as to fluctuation, diagnostic needle aspiration should be performed before incision.

C. In certain closed-space locations, such as the breast, perirectal area and distal pulp space of the finger, incision must be performed before fluctuation is apparent if extensive necrosis is to be avoided.

D. In all instances, the incision must be long enough to ensure continued drainage without premature closure of the drainage tract, and all deep extensions and loculations of the abscess must be opened widely.

4. Cellulitis should not be incised, since this opens tissue planes for more extensive spread of the infection. If organism identification is desired, needle aspiration of the area for culture is permissible.

### Systemic Management

1. If systemic symptoms are present, systemic antibiotics are indicated.

2. Local abscesses with no fever or signs of sepsis will usually respond well to drainage with no need for antibiotic therapy after drainage.

3. If the infecting organism is not yet identified, as is usually the case at the onset of therapy, clinical judgment must be relied upon to dictate an antibiotic commonly effective in the type of infection being treated. For example, cellulitis is usually a streptococcal infection and therefore should be treated empirically with penicillin, even before specific identification of the offending organism. Once the culture and sensitivity results are obtained, the appropriate antibiotic agent can be administered.

4. Always bear in mind any antibiotic sensitivity of the patient before ordering antibiotics. Cross-sensitivities between penicillin and the semisynthetic penicillins must be respected.

## STAPHYLOCOCCAL INFECTIONS

### Basic Principles

Staphylococcal infection is the most common surgical infection, since staphylococci are constantly present in man and his environment. The most important infecting staphylococcus is *Staphylococcus aureus,* which produces a hemolytic toxin and coagulase, an enzyme causing coagulation of plasma.

### Criteria for Diagnosis

1. The usual staphylococcal abscess is a skin infection which begins as an infection of a hair follicle (furuncle). These usually occur on the face, back, axillae, groins, neck and fingers.

2. Objective findings are swelling, erythema and tenderness. The abscess usually remains localized.

3. Fever and leukocytosis are absent unless extension of the infection has occurred.

4. Upon incision, the pus is usually thick, creamy, yellowish white and odorless. Those infections due to penicillin-resistant staphylococci often have a core of necrotic tissue with little liquid pus.

## Management

1. The usual staphylococcal abscess responds well to incision and drainage with no need for further therapy.

2. Local antibiotic therapy is of no value here.

3. If the abscess is extensive or systemic symptoms are present, systemic antibiotic therapy is indicated. If the organism is sensitive, the ideal antibiotic for staphylococcal infections is penicillin. However, many strains of staphylococci are resistant to penicillin since they produce penicillinase, an enzyme which destroys penicillin. For these strains, a penicillinase-resistant, semisynthetic penicillin is indicated, such as oxacillin, nafcillin or methicillin.

4. For those patients sensitive to penicillin, an alternative drug is erythromycin or cephalothin.

5. The dose of antibiotics will depend upon the severity of the infection.

6. The oral or intramuscular route will suffice for administration of antibiotics for the moderate infection, but severe septicemia will require intravenous antibiotics.

## STREPTOCOCCAL INFECTIONS

### Basic Principles

1. Most streptococcal infections are produced by *Streptococcus pyogenes,* an aerobic beta-hemolytic streptococcus. Cellulitis, erysipelas, hemolytic streptococcal gangrene and necrotizing fasciitis are examples of hemolytic streptococcal infections.

2. Less common skin infections are caused by microaerophilic streptococci, often in combination with other organisms. Burrowing ulcers are caused by microaerophilic hemolytic streptococci. Chronic progressive cutaneous gangrene (Meleney's synergistic gangrene) is caused by the combination of a microaerophilic nonhemolytic streptococcus and an aerobic hemolytic staphylococcus.

3. Anaerobic streptococci are responsible for severe fascial and muscle infections often confused with infections of clostridial origin because of gas formation.

### Criteria for Diagnosis

#### Aerobic Streptococcal Infections

1. Rapid onset
2. Diffuse involvement of skin, with marked erythema, cellulitis, lymphangitis
3. Bullae may form, containing thin, watery pus.
4. Septicemia is frequent.
5. Gangrene and necrotizing fasciitis with marked undermining of skin in more advanced infection.
6. Streptococci are identifiable in the exudate.

#### Microaerophilic Streptococcal Infections

1. The infection develops slowly.
2. Low-grade fever
3. Chronic synergistic gangrene starts as a wide area of cellulitis surrounding a central, purplish area. The central area undergoes necrosis, forming an ulcer with marked undermining of the edges. Progressive widening of the lesion occurs.
4. Burrowing ulcers produce sinus tracts through underlying tissues.

#### Anaerobic Streptococcal Infections

1. Anaerobic streptococcal infections occur in wounds of the genital, intestinal or respiratory tracts.
2. Fascial and subcutaneous infections are characterized by:
   A. Induration
   B. Foul-smelling pus
   C. Progressive tissue destruction
3. Anaerobic streptococcal myositis (1) is of slow onset, (2) produces mild toxemia, (3) has moderate wound pain and considerable gas in the tissues, and (4) the muscle is discolored but viable.
4. Identification requires anaerobic culture.

## Management

### Aerobic Streptococcal Infections

1. Local therapy of cellulitis and lymphangitis is:
   A. Moist heat
   B. Elevation
   C. Rest
2. Penicillin, oral or parenteral depending on the severity of the infection, is the drug of choice.
3. Bullae and any purulent collections are drained.
4. Hemolytic streptococcal gangrene and necrotizing fasciitis require emergency treatment, consisting of drainage of deep, longitudinal incisions and excision of necrotic fascia and skin.
5. Since necrotizing fasciitis often involves synergistic organisms, usually gram-negative rods, gentamicin should be added to the antibiotic therapy.

### Microaerophilic Streptococcal Infections

1. Local therapy of chronic progressive subcutaneous gangrene involves radical excision of the entire ulcerated area, encompassing the gangrenous border.
2. Burrowing ulcers are opened widely and radically excised, including connecting tracts.
3. Penicillin is administered parenterally.

### Anaerobic Streptococcal Infections

1. Abscesses, fasciitis and infected muscle groups should be incised and drained.
2. Large doses of parenteral penicillin are administered.

## CLOSTRIDIAL INFECTIONS
### CLOSTRIDIAL MYONECROSIS

### Definition

Clostridial myonecrosis (gas gangrene, clostridial myositis) is an invasive, anaerobic infection characterized by extensive necrosis of muscle, considerable local edema, variable degrees of gas production and severe toxemia.

### Basic Principles

1. All wounds containing devitalized muscle and decreased local oxygenation provide a susceptible environment for clostridial multiplication, since clostridia are obligate anaerobes and cannot multiply in healthy tissue. Open fractures with severe soft tissue injury and extremity wounds with arterial injury are potential sites of infection.
2. *Clostridium perfringens (C. welchii)* is the most common organism causing clostridial myonecrosis, but five other species of clostridium may be implicated.
3. The clostridia produce necrotizing exotoxins, the most lethal of which is a potent lecithinase (alpha toxin). These toxins enter the local tissues, producing edema, vessel thrombosis, tissue necrosis and death.
4. Gas production is variable, depending on the types of clostridia present.
5. Systemic symptoms and toxemia are prominent.

### Criteria for Diagnosis

1. Acute onset after an incubation period of 8 hours to 3 days
2. *Local Signs and Symptoms*
   A. Pain in the region of the wound is an early symptom and is progressive in severity.
   B. Marked edema locally
   C. Thin, brown, foul-smelling exudate, containing bacteria and red blood cells but few leukocytes
   D. The skin is initially pale and tense, becoming dusky and ecchymotic, with formation of vesicles filled with serosanguinous fluid.
   E. Affected muscles become dark red, then purplish black and finally gangrenous. Evidence of bleeding and contractility are absent.
   F. Gas and crepitation are usually present but not extensive.

G. Gram-positive rods are recovered from muscle.

3. *Systemic Signs and Symptoms*

A. Profound toxemia

B. Mild fever (101 to 102° F.)

C. Tachycardia out of proportion to the fever

D. Hypotension

E. Pale, clammy skin

F. Apprehension, progressing to disorientation and stupor

## Differential Diagnosis

1. *Clostridial Cellulitis*

A. Incubation period of 3 to 4 days

B. Gradual onset

C. Mild pain

D. Minimal edema

E. Mild systemic toxicity

F. Marked gas in the wound, with foul-smelling, brown exudate, but viable muscle not affected

G. Infection attacks injured and uninjured connective tissue, but only devitalized muscle.

2. *Streptococcal Myositis*

A. Very rare, with a 3- to 4-day incubation period

B. The clinical picture is similar to clostridial myonecrosis, but the toxicity is less, with muscle discolored but viable.

C. Gram's stain of the exudate shows abundant streptococci and leukocytes but no gram-positive rods.

3. The presence or absence of gas in the tissues is variable and not of paramount diagnostic significance.

A. Gas may represent air that entered the wound at the time of injury or it may be due to infectious agents other than clostridia (*E. coli*, anaerobic streptococci).

B. The clinical picture and Gram's stain of the exudate are the most important diagnostic criteria.

## Management

### Prophylaxis

1. Awareness of wounds susceptible to clostridial infection

2. Early, wide debridement of all devitalized tissue

3. Extensive irrigation of the wound

4. Administration of parenteral antibiotics, preferably penicillin, if the wound is severely contaminated

5. Secondary wound closure if the wound is severely contaminated

6. There is no proven value to the administration of polyvalent antitoxin.

### Treatment

1. Immediate debridement of all nonviable skin, muscle and connective tissue. The muscle must bleed and contract when pinched if it is to be allowed to remain.

2. Adequate debridement may require amputation, especially if muscle involvement is so extensive as to preclude subsequent useful function.

3. Supportive therapy, including fluid replacement and blood transfusion

4. Intravenous penicillin, 5 million units every 6 hours

5. Hyperbaric oxygen therapy, if available. Exposure of the patient to oxygen under pressure (usually 3 atmospheres) during debridement or at intervals thereafter has proven to be effective. In some cases limbs have been saved. However, only a few large medical centers are equipped for this therapy, and definitive therapy should not be delayed while arranging transfer to a hyperbaric facility.

6. The use of polyvalent antitoxin is not recommended, since its usefulness is questionable and the risk of sensitivity reactions is considerable.

## TETANUS

### Basic Principles

1. Tetanus is caused by *Clostridium tetani*, a spore-forming obligate anaerobe present in soil.

2. Tetanus-prone wounds are those wounds which provide a favorable environment for germination of tetanus

spores. Devitalized tissue, blood clots and oxygen deprivation are conducive to tetanus. Puncture wounds, open fractures and deep lacerations are examples of susceptible wounds.

3. The clinical features of tetanus are due to a neurotoxin elaborated by the bacteria which becomes fixed to the cells of the brain and spinal cord. The toxin cannot be neutralized after it has become fixed, making therapy of established tetanus extremely difficult.

## Criteria for Diagnosis

1. Incubation period of 3 to 30 days, with the average onset 6 to 10 days after injury.

2. The prodromic stage lasts 12 to 24 hours, consisting of:
   A. Headaches
   B. Restlessness
   C. Yawning
   D. Wound pain
   E. Jaw stiffness

3. The active stage consists of:
   A. Tonic and clonic spasms of skeletal muscles
   B. Trismus
   C. Spasm and tenderness of abdominal muscles
   D. Extreme irritability

4. The terminal stage consists of:
   A. High fever
   B. Urinary retention
   C. Convulsions
   D. Respiratory arrest

## Management

Prophylaxis

*Tetanus is a preventable disease.* The lethality of established tetanus (50% mortality despite vigorous therapy) makes adequate prophylaxis mandatory. Prophylaxis consists of adequate wound care and administration of appropriate immunization.

1. All wounds should be surgically debrided and all devitalized tissue and foreign bodies should be removed. Severely contaminated wounds and deep puncture wounds are tetanus-prone. If contamination is severe, secondary closure after 5 days is a safer technique than primary suture.

2. Administration of parenteral antibiotics to prevent tetanus is of questionable value, since there is no assurance that the antibiotic will be brought into contact with the tetanus spores in sufficient concentration to be effective. Antibiotics can be given to prevent infection by other infecting organisms. Antibiotics are used for prophylaxis of tetanus only when immunizing agents are contraindicated or not available.

3. The preferred agent for active immunization against tetanus is tetanus toxoid. The adsorbed (precipitated) form has been shown to stimulate higher antibody titers than the fluid form, but the promptness of antibody response to each has not been significantly different. Therefore, the adsorbed toxoid is preferred, usually in a dose of 0.5 ml. intramuscularly.

4. The preferred agent for passive immunization is homologous (human) tetanus immune globulin (TIG, HHG). This has supplanted equine and bovine tetanus antitoxin (TAT), since it carries no risk of sensitivity reaction and has a longer period of effectiveness. The usual dose is 250 units intramuscularly.

5. Active immunization requires 2 doses of adsorbed toxoid one month apart and a third dose 6 months later. Subsequent booster doses are given at 10-year intervals.

6. A history of previous immunization must include reliable assurance that an immunization schedule was completed. School children and those patients with a history of military service are usually the only ones who can be assumed to be immunized. One previous "tetanus shot" does not qualify the patient as being previously immunized.

7. *Suggested Prophylaxis for Tetanus* (adapted from "A Guide to Prophylaxis Against Tetanus in Wound Management," Bull. Amer. Coll. Surgeons, *57*:32, 1972)

*Previously Immunized Individuals:*

A. When the patient has been immunized within the past ten years, give 0.5 ml. of tetanus toxoid booster.

B. When the patient has been immunized more than ten years ago:

*(1)* To the great majority of patients only give 0.5 ml. of tetanus toxoid.

*(2)* To those patients with wounds which indicate an overwhelming possibility that tetanus will develop:

*(a)* Give 0.5 ml. of tetanus toxoid.

*(b)* Give 250 units of human tetanus immune globulin. In severe, neglected or old wounds, 500 units of human tetanus immune globulin are advisable.

*(c)* Use different syringes, needles and sites of injection for toxoid and immune globulin.

*(d)* Consider the use of oxytetracycline or penicillin.

*Individuals Not Previously Immunized:*

A. With clean, minor wounds in which tetanus is unlikely, give 0.5 ml. of tetanus toxoid (initial immunizing dose).

B. With all other wounds:

*(1)* Give 0.5 ml. of tetanus toxoid (initial immunizing dose).

*(2)* Give 250 units of human tetanus immune globulin. In severe, neglected or old wounds, 500 units of human tetanus immune globulin are advisable.

*(3)* Use different syringes, needles and sites of injection for toxoid and immune globulin.

*(4)* Consider the use of oxytetracycline or penicillin.

C. Equine antitoxin is to be used only if human tetanus immune globulin is not available within 24 hours and only if the possibility of tetanus outweighs the danger of reaction to equine tetanus antitoxin. First question the patient and test for sensitivity.

*(1)* If the patient is not sensitive to equine tetanus antitoxin, give at least 3000 units.

*(2)* If the patient is sensitive to equine tetanus antitoxin by history or test, give penicillin or oxytetracycline, not antitoxin. The danger of anaphylaxis probably outweighs the danger of tetanus. Do not attempt desensitization.

## Treatment of Established Disease

1. Debridement or excision of the primary wound, with drainage

2. Administration of human tetanus immune globulin, 3000 units intramuscularly immediately and then 500 units daily. The value of this therapy is limited if the toxin is already fixed to nerve tissue.

3. Penicillin, 5 million units intravenously every 6 hours. As noted above in paragraph 2, this is probably of limited value once the toxin is fixed, but it is useful for prevention of secondary infection.

4. Sedate the patient with an intramuscular barbiturate and keep the patient in a quiet, dark room with minimal external stimuli. Use intravenous Pentothal for control of convulsions.

5. Muscle spasms may be controlled with muscle relaxants. If the spasms are severe, muscle paralysis is indicated with curare or succinylcholine in association with institution of mechanical respiration.

6. A tracheostomy is usually necessary in the active stage to maintain an airway and to provide for respiratory support and frequent suctioning.

7. Maintain parenteral nutrition with hyperalimentation.

8. Hyperbaric oxygen therapy, if available.

# 10. SOFT TISSUE INJURIES

*Bertram E. Bromberg,* M.D.
*In-Chul Song,* M.D.

## Definition

Soft tissue injuries range from simple cutaneous abrasions or contusions to complex tissue losses with massive fat, muscle, tendon, nerve, vascular and skeletal destruction. Frequently these injuries involve, or are associated with, additional cerebral, chest, abdominal and limb trauma, thus seriously complicating an already existing life-threatening situation.

## EMERGENCY CARE

### Basic Principles

1. A rapid evaluation of the patient's injuries must be achieved and priorities of treatment established. Obviously, life-threatening situations receive immediate care, and frequently severe soft tissue damage is associated with underlying craniocerebral, chest and abdominal trauma.

2. The care of the soft tissue component in these complex injuries is frequently critical in obtaining a successful and uncomplicated result. Particularly in extremity trauma, where severe soft tissue damage is associated with underlying vascular, tendon or bone or joint injury, inadequate skin closure can jeopardize the ultimate survival of the extremity despite successful care of the deep structures.

3. In comatose or desperately ill patients, wound closure can be performed with or without anesthesia in bed. Also, in such situations minimal debridement and temporary biological coverage can be rapidly achieved.

4. In general, only abrasions, small to moderate lacerations involving the skin and subcutaneous tissue and small emergency tissue losses can be repaired in the emergency room. Unfortunately, this optimum rule is violated when the alternative is a prolonged interval before definitive repair can be achieved, due to the priority given to another life-threatening situation. Complex soft tissue injuries, particularly those involving large areas of muscle damage and soft tissue injuries of the extremities with underlying bone, joint, tendon or nerve injury, are all investigated and repaired in the operating room under appropriate anesthesia.

5. All soft tissue injuries associated with chest or abdominal trauma are repaired in the operating room.

6. *Occasionally, despite anticipated definitive operating room repair of underlying tendon, nerve, bone or joint injury, where delays are inevitable either due to the patient's general condition or priorities in the operating room, skin wounds are sutured in the emergency room after thorough preparation and irrigation.*

## Diagnosis

Diagnosis and emergency care of soft tissue injuries are directed at 4 major areas:

1. *Airway*

Airway obstruction should be suspected in soft tissue injuries about the face associated with profuse bleeding, intra-oral blood clots, injuries involving the larynx, massive hematomas of the neck, retrodisplacements of the tongue associated with mandibular fractures and retrodisplacements of the palatal structures due to maxillary fractures which compromise the airway. Careful examination of the intra-oral and head and neck areas is vital prior to specific treatment.

2. *Hemorrhage*

Obvious intra-oral or external hemorrhage can be diagnosed and treated immediately. Careful inspection of the entire body after the clothes have been removed is vital to determine the extent of bleeding wounds. Good lighting conditions are essential prior to definitive clamping of vessels

3. *Shock and Dehydration*

Although shock is not a prominent feature of most moderate soft tissue injuries, it can occur in the massive injuries where underlying muscle damage is extensive or where large avulsions have occurred. In the presence of shock, other areas such as the chest, abdomen or extremities must be investigated for underlying visceral, vascular or bony injury by careful physical examination and x-rays.

4. *Wounds*

Careful examination of all wounds should be made to determine the wound type and possible treatment which would be necessary in the presence of underlying bone, muscle, vascular, nerve or joint injuries. In addition, care should be exercised to determine the degree of contamination and extent of injury.

5. Additional diagnostic maneuvers consist of palpation of the wounds, particularly of the neck to evaluate the presence of air in the soft tissues or expanding hematomas and deviation of the trachea in relation to the injury. Penetrating wounds of the chest should be diagnosed immediately and treated to avoid the occurrence of pneumothorax. Penetrating abdominal wounds should be diagnosed immediately and covered to avoid peritoneal contamination. All serious soft tissue wounds of the extremities must be inspected with regard to underlying vascular, tendon and bone and joint injury. Thorough exploration must include the evaluation of the structural continuity of tendons, nerves and blood vessels, and all bones must be inspected for fractures. Depth of muscle damage must be established and skin margins determined. Skin fragments and tissue losses must be assessed prior to debridement. This may

necessitate the placement of key sutures in the diagnostic maneuvers in order to fully evaluate the extent of the wound.

## Management

### Initial Assessment

1. Airway obstruction secondary to wounds about the face, neck and intra-oral cavity must be treated immediately. Manual removal of blood clots and careful suctioning, followed by control of hemorrhage, are usually the only steps required.

2. Injuries involving the larynx associated with massive hematoma of the neck, mandibular fractures with tongue displacements and maxillary fractures associated with retrodisplacement of the palate may so compromise the airway that emergency tracheostomy is imperative.

3. Intubation using an endotracheal tube may be impossible in the face of severe head and neck trauma and should not be attempted.

4. Massive hemorrhage from open wounds in the extremities can frequently be secured by compression dressings and elevation. This cannot be adequately achieved in the head, neck and face regions, where direct suture or clamping is required.

5. Bleeders in all areas should be clamped promptly and meticulously under good lighting conditions while clots are removed manually and by irrigation.

6. Blind clamping can often lead to irreparable damage.

7. Conventional treatment of associated shock should be started promptly when needed by:

A. Immediate intravenous fluid administration

B. Establishment of baseline vital signs by ancillary personnel

C. Immediate performance of hematocrit determinations for a baseline and crossmatching of blood for later administration

8. Tracheal deviation may be a sign of

tension pneumothorax or neck injury and should lead to immediate establishment of chest drainage, if necessary, or tracheostomy.

9. Open wounds of the chest should be sealed immediately with grease gauze prior to definitive surgical inspection and treatment.

10. Penetrating abdominal wounds with herniated visceral contents must be covered with moist compresses while awaiting definitive care.

11. Perineal and buttock wounds may be associated with underlying genitourinary and abdominal trauma, and appropriate treatment should be administered.

12. Assuming that no major contra-indications exist to immediate treatment of the wound, the following regimen should be followed: the basis of wound treatment is the removal of all foreign material and devitalized tissue and maintenance and protection of the vascular supply to the injured parts.

13. Obvious foreign bodies should be removed, protective dressings applied, and immobilization and moderate elevation of the limbs should be provided in extremity injuries.

14. Flaps of skin that are folded upon themselves should be unfolded and placed into reasonable position so as not to further compromise their blood supply. Tacking sutures placed at key points will help to protect the underlying critical structures and maintain better tissue tension, thus preventing additional vascular compromise.

## Cutaneous Wound Repair

Timing of definitive cutaneous wound repair is important because, although the repair of moderate soft tissue injuries is seldom lifesaving, as the interval between the wounding and definitive repair increases, the possibilities of infection and less satisfactory repair increase. The following principles in the timing of wound repair are important:

1. The golden period for debridement and closure of wounds in the head and neck area can be safely extended to 24 hours.

2. Under satisfactory antibiotic coverage, where the severity of tissue damage and contamination is not great, the golden period (6 hours) can be safely extended to 10 to 12 hours or longer in areas other than the head and neck.

3. As the hours progress, consideration is always given to the degree of contamination and tissue damage to the site of the wound, leading to variations in the timing of wound closure.

4. Buried sutures are minimized in late closures, and nylon and wire are used in the skin.

5. Postoperatively, wet dressings are employed in such situations.

6. Delayed primary closure can be entertained as it is in combat injuries, and the use of temporary biological coverage, when available, is always advantageous.

7. If homografts or heterografts are used, the wounds are inspected daily for additional necrotic debris or hematoma, and further debridement is carried out as required and additional temporary coverage again applied.

8. When wounds are clinically clean and homografts or heterografts are adherent, definitive closure can be safely attained.

9. Providing that comfortable access is present and the patient's condition is satisfactory, debridement and closure of soft tissue wounds can safely be carried out simultaneously while the neurosurgeon, chest or general surgeon is caring for any lifesaving situations. The repair should be rapid and atraumatic and should add little stress and employ only key buried sutures to eliminate dead space and over-and-over continuous skin suturing. In a desperately ill patient, coordinated planning among specialties can often avoid the necessity of additional anesthetics.

10. In life-threatening situations, it is frequently necessary to obtain the quickest

possible closure and anticipate later secondary reconstruction.

11. Wounds associated with underlying visceral, bone and joint injury and those wounds with extensive muscle damage should receive the highest priority. Such major injuries should be x-rayed in 2 planes to detect the presence of foreign bodies.

## Principles of Wound Toilet and Debridement

These fundamental principles involve conscientious preparation of the wound, complete investigation of the wound and accurate and complete diagnostic evaluation, discretionary debridement, precise repair and competent postoperative care.

The following principles are followed:

1. Ample time must be given to wound preparation.

2. The surrounding integument is thoroughly cleansed with soap and water after gentle shaving.

3. No antiseptics or soaps should enter the open wounds.

4. All clots, foreign bodies and wound debris are removed and the wound is copiously irrigated with warm saline.

5. Properly designed extension incisions of the wound into skin and fascia may be necessary to afford complete exposure and inspection.

6. Tattooed dirt particles into the skin frequently require prolonged scrubbing and, on occasion, mechanical abrading.

7. Operative fields about the face and neck will frequently include the endotracheal apparatus and obviously require preparation and draping into the field.

8. Adequate protection to the cornea must be secured when preparing and operating in the facial area.

9. The need for skin graft or pedicle donor sites must be ascertained early so that proper preparation and draping are achieved.

10. Adequate debridement consists of thorough exploration, bold debridement of devitalized tissue, conservative debridement of critical facial structures, conservation of all vital structures with continued protection, repeated saline irrigations and precise hemostasis.

11. If the patient's condition is poor, continued search for elusive small foreign bodies is not warranted despite the increased chance of infection.

12. Good muscle closure must be obtained over sucking chest wounds despite bold debridement of the compromised and contaminated soft tissue.

13. Vascular continuity is restored as rapidly as possible, but tendon and nerve injury can be repaired secondarily.

14. Joint capsules should be closed promptly and liberal fasciotomies performed as necessary.

15. Adequate coverage of nerve, tendon and bone must be attained.

## Anesthesia

Anesthesia for wound repair follows these principles:

1. Local anesthesia is preferable for small lacerations and can be satisfactorily employed in infants and small children in whom the risk of general anesthesia is rarely warranted. Lidocaine, 1%, with Adrenaline (1:100,000) is generally used, although ½% lidocaine is indicated when larger amounts of anesthetic are required.

2. Local anesthesia can often be combined with intravenous medication for more extensive or prolonged procedures.

3. Premedication is not indicated along with local anesthesia when head injury is evident or suspected.

4. Block anesthesia can safely and readily be performed about the face and neck. Mental, mandibular and cervical blocks produce satisfactory anesthesia for the lower third of the face and neck, and infraorbital blocks can anesthetize the midface. The forehead and scalp can be blocked out by supraorbital and frontal blocks.

5. The upper extremities are profoundly

anesthetized by axillary and brachial blocks, and the fingers can be safely desensitized by digital blocks in the palm.

6. Spinal anesthesia is rarely employed in lower extremity emergency surgery.

7. The pain of infiltration anesthesia can be minimized if the needle is introduced into the open wound edge and the agent injected slowly.

8. Sufficient time should elapse so as to obtain the maximum hemostatic effect of the epinephrine and to decrease tissue distortion.

9. General anesthesia is employed in the more severe injury, where simultaneous or successive repairs are being performed, when more than one operative field will be employed and in markedly anxious patients.

10. Intra-oral lacerations of small size frequently require general anesthesia in infants and children.

11. Oral or nasal intubation is generally the anesthesia of choice, particularly about the face and neck, and awake intubations are indicated when there is a blood-filled upper gastrointestinal tract to minimize the danger of aspiration.

12. In cases in which bleeding into the oral cavity can be anticipated from soft tissue injuries about the face and neck, the use of a cuffed tube and the Trendelenburg position are imperative to prevent aspiration.

13. General anesthesia can be readily administered through a tracheostomy tube and the anesthetist should have the proper connecting tubes available.

## Ancillary Measures

1. Antibiotic coverage should be used in all serious soft tissue injuries.

2. Tetanus prophylaxis is used in all patients and requires the removal of devitalized tissue as well as tetanus immunization. The prophylactic procedure against tetanus as recommended by the Committee on Trauma of the American College of Surgeons is summarized in Chapter 9, p. 113.

3. The following recommendations are made with respect to transportation of these patients:

A. In soft tissue injuries about the face and neck, transportation in the prone position is favored. In the unconscious patient in whom the tongue ordinarily falls forward, rarely nasopharyngeal intubation will be required.

B. Care must be instituted in applying any type of circular bandage about the face and neck so that airway compromise does not occur.

C. Moderate elevation of the extremities during transportation is desirable.

## SPECIFIC TYPES OF SOFT TISSUE INJURIES
### ABRASIONS, CONTUSIONS AND HEMATOMAS

### Definition

Abrasions, contusions, or hematomas refer to blunt or scraping injuries of the soft tissues, sometimes associated with severe tissue loss.

### Basic Principles

As with all soft tissue injuries, the treatment depends on the extent of the injury and underlying damage. Where extensive soft tissue abrasion injuries have occurred, closure may be extremely difficult, particularly with the loss of large amounts of soft tissue or exposure of underlying bone.

### Diagnosis

Inspection of the wound is vital to determine the degree of associated injury and amount of contamination. X-rays of bone injuries may be indicated.

### Management

1. Temporary biological dressings offer a compromise until delayed primary or secondary closure can be effected.

2. Tattooed abrasions often require the use of high-speed rotary carborundum disks for particle elimination.

3. Simple contusions require little therapy, although x-ray diagnosis for underlying bony injury is still advisable.

4. Moderate hematomas respond to aspiration and pressure dressings.

5. Massive hematomas should be surgically evacuated.

## SIMPLE LACERATIONS

### Basic Principles

Simple lacerations can be adequately repaired in the emergency room under local anesthesia. When the direction of the laceration runs counter to the natural skin creases or in areas about the joints, widened and hypertrophic scarring is the inevitable result despite skillful suturing. This is frequently noted in children. No efforts should be made in the initial repair to redirect the scar by Z-plasty, even in the facial area.

### Diagnosis

The diagnosis is made essentially as noted above under Abrasions, Contusions and Hematomas.

### Management

1. The basis of good suturing is elimination of dead space by key suture placement, suturing carefully in layers (muscle, fascia, subcutaneous tissue) and the use of well-placed subdermal sutures with buried knots.

2. The amount and placement of buried suture material is strongly altered by the interval between wounding and repair and the degree of contamination.

3. Unhurried closure is the critical factor in successful management of facial scars and nowhere else is excellence in technique so rewarding.

4. Vertical and horizontal malalignments must be avoided, and one is pleasantly surprised to find that all of the parts are present as the jigsaw is reconstructed.

5. Crosshatching can be minimized by avoiding excessive skin suture tension, by early suture removal and by the use of buried subcuticular sutures.

6. Buried subcuticular sutures of 4-0 or 5-0 nylon can be left *in situ* for long periods, although in most instances additional supplemental skin sutures are necessary and are removed early.

7. Buried subdermal sutures are usually achieved with 5-0 chromic or plain catgut.

8. If there is a tendency to inversion along skin margins, undermining is a useful adjunct, along with the placement of vertical mattress sutures.

9. On the face, critical areas for accurate skin alignment are the vermilion, alar or helicoid borders, the shaved hairline and the eyebrow.

10. Skin edges must be meticulously handled, particularly on the face.

11. If forceps are employed, they should be holding tools and not pincers.

12. Minor skin adjustments can be attained by varying the depths of suture placement along the margin and altering the side upon which the knots are snugged.

13. There is little one can do to reconstruct a stellate tear. It is desirable to employ a buried subcuticular stitch to gather the apices of the several flaps, yet less than perfect approximation can be anticipated because the tips of the flaps are usually contused or crushed and often do not survive.

## AVULSION INJURIES

### Definition

Avulsion injuries involve the stripping of a segment of skin or skin and associated subcutaneous structures attached by a pedicle to the margin of the wound.

### Basic Principles and Diagnosis

These are essentially the same as above under Simple Lacerations.

## Management

1. Avulsion flaps create problems due to the degree of beveling at the edges, viability of the edges and the notorious trap-door configurations.

2. When the beveled angle is sufficient and viability is assured, a reasonable result can be anticipated by taking small superficial bites in the beveled edge and extending deeper bites at the adjacent margin.

3. When the beveled edge is thinned, cutting back to a right-angled margin and creating a right-angled mortise of the same vertical depth as the adjacent skin margin will produce a satisfactory wound.

4. It is generally not prudent to remove an extended thinned-out beveled edge and to replace it as a free graft. The segment is usually damaged and ordinarily does not survive.

5. The multiple epidermal and partial thickness of tags of tissue seen in windshield lacerations are best handled by scissor excision of the smaller and more extensively detached segments and replacement of the larger remnants. These larger remnants can be satisfactorily positioned and maintained by grease gauze dressing.

6. U-shaped or trap-door flaps create a problem which cannot be satisfactorily handled. The inevitable peripheral contracture produces an unesthetic bulge of the flap. Avoidance of hematoma formation by several well-placed deep sutures and pressure dressings is all that can be achieved.

7. Where large avulsions have occurred with accompanying tissue loss, coverage is generally obtained by split-thickness grafts taken from a suitable donor site. Grafts of moderate thickness, 0.013 to 0.018 inches in thickness, are satisfactory, although on the face, when future excision is envisaged, thin grafts are more practical because a subsequent contracture of the graft will make for an easier secondary excision.

8. The immediate use of local advancement, rotation or bipedicle or bilobed flaps is hazardous, and failure can seriously jeopardize a future reconstruction.

## WOUNDS WITH MAJOR MUSCLE DAMAGE

### Basic Principles

Soft tissue wounds involving large amounts of muscle damage receive a high priority because of the severe systemic effects of the breakdown products and the marked hypotension they produce. Evaluation of compromised muscle is frequently difficult, and, although color and bleeding are often suggestive, they are not reliable. Contractility on pinch is essentially the major characteristic of viable fibers.

### Management

1. Bold debridement of mushy, nonbleeding, noncontracting muscle is the most profound deterrent against clostridial myositis and produces little functional disability.

2. Repair is achieved by suturing the enveloping fascia and intermuscular septa, because the muscle fibers generally will not maintain any type of suture material.

## COMPLEX SOFT TISSUE WOUNDS

### Definition

Complex soft tissue wounds are integument wounds associated with open fractures or exposed bone, blood vessels, or tendons.

### Basic Principles

The ultimate uncomplicated success of any repair of underlying bone, joint, blood vessel, tendon or nerve injury is dependent upon the integrity of the overlying skin closure.

### Management

1. Closures under undue tension or employing compromised and traumatized skin edges invite disaster. Infection, struc-

tural breakdown and osteomyelitis are the inevitable sequelae.

2. Large avulsion flaps which are not unduly traumatized can be replaced as free full-thickness grafts after removal of the subcutaneous tissue, or they can be replaced as full-thickness grafts while still attached.

3. These maneuvers can be performed immediately, or they may be delayed by using temporary biological dressings if the patient's condition is deteriorating or contamination is too great.

4. The immediate or delayed use of split-thickness autograft coverage is the ideal material, but there are situations when the risk of pedicle coverage must be taken.

5. These flaps must be designed to afford the greatest margin of safety and are used in situations where split-thickness grafts are doomed to fail (e.g., exposed bone devoid of periosteum, exposed blood vessels, nerves and tendons in sites where muscle flaps cannot safely be employed).

## COLD INJURIES

*See* Chapter 18 on Frostbite.

### Basic Principles

Cold injury generally involves the exposed areas such as the face, hands and distal portions of the lower extremities. Both intracellular and vascular injury occur, and, if severe, the ultimate result is generally dry gangrene.

### Management

1. Rapid thawing at temperatures between 40 and 42°C.

2. Careful soap-and-water cleansing of the injured and surrounding areas

3. Mild elevation of the extremities

4. Immobilization and protection of the involved segments

5. Antibiotics

6. Conservative surgical debridement. Lines of demarcation should be established

before excision of necrotic tissue is pursued.

7. Immediate or delayed autografting is then performed if necessary.

8. Heparinization or the use of sympathectomy is preferred in the early treatment of cold injuries.

## BURN INJURIES

*See* Chapter 34 on Burns.

## DOG AND HUMAN BITES

### Basic Principles

Dog and human bites are relatively common injuries. Generally it is advisable to admit patients to the hospital even with small human bites. The bite wounds are contaminated with a host of mouth organisms, which frequently cause serious wound infection.

### Management

#### Human Bites

1. The wounds are left open and treated with moist saline compresses.

2. Antibiotic coverage should be instituted.

3. Elevation of the extremities is advisable.

4. Immobilization of the wound is preferred.

5. Routine tetanus prophylaxis is given.

6. If underlying nerve or tendon injury is present, the wound is debrided, but repair of these structures is carried out secondarily.

7. Delayed primary closure can be pursued after several days if clinical evaluation of the wound is satisfactory. Nylon or stainless steel skin sutures are loosely placed merely to obtain edge-to-edge approximation, and wounds are continued on saline soaks.

#### Dog Bites

1. A more aggressive approach can be employed in dog bites, although infection in these wounds is not uncommon.

2. Thorough irrigation of canine and incisor tracks should be pursued, and, although primary closure is permissible, minimal buried suture material or chromic gut is used.

3. Skin sutures should generally be of nylon or stainless steel, and wet saline dressings are applied postoperatively as in human bites.

## MISSILE WOUNDS

### Basic Principles

Primary missiles are created by the projectiles of the primary source whereas secondary missiles are the result of secondary objects being put into motion by the primary projectile. Secondary missiles, therefore, increase the degree of wounding. It is chiefly the velocity of a missile which determines its deadly effects, and modern-day weaponry is responsible for guns of unusually high velocity. Generally, weapons of low velocity are involved in civilian gunshot wounds. These wounds are therefore more localized as opposed to high-velocity wounding.

### Management

1. Emergency care is carried out as noted above (p. 115) since associated injuries are not uncommon.

2. Bold debridement is essential in high-velocity wounding and a somewhat less aggressive approach is required in low-velocity wounding. Although in recent years there has been developing a more conservative approach where life- or limb-threatening situations are not evident, prompt surgical intervention cannot be condemned if the patient's general condition is satisfactory.

3. All of the basic principles previously discussed under Emergency Care must be considered, although complete excision of the wound tract is not warranted unless obvious necrotic tissue is present.

4. Generally, delayed primary closure is indicated. The use of temporary biological dressings in the intervening period is desirable.

5. Shotgun injuries, although of low velocity, produce a severity of damage depending upon the distance of the shotgun from the target. No effort should be made to remove the shot if it is deeply embedded and only life- and limb-threatening situations are managed. Considerable soft tissue damage occurs in close-range shotgun wounding, and large skin and subcutaneous tissue losses are common. Bold and prompt debridement, particularly where considerable muscle damage has occurred, is necessary, and liberal fasciotomies must be performed in the extremities.

6. Coverage of the wound is obtained along the principles previously discussed under Emergency Care.

7. Antibiotics and tetanus prophylactic treatment are given as noted above (p. 113).

## WOUNDS INVOLVING SPECIFIC STRUCTURES
### ORAL CAVITY

### Basic Principles

For the general approach and emergency care of the patient, *see* Emergency Care, page 115. Lacerations of the lips and cheeks into the oral cavity and lacerations of the soft palate require 3-layer closures about the face, and mucous membrane can be sutured to the skin about the oral cavity and cheek area when a large amount of tissue is missing. The tongue can be used for closure about the floor of the mouth and cheek, and skin and mucous membrane can be sutured where large nasal losses exist.

### Management

1. General principles of treatment concerning airway and hemorrhage as noted under Emergency Care.

2. Careful hemostasis and evacuation of blood clots

3. The mucosa can be closed with Dexon (polyglycollate), which does not require removal, or with silk, the muscle can be closed with catgut and the skin with nylon or silk.

4. Mattress sutures should be used generously inside the mouth to prevent inversion of mucosal edges and tied with 4 to 5 knots.

5. V-excision and 3-layer closure are often the most esthetic for irregular lip wounds of small to moderate size.

6. Larger wounds of the lip may require immediate lip switch procedures.

7. Vermilion defects can be satisfactorily repaired with buccal mucosal flaps, tongue flaps or free cheek mucosal grafts.

8. Gingival disruptions should be sutured and efforts made to restore the interdental papillae by suturing from buccal to lingual through the interdental space.

9. Stensen's duct should be probed when disruption is suspected, and repair performed over a polyethylene stent anchored intra-orally for at least 10 days.

10. Tongue lacerations must be sutured with gross bites of 3-0 or 4-0 silk, tied snugly with multiple knots.

## EYELIDS—CANTHAL AREAS

### Basic Principles

Soft tissue injuries about the orbit demand careful investigation and skillful restoration. Eyelid lacerations are sutured in 3 layers: skin, muscle and conjunctiva-tarsus. Careful approximation, particularly at the gray line, will obviate the need for halving techniques. In lower eyelid losses, skin and conjuctiva can be closed as a temporary measure. However, in the upper lid, despite this type of emergency maneuver, scleral contact lenses must be employed to permit corneal protection until later reconstruction is achieved.

### Management

1. Primary treatment as noted above under Emergency Care

2. Ectropion is to be avoided at all costs and skin grafts from the upper eyelid or postauricular region should be resorted to if evidence of such a danger exists.

3. Unrepaired lacerations of the levator muscle can produce ptosis, and injuries at the medial angle can disrupt the lacrimal drainage system and the supporting canthal ligament. Restoration of the medial canthal attachment can be simply achieved by buried suturing, or, if a bony avulsion has occurred at the angle, a new hole must be drilled from across the opposite nasal bone in a more superior and posterior location and the ligament wired into position on the medial orbital wall. Generally, the lateral canthal ligament is more simply reattached by accurate suturing to the periosteum of the lateral orbital wall at the proper level.

4. Repair of the tear duct system requires meticulous care in identification and suturing over a stent. The method of injecting dye or milk into the upper punctum and picking up the liquid as it exits at the lower disruption is still employed, however, the pig-tailed probe method is probably the most effective maneuver.

## EARS

### Basic Principles

The excellent blood supply to the ear allows satisfactory repair of even the most disruptive lacerations if sufficient care is given to accurate realigning and suturing. Anterior and posterior ear skin can be approximated over cartilage for emergency closure, although an exposed residual attached ear fragment can occasionally be sutured into the postauricular skin, thereby achieving a first-stage ear reconstruction. The use of homografts or, even better, heterografts as emergency coverage has added a whole new dimension to emergency wound care in life-threatening situations, particularly in large avulsed areas or where critical structures are exposed.

## Management

1. Primary treatment as noted above under Emergency Care

2. The cartilaginous framework should be restored and sutured with 5-0 chromic catgut, although in many instances it is necessary to cut back the exposed cartilage margin to permit suture of the skin edge without tension.

3. Postauricular grafts or composite grafts from the opposite ear are good replacement sources when tissue losses have occurred.

4. Superior- and inferior-based flaps on the same side are additional areas for full-thickness replacement.

5. In some instances of full-thickness peripheral losses, burial of the anterior and posterior margins into the postauricular scalp will save a stage in a subsequent ear reconstruction.

6. Hematomas, common injuries in this area, should be aggressively treated by aspiration and finely contoured compression dressings.

## NOSE

### Basic Principles

The nose also has an abundant blood supply, and even the most jagged lacerations can be satisfactorily sutured. Layered closure is essential.

### Management

1. Basic principles of treatment as noted above under Emergency Care

2. Postauricular and composite grafts from the ear are excellent sources of repair for full-thickness losses and furnish well-contoured segments, particularly about the alae.

3. Larger full-thickness losses are best handled as secondary reconstructions, while emergency coverage is attained by split-thickness grafts or suturing skin to mucosa.

## NECK

### Basic Principles

Soft tissue wounds of the neck must be considered as grave emergencies because of the underlying critical structures which may be involved. Injuries to the laryngotracheal system can quickly cause fatal obstruction. A rapid effort to pass an endotracheal tube should be made and, if unsuccessful, immediate coniotomy or tracheostomy performed. Emphysema of the face and neck, dyspnea, dysphagia, crowing, hemoptysis and cough, all point to laryngeal injury. In addition to the respiratory tract, the pharynx and esophagus and the major vessels and nerves and thyroid gland can also be involved. If communication with the oral cavity is present, infection is a common sequela, and fatal mediastinitis frequently can occur along open fascial planes.

### Management

1. Emergency treatment as noted above under Emergency Care

2. Heavy antibiotic coverage is mandatory in these injuries.

3. Surgical exploration and repair of all critical structures are frequently painstaking and difficult procedures that are vital in soft tissue injuries of the neck to rule out major vessel, esophageal or tracheolaryngeal injury.

4. Generally there is sufficient soft tissue available to establish reasonably sound surface continuity.

5. If there is substantial soft tissue loss, muscle flaps can usually be developed to protect the deeper structures and split-thickness skin grafts can then be applied successfully.

6. If there is adjacent lower face and mandibular loss, adequate neck closure should be obtained primarily and pedicle soft tissue reconstruction and mandibular bone grafting performed secondarily.

## CHEST

### Basic Principles

Soft tissue injuries to the thoracic wall must always be inspected for possible underlying damage to the contents of the thoracic cavity. Complete debridement of all compromised and devitalized tissue must be achieved, and sound muscle closure is imperative.

## Management

1. Basic principles of treatment as noted above under Emergency Care
2. If there is substantial skin loss and the patient's condition is satisfactory, immediate split-thickness skin grafting is readily accomplished.
3. In a deteriorating situation, satisfactory temporary coverage can be provided by either homo- or heterografts. Multiple basting sutures should be utilized when grafting the mobile chest wall.
4. Where large segments of the chest wall are lost and the potential for survival exists, it may be necessary to primarily rotate and/or advance a large pedicle to obtain closure and split-thickness skin graft of the pedicle donor site.
5. No effort is made to restore the parietal pleura.

## ABDOMEN

### Basic Principles

A similar situation exists for soft tissue injuries of the abdominal wall as in the chest. Underlying visceral damage must always be considered. Surface repairs range from the use of temporary biological dressings to split-thickness autografts to pedicle coverage as a lifesaving emergency.

### Management

1. Emergency treatment as noted above under Emergency Care
2. The timing of the repair ranges from simple immediate closure to delayed primary closure with the use of temporary biological dressings or delayed autografting. Occasionally immediate autografting or the use of immediate pedicle flap coverage as a lifesaving measure without consideration of the parietal peritoneum is indicated.

3. In rare instances, primary temporary biological dressings followed by delayed autografting can be employed directly onto the visceral peritoneal surfaces where massive abdominal wall losses have occurred.

## PERINEUM

### Basic Principles

Injuries to the perineal area are often overlooked because of failure to inspect this concealed region. Hematomas are common in the female and often represent a serious injury. Ecchymosis in the perineal area should be investigated for pelvic fractures and serious retroperitoneal hemorrhage. Minimal blood accumulations can be managed conservatively. However, larger accumulations should be surgically evacuated. The male genitalia are often injured along with serious soft tissue wounding of the perineum.

### Management

1. Emergency treatment as noted above under Emergency Care
2. Skin avulsions of the proximal shaft of the penis can be handled by scrotal flaps, by employing the excess preputial skin in uncircumcised patients and, more usually, by thick split-thickness skin grafts.
3. Skin grafting is generally the method of choice, either immediately or delayed after using temporary coverage. Ordinarily the avulsed skin should not be reapplied.
4. Generally the glans penis is not involved and should not be included in the stent dressing which is so important to the "take" of the graft.
5. Hemostasis must be meticulous and interdigitating suture lines should be developed on the dorsum of the penis. Indwelling urethral catheters should be placed in all of these cases.
6. In partial amputation, grafts are again employed, whereas in total amputation, clean primary healing is essential and later reconstruction can be performed.

7. Small scrotal losses are not significant and primary suture is easily achieved.

8. Larger or complete scrotal losses require implanting of the testicles beneath the skin of the thighs, and in all of these cases the status of the rectal sphincter must be determined if there is serious associated perineal wounding.

## EXTREMITIES

### Basic Principles

Prior reference has been made to the absolute need for restoring integumentary integrity when dealing with wounds of the extremities when critical underlying structures have been injured. The margin of excess skin and subcutaneous tissue is practically nonexistent, and this situation, coupled with even mild hematoma and compartmental swelling or minimally debrided traumatized skin margins, is sufficient to cause undue tension and thereby to court disaster. This situation is best seen over the crest of the tibia, the common site of lower extremity compounding.

### Management

1. Basic treatment of emergency injuries is noted above under Emergency Care.

2. Open fractures in the lower third of the extremity are always in jeopardy because of the intrinsically poor blood supply in this area. When surrounding viable muscle can be employed over periosteum-devoid bone, some degree of protection is attained and split-thickness skin grafting can be safely performed.

3. This maneuver is frequently impossible, in which case immediate or delayed pedicle coverage must be considered, a hazardous procedure at best.

4. Bipedicle flaps and unilateral flaps, even when based proximally, are frequently in trouble because of poor mobility and marginal venous drainage.

5. Cross-leg flaps frequently solve the problem in younger individuals, but these flaps must be made to attach well beyond the bony margin, be based a considerable distance from the crest of the donor tibia and have a minimal width to length ratio of 2:1.

6. Occasionally primary cross-thigh flaps must be resorted to in order to provide immediate coverage of critical structures. These flaps can be designed even in retrograde fashion, but they must not go beyond a 1:1 width to length ratio.

7. The donor sites for both cross-leg and cross-thigh flaps must be temporarily dressed with heterografts or autografted.

8. If the general condition of the patient is poor, pigskin heterografts can be applied even to bare bone with assurance that delayed flap closure can be safely performed at a later date.

9. Generally, flap coverage, when necessary for upper extremity injury, can be obtained with somewhat more comfort and safety, although, as in the lower extremity, the rule is to employ skin grafts wherever possible.

10. Ordinarily degloving injuries require replacement with split-thickness autografts or temporary coverage and delayed autografts. The injured skin and subcutaneous tissue are generally too traumatized to be considered as a replacement.

11. When digits are involved, particularly in ring avulsions, defatted abdominal or chest tube pedicles may have to be provided.

12. Wringer injuries must be carefully inspected for vascular compromise, nerve damage and closed-compartment swelling.

13. Obvious bony injuries must be ruled out.

14. Conservative management consists of fluff compression, elevation and low-molecular-weight dextran. Surgical evacuation of progressively expanding hematomas and fasciotomies should be early considerations when necessary.

# 11. THORACIC AND CARDIOVASCULAR INJURIES

*Karl E. Karlson*, M.D.

## INJURIES DUE TO BLUNT TRAUMA

### SIMPLE RIB FRACTURE

**Definition**

A simple rib fracture is a fracture of one or more ribs occurring without significant displacement or paradoxical chest motion.

**Basic Principles**

1. The fractured rib ends rub together, causing pain which limits depth of respiration, and may be felt as crepitation.
2. A jagged rib end may penetrate the pleura and lung, resulting in pneumothorax and/or hemothorax.
3. Subcutaneous emphysema may accompany the penetration of a fractured rib into the lung.
4. Treatment is directed toward relieving pain and evacuating any hemopneumothorax.

**Criteria for Diagnosis**

1. History of injury to the chest
2. Pain on respiration, with difficulty in breathing
3. Tenderness over the fracture site
4. Crepitation on motion of the rib
5. X-ray confirmation of fracture
6. Subcutaneous emphysema and/or hemopneumothorax rarely

**Management**

1. Single fractures or multiple fractures without serious limitation of breathing may be treated on an ambulatory basis. Analgesics and intercostal nerve blocks are employed for relief of pain.
2. If physiologic impairment appears to be severe or if the patient is elderly, admission to the hospital is required.
3. *Orders:*
   A. Admit the patient.
   B. Take a chest x-ray and repeat in 6 hours.
   C. Take x-rays of the ribs.
   D. Bed rest
   E. Clear fluids may be given by mouth.
   F. Give fluids to keep I.V. lines open.
   G. Measure arterial blood gases p.r.n.
   H. Encourage the patient to breathe deeply and cough.
   I. Endotracheal suction p.r.n.
   J. Intercostal nerve block p.r.n.
   K. Complete blood count
   L. Urinalysis
   M. Analgesics—Demerol or Talwin
   N. ECG
   O. Blood enzyme determination (e.g., SGOT, LDH)

### MULTIPLE RIB FRACTURES: FLAIL CHEST

**Definition**

Flail chest results when several ribs fractured in two places produce an unstable chest wall which moves paradoxically on respiration. The sternum may also be fractured and may contribute to the paradoxical motion.

**Basic Principles**

1. Ribs fractured in two distant sites result in free fragments.
2. Free fragments of rib moving unilaterally or bilaterally result in instability of the chest wall.
3. The unstable segments of the chest wall move paradoxically on respiration. Normal respiration depends on the stability of the chest wall. As the diaphragm descends, intrapleural pressure decreases, enabling the lung to expand and air to enter the bronchi. When the stability of the

chest wall is lost, an increase in negative intrapleural pressure causes the chest wall to collapse, preventing pulmonary expansion and thereby reducing the respiratory volume. When the patient exhales, the affected chest wall moves outward, allowing exhaled air from the normal side to enter the affected lung, producing inefficient ventilation and rebreathing of exhaled air.

4. The volume of paradoxical respiration may be equal to tidal volume, necessitating a larger tidal volume and tachypnea to compensate.

5. Patchy atelectasis frequently follows decreased tidal volume, which in turn yields hypoxemia due to pulmonary arteriovenous shunting. Compensatory hyperventilation is attempted, and is a frequent finding.

### Criteria for Diagnosis

The criteria for diagnosis includes all of the signs listed under Simple Rib Fracture, above, plus the following:

1. Diffuse pain on one or both sides of the chest
2. Evidence of a fractured sternum with motion of fragments, pain and crepitation
3. Paradoxical motion of an area of the chest wall
4. Marked shortness of breath due to pain or low tidal volume
5. Cyanosis
6. Hypotension
7. Evidence of pneumothorax, hemothorax, subcutaneous emphysema (*see* below)

### Management

1. Treatment is the same as for simple rib fracture, plus stabilization of the chest wall to restore tidal volume to an adequate level for normal respiration and to reexpand atelectatic alveoli. Fixation of the ribs may be attained by grasping them with towel clamps (utilizing local anesthesia), tying the clamps together and suspending them from an I.V. stand. A simpler and more efficient method involves the use of endotracheal intubation or tracheostomy and positive-pressure ventilation, since this removes the necessity for depending upon diaphragmatic movement for respiration by forcing air into both the normal and the affected lung simultaneously.

2. *Orders:*
    A. Admit the patient to the intensive care unit.
    B. Insure an adequate airway with immediate intubation, followed by tracheostomy if necessary.
    C. Take chest x-rays.
    D. Take x-rays of the ribs.
    E. Chest tubes are inserted as necessary for pneumothorax or hemothorax.
    F. Complete blood count
    G. Urinalysis
    H. Type and crossmatch 2 to 3 units of whole blood.
    I. Keep the patient NPO.
    J. I.V.'s are necessary for maintenance fluids.
    K. Maintain the patient on a respirator with pressure or volume control.
    L. Take vital signs frequently.
    M. Measure arterial blood gases as necessary.
    N. Give routine tracheostomy care.
    O. Maintain tracheobronchial toilet.
    P. Antibiotics as indicated
    Q. Analgesics—preferably morphine sulfate
    R. ECG
    S. Blood enzyme determination

## PULMONARY CONTUSION

### Definition

Pulmonary contusion is an injury of the lung, consisting of rupture of alveoli, small vessels and small bronchi, resulting in intrapulmonary hemorrhage, usually with hemoptysis.

### Basic Principles

1. Trauma results in hemorrhage into

the alveoli and bronchi of the injured lung.

2. There is atelectasis with decreased ventilation and a decreased ventilation/perfusion ratio. There may be a pulmonary arteriovenous shunt if the injury is severe.

3. Pneumonia and lung abscess may result if severe infection supervenes.

4. An adequate airway and an adequate tidal volume are necessary to prevent and correct atelectasis.

## Criteria for Diagnosis

1. Hemoptysis following chest injury
2. Physical signs of pneumonia or "pneumonitis"
3. X-ray evidence of pulmonary "infiltrate" in an area of injury

## Management

The aim of treatment is supportive—maintaining adequate ventilation until the process resolves.

1. Admit the patient to the intensive care unit.
2. Take a chest x-ray and x-rays for rib fractures.
3. Measure arterial blood gases at frequent intervals.
4. Keep the patient NPO.
5. Maintain I.V. lines by giving restricted fluids.
6. Type and crossmatch blood as necessary.
7. Complete blood count
8. Urinalysis
9. Antibiotics
10. Take vital signs every hour.
11. Intubation, tracheostomy and respiratory assistance are provided as necessary.
12. Maintain tracheobronchial toilet.
13. ECG and blood enzyme determination

## RUPTURED TRACHEA OR BRONCHUS

## Definition

A fracture of the trachea or bronchus is usually due to injury caused by rapid deceleration. Disruption of the wall may be partial, with a small hole, or complete.

## Basic Principles

1. The airway may be interrupted, with asphyxia resulting if the trachea is totally disrupted.
2. Bronchial fracture results in atelectasis of the distal lung and pneumothorax.
3. Mediastinal emphysema and subcutaneous emphysema in the neck are common.
4. A tracheostomy may be necessary for tracheal fracture or for maintaining adequate tracheobronchial toilet. Bronchoscopy is necessary for diagnosis.
5. A closed thoracostomy is necessary in case of pneumothorax.
6. The trachea should have primary repair if possible. Bronchial repair may be delayed and done electively.

## Criteria for Diagnosis

1. Dyspnea
2. Cyanosis
3. Mediastinal emphysema and/or subcutaneous emphysema
4. Pneumothorax
5. Atelectasis distal to the injury
6. Bronchoscopy demonstrates the rupture.

## Management

1. Maintain an adequate airway with intubation or tracheostomy.
2. Take chest and neck x-rays, posteroanterior and lateral.
3. Chest tubes are inserted as necessary.
4. Maintain adequate I.V. lines.
5. Type and crossmatch 2 to 3 units of whole blood.
6. Transfer the patient to the operating room for emergency bronchoscopy and/or thoracotomy according to the diagnosis.
7. After operation, the patient should be transferred to the intensive care unit's postoperative room.
8. Give antibiotics—penicillin and streptomycin.

## RUPTURED AORTA

### Definition

Rupture of the aorta is usually due to deceleration injury. Most frequently it occurs immediately distal to the origin of the left subclavian artery and ligamentum arteriosum. It may be partial or complete.

### Basic Principles

1. Aortic wall ruptures occur immediately distal to the origin of the left subclavian artery in the majority of cases.
2. Hemorrhagic shock follows massive bleeding into the mediastinum, or it may be delayed with a tamponade from the mediastinal pleura.
3. Hemothorax may be present.
4. A widened mediastinum (chest x-ray confirmation) in the presence of hypovolemia makes the diagnosis tentative.
5. An aortogram revealing interruption of continuity of the aortic wall is diagnostic.
6. *Immediate repair of the aorta* is indicated after replacement of lost blood.

### Criteria for Diagnosis

1. History of deceleration injury
2. Hypotension
3. Hemothorax may be present.
4. Widened mediastinum maximal in the region distal to the left subclavian artery, evident on x-ray of the chest.
5. Absence of pulses in the left upper extremity may be an isolated clinical finding.

### Management

1. Insure an adequate airway.
2. Take chest x-rays, posteroanterior and lateral.
3. Type and crossmatch 8 units of whole blood.
4. Provide 2 I.V. lines with large cannulae.
5. On admission, volume replacement is indicated if shock is present.
6. Take an angiogram if necessary.

7. As soon as the diagnosis is made, transfer the patient to the operating room for an emergency thoracotomy.
8. Following operation, the patient should be transferred to the intensive care unit's postoperative room.
9. Insert chest tubes for hemothorax as soon as the diagnosis is made.

## RUPTURED DIAPHRAGM

### Definition

Rupture of the diaphragm, usually the left, is frequently accompanied by displacement of abdominal viscera into the corresponding hemithorax.

### Basic Principles

1. There is respiratory distress following injury to the thoraco-abdominal region, plus decreased breath sounds in the lower chest (usually the left).
2. Chest x-ray shows a radiopaque mass in the lower thorax which may have fluid levels and radiolucent patches because of the presence of bowel in the chest.
3. Bowel sounds may be heard in the chest.
4. Esophageal, gastric or intestinal obstruction may be present due to kinking of viscera or incarceration of viscera in the diaphragmatic tear.
5. Operation is indicated after the patient's general condition has been stabilized. Replacement of viscera into the abdomen and repair of the diaphragm may be done through either a thoracotomy or celiotomy. If there are associated injuries of the thorax or abdomen, the choice of incision is dictated by these. Operation may be delayed to time of election if the patient is *not* in acute respiratory distress.

### Criteria for Diagnosis

1. Dyspnea
2. Bowel sounds are heard in the chest, and there are decreased breath sounds.
3. X-ray of the chest shows evidence of gas-containing viscera in the chest.

4. Barium swallow shows viscera in the chest.

## Management

1. Insure an adequate airway.
2. Maintain adequate ventilation if the patient is in respiratory distress.
3. Evaluate the patient for associated injuries.
4. Take chest x-rays, posteroanterior and lateral.
5. Take additional x-rays, including barium swallow, if necessary.
6. Provide adequate I.V. lines.
7. Type and crossmatch 4 units of whole blood.
8. Volume replacement is indicated if shock is present.
9. Transfer the patient to the operating room for emergency thoracotomy if indicated after the vital signs are stable.

## SUBCUTANEOUS EMPHYSEMA

### Definition

Subcutaneous emphysema refers to air in the subcutaneous tissues.

### Basic Principles

1. Air enters the subcutaneous tissues from a tear in the lung, a rupture of the airway or an esophageal tear.
2. Pneumothorax may or may not be present.
3. Mediastinal emphysema accompanies rupture of the airway.
4. Treatment of pneumothorax by tube drainage frequently results in the arrest of subcutaneous emphysema.
5. Incision into the suprasternal notch with opening of the fascial layers or tracheostomy may be necessary if there is a rupture of the tracheobronchial tree. Repair of the tracheobronchial tree injury is indicated.
6. When the air leak into the subcutaneous tissues is arrested, subcutaneous emphysema regresses spontaneously.

## Criteria for Diagnosis

1. Crepitation of skin
2. Swelling, spreading from the site of rib fracture or wound to the suprasternal notch and neck

## Management

Treatment of subcutaneous emphysema is directed toward that of the underlying primary injury.

# INJURIES DUE TO PENETRATING TRAUMA
## PNEUMOTHORAX

### Definition

Pneumothorax refers to air in the pleural space. It may occur together with hemothorax.

### Classification

1. *Simple Pneumothorax.* This refers to air in the pleural space not under tension. The lung may not be completely collapsed.
2. *Tension Pneumothorax.* The air pressure in the pleural space is higher than atmospheric pressure, forcing the lung to collapse completely and the mediastinum to shift to the opposite side.

### Basic Principles

1. Air in the pleural space reverses the normal negative intrapleural pressure, allowing the lung to collapse.
2. The amount of air in the pleural space and the change in pressure determine the extent of collapse.
3. Evacuation of air and restitution of the normally negative intrapleural pressure allow the lung to re-expand. Occasionally this represents a lifesaving emergency procedure and must be done before a surgical consultant can be reached.
4. Obstruction of the airway (secretions, tumor, foreign body) may prevent expansion of the lung and requires bronchoscopy for diagnosis, followed by appropriate treatment of airway obstruction.

5. Tension pneumothorax must be evacuated by thoracocentesis on an emergency basis, because both lungs may be sufficiently collapsed to cause acute respiratory failure or mediastinal shift may compromise the venous return to the heart, leading to circulatory collapse.

## Criteria for Diagnosis of Simple Pneumothorax

1. Dyspnea
2. Tracheal shift toward the opposite side
3. Diminished or absent breath sounds and tympany on percussion. (These findings may be difficult to elicit in robust patients.)
4. X-ray of the chest shows collapse of the lung.
5. Thoracocentesis yields air.

## Criteria for Diagnosis of Tension Pneumothorax

Criteria for diagnosis of tension pneumothorax includes all of the above plus the following:
1. Marked shift of the mediastinum (trachea) to the opposite side
2. Severe shortness of breath
3. Cyanosis

## Management

1. Immediate insertion of chest tube if necessary. Large bore needle aspiration may be necessary while thoracostomy equipment is being assembled.
2. Take chest x-rays, posteroanterior and lateral.
3. Take a follow-up chest x-ray after the insertion of chest tubes.
4. Provide I.V. lines for maintenance fluids.
5. Since the main problem is aspiration of air, a chest tube is placed into the second or third intercostal space at the midclavicular line. Occasionally a second chest tube into the seventh intercostal space at the midaxillary line is indicated to withdraw associated fluid (blood or transudate) and to prevent loculation of air with persistent atelectasis. These tubes are connected to an underwater drainage system providing gentle suction at 17 to 20 cm. of water pressure.
6. Complete blood count.
7. Oral feedings proceed from clear fluids to regular diet as tolerated.

## HEMOTHORAX

### Definition

Hemothorax is blood in the pleural space.

### Basic Principles

1. Blood occupies the pleural space and compresses the lung, with decreased ventilation.
2. The blood may become infected, resulting in empyema.
3. Fibrothorax results if the blood is not evacuated, resulting in decreased expansion of the hemithorax during inspiration.
4. Evacuation of the blood by needle or intercostal tube is required to assess continuation of hemorrhage and to reexpand the lung.
5. If blood cannot be evacuated by tube drainage and substantial residual hemothorax remains, thoracotomy with evacuation of the blood and clots is required.

### Criteria for Diagnosis

1. Dyspnea
2. Hypotension
3. Dullness to percussion
4. Diminished or absent breath sounds
5. X-ray reveals opacification of the dependent portion or of all of the hemithorax.
6. Thoracocentesis yields blood.

### Management

1. Insure an adequate airway with immediate insertion of chest tubes if necessary. In these cases, the tube is inserted into the seventh intercostal space at the midaxillary line.

2. Treat shock if needed with necessary volume replacement.

3. Type and crossmatch 6 units of whole blood.

4. Take chest x-rays.

5. Perform an emergency thoracotomy if blood drainage continues at 200 ml./hour.

6. Transfer the patient to the intensive care unit if not to the operating room.

7. Take vital signs every hour.

8. Chest drainage. Measure the drainage every hour to assess continued hemorrhage.

9. Routine lab work

10. Analgesics

## SUCKING CHEST WOUND

### Definition

A sucking chest wound is an open wound allowing free communication between the pleural space and environmental air.

### Basic Principles

1. There is a communication between the external environment and the pleural space, allowing air to enter the pleural cavity on inspiration and escape on expiration.

2. Air in the pleural space allows the intrapleural pressure to become relatively positive and the lung to collapse.

3. Treatment is directed toward debriding and closing the hole in the chest wall and evacuating intrapleural air with needle aspiration or a tube.

### Criteria for Diagnosis

1. Presence of a wound through the chest wall

2. Sound of air being forced through a wound on inspiration and expiration

3. Blood may spurt from the wound on expiration.

### Management

1. Immediate control of the sucking wound is necessary with Furacin or Vaseline dressing and chest tubes.

2. Provide adequate I.V. lines, with treatment of shock by volume replacement if present.

3. Type and crossmatch 4 units of whole blood.

4. Take chest x-rays.

5. Transfer the patient to the operating room for emergency debridement of wounds and closure.

6. Administer antibiotics (penicillin and streptomycin) and tetanus toxoid (*see* Chapter 9).

7. Transfer the patient to the intensive care unit's postoperative room.

9. Analgesics

## LACERATION OF THE LUNG BY A PENETRATING INJURY

### Definition

A laceration of the lung is a wound of the lung with disruption of visceral pleura, alveoli, bronchi and blood vessels.

### Basic Principles

1. An instrument (missile) has penetrated the lung, disrupting visceral pleura, alveoli, bronchi and blood vessels. Hemopneumothorax results, with the possibility of continued bleeding and air leak from the lung.

2. Treatment is directed toward evacuating the pleural space with tube thoracostomy to re-expand the lung and to monitor the blood loss and air leak.

3. If the bleeding stops spontaneously, the lost blood is replaced and the air leak is observed. The air leak stops spontaneously in most patients.

4. If the bleeding or the air leak does not stop spontaneously, thoracotomy is indicated to repair or resect the injured lung.

### Criteria for Diagnosis

1. Penetrating wound of the chest

2. Pneumothorax

3. Hemothorax

4. Hemoptysis

5. Density in the lung on x-ray

## Management

1. Insure an adequate airway with immediate insertion of chest tubes if necessary.
2. Take chest x-rays.
3. Provide adequate I.V. lines.
4. Type and crossmatch 3 units of whole blood.
5. Baseline lab work
6. Transfer the patient to the intensive care unit.
7. Careful monitoring of chest-tube drainage is necessary.
8. Administer antibiotics (penicillin and streptomycin) and tetanus toxoid (*see* Chapter 9).
9. Keep the patient NPO.
10. Analgesics
11. Encourage the patient to cough. Endotracheal suction should be provided if necessary.

## CARDIAC WOUND: PERICARDIAL TAMPONADE

## Definition

A cardiac wound is a wound which penetrates one or more chambers of the heart. *Pericardial tamponade* is restriction of diastolic filling of the ventricles by blood in the pericardial sac.

## Basic Principles

1. An instrument or missile penetrates the cardiac wall, resulting in bleeding into the pericardial sac.
2. If the hole in the pericardium is small enough to limit the escape of blood from the sac, blood accumulates in the pericardium, limiting ventricular diastolic filling. Increasing venous pressure and decreasing or producing a paradoxical systemic blood pressure result.
3. Hemothorax may be present if blood escapes into the pleural space. In this case, tube thoracostomy for evacuation of blood and monitoring of blood loss is indicated. In large lacerations of the heart, immediate thoracotomy with repair of the cardiac wound may be lifesaving.

4. Pericardial tamponade is treated by increasing the atrial filling pressure with transfusion and aspirating the blood from the pericardium to relieve the tamponade. If this is unsuccessful or tamponade recurs, thoracotomy with cardiac repair is indicated immediately.
5. A traumatic ventricular septal defect or mitral insufficiency may require open repair using extracorporeal circulation. Usually intracardiac repair may be postponed to allow elective or semielective surgery. Ventricular septal defects may close spontaneously.

## Criteria for Diagnosis

1. Hypotension—"shock"
2. Pallor
3. Increased venous pressure is a constant finding if cardiac restriction is severe and can be readily demonstrated clinically by observation of the neck veins.
4. Distant heart sounds
5. Paradoxical pulse
6. Enlarged, rounded, bottle-shaped cardiac silhouette on x-ray
7. Angiogram shows a thickened pericardial shadow over the right atrium.
8. Positive echocardiogram
9. Pericardicentesis is positive for nonclotting (defibrinated) blood.

## Management if There is No Pericardial Tamponade

1. Immediately transfer the patient to the operating room.
2. Provide adequate I.V. lines and volume replacement.
3. Type and crossmatch 10 units of whole blood.
4. Take a chest x-ray if the situation is stable.
5. Insert chest tubes if not stable.
6. Perform immediate thoracotomy if the bleeding exceeds more than 200 ml./hour continuously.
7. Transfer the patient to the intensive care unit's postoperative room.
8. Administer antibiotics (penicillin and streptomycin) and tetanus toxoid.

9. Careful monitoring of vital signs
10. Analgesics
11. Routine lab work

## Management With Pericardial Tamponade

1. Perform immediate pericardicentesis with intermittent aspiration en route to the operating room.
2. Perform immediate thoracotomy if aspiration of the pericardium does not restore good cardiac output or if the tamponade recurs.
3. Provide adequate I.V. lines and volume replacement with blood, plasma or crystalloids.
4. Type and crossmatch 10 units of whole blood.
5. Transfer the patient to the intensive care unit's postoperative room.
6. Careful monitoring of vital signs
7. Administer antibiotics (penicillin and streptomycin) and tetanus toxoid.
8. Analgesics
9. Routine lab work

## LACERATION OF VEINS OR ARTERIES

### Definition

An instrument or missile may penetrate the vessels of the chest wall or mediastinum, resulting in intrathoracic hemorrhage.

### Classification

1. *Intrapericardial Laceration.* Great vessels injured inside the pericardium may result in pericardial tamponade.
2. *Extrapericardial Laceration.* Bleeding will occur into the mediastinum and/or pleural space.

### Basic Principles

1. Intrapericardial injury of the great vessels frequently results in pericardial tamponade.
2. Extrapericardial laceration results in massive bleeding into the mediastinum and/or pleural space. Mediastinal tamponade with clinical findings similar to pericardial tamponade has been noted.
3. Hemothorax is treated with tube thoracostomy.
4. Widening mediastinum is observed by x-ray examination of the chest.
5. Hypovolemia is treated by volume replacement. Operation is performed for repair of the vessel unless the bleeding ceases spontaneously.

### Criteria for Diagnosis

1. Hypotension—"shock"
2. Widening mediastinum
3. Hemothorax and/or
4. Pericardial tamponade may be seen

### Management

1. Insure an adequate airway.
2. Treat shock, if present, with adequate blood transfusion.
3. Take a chest x-ray, and insert chest tubes if hemothorax is present.
4. Take an angiogram if indicated.
5. Type and crossmatch whole blood.
6. Perform an emergency exploration and repair of the vessel if the bleeding continues.
7. Transfer the patient to the intensive care unit's postoperating room.
8. Administer antibiotics and tetanus toxoid.
9. Analgesics
10. Routine lab work

## LACERATION OF THE TRACHEA OR A BRONCHUS

### Definition

Laceration with an instrument or missile results in disruption of the wall of the trachea or a bronchus. Disruption may be complete or incomplete.

### Basic Principles

*See* Ruptured Trachea or Bronchus, page 131.

### Criteria for Diagnosis

*See* Ruptured Trachea or Bronchus, page 131.

## Management

1. Insure an adequate airway.
2. Take chest x-rays.
3. Provide adequate I.V. lines.
4. Evaluate the patient for associated injuries.
5. Type and crossmatch whole blood.
6. Perform exploration if indicated after bronchoscopy.
7. Transfer the patient to the intensive care unit.
8. Administer antibiotics and tetanus toxoid.
9. Routine lab work

## LACERATION OF THE ESOPHAGUS

### Definition

Laceration results from perforation of the esophagus with an instrument or missile; total severance of the esophagus is rare.

### Basic Principles

1. A penetrating injury of the esophagus results in escape of air and esophageal contents into the mediastinum. The perforation may be iatrogenic (as a result of esophagoscopy) or from injury.
2. Mediastinal emphysema results and hydropneumothorax may be present. Mediastinitis and empyema may result from bacterial contamination. Swallowed contrast material may leak into the mediastinum.
3. Immediate thoracotomy with repair of the esophagus is indicated when the diagnosis is made.

### Criteria for Diagnosis

1. Severe pain in the midthorax
2. Mediastinal or cervical emphysema
3. Fever
4. Pneumothorax or hydropneumothorax
5. Swallow of contrast medium escapes from the esophageal lumen. This may *not* be a constant finding even with large lacerations.

6. Esophagoscopic visualization of the injury

## Management

1. Insure an adequate airway.
2. Take a chest radiograph.
3. Insert chest tubes if pneumothorax or hemothorax is present.
4. Give I.V. fluids.
5. Gastrografin swallow with fluoroscopy (*Note:* barium is contraindicated when gastrointestinal perforation is suspected.)
6. Type and crossmatch 9 units of whole blood.
7. Perform an emergency thoracotomy with repair of the esophagus.
8. Transfer the patient to the intensive care unit's postoperative room.
9. Administer antibiotics (penicillin and streptomycin) and tetanus toxoid.
10. Analgesics
11. Keep the patient NPO.
12. Provide nasogastric or gastrostomy drainage continuously.

## LACERATION OF THE DIAPHRAGM

### Definition

An instrument (e.g., knife) or missile penetrates the diaphragm through the thoracic or abdominal route.

### Basic Principles

*See* Ruptured Diaphragm, page 132.

### Criteria for Diagnosis

*See* Ruptured Diaphragm, page 132.

### Management

1. Insure an adequate airway.
2. Take chest x-rays.
3. Evaluate the patient for associated injuries.
4. Provide adequate I.V. lines.
5. Type and crossmatch whole blood.
6. Perform a thoracotomy if

hemorrhage persists or respiratory embarrassment is severe.

7. Transfer the patient to the intensive care unit's postoperative room.

8. Administer antibiotics and tetanus toxoid.

9. Analgesics

10. Routine monitoring of vital signs

# 12. ACUTE THORACIC SURGICAL PROBLEMS

*Karl E. Karlson,* M.D.

The emergencies to be considered in this chapter are nontraumatic and do not involve the cardiovascular system primarily.

## EMERGENCIES INVOLVING THE CHEST WALL

### Definition

1. These situations commonly involve abscesses of the chest wall, usually pyogenic.
2. Empyema necessitatis
3. "Cold" abscesses, commonly tuberculous or fungal, are generally not emergencies.

### Classification

1. Subpectoral
2. Subscapular
3. Involving bone or costal cartilage

### Basic Principles

1. Determine if there is involvement of underlying ribs, pleural space and lung. Treat these accordingly.
2. Drain the abscess and allow it to granulate closed.
3. Give appropriate antibiotics after culture and sensitivity if there is a systemic component to the infection.

### Criteria for Diagnosis

1. Pain and tenderness
2. Local heat and redness
3. Swelling, fluctuance
4. X-ray examination of lungs and ribs to ascertain involvement

### Management

1. Take X-rays of the chest and ribs in appropriate views.
2. Provide sedation and analgesia.
3. Perform incision and drainage.
4. Pack the wound lightly.
5. Give appropriate antibiotics if necessary.

## EMERGENCIES INVOLVING THE TRACHEA AND BRONCHI

### Definition

1. Obstruction of the airway causes acute hypoxia and hypercapnia.
2. Aspiration of saliva, gastric contents, food, pleural fluid, etc. results in acute respiratory insufficiency or chronic recurrent pneumonia.

### Classification

1. *Obstruction*
   A. Extrinsic due to a compressing mass
   B. Intrinsic due to a foreign body, benign or malignant tumor, inflammatory edema or stricture.
2. *Aspiration*
   A. Congenital tracheo-esophageal fistula
   B. Acquired tracheo-esophageal fistula, commonly due to carcinoma of the esophagus
   C. Obstruction of the esophagus or regurgitation into the esophagus with spillover into the trachea
   D. Incompetent swallowing reflex with aspiration into the trachea
   E. Mental obtundation with regurgitation of gastric contents

### Basic Principles

1. Obstruction of the airway must be relieved:
   A. Endoscopy with removal of the foreign body or tissue causing the obstruction
   B. Tracheostomy if the obstruction is at the larynx or upper cervical trachea

C. Emergency thyroidectomy (possible upper sternal split incision) for a substernal thyroid compressing the trachea. Emergency placement of an endotracheal tube is the preliminary step to ensure an airway.

2. Aspirated material is suctioned from the tracheobronchial tree by nasotracheal suction or bronchoscopy. Further aspiration is prevented if possible by correction of the basic problem.

A. If there is an obstruction of the esophagus, a tube is inserted into the esophagus to aspirate it continuously until further therapy can be done.

B. Esophageal obstruction or tracheo-esophageal fistula is corrected surgically if possible.

C. Tracheo-esophageal fistula due to carcinoma of the esophagus may occasionally be effectively closed with an indwelling funnel-shaped esophageal tube passed through the tumor into the stomach and fixed to the stomach at the lower end.

## Criteria for Diagnosis of Obstruction of the Airway

1. *Acute:* choking, struggle to breathe, cyanosis
2. *Chronic or partial:* wheezing, increased airway resistance and work of breathing
3. Tachypnea, hypercapnia
4. Cyanosis, hypoxemia
5. Repeated respiratory infections from recurrent aspiration

## Management

1. *Obstruction*

A. Endoscopy is necessary to make the diagnosis and to remove a foreign body or secretions.

B. Endoscopic removal of sufficient tumor or stricture, if possible, is done to restore the airway.

C. Perform a tracheostomy for tumors or strictures in the larynx or high trachea.

2. *Aspiration*

A. Maintain the patient in a sitting or semi-sitting position.

B. Nasotracheal suction

C. Use bronchoscopy for tracheobronchial toilet if suction with a catheter is inadequate.

D. Place an indwelling catheter into the esophagus for continuous aspiration if there is pooling of fluid in the esophagus which spills over into the trachea.

E. Provide antibiotic and ventilation therapy for pneumonia if present.

F. Provide appropriate treatment for lung abscess, esophageal tumor or obstruction if present.

G. Early aspiration may be treated with steroids parenterally, followed by ventilatory support and antibiotics.

## EMERGENCIES INVOLVING THE LUNGS AND PLEURA

### SPONTANEOUS PNEUMOTHORAX

#### Definition

Spontaneous pneumothorax is partial or complete collapse of the lung due to entry of air into the pleural space from ruptured visceral pleura in a normal individual. The primary process in the lung is usually a small asymptomatic bleb on the lung surface.

#### Classification

1. *Simple Pneumothorax.* This is collapse of the lung without increase in pressure in the pleural space.

2. *Tension Pneumothorax.* Pressure in the pleural space becomes positive, with complete collapse of the lung, depression of the hemidiaphragm, shift of the mediastinum toward the opposite side and widening of the interspaces.

#### Basic Principles

1. Evacuate the air from the chest, first by thoracocentesis for diagnosis.

2. If pneumothorax is more than minimal, a closed thoracostomy tube is placed with underwater seal drainage and mild suction.

3. If tension pneumothorax exists, immediate needle aspiration or open thoracostomy may be lifesaving to relieve compromise of respiration and cardiac output. This must be followed by closed thoracostomy drainage.

4. The lung must be expanded before hydrothorax and fibrin "peel" develop, which trap the lung in the collapsed state.

5. If the lung does not expand because a continuing bronchopleural fistula is present, thoracotomy with closure of the fistula and re-expansion of the lung should be done after a delay of not over 7 to 10 days.

6. Pneumothorax complicating diffuse obstructive emphysema is treated with closed thoracostomy tube drainage, often with two or three tubes simultaneously, to evacuate all intrapleural air and allow expansion of the lung. Thoracotomy is avoided if possible because persistent air leak after attempts at resection of blebs or closure of fistulae are common.

## Criteria for Diagnosis

1. Acute pain in the chest
2. Shortness of breath
3. Tympany on percussion
4. Decrease or absence of breath sounds
5. X-ray reveals the collapsed lung.
6. Tension pneumothorax is suspected from extreme shortness of breath, shift of the mediastinum (trachea) toward the opposite side and widening of intercostal spaces.

## Management

1. Evaluate the patient. If there is no serious distress (cyanosis, tachypnea, hypotension), an x-ray of the chest may be obtained. Clinical diagnosis suffices for starting treatment if there is any question of compromise of ventilation or cardiac venous return. It need not await x-ray confirmation.

2. Minimal asymptomatic pneumothorax may be treated with simple needle aspiration, sedation and close observation. Reaccumulation of air expanding the pneumothorax or where symptoms of respiratory or cardiac restriction are noted requires tube thoracostomy for safe, reliable management. Repeated needle aspiration is usually inadequate and may be dangerous.

3. If evidence of tension pneumothorax exists, immediate aspiration of air with a large bore needle, using local anesthesia (½% Xylocaine infiltration), is mandatory.

4. Under local anesthesia, insert a closed thoracostomy drainage tube through the second anterior interspace into the apex and attach it to underwater seal and suction (—15 cm. of water).

5. Provide sedation, analgesics and supportive therapy.

## BRONCHOPLEURAL FISTULA

### Definition

A bronchopleural fistula is a fistulous communication between the bronchial tree and the pleural space.

### Classification According to Common Etiology

1. *Spontaneous:* manifest or spontaneous pneumothorax with persistent air leak

2. *Infectious:* from infection, such as a lung abscess with a break through the visceral pleura

3. *Neoplastic:* carcinoma eroding from the bronchus to the visceral pleura with fistula formation

4. *Postoperative:* persistent air leak after pulmonary resection or from a leak of bronchial closure

### Basic Principles

1. The fistula may close spontaneously if the lung can be re-expanded with suction applied to the thoracostomy tube.

2. The underlying condition must heal or be treated surgically by pulmonary resection (and decortication if necessary) or suture of the bronchial leak.

## Criteria for Diagnosis

1. Development of pneumothorax
2. Persistent air leak after thoracostomy tube drainage of pneumothorax or after pulmonary resection
3. Expectoration of pleural fluid (increase of sputum)
4. Fluid level in hydrothorax or empyema in the absence of thoracocentesis
5. In questionable cases, radiographic confirmation can be obtained by the appearance of dye in the pleural cavity after intrabronchial instillation.
6. Tube drainage of the pleural space will deal adequately with hydropneumothorax or pyopneumothorax and will convert an emergency situation into an elective one.

## Management

1. Place a thoracostomy drainage tube in the 7th intercostal space at the midaxillary line. This tube should have many holes and should be placed to drain both the apex (air) and the base (fluid). In some cases, two tubes may be preferred.
2. Take chest x-rays to determine expansion of the lung and underlying pulmonary pathology.
3. Postural drainage is necessary if sputum is excessive.
4. Bronchoscopy is needed for diagnosis and aspiration of bronchial plugs.
5. Obtain a bronchogram if necessary to outline the pathology in the lung and to determine the site of the fistula.

### ACUTE PLEURAL EMPYEMA

## Definition

Acute pleural empyema is pus in the pleural space

## Classification

1. Acute
2. Chronic
3. Postoperative
4. Pyogenic (gram-positive and gram-negative)
5. Pneumococcal
6. Tuberculous
7. Mycotic, parasitic, etc.

## Basic Principles

1. Pus (infected fluid) must be evacuated, allowing the lung to expand to the chest wall
2. Thoracocentesis is adequate drainage only if all of the pus can be removed.
3. Most cases require dependent closed thoracostomy tube drainage.
4. If the pus cannot be evacuated adequately and the empyema becomes chronic with the lung trapped by fibrin, open drainage with rib resection may be indicated.
5. Thoracotomy with excision of the intrapleural abscess and decortication may be done electively, as may thoracoplasty to obliterate a residual pleural space.
6. Appropriate antibiotic therapy is given systemically from the time of diagnosis.
7. Tuberculous empyema (pure culture) may be treated by aspiration and antibiotics.

## Criteria for Diagnosis

1. Fever
2. Dullness to percussion
3. Decreased breath sounds
4. Dependent opacification of the pleural space on x-ray
5. Thoracocentesis reveals turbid fluid containing bacteria and/or pus cells.
6. Presence of bronchopleural fistula

## Management

1. X-ray of the chest (posteroanterior and lateral)
2. Thoracocentesis with smear and culture of the fluid
3. Appropriate antibiotics systemically
4. A large (No. 40 French) chest tube is inserted with local anesthesia for dependent underwater drainage and suction.

### INFECTED PULMONARY CYSTS

## Definition

An infected pulmonary cyst is an infection of intrapulmonary cystic structure, as contrasted to pleural empyema.

## Classification

1. Congenital cyst of the lung which becomes infected
2. Infected bulla of emphysema

## Basic Principles

1. Recognize that an infected cyst or bulla is not empyema.
2. Treat the patient with antibiotics, bronchoscopy and tracheobronchial toilet.
3. Avoid drainage if possible.
4. Resect when the patient's condition is stable.
5. Noninfected cysts rarely enlarge sufficiently with increased tension to compress a functioning lung and produce acute respiratory distress. If this should occur, emergency lobectomy would be indicated, removing the cyst and allowing the normal lung to expand.

## Criteria for Diagnosis

1. Differential diagnosis of infected pulmonary cysts from empyema is most important.
2. An infected cyst or bulla is generally spherical on x-ray. Empyema is triangular or conforms to the chest wall.
3. Pleural thickening may be absent with infected cysts.
4. An air–fluid level is common in infected cysts.
5. Bronchography or pulmonary angiography may outline the cyst and prove its intrapulmonary position.

## Management

1. X-ray of the chest (posteroanterior and lateral)
2. Bronchogram or angiogram if necessary to confirm the diagnosis
3. Encourage coughing and expectoration.
4. Bronchoscopy
5. Give antibiotics according to the sputum culture.

# LOBAR OBSTRUCTIVE EMPHYSEMA

## Definition

Lobar obstructive emphysema is marked diffuse emphysema of a lobe of the lung, associated in many cases with softening of the bronchial rings.

## Classification

1. Overexpansion of the single involved lobe without infection
2. Bilobar involvement is rare.
3. Lobar obstructive emphysema must be distinguished from overexpansion of the lung due to partial bronchial obstruction due to a foreign body, bronchial edema or tumor.

## Basic Principles

1. An abnormal emphysematous lung inflates but does not deflate.
2. An emphysematous lobe compresses the normal lung.
3. The abnormal overdistended lobe is removed, allowing the normal compressed lung to re-expand and ventilate normally.

## Criteria for Diagnosis

1. Usually occurs in infancy (shortly after birth)
2. Respiratory distress, wheezing, cyanosis
3. Hyperresonance and decreased breath sounds over the involved overexpanded lobe
4. X-ray of the chest shows a radiolucent area of the lung field with adjacent evidence of a compressed lung. Mediastinal shift to the opposite side is common.
5. A foreign body or other partial obstruction of the bronchus should be excluded by bronchogram and, if necessary, by bronchoscopy.

## Management

1. Admit the patient to the hospital.
2. Oxygen by nasal catheter
3. Posteroanterior and lateral x-rays of the chest

4. Preoperative medication

5. Bronchogram under appropriate anesthesia

6. Thoracotomy and resection

## LUNG ABSCESS

### Definition

A lung abscess is a localized collection of pus in the substance of the lung.

### Etiology

1. Aspiration of infected material
2. Septic emboli
3. Carcinoma
4. Pneumonia, particularly staphylococcal

### Basic Principles

1. Establish the sensitivity of the predominant pathogenic organisms to antibiotics and treat accordingly.

2. Bronchoscopy is necessary for diagnosis of carcinoma or foreign body and aspiration of purulent bronchial secretions, including mucus plugs in a bronchus-draining abscess. Repeat bronchoscopy, if necessary.

3. Postural drainage should only be done after consultation with a thoracic surgeon, since conversion of a simple abscess to an empyema may result from poorly timed drainage.

4. If severe sepsis continues after the above therapy, tube drainage of the abscess is occasionally necessary.

5. If the abscess cavity persists over 2 months and produces sputum or hemoptysis, lobectomy may be indicated to remove the destroyed lung.

6. Staphylococcal abscesses and cysts in infants are treated with antibiotics alone. Tube thoracostomy is used only if pyopneumothorax occurs.

### Criteria for Diagnosis

1. Persistent fever
2. Purulent sputum
3. Cavitation with a fluid level in the area of consolidation of the lung, as seen by posteroanterior and lateral chest x-rays
4. Hemoptysis

### Management

1. Posteroanterior and lateral chest x-rays
2. Smear and culture of the sputum
3. Postural drainage
4. Bronchoscopy, repeated if necessary
5. Antibiotics according to the sensitivity of the organisms present
6. Rarely, tube drainage of the abscess after the above therapy is shown to be ineffectual
7. Lobectomy for persistent symptomatic cavities

## HEMOPTYSIS

### Definition

Hemoptysis is bleeding from the lungs.

### Classification According to Volume

1. Blood-streaking
2. Moderate hemoptysis, 100 to 600 ml. per 24 hours
3. Massive pulmonary hemorrhage, over 600 ml. in 24 hours

### Basic Principles

1. Moderate hemoptysis of 100 to 600 ml. or less per 24 hours will stop spontaneously in most cases.

2. Pulmonary hemorrhage of 600 ml. or more per 24 hours will usually not stop spontaneously.

3. Aspiration pneumonia is certain to follow if the patient is unable to clear his tracheobronchial tree by coughing.

4. Before operation is undertaken, bronchoscopic determination of the source of the bleeding is necessary.

5. Tracheostomy may be needed to allow adequate aspiration of the blood.

6. An endobronchial tube capable of obstructing one bronchus may be required to confine the blood to one lung until the operation can be done.

7. Pulmonary function must be adequate to sustain the patient after resection. If feasible, pulmonary function tests should be done to determine the risk of pulmonary resection.

8. Emergency pneumonectomy is to be avoided because the risk is high.

### Criteria for Diagnosis

1. Expectoration of bloody sputum or coughing of blood

2. Rule out hematemesis or bleeding from the nasal or oropharyngeal area.

3. Chest x-rays should be taken to possibly localize the lesion in the lung.

4. Bronchoscopy is necessary during bleeding to determine which lobe the blood is coming from and also to determine the presence of lesions such as carcinoma.

5. Immunologic and culture studies are done to determine the presence of tuberculosis, fungal or bacteriological infection and antibiotic sensitivity.

### Management

1. Sedation

2. Reassurance

3. Posteroanterior and lateral chest x-rays

4. Pulmonary function tests

5. Bronchoscopy

6. Blood transfusion as indicated

7. Tracheostomy if necessary for tracheobronchial toilet

8. Emergency lobectomy is done if bleeding is more than 600 ml. per 24 hours. Pneumonectomy is performed only if spontaneous cessation of bleeding is extremely unlikely.

## EMERGENCIES INVOLVING THE ESOPHAGUS

### CHEMICAL BURNS OF THE ESOPHAGUS

### Definition

A chemical burn of the esophagus is an inflammatory reaction and/or necrosis of the mucosa of the esophagus by strong alkali or acid.

### Classification

#### According to Agent

1. Alkali burns, which cause strictures of the esophagus

2. Acid burns, which cause strictures of the prepyloric area of the stomach

#### According to Depth of Burn

1. First-degree burns with erythema and edema

2. Second-degree burns with blisters and superficial ulceration

3. Third-degree burns with eschar formation and deep ulceration

### Basic Principles

1. The burn must be demonstrated by esophagoscopy.

2. Esophageal perforation may occur acutely.

3. Steroids are given after visual diagnosis to aid in prevention of stricture.

4. Dilation of the esophagus is done over a guide or string if stricture occurs. This should be delayed until the burn heals, or after a minimum of 2 weeks.

5. If dilation is not successful in providing a very adequate lumen, an esophageal bypass should be performed.

### Criteria for Diagnosis

1. History

2. Examination of the mouth and pharynx. Most patients have burns of the mouth, although occasionally a patient will have burns of the esophagus without mouth burns.

3. Esophagoscopy

### Management

1. The mouth may be washed well with water.

2. Sedation

3. Examination of the mouth

4. Esophagoscopy to visualize the burn. Do not attempt to pass the esophagoscope beyond the burned segment.

5. If no burn is demonstrated by esophagoscopy, no therapy is indicated.

6. If a burn is seen, prednisone, 1.5 mg./kg. per day in 4 divided doses up to 25 mg. every 6 hours for adults, is given. This dose is continued for 2 weeks; then the dose is tapered so that prednisone is discontinued at 6 weeks postburn.

7. Antibiotics should be given in conjunction with steroids.

8. Have the patient swallow a string with a bead on the end of it.

9. Esophagogram at 2 weeks after the burn

10. Dilation of the esophagus over a string may be started at 2 weeks after the burn if indicated for stricture.

# SPONTANEOUS RUPTURE OF THE ESOPHAGUS

## Definition

Spontaneous rupture of the esophagus is rupture of a normal esophagus, usually associated with severe vomiting.

## Classification

1. Rupture of the lower third of the esophagus. The distal 5 to 10 cm. of the esophagus make up the weakest part of the esophagus and the vast majority of spontaneous ruptures occur here.

2. Rupture of the middle third of the esophagus is rare.

3. Ruptures including the wall of the stomach are frequently associated with severe bleeding.

## Basic Principles

1. High internal pressure causes the esophageal wall to tear at the weakest point.

2. The diagnosis is strongly suspected by the history and demonstration of air in the mediastinum or pleural space.

3. Differential diagnosis is acute myocardial infarction, perforated ulcer, pancreatitis, dissecting aneurysm or spontaneous pneumothorax, among others.

## Criteria for Diagnosis

1. History of vomiting. The initial vomitus is often nonbloody and followed by hematemesis.

2. Sudden severe substernal or epigastric pain

3. Mediastinal and cervical subcutaneous emphysema may be present.

4. Hydropneumothorax, with gastric contents in the pleural space

5. X-ray studies are confirmatory. Posteroanterior and lateral chest x-rays show mediastinal emphysema and/or hydropneumothorax. If necessary, contrast medium introduced into the esophagus may demonstrate the leak.

## Management

1. Examination for subcutaneous emphysema in the neck and pneumothorax

2. Posteroanterior and lateral chest x-rays; possible Gastrografin swallow

3. Admit the patient to the hospital.

4. Nasogastric suction

5. Sedation and analgesics

6. Closed thoracostomy tube drainage for pneumothorax

7. Emergency thoracostomy and primary repair of the esophagus

# FOREIGN BODIES IN THE ESOPHAGUS

## Definition

A foreign body in the esophagus is a swallowed object which does not pass through the esophagus into the stomach.

## Classification

1. *Normal esophagus:* the foreign body is generally sharp and catches on the mucosa or is too large to pass the level of the aorta or cardia.

2. *Abnormal esophagus:* usually a bolus of food (e.g., meat) does not pass a benign stricture or carcinomatous obstruction.

## Basic Principles

1. The foreign body obstructs or perforates the esophagus.

2. Esophagoscopy is essential for diagnosis and treatment (removal).

3. If the foreign body cannot be removed by esophagoscopy or laceration is present in the esophagus; emergency thoracostomy is required.

## Criteria for Diagnosis

1. History of swallowing an object
2. Complaint of feeling something stuck in the esophagus
3. Inability to swallow
4. Pain, which may become severe and associated with fever and mediastinal emphysema if the esophagus is perforated
5. Lipiodol or Gastrografin swallow to demonstrate the obstruction. When the diagnosis is in doubt, the swallowing of a barium-coated marshmallow will demonstrate the site of narrowing.
6. Esophagoscopy

## Management

1. Posteroanterior and lateral chest x-rays
2. Admission to the hospital
3. Sedation
4. Esophagoscopy
5. Thoracostomy, if necessary, as above under Spontaneous Rupture of the Esophagus

## PERFORATION OF CARCINOMA OF THE ESOPHAGUS

### Definition

Carcinoma of the esophagus may become necrotic, ulcerate and perforate into the mediastinum, pleural space or trachea.

### Classification

Perforation may be:
1. Mediastinal, with mediastinal emphysema and mediastinitis
2. Pleural, with esophagopleural fistula
3. Tracheal, with tracheo-esophageal fistula

## Basic Principles

1. Treat complications with drainage of the mediastinum or pleural space.
2. Treat infection with appropriate antibiotics.
3. Cervical esophagostomy and gastrostomy are necessary to divert saliva and allow feeding.
4. A tumor is categorically unresectable.

## Criteria for Diagnosis

1. Pain from mediastinitis or pleurisy
2. Severe coughing on swallowing with a tracheo-esophageal fistula
3. Endoscopy: esophagoscopy to demonstrate ulcerated carcinoma; bronchoscopy to confirm tracheal involvement
4. Posteroanterior and lateral chest x-rays to show mediastinitis or pneumothorax (hydropneumothorax)
5. Contrast-medium swallow to demonstrate the fistula

## Management

1. Hospitalize the patient.
2. Posteroanterior and lateral chest x-rays
3. Esophagoscopy and bronchoscopy
4. Closed thoracostomy tube drainage if hydropneumothorax is present
5. Use of an indwelling tube to bypass the obstruction (e.g., Celestin tube).

## ESOPHAGEAL ATRESIA AND TRACHEO-ESOPHAGEAL FISTULA

*See* Chapter 36, Pediatric Surgical Emergencies.

# 13. NONTRAUMATIC CARDIAC AND THORACIC VASCULAR EMERGENCIES

*Karl E. Karlson,* M.D.

## CARDIAC AND THORACIC VASCULAR EMERGENCIES IN THE INFANT AGE GROUP

### EMERGENCIES ASSOCIATED WITH CYANOSIS

#### Definition

1. Central cyanosis occurs when there is at least 5 gm./100 ml. of reduced hemoglobin in the capillary blood.
2. Peripheral cyanosis has normal arterial saturation, but peripheral stasis results in cyanosis and mottling of the skin.

#### Classification

1. Central cyanosis results from intracardiac or intrapulmonary venous-to-arterial shunts.
   A. *Cardiac lesions* associated with cyanosis may have *increased* or *decreased* pulmonary blood flow.
      *(1)* Cyanosis with *increased* pulmonary blood flow:
         *(a)* Transposition of the great arteries
         *(b)* Total anomalous pulmonary venous drainage
         *(c)* Hypoplastic left heart syndrome
         *(d)* Truncus arteriosus
      *(2)* Cyanosis with *decreased* pulmonary blood flow:
         *(a)* Tricuspid atresia
         *(b)* Pulmonary stenosis or atresia with intact ventricular septum
         *(c)* Tetralogy of Fallot
         *(d)* Ebstein's disease
   B. *Pulmonary* lesions associated with cyanosis:
      *(1)* Pneumothorax, hemothorax, empyema
      *(2)* Lobar obstructive emphysema
      *(3)* Pneumonia
      *(4)* Diaphragmatic hernia
      *(5)* Tracheo-esophageal fistula
      *(6)* Atelectasis
      *(7)* Hyaline membrane disease
2. Cyanosis may also result from methemoglobinemia or central nervous system depression.
3. Peripheral cyanosis results from vasomotor instability as in sepsis and shock.

#### Basic Principles

1. Differentiate pulmonary causes of cyanosis from cardiac causes.
2. Pulmonary emergencies are discussed in Chapter 12, Acute Thoracic Surgical Problems.
3. If the patient is thought to have a cardiac problem, consultation with a cardiologist is required, and cardiac catheterization is probably necessary for diagnosis.
4. Emergency operation is indicated in many cyanotic infants, but cardiac catheterization must be done first to establish the diagnosis.

#### Criteria for Diagnosis

1. Cardiac cyanosis, worse on crying or exercise
2. Cardiac cyanosis does not disappear on oxygen therapy.
3. A cardiac lesion is frequently, but not always, associated with murmur.
4. Pulmonary cyanosis frequently improves with the deep breathing of activity and oxygen administration.
5. Cyanosis of central nervous system etiology is associated with a weak, shallow breathing pattern, generalized inactivity and depression.
6. Low arterial $pO_2$ with breathing of 100% oxygen will indicate venous-to-arterial shunt.

7. Chest x-ray shows abnormalities of the heart or lungs, which give clues to the diagnosis.

## Management

1. Immediate workup for cause of cyanosis.
2. Give oxygen only after workup has started, because deterioration may occur during oxygen administration.
3. If it is cardiac cyanosis, the cardiologist will continue the care; if pulmonary cyanosis, continue oxygen and treat the underlying pathology.

## EMERGENCIES ASSOCIATED WITH CARDIAC FAILURE

### Definition

These emergencies are due to the inability of the heart to provide adequate cardiac output.

### Classification

1. Left heart failure is associated with pulmonary congestion and edema. Frequently right heart failure is also present.
2. Right heart failure is associated with distended neck veins, enlarged liver and peripheral edema.

### Basic Principles

1. Inadequate cardiac output results in increasing atrial pressures and venous hypertension.
2. Treatment is directed toward emergency measures to increase the ability of the heart to do work and to relieve the congestion of the lungs.
3. Further investigation of the cause of the failure must be undertaken.

### Criteria for Diagnosis

1. *Left Heart Failure*
   A. Dyspnea
   B. Rales
   C. Pulmonary congestion or edema on x-ray
2. *Right Heart Failure*

A. Increased venous pressure
B. Distended neck veins
C. Enlarged tender liver
D. Puffiness of the eyes
E. Dependent edema

## Management

1. Call a cardiologist.
2. The patient lies in a semi-sitting position.
3. Administer 40% oxygen by hood or tent.
4. Give digoxin orally, 0.05 mg./kg. in 4 divided doses in 24 hours, to digitalize.
5. Give diuretics such as ethacrynic acid, 1 mg./kg. intravenously.
6. Emergency operation may be indicated after intensive treatment and precise diagnosis in the following:
   A. Transposition of the great arteries
   B. Patent ductus arteriosus
   C. Coarctation of the aorta
   D. Tetralogy of Fallot
   E. Ventricular septal defect
   F. Pulmonary stenosis or atresia
   G. Total anomalous pulmonary venous return
   H. Tricuspid atresia

## CARDIAC AND THORACIC VASCULAR EMERGENCIES IN THE ADULT AGE GROUP
### CARDIOGENIC SHOCK

### Definition

Cardiogenic shock is suboptimal cardiac output, resulting in insufficient organ perfusion to sustain function.

### Classification

Classification of shock is on the basis of cardiac failure, usually myocardial infarction.

### Basic Principles

1. Increase tissue perfusion by measures which increase cardiac output.
2. Administer an inotropic drug to increase the myocardial work capacity.

3. Relieve intensive vasoconstriction.

4. Increase oxygenation of blood as necessary.

### Criteria for Diagnosis

1. Evidence of decreased organ perfusion, such as decreased urine output (less than 25ml./hour), and mental confusion.

2. Increased central venous pressure and/or left atrial pressure (Swan-Gantz catheter in pulmonary wedge position)

3. Hypotension

4. Evidence of heart failure, such as orthopnea, rales, venous distention, enlarged liver, peripheral edema

5. Evidence of adrenergic overactivity, such as cold sweat, mottled skin, tachycardia

### Management

1. Administer 40% oxygen.

2. Digitalize the patient as above.

3. Give epinephrine or isoproterenol, 2 mg. in 500 ml. of dextrose and water I.V., in sufficient volume to improve cardiac output (2 to 8 mcgrs./minute).

4. Levophed, 10 mg., plus Regitine, 10 mg. in 500 ml. of dextrose and water given slowly I.V. may be effective as an antihypotensive agent if epinephrine or isoproterenol fails.

5. Give morphine in small doses for pain.

6. Give diuretics such as ethacrynic acid, 20 to 40 mg., if pulmonary edema is present or urine output is less that 25 ml./hour.

7. Monitor arterial pH, $pO_2$ and $pCO_2$, and central venous pressure and left atrial pressure if possible.

8. Sodium bicarbonate is indicated for metabolic acidosis, 0.5 mEq./kg./0.1 pH decrease below 7.4.

9. Provide ventilation therapy if hypoventilation is present.

10. Atropine or cardiac pacing for bradycardia if necessary

11. Administer intravenous fluids if the left atrial pressure is low (less than 15 mm. Hg).

12. An assist device, such as an intra-aortic balloon pump, is indicated if shock persists.

13. Emergency coronary angiography and myocardial revascularization should be considered early in the course (less than 6 hours).

## ACUTE CORONARY INSUFFICIENCY

### Definition

Acute coronary insufficiency is acute myocardial ischemia.

### Classification

1. Impending myocardial infarction

2. Myocardial infarction without cardiac failure

3. Myocardial infarction with cardiac failure

### Basic Principles

1. Impending infarction or early infarction (less than 6 hours) are amenable to prompt myocardial revascularization, and reversal of ischemia is expected in the majority of cases.

2. Prompt cardiac catheterization and coronary angiography must be performed before operation is decided upon.

3. Uncontrollable arrhythmias are an indication for consideration of myocardial revascularization and/or infarctectomy.

### Criteria for Diagnosis

1. *Impending myocardial infarction:* angina unrelieved by usual treatment, progression of intensity of angina, angina decubitus, severe angina as the first episode; ECG signs of ischemia

2. *Myocardial infarction:* ECG changes of myocardial damage, with appropriate enzyme changes.

3. *Myocardial infarction with cardiac failure:* as above plus dyspnea or orthopnea and/or signs of clinical shock

## Management

1. Call a cardiologist and cardiac surgeon.
2. Sedation and bed rest
3. Give digitalis, oxygen, diuretics and inotropic drugs as indicated: digoxin, 0.5 mg. t.i.d. orally as a loading dose (or 1.0 mg. I.V. slowly), ethacrynic acid, 50 mg. I.V. (0.5 to 1.0 mg./kg.).

# CARDIAC ARREST

## Definition

Cardiac arrest is the sudden disappearance of signs of cardiac activity usually associated with arrest of respiration.

## Classification

1. Asystole
2. Ventricular fibrillation
3. Minimal cardiac activity without effective circulation

## Basic Principles

1. Circulation and respiration are inadequate.
2. Adequate circulation must be restored promply by external cardiac massage.
3. Respiration must be restored by artificial ventilation.
4. Intrinsic cardiac rhythm and adequate cardiac output must be restored.
5. Metabolic acidosis occurs quickly with inadequate tissue perfusion and must be corrected.

## Criteria for Diagnosis

1. Apnea
2. Syncope, loss of consciousness, dilating of pupils
3. Absent pulse
4. Absent heartbeat
5. ECG for diagnosis of ventricular fibrillation

## Management

1. Institute external cardiac compression immediately. Adequacy is judged by feeling an adequate pulse, constriction of previously dilated pupils, regaining of consciousness, spontaneous breathing and achieving a blood pressure above shock levels (above 90 mm. Hg systolic).
2. Insert an airway and ventilate with oxygen, or do mouth-to-mouth resuscitation.
3. Administer sodium bicarbonate I.V. to restore the pH of blood to 7.4 or give it every 10 minutes in 1-ampule (44.6 mEq.) doses.
4. If effective cardiac action is not restored quickly, give epinephrine, 0.5 mg. by intracardiac or I.V. injection every 5 minutes.
5. Take an ECG.
6. Perform external defibrillation with 100 to 400 watt-seconds of D.C. shock if ventricular fibrillation is present.
7. Doses of lidocaine, 50 mg. I.V., are repeated 2 or 3 times if ventricular fibrillation persists or extrasystoles are frequent (over 6/minute). Then start an I.V. drip of not more than 300 mg./hour.
8. Only if external cardiac compression is ineffective and proper facilities are available should the chest be opened and internal cardiac compression instituted.
9. Maintain circulation after the heartbeat is restored with I.V. epinephrine (2 mg. in 500 ml. of dextrose and water) given by microdrip in sufficient volume to maintain blood pressure over 100 mm. Hg systolic. *See* Cardiogenic Shock, above.
10. *See also* Chapter 7, Cardiopulmonary Resuscitation.

# RUPTURED THORACIC AORTIC ANEURYSM

## Definition

A ruptured thoracic aortic aneurysm is rupture of the wall of the aorta at the site of a previously existing aneurysm.

## Classification

1. *Extrapericardial:* bleeding is into the mediastinum and/or pleural cavity.

2. *Intrapericardial:* bleeding is into the pericardial sac, with acute pericardial tamponade.

## Basic Principles

1. The hemorrhage must be stopped.

2. Repair of the aortic wall is impossible (unless the aneurysm is saccular).

3. The aneurysm must be resected and the aorta reconstituted with a prosthetic graft.

4. Preoperative preparation involves restoring blood volume, ensuring adequate cardiac output and achieving adequate urine flow.

5. Hemothorax is evacuated by closed thoracostomy tube drainage if ventilation is compromised and operation is not imminent.

6. Pericardial tamponade is relieved during the preoperative period by pericardicentesis.

## Criteria for Diagnosis

1. Acute onset of chest or back pain

2. Hypotension

3. Widened mediastinum or pleural fluid on chest x-ray

4. Evidence of cardiac tamponade

5. Anemia

6. An aortogram demonstrating the aneurysm

7. There may be a history of thoracic trauma.

## Management

1. Surgical resection with replacement of the involved aortic segment is the treatment of choice if there are no significant contraindications.

2. Admit the patient to the intensive care unit.

2. Type and crossmatch whole blood, and transfuse when the blood becomes available.

3. Infuse 1000 ml. of Ringer's lactate I.V. through a large bore needle, followed by plasma until blood becomes available.

4. Insert a central venous pressure catheter.

5. Strictly record fluid intake and output.

6. Give an analgesic for pain.

7. Take chest x-rays, posteroanterior and lateral.

8. Perform thoracocentesis, followed by closed thoracostomy tube drainage, if a large hemothorax is present.

9. Pericardicentesis is indicated if tamponade is suspected.

10. Transfer the patient to the operating room as soon as blood volume is restored or immediately if bleeding is massive.

# ACUTE DISSECTING ANEURYSMS

## Definition

An acute dissecting aneurysm is a tear of the aortic intima, with subsequent dissection of the hematoma in the wall of the aorta.

## Classification

1. *Location of the Site of the Intimal Tear*

A. In the ascending aorta—68 per cent

B. In the arch—12 per cent

C. In the descending aorta—20 per cent

2. *Level of Dissection in the Aortic Media*

A. Inner third of the intima—probably heals

B. Outer third of the intima—saccular aneurysm develops or rupture occurs.

## Basic Principles

1. Dissection is propagated by the force exerted by the pulse wave in proportion to the steepness of this wave.

2. Alteration of the pulse wave to decrease the slope of the curve is necessary so that dissection will not continue.

3. If complications requiring operation do not occur, the intramural hematoma will organize and the aortic wall will heal.

4. Early aortography is indicated to

confirm the diagnosis if the patient is stable.

5. Emergency operation should be done without aortography if necessary, if the patient is deteriorating rapidly in face of indications for operation.

## Criteria for Diagnosis

1. Acute chest or back pain
2. Widening of the mediastinum and calcification of the aorta on x-ray
3. History of hypertension
4. Diminished or absent pulses in an aortic arch vessel
5. Aortic insufficiency
6. Congestive heart failure
7. Stigmata of Marfan's syndrome
8. An aortogram to demonstrate false channels in the aortic wall

## Management

1. Management is primarily operative on an·emergency basis if the dissection is complicated by aortic valve insufficiency, leakage of the aneurysm, partial or total occlusion of a major branch of the aorta, or if the symptoms of uncomplicated dissection are not relieved by nonoperative therapy.

2. Operation involves resection of the aorta involved with the intimal tear and repair, usually with insertion of a prosthetic graft.

## Medical Therapy

1. Careful monitoring of the ECG, blood pressure and urine output
2. Systolic blood pressure is reduced with Arfonad to 100 to 120 mm. Hg. If this level of blood pressure does not control the symptoms, the blood pressure may be lowered further as long as mental status and urine output remain satisfactory (25 ml./hour).
3. Reserpine, 0.5 to 2.0 mg. I.M. every 4 to 6 hours, or Inderal, 1 mg. I.M. every 4 to 6 hours
4. Guanethidine, 25 to 50 mg. b.i.d. orally
5. Posteroanterior and lateral chest x-rays
6. An aortogram when pain is relieved.

# 14. ABDOMINAL TRAUMA

*Gerald W. Shaftan*, M.D.

## Definitions

1. *Abdominal trauma* is any injury to the body which may have produced damage to intra-abdominal or retro-peritoneal structures.

2. *Exploratory paracentesis (abdominal tap)* is a diagnostic study performed by the insertion of a needle into the abdominal cavity and the aspiration of contents free within the peritoneal cavity.

3. *Diagnostic peritoneal lavage* is the instillation intraperitoneally of fluid with its subsequent aspiration to permit evaluation of intraperitoneal contamination by blood, bile or gastric or intestinal contents.

## Basic Principles

1. Prior to the treatment of patients with abdominal injury, the effectiveness of ventilation must be assessed, since injuries to the thoracic bony cage are frequently associated with abdominal trauma. If there is a question about the adequacy of the airway, endotracheal intubation, preferably with a cuffed tube, is immediately indicated. Not only will this permit the evacuation of secretions from the bronchial tree and lung, but it also provides for the easy administration of partial or complete assisted ventilation as necessary.

2. Resuscitation is carried out with balanced salt solution, which is given rapidly until blood is available (typing and crossmatching of blood having been done at the time of initial venous cannulation). We arbitrarily will administer up to 2 liters of crystalloid and/or colloid solution prior to beginning transfusion. By that time, in most instances, type-specific crossmatched blood is available. The use of uncrossmatched type O Rh negative blood is rarely needed for resuscitation, except in the instance of major vascular injury with massive hemoperitoneum. If after 2 liters of fluid have been given the patient does not stabilize his vital signs or elevate his central venous pressure into the rage of 12 to 15 cm. of water, blood is started.

3. Nasogastric intubation, preferably with a No. 18 French plastic sump-type tube, if possible, is done in every instance of actual or suspected abdominal trauma. This not only permits the stomach to be emptied, ensuring against aspiration of vomitus, but may also be diagnostic of gastric or duodenal injury if blood, in some quantities, is present in the gastric contents. An indwelling urethral catheter also is placed.

## Criteria for Diagnosis

1. The recognition of abdominal trauma may be obscured at times by other obvious thoracic, cranial, facial and extremity injuries, especially in the obtunded patient. The multiple injury patient is therefore considered to have sustained abdominal trauma until this contention is disproven.

2. History alone may be unreliable, especially in the drunk, comatose or semicomatose patients.

3. Penetrating-type wounds to the abdomen may be obvious; however, abdominal injury may be sustained from missile or stab wounds where, in our experience, the point of entrance has ranged from the neck down to the lower third of the thigh. Thorough physical examination, including inspection of the back and buttocks, must be done to rule out a penetrating injury.

4. Blunt or nonpenetrating-type abdominal trauma is more difficult to diagnose and should be suspected from

history or from signs of physical violence such as ecchymosis or abrasions on the abdominal or flank skin.

5. *The recognition of the necessity to perform exploratory celiotomy is of primary importance.*

A. Clinical assessment is based upon the same criteria used at judging the need for operation in inflammatory or intraperitoneal disease.

B. The signs of peritoneal irritation (generalized tenderness or regional abdominal tenderness away from the missile wound, rebound tenderness, abdominal wall spasm and/or progressive diminution in bowel sounds or their total absence) are prime indications for exploration.

C. The loss of bowel sounds is perhaps the most reliable index of intra-abdominal injury, especially when the patient is not in severe shock or the hypoactive or absent bowel sounds persist after initial resuscitation has been completed.

D. Peritoneal tap or exploratory paracentesis is valuable in the earlier assessment of these patients, since blood or bile may produce peritoneal irritation later.

(1) An exploratory paracentesis (and lavage if necessary) is done in all instances in which clinical signs do not demand abdominal exploration.

(2) The prognostic value of the peritoneal tap is only in its positive findings.

(3) Failure to obtain fluid from the paracentesis needle has *no negative prognostic significance and should be ignored.*

(4) A flexible 15-gauge Teflon needle (Becton-Dickenson #01-0049) with 4 side holes near the tip and a short bevel obturator is inserted in the midline 2 cm. below the umbilicus.

(a) The needle and obturator are advanced slowly until the point of the obturator can be felt to just penetrate the peritoneum.

(b) The Teflon sheath is then advanced over the obturator rather than pushing the entire needle into the peritoneal cavity and withdrawing the obturator.

(c) Once the needle has been passed into the abdomen and the obturator removed, the patient's position or the direction of the needle may be changed to reach various parts of the abdominal cavity.

(5) Positive aspiration, that is, removal of 0.1 ml. of blood or the appearance of bile or gastric or intestinal contents in the aspirating syringe, is considered a positive tap.

(6) If the diagnostic abdominal tap is not productive, instill 1 liter of 1.5% Dianel or normal saline into the usual adult abdominal cavity, with lesser amounts used for smaller adults or children, and aspirate 3 aliquots.

(7) Frankly bloody or bile-stained return is always an indication for operation. Pink lavage return is presently an indication for celiotomy, but it is a frequent finding that such minor bleeding results in unnecessary exploration, especially with penetrating abdominal trauma.

(8) Technical considerations in the placement of the tap or lavage needle include:

(a) *The avoidance of scars* in areas of previous surgery

(b) Care taken in the insertion of the needle when bowel distention is evident

E. Shock, persistent and unexplained, or recurrent shock after initial resuscitation is another indication for abdominal exploration.

(1) There is no other area of the body except the peritoneal cavity or the retroperitoneum into which large quantities of circulating volume can be sequestered without clinical or radiographic evidence of their presence.

(2) Increase in abdominal girth occasionally will signify bleeding within the abdominal area, but it is wiser to explore

those patients with shock, especially following blunt abdominal trauma, immediately without waiting for such objective evidence.

F. Ancillary signs may indicate the need for operation. These include:

(1) Gastric bleeding either in vomitus or from the nasogastric tube

(2) Proctorrhagia or blood on the rectal examining finger

(3) The appearance of free intraperitoneal air under the diaphragm on upright chest film or against the parietes on the lateral decubitus film of the abdomen

6. The technique of assessment of operative need in abdominal trauma described above requires no other evaluation except routine chest and abdominal films.

A. The technique does require repetitive examination at half-hourly and then hourly intervals.

B. Confidence of the absence of significant intra-abdominal injury by repeated negative examinations permits the gradual lengthening of the interval between observations.

7. Laboratory studies, although necessary, provide little useful information.

A. The level of the white blood count has been notoriously misleading in our experience.

B. Routine urinalysis is essential to complete preoperative work-up, but it is rarely of prognostic value in assessing the need for operation.

(1) Hematuria makes intravenous pyelography and cystography mandatory.

(2) Proteinuria is often a reflection of temporarily diminished renal blood flow and urinary output secondary to shock rather than specifically indicative of intra-abdominal injury.

C. Routine x-ray for the establishment of the need for abdominal exploration in acute abdominal trauma is almost useless except:

(1) The presence of free in-

traperitoneal air always demands exploration.

(2) X-ray is valuable in demonstrating the presence of fractures and the location of retained missiles.

(3) Drip pyelography provides better contrast visualization than a standard IVP, both of the renal parenchyma and the excretory system.

(a) In cases of suspected renal injury, give an initial dose of 50 ml. of 50% Hypaque or Renograffin 60 and then follow with an infusion of 250 ml. of 25% Hypaque or Renograffin 30, which is kept running while the patient is transferred to the x-ray department.

(b) Nephrotomography can be done as a comparatively safe and easy technique for the determination of renal parenchymal lesions.

(c) When the nephrotomography is suggestive of extensive parenchymal damage or where hematuria continues with the patient at bed rest in excess of 96 hours, selective renal angiography may be performed to confirm devitalization of renal tissue.

(4) Other roentgenographic studies which may be done include contrast visualization of the inferior vena cava and percutaneous retrograde aortography, as well as selective intra-abdominal arterial visualization.

## Management

1. Once the need for operation is confirmed, little purpose is served in delaying exploration for ancillary studies, with the exception of intravenous pyelography if there is evidence of hematuria.

2. All patients for surgery have at least 2 venous lines placed (one is a central venous catheter).

3. Insert a nasogastric tube.

4. Catheterize the bladder for serial measurements of urinary output.

5. Resuscitation should have been accomplished in all but the most desperately ill patient.

A. A minimum of 3 units of whole blood should be available in the operating suite.

B. A second sample of blood for crossmatching and typing should be sent to the blood bank in case additional blood is needed emergently during the operation.

6. Proven concomitant thoracic injury usually warrants the placement of a prophylactic thoracostomy tube on the injured side in the 5th intercostal space in the midaxillary line prior to anesthesia and controlled ventilation.

A. The tube will provide security against the rapid, unexpected development of a tension pneumothorax or warn of sudden massive thoracic hemorrhage.

B. Bilateral tubes are occasionally needed when both hemithoraces are involved.

C. Suspected thoracic injury may also require thoracostomy-tube insertion.

7. The need for consultation should be anticipated and requested on the basis of initial evaluation (i.e., cardiologist for abnormal ECG findings, urologist when hematuria is present, etc.).

8. Fractures should be splinted so that abdominal preparation and draping will not be compromised but so that immobility of the bone ends will still be maintained.

A. If fracture immobilization is inadequate, compounding may occur during anesthesia induction or when the patient starts to awaken.

B. Molds, temporary plaster casts or pneumatic splints are better than traction splints if possible. Femoral shaft fractures still require Thomas-splint traction, but this can be fixed traction through adhesive skin traction rather than a foot clove hitch.

9. Visual ECG monitoring should be used throughout the operative and postoperative period.

10. The abdomen should be explored through a midline incision.

A. With the midline incision the abdomen can be easily opened with minimal bleeding, and the incision can be extended around the umbilicus up to the xiphoid or down to the pubis and into either thoracic cavity by oblique incisions across the rib margin.

B. It is simple to close this type of incision either with buried sutures for the single fascial layer (linea alba) or through-and-through retention-type sutures.

C. Mass abdominal wall closure with heavy monofilament steel or No. 2 Tevdek in figure-of-eight fashion over wound splints is used in the unconscious patient, in those patients who are drunk, with the possibility of postoperative delirium tremens, or in the narcotic addict.

11. On opening the peritoneal cavity, there are two priorities:

A. To control bleeding

B. To prevent further spillage of intestinal contents

12. Blood present in the peritoneal cavity should be rapidly evacuated.

A. Two suction lines are appreciated here, since one is usually being cleaned of clots. It is advisable to suction the blood with the cupped palm thrust deeply into the peritoneal cavity, gutters or pelvis.

B. Manual removal of large quantities of clots is often preferable and expeditious.

13. Hemorrhage from the spleen or kidney can be quickly controlled by compressing the respective pedicle between the thumb and fingers.

14. Massive hemorrhage from the retroperitoneum or pelvis as well as from the liver can be reduced by occluding the aorta at the diaphragmatic hiatus.

15. A systematic search for injury of the gastrointestinal tract is done.

A. If perforations are found, they should be temporarily closed with intestinal Allis or Babcock clamps.

B. Areas of ecchymosis, especially along the retroperitoneal border of the duodenum, ascending and descending colon and rectosigmoid, should be opened and the bowel wall explored.

C. Hemorrhage at the mesenteric

border of the bowel should be explored to determine whether bowel injury has occurred.

D. The lesser peritoneal sac is always opened in blunt abdominal trauma to visualize the pancreas at the point where it crosses the spine.

16. After bleeding and gastrointestinal leakage have been stopped, the abdomen is irrigated with copious amounts of room-temperature saline to dilute the bacterial contamination or chemical irritation from gastric or pancreatic leakage.

17. Repair or removal of bleeding solid viscera is accomplished first, delaying the repair of the gastrointestinal tract until this has been done.

18. Reinspect the area of vascular repair or organ removal again for additional bleeding points prior to closure.

19. No attempt is made to drain the general peritoneal cavity which has been contaminated with intestinal contents.

. A. In the instance of severe contamination, one or more small-caliber polyethylene catheters are placed through the abdominal wall for the instillation of kanamycin, 100 ml. of a 1% solution every 6 hours, following full recovery from anesthesia.

B. Drainage for localized abscess collections, persistent minor bleeding or for the evacuation of subsequent necrotic material or pancreatic juice is done with a soft, rubber sump drain together with one or more large Penrose drains.

20. Antibiotic use depends on the type of management.

A. Antibiotics are not used if operation is not planned for fear of masking the signs of development of intraperitoneal infection.

B. As soon as the need for operation becomes evident, we use intravenous penicillin and tetracycline both preoperatively and for the first 48 hours postoperatively.

*(1)* The first infusion bottle contains 10 million units of aqueous penicillin G and 0.5 gm. of tetracycline.

*(2)* This dose is maintained so that 30 million units of penicillin and 1.5 gm. of tetracycline are given each 24 hours.

*(3)* At the end of 48 hours, the antibiotic combination is either stopped or changed to an organism-specific antibiotic or antibiotic combination, depending upon the culture and sensitivity reports of the intraperitoneal contents.

C. Missile wounds not operated upon are treated by local debridement and drainage, without systemic antibacterial agents.

## INJURIES TO THE GASTROINTESTINAL TRACT

### Basic Principles

R. D. Williams has shown that blunt trauma to the gastrointestinal tract is due to a shearing force between the extra-abdominal injuring agent and the spinal column. The concept of pneumatic blowout probably does not exist except where a loop of intestine is entrapped in a hernial sac or in another closed-loop phenomenon. Penetrating trauma, of course, can injure any part of the gastrointestinal system.

All injuries of the gastrointestinal tract must be repaired, whether they be transmural, serosal or mesenteric vascular.

## STOMACH

### Basic Principles

Penetrating injuries of the stomach may occur in any area. It is essential to inspect the dorsal (or posterior) aspect of the stomach for a continuation of the knife or bullet wound even though the ventral (or anterior) wound may appear superficial. Blunt injuries of the stomach are rarely noted and would probably represent "closed-loop" blowout injuries in the presence of gastric distention.

### Criteria for Diagnosis

1. Gastric injury may be suspected preoperatively by the presence of blood in the vomitus or nasogastric aspirate.

2. At exploration, wounds of the anterior wall are generally easily appreciated.

3. Hematomas in the region of the greater or lesser curvature should alert the surgeon to the possibility of underlying gastric wall perforation. In these instances, the mesentery or omentum should be carefully dissected away from the gastric wall to ensure that there is no occult injury.

4. Occasionally gastrotomy will be necessary to identify high-lying injuries, especially at the cardio-esophageal junction.

5. The lesser peritoneal sac should always be opened to inspect the posterior gastric wall if there is question of upper abdominal blunt or penetrating injury or where free intraperitoneal air was visualized preoperatively without obvious gastric perforation.

## Management

1. Gastric contents spilled into the peritoneal cavity are meticulously washed out with large quantities of room-temperature saline solution.

2. The gastric wound is debrided as necessary and hemostasis obtained either with ties on individual bleeding vessels or with the use of the Bovie coagulating current.

3. The wounds are closed with a single layer of interrupted sutures of 00 or 000 nonabsorbable suture material.

4. Postoperatively, gastrointestinal suction is continued until adynamic ileus has subsided.

5. Progressive feeding may be started after bowel function has returned.

## Complications

1. Leakage from gastric repair is unusual.

2. Infection in the subphrenic spaces or pelvic area may occur due to contamination from gastric spillage.

## DUODENUM
## Basic Principles

Blunt injuries to the duodenum are often occult and recognized late in the patient's course. The lowest reported mortality in a large series of duodenal injuries was 23 per cent. Most of the deaths, however, are due to associated injuries and not to the duodenal injury *per se.* Unlike the stomach, blunt injury to the duodenum is seen as frequently as is penetrating injury to this structure. Intramural hematoma of the duodenum is an unusual entity which recently has been recognized with increased frequency.

## Criteria for Diagnosis

1. As with gastric trauma, duodenal injury may be suspected preoperatively by the presence of blood in the nasogastric aspirate or the presence of free air in large quantities under the diaphragm.

2. Retroperioneal rupture of the duodenum cannot be easily diagnosed preoperatively. X-rays may rarely reveal free air superimposed on the gastric outline within the lesser sac or in the perirenal fat, making visualization of the right kidney especially distinct.

3. The presence of bile-stained fluid on paracentesis or in the lavage return suggests duodenal injury.

4. The diagnosis of duodenal hematoma is suspected from:

A. A syndrome triad of:

*(1)* A history of upper abdominal trauma

*(2)* Increasing gastric distention

*(3)* Bilious vomiting

B. A tender mass is often palpable in the right upper quadrant.

C. X-ray demonstration of partial or near-total obstruction of the second or third portion of the duodenum with proximal duodenal and gastric dilatation and a coil-spring appearance of the mucosa immediately proximal to the obstruction confirms the diagnosis.

5. At exploration, hematomas in the region of the duodenum must be thoroughly explored.

A. A Kocher maneuver will expose

the posterior aspect of the second and third portions of the duodenum.

B. The fourth portion of the duodenum may be inspected by incising the lateral peritoneal reflection of the ascending colon to the hepatic flexure and mobilizing the ascending and proximal transverse colon superiorly and medially (Cattell maneuver).

## Management

1. Management of duodenal injury depends upon:
   A. Location
   B. Size
   C. Associated structures
2. Isolated knife wounds of the duodenum are closed with a single layer of inverting Lembert sutures of fine nonabsorbable material.
3. Gunshot wounds and blunt traumatic perforations require debridement of the wound edges and primary closure, avoiding stricture by a transverse or oblique suture line.
4. Extensive loss requires procedures tailored to the individual patient's injury.
5. Concomitant injury of the pancreas *rarely* may necessitate pancreato-duodenectomy.
6. The common bile duct should be probed in extensive injuries, especially those that involve the distal part of the first and the second portions of the duodenum, to rule out disruption of the duct.
   A. A T tube is always placed for drainage if the common bile duct is opened.
   B. In the event that the common bile duct has been severed, the distal common duct is ligated and choledochoduodenostomy or an implantation of the divided proximal common duct into the isolated Roux-Y loop used for the duodenal repair is done.
7. Repairs of the duodenum are always drained by the placement of multiple large Penrose drains in the vicinity of, but not at or on, the duodenal suture line. This is especially true if there is associated pancreatic injury when sump-catheter drainage is added to the Penrose drainage.

8. Intramural hematoma of the duodenum is treated by incision of the serosa overlying the intramural clot and the evacuation of the clot if possible.
   A. The posterior wall of the duodenum and the submucosal layer underlying the clot must be carefully inspected for true rupture.
   B. If there is no duodenal lumen leakage, simple incision *without* closure will suffice to relieve the symptomatology.
   C. Penrose drains are placed close to, but not on, the area of injury.

## Complications

The prime complication is fistula formation. Prevention is difficult.

1. Careful suturing following meticulous debridement and avoidance of tight anastomotic closures obviously will reduce the incidence of fistulae.
2. Decompression of the duodenum may serve to lessen the internal tension on the anastomosis. This is done by:
   A. Drainage of the proximal duodenum by nasogastric or gastrostomy sump tube through the pylorus
   B. Direct duodenostomy drainage with a small-caliber Foley catheter placed through a stab wound in the first portion of the duodenum

## SMALL INTESTINE

### Basic Principles

Penetrating injury of the small intestine is the most common form of intra-abdominal trauma. These injuries are usually multiple and frequently clustered in a short segment. Blunt trauma injuries of the small intestine usually occur not at the point of attachment of the intestine but where it crosses the vertebral column. Injury, therefore, is found frequently just distal to the ligament of Treitz, 8 to 10 inches beyond that point or 5 or 6 inches proximal to the ileocecal valve. In loops which are partially obstructed by incarceration in hernial sacs or enclosed tight loops due to adhesive bands, "blowout" perforation is possible.

## Criteria for Diagnosis

1. Preoperative diagnosis is rarely specific for small bowel injury, usually indicating early peritonitis.

2. Radiography infrequently shows free intraperitoneal air, although there may be an evident increase in intraperitoneal fluid with separation of gas-filled loops of intestine and loss of properitoneal fat stripes.

3. At operation, it is essential to explore the entire circumference of the small intestine from the duodenum down to the ileocecal valve, with special attention to incarcerated hernial loops which must be extracted and visualized.

4. The axiom with penetrating wounds is that the number of perforations must be even, but this is only a "rule of thumb," realizing that it is occasionally incorrect.

5. When penetration is tangential (as with the stomach and duodenum), the presence of a mesenteric hematoma requires careful dissection to visualize the bowel wall at and surrounding the area of ecchymosis.

   A. Hematomas of the bowel without perforation are not always benign, for in some instances they have gone on to subsequent perforation.

   B. Large intramural hematomas may serve as a leading point for postoperative intussusception.

6. The mesentery must be inspected not only for patency of the vasculature but also for defects which will permit postoperative internal herniation.

## Management

1. Small perforations or transections involving less than one half of the circumference of the small intestine, after debridement, may be closed with interrupted Lembert sutures of 0000 nonabsorbable material.

2. If the entire circumference is transected or where there are multiple perforations within a relatively short segment, formal resection and reanastomosis, utilizing closed technique with anastomotic clamps, are done.

3. Similar resection is carried out when primary closure of long longitudinal tears will produce bowel stricture or where there is evident loss of circulation and bowel viability.

4. Postoperatively, nasogastric suction and intravenous fluids are maintained until evidence of ileus has completely subsided.

5. Drainage is not used.

6. Intraperitoneal antibiotic instillation (kanamycin) may be of value in preventing localized sepsis.

## Complications

1. Leakage and fistula formation with intraperitoneal sepsis are the primary complications.

2. If the fistulae are small and into the wound, they may be treated nonsurgically.

3. In most instances it is preferable to reexplore the abdomen, resect the area of breakdown, drain and irrigate the sites of loculated infection and reclose the abdominal wound using the figure-of-eight wound closure over plastic splints as previously described.

## LARGE INTESTINE

### Basic Principles

Injuries of the colon and intraperitoneal rectum now have an improved survival rate, undoubtedly due to superior resuscitation and the early use of antibiotics. As with the stomach, blunt injuries of the colon are rare; most injuries of the colon are penetrating-type injuries. One unusual type of nonpenetrating injury to the colon occurs with sudden pneumatic distention as the result of compressed-air instillation into the anus. Additionally, pneumatic "blowout" may occur when the colon is present in a hernial sac or from improper placement of a seat belt.

## Criteria for Diagnosis

1. The need for operation, as with the small intestine, is usually evident, although the site of injury may not be recognized until celiotomy.

2. Proctorrhagia, blood on the examining finger or, more rarely, sigmoidoscopic evidence of perforation assists in a preoperative diagnosis.

3. Contrast studies of the colon should never be necessary.

4. At operation, the colon must be inspected thoroughly, elevating the retroperitoneal structures or dissecting the mesentery in areas where there is hemorrhage or ecchymosis.

    A. Both the hepatic and splenic flexures must be thoroughly visualized where there has been peritoneal penetration in the upper abdomen.

    B. This may require extension of the wound and freeing of the flexures to bring them into the wound.

    5. *As with the remainder of the gastrointestinal tract, mesenteric hemorrhage presupposes bowel wall damage until proven otherwise.*

## Management

1. Small single wounds of the colon with minimal peritoneal soilage, after debridement of the edges, may be closed primarily with a single layer of inverting Lembert sutures of fine nonabsorbable material.

2. Multiple perforations or extensive destruction of the colonic wall require resection.

3. If peritoneal soilage is minimal and other extensive organ injuries are absent:

    A. On the right side, resection is accomplished without proximal colostomy.

    B. Left-sided or sigmoid resection and anastomosis are usually accompanied by a proximal diverting transverse colostomy.

    C. Diverting colostomy is also used when numerous sigmoid or rectosigmoid perforations have been repaired.

    D. Cecostomy, except in the case of cecal injury, has no place in the management of other colon injuries.

    E. Decompression of the proximal limb of the diverting colostomy is usually done after 48 hours, although in some instances it may be accomplished by suturing a large-caliber catheter into the proximal limb immediately after abdominal wound closure.

4. Exteriorization of colon injuries or bringing out the proximal and distal ends of the resected bowel should be done in the critically ill patient or where primary anastomosis is not accomplished.

5. Postoperatively, intravenous antibiotics are continued for 48 hours.

6. Depending upon the sensitivity of the culture of the intraperitoneal organisms, type-specific antibiotics are started as soon as they are available.

## Complications

1. Major complications are related to infection. This may be due to:

    A. Anastomotic disruption with leakage. This may occur particularly when there is:

        *(1)* Lack of meticulous closure after debridement

        *(2)* Failure to use proximal diversion with difficult or insecure closures

    B. Missed perforation

    C. Failure to scrupulously remove all fecal contamination from the peritoneal cavity

2. When colon injury is combined with hepatic trauma or retroperitoneal hemorrhage, the problems of infection are multiplied.

3. The surgeon must be prepared to reexplore the peritoneal cavity and drain areas of sepsis as soon as he suspects the occurrence of the complication.

## EXTRAPERITONEAL RECTUM

### Basic Principles

Wounds of the extraperitoneal rectum are exclusively of the penetrating type, whether from outside of the body or through the intra-anal route.

## Criteria for Diagnosis

1. History of a penetrating wound that might have injured the rectum
2. Blood on the rectal examining finger
3. Occasionally the palpation of a defect in the rectum
4. Proctoscopic visualization of the rectal wall penetration is necessary for confirmation.
5. Abdominal peritoneal signs are absent and exploratory paracentesis is nonproductive unless other intraperitoneal organs have been damaged.

## Management

1. Management of these lesions is simply the true diversion of the fecal stream by the construction of a double-barrelled transverse colostomy.
2. At operation (which is only done for colonic diversion), no peritoneal soilage is noted.
3. A catheter may be placed in each limb and secured with purse-string sutures; the proximal limb catheter is for decompression of the gastrointestinal tract and the distal catheter is for the instillation of a continuous slow drip of 1% kanamycin solution to sterilize the distal colon.
4. Local wound care must be given for the inevitable infected missile tract.
5. In general, the colostomy is ready to be closed in 6 to 8 weeks. There must be radiographic as well as proctoscopic visualization of the rectal wall closure prior to re-establishment of colon continuity.

## Complications

1. Primarily perineal and pararectal sepsis
2. These are adequately handled by appropriate drainage.
3. The initial use of pararectal drains has not avoided these complications.

## INJURIES TO THE SPLEEN

### Basic Principles

The spleen is the intra-abdominal structure most frequently injured in blunt trauma. Fewer than 10 per cent of our splenic injuries occur as a result of penetrating-type trauma. Classically, injuries of the spleen have been associated with fractures of the lower left ribs, but some doubt this association. Delayed rupture of the spleen is seen with a subcapsular hematoma due to blunt injury that continues to enlarge by osmotic ingress of fluid (in the same fashion as a subdural hematoma) and eventually ruptures the splenic capsule. This may occur in 2 to 60 days after the initial splenic injury. Selective celiac angiography may give a clue to the possibility of delayed splenic rupture.

## Criteria for Diagnosis

1. History of blunt or penetrating abdominal trauma to the left upper quadrant
2. Shock, associated with abdominal signs or postive paracentesis or lavage
3. Occasionally with localized splenic rupture, bleeding may be minimal and confined to the left upper quadrant.
   A. Shock is not evident.
   B. Exploratory paracentesis may be negative.
   C. Lavage, however, is generally confirmatory of intra-abdominal bleeding.
4. An enlarged splenic shadow on abdominal flat film, the demonstration of the deviation of the gastric bubble or serration of the greater curvature of the stomach on contrast visualization is strongly suggestive of splenic injury.
5. At operation, splenic rupture or subcapsular hematoma of the spleen can usually be diagnosed either by palpation or by inspection.
6. Localized bleeding confined to the left upper quadrant is splenic in origin until proven otherwise.

## Management

1. Because of the ease of removal and the fear of recurrent bleeding, all lacerations or subcapsular hematomas of the spleen are treated by splenectomy.

2. It is advisable, where possible, to do the splenectomy by careful anatomical dissection of the hilus with individual ligation of the splenic artery and vein.

A. The splenic pedicle is grasped between the thumb and forefinger to stop major bleeding.

B. The short gastric vessels are divided between clamps.

C. The spleen is mobilized by dividing the lienorenal and lienocolic ligaments and the attachment to the diaphragm (lienodiaphragmatic ligament) if any.

D. The splenic pedicle and the tail of the pancreas are then visualized by reflecting the spleen medially.

E. Splenic vessels are dissected from the tail of the pancreas, with care being taken not to injure pancreatic parenchyma, and individually doubly ligated and divided.

F. The splenic bed is irrigated, small bleeding vessels in the area are controlled either with ties or Bovie coagulating current, and a soft, rubber sump catheter is placed into the splenic bed prior to abdominal closure.

## Complications

1. Major complications are missed diagnosis and delayed rupture of the spleen.

2. Late problems of infection can be avoided by meticulous attention to hemostasis in the area.

3. Inadvertent pancreatic damage in many instances may be due to the initial trauma rather than to the surgical manipulation.

A. If the drainage from the sump catheter in the splenic bed shows an elevated amylase, the catheter should be retained in the space for longer than the usual 5 days.

B. The pancreatic leak eventually will subside, permitting the removal of the sump catheters.

C. Occasionally, despite the presence of the sump catheters and other rubber tissue drains, subphrenic collections of pancreatic fluid or infection do occur and will require additional surgical drainage.

## LIVER INJURIES

### Basic Principles

Mortality from liver injuries has decreased during the past 25 years because of prompt recognition, adequate resuscitation and better concepts of repair. As the largest organ in the abdominal cavity, the liver is most frequently injured by penetrating trauma. It is the second most common injury in most series of blunt abdominal trauma. Blunt trauma to the liver, however, carries a far higher mortality than penetrating trauma, undoubtedly due to the more extensive hepatic destruction.

### Criteria for Diagnosis

1. Blunt or penetrating trauma to the right side of the abdomen, usually associated with shock, frequently seen in conjunction with peritoneal signs, and almost always accompanied by a positive peritoneal tap or lavage, is sufficient to make the diagnosis of hepatic injury.

2. The specific diagnosis is of lesser importance than the need for abdominal exploration.

3. Celiac angiography, splenoportography and hepatic scans are unnecessary in the usual patient with hepatic trauma.

### Management

The management of the hepatic wound depends in large measure on the nature, extent, location and multiplicity of the wound, and on the associated injuries.

1. Nonbleeding simple wounds of the liver should not be interfered with.

A. Adequate drainage with a large Penrose drain down to the region of the injury will suffice for management.

B. If the nonbleeding wound is central in location, additional Penrose drains should be used.

C. Suturing of the nonbleeding wound, especially suturing which will close the hepatic capsule, should be scrupulously avoided; it frequently will precipitate hemorrhage or intrahepatic abscess.

2. Simple wounds which are actively bleeding are treated by the placement of deep simple sutures.

A. Sutures of chromic catgut on long malleable blunt needles are placed in chevron fashion parallel to the wound.

(1) The sutures are placed parallel to the wound in order that the wound itself will not be closed, avoiding the complication of internal "explosion" fracture of the liver.

(2) It cannot be emphasized too strongly that the wound of the liver must never be closed in order to tamponade intrahepatic bleeding.

B. Care must be taken not to tie these sutures too tightly, to prevent their cutting through the hepatic capsule.

C. An alternative is to tie the sutures over a bolster of Gelfoam or omentum.

D. The use of hemostatic agents such as Gelfoam, Oxycel and Surgicel should be avoided if possible because of prolonged morbidity from their use.

3. Extensive fracture wounds of the liver, either due to blunt trauma or high-velocity missile injury, require initial control of the hemorrhage and then debridement of the devitalized and damaged tissue.

A. Hemostasis is of primary importance.

(1) Control of bleeding is accomplished initially by the Pringle maneuver, which is compression of the porta hepatis between the thumb and the forefinger which is placed in the foramen of Winslow. This effectively occludes arterial and portal inflow to the liver.

(2) Replacing the fingers with a rubber-shod intestinal clamp frees the surgeon's hands. In order to control the bleeding which refluxes into the liver from the inferior vena cava, it is necessary to occlude the vena cava both above and below the liver. This is easily accomplished below the liver by dissecting the vena cava caudal to the fourth portion of the duodenum and passing an umbilical tape around it. The aorta must then be occluded at the diaphragmatic hiatus before the inferior vena cava is occluded with the umbilical tape.

(3) Isolation of the suprahepatic inferior vena cava either below the diaphragm in the child or above through an incision on the diaphragm in the adult will complete the vascular isolation of the liver. Extension of the incision as a right thoracostomy facilitates both vascular control and resection.

(4) Such total vascular occlusion can be well tolerated apparently for upward of 15 minutes during normothermia and can probably be extended to 60 minutes with hypothermia which includes even local hepatic and renal cooling.

(5) The insertion of a large intraluminal bypass catheter between the suprarenal vena cava and the suprahepatic vena cava has been used, avoiding the need for aortic cross-clamping and permitting blood flow to the extremities and kidney to continue while excluding the hepatic circulation.

B. There are two types of hepatic resection—resectional debridement and anatomical lobectomy.

(1) In resectional debridement, there is:

(a) Accurate control of bleeding

(b) The prevention of later septic complications by the removal of necrotic liver tissue, providing better drainage

(c) Prevention of biliary fistula by individual ligation of the bile ducts

(2) Lobar resection in case of extensive damage to one aspect of the liver is carried out along the anatomical vascular divisions (Fig. 14-1).

(a) For the right lobe, from a point from the right of the gallbladder fossa to the right of the vena cava

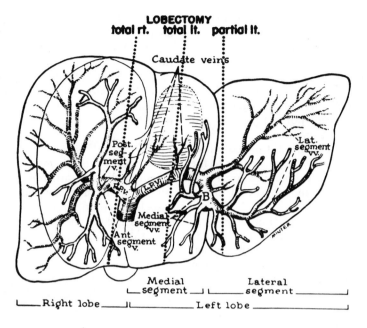

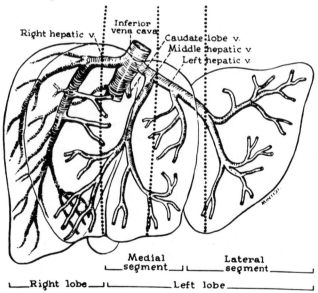

Fig. 14-1. Anatomic representation of the portal venous system *(above)* and the hepatic venous system *(below)* with relation to the planes of hepatic lobar resection. Note that the umbilical portion *(B)* of the left portal vein *(A)* lies immediately in the plane of the ligamentum teres so that resection must lie to one side of this vein. (Braasch, J. W.: Surg. Clin. N. Amer. 6:747, 1958)

*(b)* For the left lobe, from the left of the gallbladder fossa to the left of the vena cava

*(c)* Resection of the left lateral lobe, whose true anatomical plane is in the line of the falciform ligament, should be carried out to the *left* of the ligament so that the umbilical portion of the left hepatic vein is not damaged.

*(d)* Extended right or left lobectomy, when necessary, begins either to the right or left of the gallbladder fossa and goes down to the opposite side of the inferior vena cava.

*(e)* In lobar resection for trauma, do not ligate the branches of the hepatic artery in the porta hepatis at the outset, because resection of injured liver may not require complete lobectomy.

*(f)* Resection of the liver is most simply accomplished by the so-called finger-fracture technique. This involves incision of the hepatic capsule, and then the hepatic parenchyma is squeezed and morcellated between the thumb and forefinger. As the large vessels and bile ducts are encountered, they are doubly clamped, divided and ligated with nonabsorbable sutures.

*(g)* Definitive management of the massive simultaneous injury to the right and left lobes of the liver is insoluble. We use local debridement, deep hemostatic sutures and extensive drainage, including choledochostomy with T-tube insertion.

C. After debridement, the control of hepatic hemorrhage may require ligation of the hepatic artery to the bleeding lobe, which can be done without hepatic parenchymal necrosis. This may also be advantageous in the control of hematobilia from a deep-seated source.

4. Drainage of the liver should be extensive.

A. The number of drains increases as the multiplicity of wounds increases.

B. The size, caliber and type of drain increase up to and including one or more soft, rubber sump-type drains and multiple Penrose drains as the degree of injury increases.

C. We have discontinued the insertion of T tubes for drainage, except for massive or central injuries, and feel that we have lost only the ability to visualize clinically evident fistulae and their eventual closure.

## Complications

1. Infection is the most common complication directly attributable to hepatic trauma alone; more than half of these have associated colon injury.

A. Even in the absence of a source of infection, hepatic wounds, especially where debridement has been incomplete, are prone to develop abscess formation.

B. Recognition must be prompt, and drainage of subphrenic, subhepatic and intrahepatic collections must be expeditious and adequate.

C. We use large bore semirigid catheters and sumps for evacuation of such collections.

*(1)* The drainage tube exits through a stab wound in a dependent portion of the abdominal cavity by the shortest possible route.

*(2)* Occasionally this involves resection of the twelfth rib for adequate placement.

2. Persistent biliary fistulae are rarely seen following simple injuries to the liver.

3. Bile drainage following resection may persist for upward of several weeks, but almost all fistulae will eventually close spontaneously.

4. Recurrent hemorrhage is a rare complication now that we have discontinued the use of gauze packs and local hemostatic agents.

5. Hematobilia is an unusual type of bleeding after hepatic injury.

A. It is characterized by a triad of jaundice, biliary colic and upper gastrointestinal bleeding.

B. Usually it occurs one to three weeks following the initial hepatic injury.

C. Selective celiac angiography or splenoportography may be helpful preoperatively in identifying the area of bleeding.

D. Suspicion of the diagnosis requires immediate re-exploration and control of the site of hemorrhage.

E. This will often require anatomical lobar resection as described previously.

F. Simple decompression of the extrahepatic biliary system will only identify, and not treat, this intrahepatic hemorrhage.

## INJURIES TO THE EXTRAHEPATIC BILIARY TREE

### Basic Principles

Blunt injury to the gallbladder and extrahepatic biliary system is rare. Penetrating injury, contrariwise, associated as it often is with vascular damage to the other structures in the portal triad and the underlying vena cava, is often fatal before surgical intervention is possible. If a patient has survived the initial period and resuscitation and recognition are accomplished promptly, subsequent repair is comparatively simple and mortality should be low.

### Criteria for Diagnosis

1. Diagnosis is based primarily on the findings of signs of peritoneal irritation and/or positive paracentesis or lavage.

2. Bile alone does not produce severe chemical peritonitis early after leakage into the coelom.

3. Retroperitoneal biliary leakage may not be recognized even on peritoneal lavage, and diagnosis in such injuries will depend upon:

A. Evidence of increasing biliary obstruction

B. The appearance of bile in the urine

C. Decrease in the brown coloration of the stool to the point of the characteristic clay color of total ductal obstruction

4. When signs of obstructive jaundice appear in the posttrauma patient, extrahepatic biliary injury must be presumed until exploratory celiotomy disproves this contention.

5. Injury of the common hepatic or common bile duct is usually accompanied by the presence of a mixture of blood and bile in the peritoneal cavity.

6. Bile-staining in the region of the hepatoduodenal ligament or in the region of the cystic duct or gallbladder should alert the surgeon to the possibility of subserosal or retroperitoneal extravasation.

### Management

1. The preferable management for blunt or penetrating injuries of the gallbladder is cholecystectomy. In rare instances when the patient's condition is critical, simple tube cholecystostomy and closure of a penetrating wound may suffice as an interim procedure.

2. With injury to the extrahepatic bile ducts, suspected by bleeding or bile leakage from the portal area or retroperitoneal extravasation, primary control of the portal triad should be obtained before the area is dissected.

A. This may be initially controlled by the Pringle maneuver.

B. It can be definitively controlled by passing a tape around the hepatic artery, portal vein and common bile duct structures as far distally as possible and around the portal structures in the hilus of the liver.

C. After such control of the hepatoduodenal ligament, the extrahepatic duct and cystic duct together with the portal vein and hepatic artery are explored.

D. Defects in the vascular structure are repaired using standard vascular technique with 6-0 arterial silk or Dacron.

E. If the cystic duct is transected, only cholecystectomy need be done with ligation of the distal duct.

F. Linear laceration or transection of the common bile or hepatic duct is repaired primarily with fine nonabsorbable suture material.

*(1)* The duct is drained with a short-limbed T tube placed through a stab wound above or below the region of repair.

*(2)* One limb of the T tube should pass for a short distance through the anastomosis if the repair encompasses more than 50 per cent of the diameter of the duct.

G. Defects in the duct up to 1.5 cm. in size may be repaired primarily, after debridement, by mobilizing the duodenum and pancreas cephalad.

H. In most instances, however, the distal end of the divided duct should be ligated and the proximal end implanted into the isolated limb of a Roux-Y anastomosis by an end-of-duct-to-side-of-jejunum technique.

3. Postoperatively, fluid replacement should be generous since late chemical peritonitis from extravasated bile may be anticipated. Even in the absence of gastrointestinal tract injury or evident contamination, a combination of penicillin and tetracycline is given prophylactically.

### Complications

1. Biliary fistula is the only complication other than infection which may be anticipated. In general, these fistulae will close spontaneously.

2. Late stricture of an anastomosis is handled in identical fashion to those following elective biliary tract surgery.

## INJURIES TO THE PANCREAS
### Basic Principles

Pancreatic trauma undoubtedly occurs with much greater frequency than is appreciated from surgical reports alone. Blunt injury to the pancreas is frequently evidenced only by a transient rise in serial serum amylase determinations. If it is unaccompanied by clinical signs, it may be of only academic importance. There may, however, be late clinical manifestations of traumatic pseudocyst of the pancreas.

### Criteria for Diagnosis

1. Injury of the pancreas may be diagnosed preoperatively by a rapid rise in the serum amylase, usually within 1½ to 2 hours following trauma.

2. When accompanied by clinical signs or if persistent, this constitutes an indication for exploration.

3. In all instances of blunt trauma to the abdomen or penetrating trauma in this region, the lesser sac should be opened for inspection of the pancreas.

4. Edema, fat necrosis, hemorrhage in the vicinity of the pancreas or obvious transection or leakage of pancreatic juice confirms the injury.

### Management

The treatment obviously varies with the severity and location of the damage.

1. Complete transection of the pancreas through the body or tail is treated by:

A. Excision of the distal pancreas

B. Ligation of the main pancreatic duct

C. Closure of the proximal end of the pancreas with nonabsorbable sutures

D. Adequate drainage of the area

2. Partial transection of the pancreas, not involving the main pancreatic duct, may be treated by simple drainage, with a few nonabsorbable sutures utilized to partially reapproximate the pancreatic parenchyma. An omental patch may be used under the mattress sutures to prevent them from pulling through the pancreatic tissue.

3. In the head of the pancreas, extensive damage with destruction of the main pancreatic duct and/or extensive duodenal injury may require pancreaticoduodenectomy.

4. Injury to the pancreas, probably more than injury to any other organ, requires extensive drainage.

A. This is done both with sump tubes and large-caliber Penrose drains.

B. Use two or more sump tubes and as many as five or six Penrose drains in extensive injuries about the head and prox-imal body of the pancreas.

C. The purpose of the drainage is for control of the pancreatic fistula which is almost inevitable in these patients.

D. Even simple contusion of the pan-creas with slight ecchymosis or edema sur-rounding it requires drainage to diminish subsequent development of pseudocyst.

## Complications

Fistula and pseudocyst formations are the major complications following pan-creatic trauma.

1. Fistulae, in general, are unavoidable after ductal rupture.

A. The egress of pancreatic fluid may be sufficiently controlled so that general-ized chemical peritonitis from the effects of trypsin and lipase is not seen.

B. With time, most, if not all, fistulae will close.

C. On rare occasions it is necessary to implant a fistulous tract into an isolated Roux-Y loop.

2. Pseudocysts are almost always the result of unrecognized traumatic injury to the pancreas or inadequate drainage of recognized injury.

A. When recognized early, simple sump-catheter drainage of the pseudocyst will suffice.

B. Gastrocystostomy and enterocys-tostomy are done when the wall is suf-ficiently fibrous, and they will provide for internal drainage and eventual obliteration of the pseudocyst.

## INJURIES TO THE GENITOURINARY SYSTEM
### KIDNEY

## Basic Principles

Blunt trauma, usually secondary to flank injury or abdominal crush, repre-sents the usual cause of renal paren-chymal damage. Indirect injury by accel-eration or deceleration forces will occa-sionally produce kidney injury, especially when the kidney is in an ectopic location or when the kidneys are the site of con-genital malformations, tumors or obstruc-tive disease. The kidney, of course, may also be penetrated by a missile or knife. Renal injuries frequently are seen in com-bination with other intra-abdominal trauma, and the finding of renal injury should *alert* the surgeon to that possibility rather than *allay* his suspicion.

## Classification

The injury to the kidney may be divided by degree into:

1. *Contusion*

2. *Laceration,* which may involve only the parenchyma or the collecting system alone or a combination of both

3. *Avulsion,* when the kidney is either wholly or partially torn from the renal pedicle

## Criteria for Diagnosis

1. Hematuria, which may range from microscopic to gross bleeding with the passage of clots, is a constant finding in all renal injuries except in the rare instance of avulsion at the ureteropelvic junction.

2. Combined with a history of trauma, hematuria demands urologic investigation.

3. Occasionally there may be a palpable mass felt in the flank, and rarely bloody urine may drain from a penetrating flank wound.

4. Excretory urography is an urgent ex-amination when renal injury is suspected.

A. Intravenous pyelography should be done preoperatively in every patient with hematuria except in the exceptional instance where resuscitation is impossible without operation.

B. The technique of drip excretory urography and nephrotomography is described elsewhere.

5. Angiography has increasing use in the evaluation of the injured kidney. It should be done:

A. When hematuria continues after 96 hours of treatment with bed rest

B. Where nephrotomography is suggestive of parenchymal damage

C. It has in large measure replaced the use of retrograde pyelography in the evaluation of the "silent kidney" following trauma.

## Management

1. The management of most renal injuries is conservative. Ninety per cent of blunt injuries will respond to the following regimen:

A. Bed rest which is continued for 10 days if the patient responds with subsidence of clinical and laboratory signs

B. Replacement of blood loss

C. Maintenance of urinary output by adequate fluid administration

2. In patients with renal injury who fail to stabilize their vital signs after 3 units of blood have been given, exploration is warranted.

3. Penetrating injuries will evidence the need for surgical intervention much more readily, usually with signs of hemoperitoneum on tap or lavage:

A. If evidence of intraperitoneal bleeding, continued extraperitoneal bleeding or urinary extravasation is absent, selective conservatism with close observation may also be practiced in renal trauma.

B. When exploratory operation is indicated, this is best performed through the transperitoneal route. This allows easy access to the renal vessels and thorough exploration of the other intraperitoneal structures which may be damaged.

C. Large perirenal hematomas, when found, should be opened for evidence of controllable bleeding.

D. Ligation of individual bleeding points in the kidney, with debridement of necrotic, pulpified or avulsed renal parenchyma, will lead to salvage of usable portions of the kidney.

E. Nephrectomy should be reserved only for the totally pulpified kidney or where the main pelvis has been irreparably damaged.

F. Renal vascular laceration may not necessitate nephrectomy, although in the multiple injury patient where a good functioning kidney is present on the opposite side, it may be expeditious for control of bleeding and thus represents better over-all management.

## Complications

Primary complications of renal injury are delayed bleeding, urinary extravasation and abscesses.

1. When bleeding recurs following the cessation of conservative management, a second trial of bed rest will frequently allow the bleeding to stop. Rebleeding, however, is an indication for more detailed renal evauation such as nephrotomography or selective renal angiography, for it indicates more serious renal parenchymal damage than initially anticipated.

2. Areas of urinary extravasation which are evidenced as a mass, signs of flank tenderness and systemic toxemia may be definitively diagnosed by retrograde pyelography and require surgical drainage.

3. Surgical drainage also is required in abscesses of the kidney and the perinephric region.

## URETER

### Basic Principles

Disruption of the ureter is usually the result of penetrating injury. Only occasionally will blunt forces, usually of a change-in-momentum type, result in disruption of this structure. Partial or complete division of the ureter always leads to extravasation of urine. Occasionally bilateral injuries may occur.

### Criteria for Diagnosis

1. Diagnosis is based on the history of the injury, rarely the drainage of urine from the penetrating wound or the palpation of a cystic collection in the flank (uroma).

2. Urine may initially show red cells but can be completely normal.

3. When damage to the ureter is suspected, an excretory urogram should be done after a preliminary cystogram has been performed.

4. At the time of abdominal exploration, hematoma in the retroperitoneum requires visualization of the ureter, especially if the penetrating wound is in the vicinity of the normal ureteral path.

## Management

1. Repair of complete transections may be either by ureteroureterostomy, ureteroneocystostomy or transureteroureterostomy (that is, implantation of the proximal ureter into the opposite ureter).

2. Partial transection which is noted at operation should be repaired with fine chromic interrupted sutures.

3. We no longer use a longitudinal ureterotomy above the line of anastomosis or repair of the ureter for drainage, but place our Penrose catheter down to the line of anastomosis.

## Complications

Urinary fistulae from ureteral injuries usually will close if the anastomotic line is not constricted. Revision of ureteral repair may be necessary in some instances. This should be accomplished before irreparable damage to the kidney occurs.

## BLADDER

### Basic Principles

Injuries of the bladder are primarily due to blunt injury, although penetrating wounds are not uncommon.

### Classification

Bladder injuries are arbitrarily divided into contusions and ruptures, the latter being either intraperitoneal and extraperitoneal. Contusions of the bladder are seen frequently and probably account for the vast majority of hematuria noted following lower abdominal trauma. Symptoms, treatment and prognosis differ greatly according to the site of rupture.

## Criteria for Diagnosis

1. There is usually a clear history of trauma to the lower abdomen, although in intoxicated patients this is frequently absent.

2. Even with rupture of the bladder, the patient may be able to void freely.

3. Most extraperitoneal ruptures are associated with fracture of the pubic bones.

4. There is tenderness in the lower abdomen.

5. If there is intraperitoneal rupture, there may be signs of peritoneal irritation and urine may be obtained on peritoneal tap.

6. The instillation of a measured volume of sterile fluid into the bladder and the return of this measured fluid does *not* rule out the diagnosis of ruptured bladder.

7. Rupture of the bladder is confirmed only by retrograde cystography.

A. Extravasation of the dye into the peritoneal cavity or into the perivesical space is diagnostic.

B. We consider overdistention of the bladder with dye to visualize small lacerations as unnecessary.

C. If extravasation is not visualized with 150 ml. of dye, simple catheter drainage for 10 days will suffice for treatment.

## Management

1. In both types of rupture, urinary diversion by suprapubic cystostomy is essential.

2. In intraperitoneal ruptures, the tear in the bladder should be repaired with interrupted sutures of 0 chromic catgut.

3. In extraperitoneal ruptures, this is not necessary, but the perivesical space should be adequately drained with large Penrose drains.

## Complications

1. With good drainage, most ruptures of the bladder, whether due to penetrating or blunt injury and with intraperitoneal or extraperitoneal leakage, should do well.

2. Extensive extravasation into the perivesical space with subsequent infection may require prolonged drainage. Osteitis pubis is a rare complication.

3. Disturbances in the dynamics of micturition following bladder rupture are occasionally noted.

## INJURIES TO THE FEMALE REPRODUCTIVE SYSTEM

### Basic Principles

Injuries of the uterus, fallopian tubes and ovaries are unusual. Most of these injuries in the nonpregnant uterus or in the tubes or ovaries are caused by penetrating-type trauma. In the gravid uterus, rupture has been produced by blunt trauma. Cystic tumors of the ovary have been similarly ruptured by nonpenetrating forces. We find that most pregnant patients who have exploratory celiotomy for abdominal trauma *other than to the uterus* will abort. The administration of large doses of progesterone in an effort to avoid such abortion has rarely been successful in retaining the fetus.

### Criteria for Diagnosis

1. A history of lower abdominal penetrating or blunt injury, together with shock and a positive paracentesis, demands exploratory celiotomy.

2. Diagnosis is made at operation.

### Management

1. Injuries of the adnexa may be treated by excision of the ovary and of the tube if necessary.

2. Penetrating wounds of the uterus, if clean, should be closed by simple interrupted 0 chromic sutures.

3. In ragged gunshot wounds, minimal debridement of only the muscular wall should be done, and an attempt must be made to close the defect.

4. Rupture of the pregnant uterus should be handled in a similar manner. Hysterectomy is reserved for those instances:

A. When bleeding cannot be controlled by suture technique

B. When there is massive destruction in the lower uterine segment

5. Almost without exception, all injuries of the uterus in pregnancy will go on to abortion or spontaneous delivery within 48 hours. To avoid the contractile forces on a recently sutured uterine wound, delivering the child by cesarean section is sound judgement. This is especially true during the later part of the third trimester when a viable child can be anticipated.

### Complications

Complications include recurrent bleeding, abortion and infection.

1. Problems with abortion or spontaneous delivery have been discussed above.

2. Recurrent bleeding may require emergency reoperation for control of hemorrhage.

A. Sometimes this control is possible by incontinuity ligation of the internal iliac arteries.

B. In most instances total hysterectomy is the most expeditious procedure and avoids some of the complications associated with hypogastric artery ligation.

3. When total hysterectomy is done in the presence of evident contamination from other organ injury, the vaginal wall is left open to permit drainage through this structure if pelvic abscess supervenes.

## VASCULAR INJURY
### AORTA
### Basic Principles

With the increased rapidity in transport of accident victims to the hospital, improved techniques for resuscitation and everyday familiarity with the techniques of vascular repair, lacerations of the abdominal aorta, once an autopsy room demonstration, now represent a real surgical salvage. The injuries are primarily penetrating, although occasionally blunt trauma may produce subintimal tears and hemorrhage.

## Criteria for Diagnosis

1. The diagnosis is made at operation, which must be immediate without awaiting full resuscitation.

2. Based on the history of penetrating trauma and the finding of unremitting shock, operation is carried out even in the face of a negative paracentesis.

3. Diagnosis and treatment now progress simultaneously.

## Management

1. Massive hemoperitoneum and retroperitoneal bleeding demand immediate proximal control of the aorta by cross-clamping at the diaphragmatic hiatus.

2. Distal control is obtained subsequently.

3. The aorta is rapidly exposed by incision of the posterior parietal peritoneum and the injury is identified.

4. Occlusion can then be moved to a more distal area to provide renal and intestinal perfusion.

5. Combined injuries involving the inferior vena cava are not infrequent.

6. Knife wounds of the aorta may be repaired with simple continuous arterial 5-0 or 6-0 silk or Dacron.

7. The posterior wall of the aorta cannot be easily visualized by rotating the aorta, so that it is advantageous to enlarge the proximal laceration in order to see the posterior wall. If there is a laceration, this should be repaired transluminally.

8. Small-caliber bullet wounds may similarly be repaired by debridement of the wall and primary closure or repair with an autologous venous or Dacron patch.

9. In most instances of major loss, replacement with a small segment of prosthetic-tube graft is preferable unless there is contamination from associated bowel injury.

## Complications

Complications are the same as in any aortic vascular surgery, that is, leakage at the anastomotic line, enteric fistulization, usually with exsanguination before repair can be accomplished, and infection. Thrombosis of the aorta has not been noted except in the instance of subintimal hemorrhage with complete narrowing of the aortic lumen.

## INFERIOR VENA CAVA

### Basic Principles

Injuries of the inferior vena cava may be divided into three areas: the infrarenal portion, the suprarenal portion and the intrahepatic portion. The mortality increases as the injury progresses centrally. Injuries are invariably penetrating in type, varying from a small laceration of the anterior wall or avulsion of a lumbar vein down to blast destruction of the suprarenal vena cava. Injuries in the intrahepatic portion may also be due to blunt trauma, with avulsion of the hepatic veins extending as lacerations at their vena caval entrance. It is only in recent years with the four-vessel occlusion technique of Heaney, and especially with the use of intraluminal bypass catheters, that any survivals have been reported when this area was traumatized.

### Criteria for Diagnosis

1. Diagnosis is made at operation with the finding of either massive hemoperitoneum without evident organ injury or of retroperitoneal hematoma in the vicinity of the vena caval course.

2. Occasionally, the vena caval injury is discovered embarrassingly late when sudden, massive bleeding occurs during the repair of a hepatic, pancreatoduodenal or intestinal injury.

3. The old dictum that retroperitoneal hematomas are not explored unless they are expanding is not valid and is dangerous.

A. The previously expressed fear of disturbing an established hematoma and thereby producing massive bleeding is not consonant with our current vascular surgical practices.

B. It is far preferable to find and

repair bleeding at the time of initial exploration than to re-explore a patient in shock when the occluding clot undergoes spontaneous lysis or is pushed out when the central venous pressure is elevated during postoperative coughing.

## Management

1. *Infrarenal Vena Cava*

A. As in all vascular surgical procedures, direct pressure may be applied to the area of bleeding while proximal and distal control is obtained either with vascular clamps or with umbilical tapes.

B. It may be necessary to temporarily occlude or tie the lumbar veins in the vicinity of the injury.

C. Repair is carried out with 6-0 vascular silk or Dacron suture.

D. Ligation and division of the lumbar veins and rotation of the vena cava may be necessary if a posterior laceration needs to be repaired.

E. Alternatively, a posterior laceration may be repaired intraluminally by enlarging the anterior wound and sewing the vena cava from within.

F. In the case of a ragged laceration, the vena cava must be debrided to clean viable venous wall which may require the application of an autogenous saphenous venous patch to prevent constriction of the vena cava.

G. Massive destruction of the infrarenal vena cava may be treated by ligation of the vena cava above and below the area of injury, utilizing umbilical tape and transfixion sutures, as well as ligation of the feeding lumbar veins.

2. *Suprarenal Vena Cava*

A. Small, simple lacerations of the suprarenal vena cava may be repaired without complete proximal and distal control by the use of a partially occluding clamp.

B. If it is necessary to occlude the renal venous effluent, the aorta or at least the renal arteries should be similarly occluded to prevent renal parenchymal engorgement.

C. Although there have been survivals from ligation of the suprarenal vena cava, it is preferable to repair the cava here if possible.

D. Such restoration of caval continuity can be accomplished either with:

*(1)* A saphenous venous patch

*(2)* A tailored tube made from an opened length of saphenous vein divided in half and sutured together

*(3)* A segment of the infrarenal vena cava which is ligated and the excised portion used to replace the destroyed suprarenal section

E. An intraluminal bypass cannula may facilitate repair.

3. *Intrahepatic Vena Cava*

A. In general, this injury is seen accompanying hepatic trauma.

B. Rapid control of the bleeding, both from the vena cava and from the liver, must be accomplished by the vascular isolation techniques described under massive hepatic injury, page 168.

C. The injured lobe (or the right lobe where hepatic injury is not evident) is rapidly resected down to the vena cava, and avulsed hepatic veins are ligated with figure-of-eight sutures of fine vascular nonabsorbable material.

D. The vena caval tear is closed with continuous simple sutures as used in all cardiovascular closures.

4. Postoperatively, a loading dose of 1000 ml. of low-molecular-weight dextran is infused, repeating this dose of low-molecular-weight dextran on the first and second postoperative day. Twenty-four hours after operation, we begin systemic heparinization, which is continued for 10 days and then gradually tapered off over a 48-hour period.

## Complications

Complications are the same as in any venous vascular surgery, that is, thrombosis, embolization and recurrent bleeding.

1. Our regimen of low-molecular-weight dextran, followed by hepariniza-

tion, has reduced the latter two problems.

2. Rebleeding is invariably due to missed posterior injury.

## OTHER MAJOR VESSEL INJURY

### Basic Principles

Injuries of the celiac axis, superior mesenteric artery, renal vessels and portal veins have been experienced and represent potentially salvageable lesions.

### Criteria for Diagnosis

This is invariably made at operation by the careful dissection of areas of hematoma in the retroperitoneum and isolation of these major vascular trunks as necessary.

### Management

1. As with injuries of the aorta and vena cava, repair is accomplished by standard vascular techniques with fine suture and suture material.

2. Depending on the vessel and its location, bleeding may be treated either by:

A. Ligation (as with lacerations of the external or common iliac vein when damage is extensive)

B. The placement of an autologous venous patch or tube grafts (as in zones one or two of the superior mesenteric artery)

C. Reimplantation may also be done (as in portacaval end-to-side anastomosis when the proximal portal vein is destroyed).

### Complications

Besides those noted above, injury of these major tributary vessels may develop subsequent arteriovenous fistulae. When diagnosed postoperatively, with the aid of selective angiography, standard vascular repair can be accomplished at a later date. Thrombosis of the repair with loss of bowel or organ viability may require subsequent resection.

## RETROPERITONEAL HEMATOMA

### Basic Principles

Retroperitoneal hematoma not related to the duodenum, pancreas, kidneys, aorta or vena cava, which have been discussed previously, is almost invariably due to blunt trauma to the pelvis. This entity, when extensive, is the "bête noire" of the trauma surgeon. Theoretically, the pelvic retroperitoneal space and its proximal extension to the lower border of the kidney will hold about 4 liters of blood; it is not unusual for us to see patients who require replacement in excess of 10 liters of blood with pelvic fracture and retroperitoneal hematoma being the only finding at exploratory celiotomy.

### Criteria for Diagnosis

1. Blunt trauma to the pelvis, usually with comminuted fracture of the pelvis, is the most common associated finding in massive retroperitoneal hematoma.

2. The term "massive" is used here because small retroperitoneal hematomas almost certainly escape exploration because they produce neither symptoms nor shock.

3. The massive retroperitoneal hematoma may exhibit signs of peritoneal irritation, although these are frequently late in development.

4. External flank ecchymosis (Grey-Turner sign) is rarely seen early.

5. Paracentesis or lavage is usually positive; occasionally the paracentesis needle is actually within the retroperitoneal hematoma.

### Management

1. We arbitrarily utilize 3 liters of transfusion as the point at which we will perform exploratory celiotomy in the absence of peritoneal signs or positive paracentesis or lavage.

2. If the patient requires more than 6 units of whole blood in addition to other resuscitative fluids, we will attempt an inferior vena cavagram and retrograde aortography prior to exploration if the patient's condition permits such delay.

A. On rare occasions this has provided us with significant information to assist in the localization of bleeding at operation.
in the localization of bleeding at operation.

B. Most times, like the treatment, it is an exercise in futility.

3. On exploring the abdomen, identify the major organs and vessels that could be the source of bleeding in the retroperitoneum.

4. Exploration is carried out down past the external iliac vessels bilaterally.

5. Fractures of the pelvis are reduced manually if there is marked displacement since this will frequently control significant venous hemorrhage.

6. If bleeding persists after major vessel or organ injury in the pelvis has been ruled out and the fractures have been reduced as anatomically as possible, bilateral incontinuity ligation of the internal iliac arteries is done. In some instances this has provided sufficient control of the arterial inflow to the area to slow and eventually stop the hemorrhage.

7. If bilateral incontinuity ligation is not successful, packing with head rolls is the last recourse. These are brought out through the wound and are removed gradually after the fifth to seventh day.

## Complications

1. Futile operation is the most significant complication of retroperitoneal hematoma. Better means of diagnosis and hemostatis of bleeding are needed.

2. Repeated bleeding is often seen. Control at reoperation is often as useless as the initial hemostasis. Drug-induced systemic hypotension may have value here.

3. Infection of the retroperitoneal hematoma is a constant accompaniment of head-roll packing and must be treated by maintained adequate drainage.

## INJURIES TO THE ABDOMINAL WALL

### Basic Principles

Abdominal wall trauma may simulate many of the signs of intraperitoneal injury. There may be a palpable mass, peritoneal signs may be present, especially paralytic ileus, and there is abdominal tenderness, abdominal wall spasm and even rebound tenderness. Diagnosis of intra-abdominal injury in such instances is difficult, and unnecessary negative celiotomies are unfortunate but unavoidable. In this instance, even such staunch advocates of selective conservatism as our group believe that "look and see is better than wait and see."

# 15. GASTROINTESTINAL BLEEDING

*Bernard Gardner,* M.D.

## GASTROINTESTINAL BLEEDING

### Definition

Gastrointestinal bleeding is hemorrhage into the gastrointestinal tract occurring at any point from the mouth to and including the anus, manifested by blood or blood products in vomitus, gastric aspirate or stool.

### Classification

Gastrointestinal bleeding may be divided into massive (over 40% of calculated blood volume) or nonmassive gastrointestinal bleeding. Either of these may come from the upper or lower gastrointestinal tract.

### Basic Principles

1. The differentiation between upper and lower gastrointestinal tract bleeding is important since the over-all plan of management may differ as well as the ultimate treatment goal.

2. The most common lesions responsible for upper gastrointestinal tract bleeding are:

    A. Gastroduodenal ulceration (70%)

    B. Esophageal varices (20%)

    C. Acute gastritis (5%)

    D. Miscellaneous causes (i.e., gastric cancer, hiatus hernia, gastric or esophageal lacerations, gastric tumors)

3. In almost all cases of massive lower gastrointestinal tract bleeding, the cause is diverticulosis. Rarely small intestinal tumors, particularly hemangiomas, may bleed massively.

4. Bleeding may also be seen as part of systemic problems such as primary coagulation defects and secondary coagulation defects due to drug ingestion or uremia. Less servere bleeding frequently accompanies diverticulitis of the colon, colonic tumors and ingestion of aspirin, but, in our experience, these seldom threaten the patient's life. Rectal hemorrhoids rarely may bleed extensively.

### Criteria for Diagnosis

1. Gastrointestinal bleeding may present as vomiting of red blood or coffee-ground material, or as passage of a bloody stool varying in color from bright red to wine-colored to black.

2. Hematemesis is always a sign of a lesion in the esophagus, stomach or upper intestine. When blood is acted upon by gastric juice, it becomes brown, but, when bleeding is massive, the vomitus may be bright red despite high gastric acidity. If the history clearly indicates that the initial vomiting was nonbloody, a gastric or esophageal laceration should be suspected. This is important since these lacerations are high on the lesser curvature and must be searched for at operation or they will be missed, leading to catastrophic postoperative bleeding.

3. Passage of a black or tarry stool, often foul smelling, is a sign of upper gastrointestinal tract bleeding, although the bleeding from right colonic disease may, on occasion, be quite dark.

4. Bright-red rectal bleeding may occur with upper gastrointestinal tract lesions, but this implies massive hemorrhage. In these cases, associated systemic signs of hypovolemia will be present (e.g., tachycardia, syncope, hypotension). In the absence of these signs, the red rectal bleeding must be assumed to be of colonic or rectal origin. Formation of the stool occurs in the left colon, so that the presence of recognizable brown stool with the blood points to a descending colon or rectal

origin. In massive diverticular bleeding, the usual finding is the passage of a wine-colored stool.

5. History and physical examination may elicit associated conditions that can cause gastrointestinal bleeding. This will include excessive alcoholic ingestion, the presence of spider angiomas, collateral peripheral venous-pattern (caput medusae) ascites, jaundice or hepatomegaly. Although ulcers frequently occur in the cirrhotic patient, massive hemorrhage associated with jaundice and ascites is almost always due to esophageal varices. Primary or secondary coagulation disorders must also be considered as an underlying cause.

## MASSIVE GASTROINTESTINAL BLEEDING—DIAGNOSIS UNKNOWN

### Basic Principles

1. Stabilization and restoration of the blood volume should precede all efforts at diagnosis. Occasionally it may be necessary to operate without further diagnostic procedures, and rarely bleeding may be so massive that not even a history should be obtained prior to operation.

2. Bleeding may be arteriolar, arterial (i.e., gastroduodenal artery), major arterial (aortoduodenal fistula) or venous under elevated pressure (variceal). The rate of bleeding, therefore, is the best guide to indicating the necessity for operation and must be estimated early by indirect means such as the rate of reinfusion of blood and fluid to maintain blood pressure and the rate of loss from an indwelling nasogastric tube. In these cases, diagnosis and management are carried out simultaneously.

### Management

The progressive hourly management of the massive bleeder is outlined below.

#### Initial Hour

1. Insert 2 large bore cannulae (17-

gauge or larger) for blood and fluid administration, preferably in the upper extremities.

2. Draw blood for hematocrit and type and crossmatch 8 units of blood.

3. Start intravenous infusion with a plasma substitute (expander).

4. Measure blood pressure and pulse.

A. If systolic blood pressure is below 60 mm. Hg, it may be necessary to infuse or transfuse under pressure or to use uncrossmatched type-specific blood.

B. If blood pressure fails to respond to 1 liter of fluid replacement in 10 minutes, prepare the patient for immediate operation.

C. If systolic blood pressure is over 60 mm. Hg:

(1) Insert a nasogastric sump tube and irrigate with iced saline. Usually the blood-tinged fluid will become more dilute with the saline and often clear.

(2) Obtain a more careful history and do a complete physical examination.

(3) Emergency surgery will be indicated if the rate of bleeding is greater than 2 units per hour (necessary to maintain blood pressure). The presence of jaundice and ascites, however, *contraindicates* immediate operation, and the Sengstaken-Blakemore tube is used to tamponade the bleeding varices (*see* p. 184).

### If the Bleeding Has Stabilized Within the First Treatment Hour

1. Insert a Foley catheter to monitor urinary output. This serves as a reflection of tissue perfusion.

2. Insert a central venous cannula to monitor right atrial pressure as a reflection of filling of the venous capacitance system.

3. Get hematocrit results.

4. Transfuse the patient until the central venous pressure rises.

5. When bleeding has significantly decreased and less than 3 units of blood have been transfused in 8 hours, continued monitoring is instituted. This includes frequent measurements of the central venous

pressure, blood pressure and pulse and repeated aspirations of the gastric contents. Hematocrits are repeated every 2 hours to evaluate the balance between vascular refilling and transfusion. Each subsequent unit of blood is expected to raise the hematocrit by 1.5 to 3.0 per cent when it is below 30 and if bleeding is not persisting.

We do not perform a GI series within the first 24 hours in an unstable patient because it seldom influences the need for operation or alters the management. The differentiation between gastric and duodenal ulceration is not vital at this point and is often difficult to evaluate when blood clots are present in the stomach.

A. When the gastric aspiration is clear, a drip of iced milk is started via the nasogastric tube. Continued neutralization of gastric acidity is important in preventing further hemorrhage.

B. Sedation with barbiturates is vital in the management of the ulcer patient and must be carried to the point of mental obtundation to obviate the cephalic phase of gastric secretion.

C. Intramuscular anticholinergics are used in high doses to neutralize vagal activity (Pro-Banthine, 30 mg. every 3 to 4 hours).

D. If by 24 hours the bleeding has ceased or slowed significantly so that restoration of normal hemodynamics is not a problem, other diagnostic procedures are performed.

*(1)* GI series or barium enema to delineate the source of hemorrhage

*(2)* Celiac or mesenteric angiography may demonstrate a leak of contrast material into the gastrointestinal tract if bleeding is over 4 ml./minute. On occasion, less common causes of bleeding have been demonstrated by this means (small intestinal hemorrhage). In some instances, emergency arterial catheterization has been successfully employed to infuse Pitressin into the bleeding vessel, with subsequent cessation of hemorrhage. The

venous phase of the angiogram may demonstrate the portal venous system.

E. Hematocrit is followed every 8 to 12 hours during the second hospital day.

F. Stool guaiacs are performed and should demonstrate gradual diminution of bleeding. Change in character of the stool from black to dark brown is a helpful sign.

6. *Ancillary diagnostic measures* are indicated at this time, assuming qualified consultants are available who may perform them under these emergency conditions.

A. *Esophagoscopy.* In experienced hands, esophagoscopy is the most effective method of diagnosing esophageal variceal bleeding with minimal morbidity. The procedure may be carried out in a well-equipped emergency department.

B. *Sigmoidoscopy.* Sigmoidoscopy without preparation is of value in determining the character of the stool in the rectum, the character and extent of colonic bleeding and occasionally the visualization of rectal or colonic lesions. In emergency situations we prefer to use the Sims position, which is easier for the patient than the Bouie or lithotomy position.

C. *Measurement of Splenic Pulp Pressure.* In the hands of the experienced consultant, and when the differential diagnosis is critical, measurement of splenic pulp pressure will reflect portal pressure and can be performed at the bedside with minimal morbidity. Corrected pressures above 30 cm. of water strongly imply variceal hemorrhage while those below 25 cm. of water tend to rule out this source of hemorrhage. In our experience, complications of splenic tear or injury are minimal (below 5%). We prefer, however, to reserve this test for a time when the patient can be moved to the radiology department. Under the latter circumstances, the test can be combined with splenic portography for direct visualization of the portal bed and varices. Although the portal vein is not always visualized, failure to see the varices makes their presence unlikely. A radiologist experienced with splenic portography is vital.

7. If esophageal varices are suspected and the bleeding, though stabilized, persists, as indicated by continued aspiration of blood and the need for additional transfusion, the Sengstaken-Blakemore tube should be tried to control the hemorrhage.

A. The tube is introduced through the nares into the stomach and an attempt is made to aspirate the gastric contents.

B. The gastric balloon is inflated with 100 ml. of air and firm pressure is exerted at the cardio-esophageal junction. This can be accomplished by attaching a 2-lb. weight over a pulley to the tube (a 500-ml. I.V. bottle containing fluid will serve).

C. In the presence of gastric varices (a frequent cause of variceal bleeding), there will be cessation of bleeding and failure to aspirate blood from the gastric lumen.

D. Use of this tube is dangerous because of its tendency to produce gastro-esophageal erosion and the danger of filling up of the proximal esophagus with blood or secretions. A sump nasogastric tube is always used to aspirate the proximal esophagus to avoid fatal aspiration.

E. When the Sengstaken-Blakemore tube is used for more than 18 hours, a tracheostomy or endotracheal tube is passed to obviate aspiration. It may be necessary to inflate the esophageal balloon if bleeding persists.

F. Once the tube is inflated and if it is successful in producing tamponade, it is not deflated for at least 24 hours. Subsequent reinflation may be necessary.

G. Stabilization of the patient is usually achieved so that elective shunting may be performed days or weeks later with lower mortality. Emergency shunting (during active bleeding) has a mortality of over 80 per cent in our experience.

## Indications for Operation

1. *If bleeding has not stabilized* within the first treatment hour, or if the patient requires massive transfusion without evidence of stabilization of either blood pressure or bleeding, emergency operation is performed. Preparation for surgery includes rapid transfusion until a rise in central venous pressure is demonstrated and urine output is obtained. This almost always can be achieved even in the face of continued hemorrhage.

2. *If there is evidence of continual bleeding,* that is, failure of maintenance of the blood pressure and central venous pressure with transfusion in excess of 3 units/ 8 hours or 4 units/24 hours except where variceal bleeding is suspected, operation should be performed.

3. *Delayed early operation* is indicated in case of the following:

A. An ulcer crater is demonstrated on the GI series.

B. Persistent bleeding necessitates transfusion at a rate exceeding 6 units/48 hours to maintain hematocrit or vital signs.

C. There is persistent pain indicating an active penetrating ulcer with unneutralized acid.

D. Massive rebleeding occurs after it has clearly ceased.

After 48 hours, a Sippy or Andresen regimen diet is instituted.

4. *In the late phase* (after 48 hours), operation is indicated in the face of:

A. Persistent slow bleeding as manifested by continued stool guaiacs of 3 to 4+ or slowly dropping hematocrit

B. Persistent pain in the face of adequate antiulcer treatment

C. Rebleeding.

## Summary of Orders

1. Two large bore intravenous cannulae
2. Draw 10 units of blood for cross-matching.
3. Infuse plasma or albumin.
4. Insert a Foley catheter.
5. Insert a central venous line.
6. Measure blood pressure and pulse every 15 minutes until stable, then every 1/2 hour.

7. Obtain adequate history and physical examination.

8. Notify the surgeon, gastroenterologist and radiologist. Obtain consultation for esophagoscopy, splenic portography and sigmoidoscopy.

9. Consider the Sengstaken-Blakemore tube for bleeding varices.

10. Use milk drip if bleeding has ceased.

11. Repeat hematocrit every 2 hours.

12. Seconal, 100 mg. I.M. every 6 hours for sedation

13. Pro-Banthine, 30 mg. I.M. every 4 hours

## SPECIAL PROBLEMS IN THE UNDIAGNOSED BLEEDING PATIENT

### *Poor-Risk Patients*

#### Definition

Poor-risk patients are elderly patients or those with associated debilitating disease.

#### Basic Principles

Patients who have advanced arteriosclerosis or chronic renal, pulmonary or cardiac disease, etc. have borderline perfusion of vital organs, decreased oxygenation, depressed metabolism, alterations of their body fluid spaces or acid–base imbalance and therefore do not tolerate continued severe hemorrhage. Under these circumstances, indications for surgery are relaxed and *earlier* operation is frequently indicated. Mortality from severe hemorrhage is limited in most series to patients over 40 years of age, with the greatest mortality in those over 60 years of age.

#### Criteria for Diagnosis

Advanced age, electrocardiographic changes, pulmonary disease on chest x-ray, alteration of serum electrolytes or an increased blood-urea nitrogen or blood sugar are indicators of patients who fall into this category. Many of these simple tests can be performed within hours of admission to the hospital.

## Management

1. Achieve stabilization as above within 1 hour.

2. ECG

3. Chest x-ray

4. Serum electrolytes, blood-urea nitrogen, blood glucose

5. If indications of severe associated disease are present, the patient will not withstand continued bleeding or rebleeding. Operation should be performed if bleeding persists after 3 units of blood have been given or 36 hours have elapsed.

### *Severe Lower Gastrointestinal Tract Bleeding*

#### Definition

Severe lower gastrointestinal tract bleeding is massive bleeding occurring from a lesion distal to the ligament of Treitz. Ninety per cent of massive colonic hemorrhage is secondary to diverticulosis.

#### Basic Principles

Although colonic bleeding may be life-threatening, the rate of bleeding is usually slow and the duration is prolonged so that surgery is rarely necessary within the first 24 hours. The localization of the bleeding lesion at operation is more difficult in lower bowel than in gastroduodenal bleeding, and the choice of operation will depend on the location of the lesion. It is therefore desirable to obtain a barium enema and sigmoidoscopy within 48 hours so that a decision can be made before operation. With definition of the site of hemorrhage, a localized resection is adequate in colonic bleeding. Without a diagnosis, or, if multiple diverticula alone are found, subtotal colectomy with ileosigmoidostomy is our operation of choice.

#### Criteria for Diagnosis

1. There is no blood on gastric aspiration and there has been no hematemesis.

2. The bleeding is extensive from the rectum but there are no systemic signs of hypovolemia (syncope, tachycardia, etc.).

3. Brown stool can be recognized with the blood (lesion is in or distal to the left colon).

4. Sigmoidoscopy discloses a lesion.

5. Inferior and superior mesanteric angiograms are performed.

6. Barium enema is performed and will provide evidence of diverticula in 80 per cent of cases.

## Management

1. Stabilize the patient as with upper gastrointestinal tract bleeding.

2. Sigmoidoscope the patient without preparation.

3. Order angiograms to demonstrate bleeding site before barium enema.

4. Order a barium enema if the patient will tolerate it. An air-contrast study should be performed to demonstrate polyps if possible.

5. In most cases, operation will be elective since the patient usually stops bleeding.

6. If no diagnosis is apparent or can be found at emergency operation, subtotal colectomy is done.

*The Jaundiced and*
*Ascitic Patient*

## Basic Principles

Although in some series of cirrhotics, gastroduodenal ulcer bleeding is more common than variceal bleeding, in our experience, hemorrhage in the jaundiced and ascitic patient is almost always due to varices. Every possible means should be employed to avoid emergency operation since these patients are in impending hepatic failure. Many anesthetic agents markedly reduce hepatic blood flow and, when associated with hypotension or hypovolemia, result in postoperative hepatic failure. Bleeding disorders are commonly associated with severe cirrhosis, and emergency operation leaves inadequate time to prepare for the restoration of reduced clotting factors which may precipitate or prolong bleeding.

## Criteria for Diagnosis

1. Scleral icterus

2. Protuberant abdomen with fluid-wave succussion splash or shifting dullness

3. The patient may be semicomatose or may demonstrate asterixis.

## Management

1. Stabilize the patient as above.

2. Use the Sengstaken-Blakemore tube, which controls variceal hemorrhage in over 90 per cent of our patients, although gastric bleeding may resume on deflation of the balloon (gastric or esophageal) or removal of the tube.

3. Intra-arterial celiac or hepatic infusion of Pitressin has been associated with cessation of bleeding at some institutions. Catheterization is easily performed under fluoroscopic control by the Seldinger technique.

4. If bleeding can be stopped, a regimen of strict bed rest, high-caloric diet, vitamins, salt restriction, aldosterone antagonists, etc. is instituted.

5. Elective operation is performed when the jaundice and ascites have disappeared and the prothrombin time is normal.

*Aortoenteric Fistula*

## Definition

An aortoenteric fistula is bleeding from the aorta or one of its major branches into the gastrointestinal tract. This is always preceded by previous aortic surgery or aortic aneurysm.

## Basic Principles

Aortoduodenal communication, the most common aortoenteric fistula, may occur from rupture of an aneurysm into the duodenum by erosion or, from a false aneurysm developing at the upper anastomosis of an aortic graft. Although initial hemorrhage may be mild, every effort should be directed at determining if a prosthetic graft has been placed, since rapid, fatal bleeding is a common sequela of this complication. The presence of a pulsatile abdominal mass in a patient with gastrointestinal bleeding should suggest the possibility of fistulization, indicating emergency operation.

### Criteria for Diagnosis

1. History of previous aortic surgery
2. History and physical findings of an aortic aneurysm
3. Rarely penetrating trauma will antedate the bleeding episode by days or even months.

### Management

1. Stabilize the patient as above.
2. Crossmatch 10 units of blood. These patients òften have a massive exsanguination during induction of anesthesia.
3. A central venous pressure line and a Foley catheter are essential.
4. Emergency operation

## NONMASSIVE GASTROINTESTINAL BLEEDING—DIAGNOSIS UNKNOWN

### Basic Principles

A large number of systemic and gastrointestinal diseases may precipitate gastrointestinal hemorrhage. The bleeding may be acute or chronic, but, since it is not massive, there is sufficient time for a careful work-up. It is important to determine the occurrence and course of previous episodes and results of prior diagnostic tests (admissions to other hospitals). The most life-threatening conditions are those associated with defects in the blood clotting mechanism and gastrointestinal lesions. Adequate hematologic consultation and scanning tests, including platelet count, prothrombin time and fibrinogen levels, will be helpful. Upper and lower gastrointestinal series will help diagnose most lesions. The chance of making the diagnosis at operation if all tests are negative is under 10 per cent.

Continued monitoring of hematocrit and occult blood in the stool will indicate if bleeding is persisting, subsiding or increasing. Occasionally, mild gastrointestinal bleeding may terminate in a massive bleeding episode. If there is doubt about the degree of bleeding, it is safest to treat the patient as a massive bleeder until he is clearly stable.

### Criteria for Diagnosis

1. Complete history and physical examination
2. Sigmoidoscopy
3. Radiographic Examinations
    A. Upper GI series
    B. Small bowel follow-through
    C. Barium enema
4. Prothrombin time, prothrombin consumption, partial thromboplastin time, fibrinogen levels, clotting time and evidence of clot lysis
5. Hematologic consultation for special studies
6. Fluorescein string test. This is performed by the passage of a string labeled with distance markers through the mouth and the injection of fluorescein intravenously. Staining of the string with fluorescein will suggest the level of the lesion.
7. A similar test is done by the injection of radioactive-chromium-labeled red cells into the patient and sampling at different levels with a long intestinal tube.

Both this test and the tests in paragraph 6 are not done routinely since yields of positive results have been below 5 per cent in our experience.

8. Celiac angiography with demonstration of a leak of contrast material into the bowel has been successful in the more massive bleeders (4 ml./minute) and unsuccessful in the others. Occasionally early venous pickup of the dye has given a clue to the level of bleeding (vessel of involvement).
9. Fiberoptic examinations of the colon and stomach are being used more frequently and may be of value, particularly in small colonic lesions now beyond the reach of a standard sigmoidoscope.

## Management

1. The patient is monitored by measurement of vital signs until stable.
2. Daily stool guaiac (occult blood) and hematocrit
3. Complete diagnostic work-up
4. Obtain special consultations.
5. If no diagnosis is obtained, avoid operation unless bleeding persists or recurs.

# GASTROINTESTINAL BLEEDING— DIAGNOSIS KNOWN

## DUODENAL ULCER

## Definition

A duodenal ulcer is mucosal erosion of the duodenum, usually associated with high gastric acidity.

## Basic Principles

The ulceration usually occurs in the first part of the duodenum. Anterior ulcers may bleed but frequently perforate if they are deeply penetrating. Posterior ulcers often overlie the gastroduodenal artery, and perforation into this vessel is associated with hemorrhage. Clotting of the vessel is the rule, so that bleeding may be continuous or intermittent. Dissolution of the clot due to continued bathing of the ulcer with hydrochloric acid leads to continued massive hemorrhage. In minor bleeding episodes, neutralization of gastric acidity by specific treatment can be obtained before the hemorrhage becomes life-threatening, and these episodes often resolve without difficulty.

In bleeding from the main gastroduodenal artery, hemorrhage may be so severe as to preclude attempts at non-operative therapy.

## Criteria for Diagnosis

1. Previous history of ulcer disease proven on x-ray
2. Present or previous symptoms of epigastric burning or pain occurring 1 to 1½ hours after meals and at night, classically relieved by ingestion of antacids or food

3. An upper GI series demonstrating deformity or crater formation in the duodenal bulb. Interpretation by an experienced radiologist is helpful.
4. Gastroscopy performed by an experienced endoscopist may reveal the bleeding ulcer. However, this is not generally used for duodenal ulcer disease.

## Management

1. Management of the massive bleeding duodenal ulcer is the same as indicated for massive hemorrhage, page 182.
2. For persistent or intermittent bleeding, neutralization of gastric acidity is attempted by the use of a continual drip of iced milk, supplemented with antacids.
3. For the mild bleeder, oral intake is started utilizing an Andresen or similar regimen with multiple feedings of milk or cream, with the use of antacids interspersed throughout.
4. Sedation of the patient is helpful during the bleeding episode in order to prevent apprehension during the multiple manipulations which are done by the physician and nursing personnel. Phenobarbital in a dose of 60 mg. every 6 hours is helpful, but this dose should be increased to the point of mental obtundation in the severe bleeder.
5. Regular oral intake should be divided into multiple feedings throughout the day as tolerated by the patient. An attempt should be made to avoid long periods without something in the stomach to neutralize gastric acidity. Antacids can be used intermittently for this purpose.
6. Anticholinergics are used frequently for vagolytic activity and reduction of the cephalic phase of gastric secretion. Pro-Banthine in a dose of 30 mg. 3 times a day may be beneficial and should be used to the point where dryness of the mouth and mucous membranes is noticed by the patient.
7. Hematocrits, stool guaiacs and repeated evaluations of vital signs and the overall condition of the patient should be monitored frequently throughout the day

during the bleeding episode. As the bleeding subsides, daily hematocrits and stool guaiacs will indicate persistent slow bleeding which may represent a significant problem during this hospitalization. The appearance of a second massive hemorrhage following an interim period of quiescence is an ominous sign, usually considered an indication for immediate operation.

8. If an upper GI series has not been performed or was inadequate, it is ordered or repeated at this time.

9. Analysis of total overnight gastric acid production as well as response to Histalog may be performed during the quiescent phase in order to ascertain the possible presence of a gastrin-producing tumor.

10. Consultation is usually indicated at this time in order to determine whether operative or nonoperative treatment is best suited to the definitive management of the ulcer diathesis.

## GASTRIC ULCER

### Definition

A gastric ulcer is mucosal erosion of the stomach, usually unrelated to gastric acid levels. Ulceration of the stomach may be secondary to several known and unknown causes.

### Classification

Among the etiologies considered are a breakdown of the mucosal protective barrier by alteration of gastric mucus production, changes in the vascular supply to the mucosa, hyperacidity in association with duodenal ulcer, gastric stasis secondary to duodenal ulcer with obstruction, reflux of bile, or in association with head injuries, intracranial tumors or burns (*see* Stress Ulcers, below).

### Basic Principles

The bleeding from gastric ulceration is due to mucosal vessels, submucosal arterioles or, when the ulcer is deeply penetrating, due to ulceration of major branches to the stomach such as the left gastric vessels. The prognosis of hemorrhage is related to the size of the eroded vessel, and the overall mortality for massive hemorrhage from gastric ulcer is higher than equivalent hemorrhage from duodenal ulcer. This is due to the fact that only rarely is gastric hyperacidity a primary cause and treatment directed at neutralization of gastric acid is consequantly often unsuccessful.

### Criteria for Diagnosis

1. A previous history proven by gastrointestinal x-rays demonstrating the gastric ulcer

2. A history compatible with postprandial pain occasionally relieved by the use of antacids. Although hyperacidity is not a primary cause of most gastric ulcers, the pain secondary to ulceration is accentuated by levels of acid produced by secretagogues and neutralization often produces relief of pain.

3. Gastroscopy demonstrating the ulcer should be performed by an experienced gastroscopist.

4. Upper GI series demonstrating gastric ulceration. This may be difficult during the acute bleeding episode if large clots are present in the stomach. On these occasions, gastric lavage through an Ewald tube may successfully prepare the stomach for diagnosis by barium-contrast x-ray.

### Management

1. For massive hemorrhage from gastric ulcer, the treatment is similar to that noted above.

2. For less severe hemorrhage, monitor daily hematocrits and stool guaiacs as for duodenal ulcer.

3. After confirmation by GI series, early operation is recommended, preferably when the bleeding has ceased but during the same hospitalization.

4. An attempt at neutralization of gastric acid by use of antacids and divided diet

(6 small feedings) is often used for gastric ulcers and will promote healing in some small ulcers.

5. With small ulcers of the stomach, a nonoperative treatment may be used, but repeat GI series should be obtained in 4 weeks in order to confirm healing. Failure to heal is an indication for operation.

6. Operation for gastric ulceration is usually recommended for the following reasons:

A. Healing is by mucosal coverage of the ulcer bed and does not involve the full thickness of the gastric wall. Recurrence of ulceration is therefore common and operation is necessary in over half of patients with gastric ulcer originally treated nonoperatively.

B. Malignancy cannot be ruled out and there is a 10 per cent error in the diagnosis of benign gastric ulcer.

C. Ulcers appearing benign but which are in fact malignant have a survival rate threefold higher when adequately excised than those lesions which are obviously malignant.

D. Complications of gastric ulcer such as perforation, bleeding and obstruction have a higher mortality than the same complications of duodenal ulcer.

E. Operation for gastric ulcer is uniformly successful in relieving the symptoms. It is technically easier and with a lower mortality than a similar operation for duodenal ulcer, since the duodenum is free of disease. Recurrence of ulceration is unusual following gastrectomy for gastric ulcer.

## STRESS ULCERS

### Definition

A stress ulcer is a mucosal erosion occurring in the stomach or the duodenum, associated with sepsis, severe trauma, intracranial tumors or injury and burns. The etiology is unclear.

### Basic Principles

Stress ulcers are rarely seen initially in the emergency department since they usually occur later in the patient's course. They may be associated with postoperative sepsis and are occasionally seen with other conditions. The ulcerations may be single or multiple and located either in the stomach or duodenum. Bleeding may be massive or mild and is associated with a high mortality due to the presence of the primary disease. As noted above, the etiology is unknown, although some investigators feel that back-diffusion of hydrogen ions across the gastric mucous membrane is in some way related to the breakdown of the mucosal barrier. In those conditions frequently associated with stress ulceration, the prophylactic use of continuous antacid therapy is recommended.

### Criteria for Diagnosis

1. Massive upper gastrointestinal tract bleeding occurring in a severely ill patient either postoperatively, posttrauma or in association with sepsis, intracranial tumors or burns

2. Gastroscopy will frequently demonstrate multiple ulcerations.

3. GI series is usually unsuccessful in demonstrating the lesions since they are frequently superficial and multiple.

### Management

1. A high index of suspicion should be maintained in all critically ill patients, especially those in the specific groups who may develop these stress ulcerations.

2. Continual use of intragastric antacids is recommended as a prophylactic procedure in those patients with postoperative sepsis or severe injury.

3. Nonoperative or operative treatment will depend on the degree of hemorrhage and whether it can be controlled. There is considerable feeling among surgeons that early operation will produce a lower overall mortality in these patients. There is, however, a reluctance to reoperate on patients having undergone serious

procedures in association with postoperative sepsis.

4. Management is as for acute hemorrhage as noted above (p. 182) and is to include careful monitoring of fluids, blood, venous pressure, hematocrits and stool guaiacs, the use of a nasogastric tube to determine continued bleeding and response of the patient to transfusion.

5. If it is apparent that hemorrhage is massive, early operation should be performed, and the operation recommended is a subtotal or near-total gastrectomy. Lesser procedures involving vagotomy and drainage have been associated with rebleeding in a large percentage of patients.

## ESOPHAGEAL VARICES

### Definition

An esophageal varix is variceal enlargement of the veins in the submucosa of the esophagus, usually secondary to increase in portal venous pressure, with ulceration of the overlying mucosa permitting hemorrhage.

### Basic Principles

Esophageal varices secondary to increases in the portal venous pressure occur in association with diseases of the liver and hepatic circulation. Hepatic vein thrombosis usually produces ascites rather than esophageal variceal bleeding, since the liver is an expansile organ which can retain a significant amount of delivered blood. With certain parenchymal diseases such as schistosomiasis, variceal hemorrhage can occur. The most common cause is portal cirrhosis secondary to ingestion of large amounts of alcohol over a long period of time. The alcohol has a direct toxic effect on the liver cells, with secondary scarring and compression of the portal circulation within the liver parenchyma. Portal hypertension occurs and values exceeding 30 cm. of water pressure in the portal circulation can be associated with significant hemorrhage. Extrahepatic block of the portal circulation can also be associated

with variceal bleeding. Veins draining the esophagus and upper portion of the stomach empty into the coronary vein, which then empties into the portal vein or the most distal portion of the splenic vein just prior to its junction with the superior mesenteric vein to form the portal vein.

Definitive treatment for massive hemorrhage entails the performance of a shunting procedure which reduces the pressure in the portal system by anastomosing it to the systemic venous circulation via either the renal vein, superior mesenteric vein or directly to the inferior vena cava. This should be associated with a significant drop in the portal pressure to levels at which bleeding is unlikely to occur. Selection of patients for performance of shunts depends on the degree of liver damage, since the overall prognosis of the patient often is dependent on the disease with its extensive parenchymal hepatic damage rather than on the bleeding. It is our policy to perform shunt procedures only on those patients that demonstrate active variceal hemorrhage, avoiding prophylactic shunting in those patients who have portal hypertension and cirrhosis without bleeding.

### Criteria for Diagnosis

1. History of previous liver disease
2. History of substantial alcoholic intake over a long period of time
3. Physical examination demonstrating evidence of collateral circulation (caput medusae); the presence of hepatosplenomegaly, liver palms, spider angiomas, jaundice, ascites, etc.
4. Esophagoscopy by an experienced endoscopist may demonstrate the presence of varices in 80 per cent of patients with the disease.
5. Esophagogram included in an upper GI series may demonstrate the presence of varices at the time of bleeding in over half of the patients.
6. Direct puncture of the spleen and measurement of splenic pulp pressure reflects portal hypertension directly after

correction for the height of the needle above the portal vein. The normal portal pressure should be very slightly above systemic venous pressure. Levels over 30 cm. of water are often associated with hemorrhage.

7. Direct injection of dye through the splenic pulp will yield a splenic portogram which may directly demonstrate the presence of varices by reflux of the dye through the coronary circulation around the esophagus and upper stomach.

8. A Sengstaken-Blakemore tube has been used as a diagnostic test for patients with upper gastrointestinal tract bleeding, since those bleeding from the lower portion of the stomach or duodenum will continue to bleed through the central lumen of the tube with the gastric balloon inflated. This test is not absolutely diagnostic since it depends on correct placement of the tube and adequate inflation of the gastric balloon producing sufficient compression to stop the variceal hemorrhage.

9. Tests of liver function may confirm the presence of significant liver disease in association with upper gastrointestinal tract bleeding. The incidence of gastro-duodenal ulceration is higher in patients with portal cirrhosis, so that the presence of liver disease *per se* does not rule out this possibility. It is extremely unusual, however, to have gastroduodenal ulceration as the cause of massive hemorrhage in patients with jaundice or ascites, who are almost always bleeding from esophageal or gastric varices. The Bromsulphalein test will be abnormal in any condition with decreased liver perfusion and, therefore, is unreliable in the bleeding patient.

## Management

1. Treatment for massive esophageal variceal bleeding is noted above, page 184.

2. Where liver decompensation is a significant factor, early operation is avoided by the use of supportive measures, including blood, parenteral fluids, the Sengstaken-Blakemore tube for variceal occlusion, complete bed rest, Aldactone and salt restriction for control of ascites, high-caloric diet, etc.

3. Careful monitoring of the patient is vital for survival, as noted above.

4. In the presence of ascites and jaundice, operation is restricted to those patients who may be dying from massive hemorrhage. Early operation may be performed in those nonjaundiced, nonascitic patients with a diagnosis of portal cirrhosis in whom the site of bleeding is unclear.

5. Choice of operation depends on the experience of the operating surgeon. It may include:

A. Emergency shunting of the portal circulation to the systemic circulation

B. Ligation of the esophageal varices directly through a transesophageal and gastric approach as a preliminary stage prior to definitive shunting

C. Upper gastrointestinal devascularization by ligation and division of the blood supply of the lower esophagus and upper stomach

D. A series of specialized shunting procedures other than the standard portacaval, mesocaval or splenorenal shunts

All emergency procedures are associated with a high mortality, usually exceeding 50 per cent and over 80 per cent in the experience of our institution.

## GASTRITIS

### Definition

Gastritis is multiple erosions of the stomach secondary to the corrosive effect of chemicals or a breakdown of the gastric defensive barrier by the use of particular drugs.

### Basic Principles

Gastritis may be caused by the ingestion of toxic chemicals such as alcohol, specific caustics, cleaning fluid, etc. In addition, the use of certain drugs such as aspirin and corticosteroids has been associated with increased incidence of gastritis. It has been hypothesized that the aspirin produces a defect in the gastric mucus which prevents adequate protection of the gastric lining from the normal secretion of hydrochloric acid and pepsin. Back-diffusion of hydrogen ions may be an important contributing factor.

## Criteria for Diagnosis

1. A history of ingestion of large amounts of aspirin, the continued administration of corticosteroids or an acute history of ingestion of a caustic chemical or alcohol
2. Hematemesis and severe vomiting
3. Previous history of similar attacks
4. Presence of blood in the gastric aspirate
5. An upper gastrointestinal series may demonstrate the diffuse superficial mucosal ulcerations and the lack of an associated deep ulcer or the presence of varices.
6. Gastroscopy using the fiberoptic technique will reveal the mucosal ulcerations in most patients.

## Management

The specific treatment of erosive gastritis depends on the exact etiology.

1. Those cases associated with the ingestion of caustic chemicals should be treated with specific antidotes directed at neutralizing the effects of these chemicals on the stomach.
2. Lavage of the stomach should be reserved for the experienced surgeon, since very caustic materials may be associated with perforations of the stomach and lavage can be dangerous under these circumstances.
3. In the vast majority of cases, alcohol is the agent responsible, and withdrawal of the agent, associated with the use of gastric aspiration of acid, usually produces spontaneous relief of the symptoms.
4. Rarely the hemorrhage may be massive enough to warrant the treatment noted above for massive upper intestinal hemorrhage.

5. In those cases where the patient is stable and not vomiting, and where bleeding is not massive, the immediate institution of a milk drip with the use of antacids will successfully resolve the situation.
6. Occasionally elderly patients using large doses of aspirin present with massive gastrointestinal hemorrhage which subsides spontaneously on withdrawal of the drug.
7. Supportive treatment should be directed at restoring blood volume, maintaining stability of the patient by the use of parenteral fluids, early nasogastric aspiration followed by oral antacids and allowing sufficient time for the hemorrhage to stop.

## HIATAL HERNIA

### Definition

A hiatal hernia is herniation of a portion of the stomach through the diaphragmatic hiatus (sliding esophageal hernia) or through a separate para-esophageal defect in the diaphragm, with the result that a portion of the stomach is displaced into the thoracic cavity.

### Basic Principles

Hiatal hernias may be of the sliding or para-esophageal type. Gastrointestinal bleeding in association with the more common sliding hernia is never seen without the association of concomitant esophagitis and reflux. Para-esophageal hernias may bleed when the herniated portion of the stomach has compromised its blood supply or if an associated ulcer is present in that portion of the stomach.

### Criteria for Diagnosis

1. A history of recurrent reflux with symptoms of acid esophagitis (heartburn particularly related to position such as lying flat in bed or stooping)
2. An upper gastrointestinal series will usually demonstrate the presence of the hiatal hernia when Trendelenburg views are taken to see the fundus of the stomach.

The use of concomitant abdominal pressure will also yield a high incidence of positive findings of hiatal hernia in these studies.

3. Esophagoscopy is used to view the gastroesophageal junction and associated esophagitis. Frequently biopsy of the esophagus is necessary to document very severe esophagitis which may not be clearly evident on esophagoscopy. The esophagus may be shortened so that the gastroesophageal junction is reached before the normal level of 40 cm. from the upper incisors. Direct visualization of reflux into the esophagus can often be seen at esophagoscopy. Rigid tube esophagoscopy will be of little value in patients with paraesophageal hernias since the gastroesophageal junction is in the normal position in these patients.

## Management

The treatment of hiatal hernia depends on the underlying symptoms. Bleeding is usually mild, and hiatal hernia represents a very rare cause of massive hemorrhage in spite of the common occurrence of the disorder. Initial treatment is directed at neutralization of gastric acidity by use of milk and antacids with multiple feedings or a Sippy-type diet. When the initial symptoms are controlled, diagnosis is confirmed and an attempt is made to evaluate the presence and extent of associated reflux.

Definitive repair consists of restoring the normal position of the cardio-esophageal junction below the diaphragm and ensuring its position by adding a fundal plication (Nissen or Belsey).

## GASTROESOPHAGEAL LACERATION

## Definition

A gastroesophageal laceration is a tear in the lower portion of the esophagus or upper portion of the stomach, usually secondary to increased intragastric pressure during the act of vomiting.

## Basic Principles

Tears of the lower esophagus or upper stomach have been referred to in literature under various eponyms, the most common of which is the Mallory-Weiss syndrome. The tears are caused by massive increase of intragastric pressure during vomiting, especially after eating large meals. They are frequently located on the lesser curvature of the upper portion of the stomach in the vicinity of the left gastric vein, which may bleed massively if injured. Unless considered preoperatively, the tear may be missed entirely at operation. A long gastrotomy is necessary to visualize this portion of the stomach, with inversion of the esophagus into the lumen of the stomach in order to see the area for repair.

## Criteria for Diagnosis

1. Classical history of vomiting of non-bloody material followed by hematemesis should lead the examiner to suspect this diagnosis.

2. Upper gastrointestinal x-rays usually do not demonstrate the lesion successfully. We have had experience with large tears of the esophagus or stomach without any extravasation of Gastrografin or barium on upper GI series.

3. Endoscopy may be equally unsuccessful in visualizing this area of the stomach.

4. Recent use of celiac angiography has successfully delineated the bleeding point in the vicinity of the upper portion of the lesser curvature of the stomach, confirming the diagnosis.

## Management

1. Treatment is directed at the correction of the blood volume deficits as noted above in the handling of the upper intestinal bleeder.

2. Occasionally the use of the Sengstaken-Blakemore tube with inflation of the gastric balloon has produced sufficient tamponade to control bleeding in this syndrome.

3. If the patient is stabilized with the use of supportive measures, no operative treatment is necessary.

4. The associated finding of upper abdominal peritoneal signs indicates free perforation and necessitates early operation.

5. In most cases, operation is reserved for those patients who cannot be controlled nonoperatively, i.e., in whom bleeding is massive.

6. Operation usually consists of gastrotomy and oversewing of the gastroesophageal tear and associated vessels. The prognosis is good if the diagnosis is made early. In those cases where the diagnosis is missed, disastrous postoperative bleeding frequently occurs.

## DUODENAL DIVERTICULA

### Definition

A duodenal diverticulum is an outpocketing of the full thickness of the duodenum (true diverticulum) or the mucosa of the duodenum through a defect in the duodenal wall (false diverticulum).

### Basic Principles

Duodenal diverticula are commonly found on upper gastrointestinal x-rays and are usually asymptomatic. Rare cases of hemorrhage from duodenal diverticula have been diagnosed and treated. These diverticula occur commonly in two locations. The first is on the medial aspect of the second portion of the duodenum buried in the head of the pancreas. This particular location is extremely dangerous to handle operatively, leading to major complications (i.e., pancreatic fistula, injury of the common bile duct, etc.). The other common location is on the posterior surface of the duodenum along the intraduodenal portion of the common bile duct, in which case a common wall may exist between the common bile duct and the diverticulum. These are usually asymptomatic and are diagnosed occasionally at operations involving the biliary tract with instrumentation of the common bile duct

during which the diverticulum may be perforated.

### Criteria for Diagnosis

1. Upper gastrointestinal x-rays are the only definitive method of diagnosing these usually asymptomatic lesions.

2. They may be suspected in the presence of repeated undiagnosed gastrointestinal hemorrhage and in rare cases they represent the etiology of such a condition.

### Management

Surgical management of these diverticula should be avoided under most circumstances, and all attempts at supportive nonsurgical treatment of upper gastrointestinal bleeding from these sources should be carried out. On rare occasions, recurrent hemorrhage necessitates operation with a direct attack requiring resection. It should be recognized that the mortality of such an operation may be high and this should temper the surgeon's aggressiveness.

## SMALL INTESTINAL TUMORS

### Definition

Tumors of the small intestine are neoplastic growths in the wall or mucosal surface of the small intestine.

### Basic Principles

These lesions occurring in the small bowel are most commonly of the lymphoma group or carcinoids. Primary cancers of the small bowel are extremely rare, and those lesions proving to be carcinomas are often metastatic from other areas. Bleeding from small intestinal tumors is rare, the most common presentation being intermittent obstruction due to intussusception.

### Criteria for Diagnosis

1. Small bowel gastrointestinal series. These lesions may be small and they are difficult to detect.

2. Those lesions producing bleeding are often of the angioma group and do not usually present as space-occupying defects. These lesions may be multiple throughout the small intestine, and the diagnosis may be impossible to make without an operation.

3. A search should be made for the presence of angiomas elsewhere on the mucous membranes of the patient.

4. Use of special tests for the diagnosis of the level of gastrointestinal bleeding such as radioactive-chromium labeling of the blood with pickup by a long intestinal tube, the use of a fluorescein dye picked up in a similar manner, etc. have rarely been successful in our experience.

5. The use of mesenteric artery angiography may be successful if the bleeding is of sufficient magnitude to demonstrate leakage of the dye into the lumen of the small intestine.

## Management

Although this is an extremely rare cause of massive hemorrhage, it may be responsible for repeated milder types of gastrointestinal bleeding. In the presence of angiomas elsewhere in the body, an attempt may be made at definitive bowel resection. These lesions are often multiple throughout the small intestine, however, and large resections should be reserved for the most serious cases. If the tumor can be diagnosed on x-ray, resection is the treatment of choice.

## MECKEL'S DIVERTICULUM

### Definition

Meckel's diverticulum is a true diverticulum of the distal ileum, representing a remnant of the omphalomesenteric duct or yolk sac.

### Basic Principles

Bleeding from Meckel's diverticulum in the adult is a very rare cause of gastrointestinal hemorrhage. The presenting complaint usually involves intestinal obstruction, with a loop of bowel caught between the obliterated omphalomesenteric duct to the umbilicus and the diverticulum. On rare occasions symptomatic inflammation of the diverticulum may occur, simulating acute appendicitis. It also may be the site of ectopic gastric mucosa or pancreas (Meckel's diverticulum in children is discussed in Chap. 36, Pediatric Surgery).

### Criteria for Diagnosis

X-rays of the small intestine may reveal an outpocketing in the distal ileum. Rarely these may contain pancreatic rests or carcinoid tumors which may present with bleeding or other symptoms. The diagnosis is otherwise made at operation.

### Management

Treatment is the same as for other causes of massive intestinal hemorrhage. The lesion should be searched for at operation, especially when a definitive cause of the bleeding cannot be located preoperatively.

## CANCER OF THE COLON

### Definition

Cancer of the colon is a malignant growth involving any segment of the colon or rectum.

### Basic Principles

Cancer of the colon or rectum often presents with gastrointestinal hemorrhage, manifested by bright-red rectal bleeding. Seventy-five per cent of these lesions are within view of the sigmoidoscope and this, therefore, is a vital examination in all patients with rectal bleeding. Usually these lesions do not bleed massively; therefore, supportive treatment will allow sufficient time for a diagnosis to be made.

### Criteria for Diagnosis

1. Rectal examination
2. Sigmoidoscopic examination
3. A history of recent change in bowel

habits or the chronic history of weight loss and intermittent abdominal pain with or without rectal bleeding

4. Occasionally an abdominal mass may be palpated.

5. Barium enema examination

6. Rarely the diagnosis is made at operation. In the vast majority of cases, preoperative diagnosis can be easily ascertained by examinations.

## Management

1. The treatment for massive hemorrhage is as noted above, page 182.

2. Minor degrees of rectal bleeding can be handled with supportive treatment directed toward re-establishing the patient's blood volume and thereby allowing deliberate evaluation to make a preoperative diagnosis.

3. As with all lesions of the colon, proper preoperative preparation of the colon is necessary, involving cleansing enemas and the establishment of a low residue of material in the colon. Occasionally, the use of intestinal antibiotics is required prior to resection.

4. Definitive treatment involves wide resection of the tumor and its lymph-node bearing mesentery.

5. On rare occasions in elderly or debilitated patients, fulguration of the lesion from the rectum can be performed rather than definitive resection.

## POLYPS OF THE COLON AND RECTUM

### Definition

Polyps of the colon or rectum are benign neoplastic growths of the mucosa of the colon or rectum.

### Classification

Colonic and rectal polyps can be divided into two main groups: adenomatous polyps and villous adenomas. These lesions may be multiple or single and may be associated with carcinomas of the colon and rectum.

## Basic Principles

Because of the variety and multiplicity of these lesions, a complete evaluation of the entire colon prior to definitive treatment is necessary. Varying opinions exist as to the type of treatment used for these lesions.

## Criteria for Diagnosis

1. A history of bright-red rectal bleeding or differentiation of the blood from surrounding stool indicates a lesion on the left side of the colon or rectum.

2. Rarely these lesions may extrude through the anus if they are present on a long stalk.

3. Rectal examination on every patient

4. Sigmoidoscopic examination is vital because the majority of lesions are located within 25 cm. of the anus.

5. Barium enema examination should be performed and should include an evacuation study of the colon followed by air-contrast visualization. These special studies will delineate the mucosa of the colon and small lesions. It is necessary to have the colon properly cleansed in order to obviate confusion of the lesions with fecal matter.

6. Use of the fiberoptic colonoscope has facilitated visualization of longer segments of the colon and made the diagnosis of colonic polyps easier.

7. The presence of large quantities of mucus may indicate an underlying villous adenoma.

8. Intermittent diarrhea may be a heralding sign of colonic polyp.

## Management

1. A massive hemorrhage is rare with colonic polyps but, if present, should be treated as noted above, page 182.

2. Supportive treatment is advisable in order to allow sufficient time for thorough examination of the colon in order to delineate all associated lesions and polyps.

3. Adenomatous polyps larger than 2 cm. in size are best treated by excision. This can be performed through the

sigmoidoscope if the lesions are located below the peritoneal reflection. For those lesions above the peritoneal reflection, it is safer to perform transabdominal excision.

4. As with all colonic operations, proper preoperative preparation of the colon is vital.

5. Villous adenomas of the colon and rectum are associated with a high incidence of cancer. These may be *in situ* carcinomas or early mucosal lesions as well as infiltrating carcinomas. For those lesions not infiltrating the muscle of the colon or rectum, wide local excision is usually adequate. Where colonic wall infiltration is evident, the lesions should be treated as carcinomas, including abdominal perineal resection if necessary.

6. Patients with solitary lesions smaller than 1.5 cm. in size may be observed intermittently with repeated sigmoidoscopic and barium enema examinations since they are unlikely to have a cancer. The incidence of cancer in lesions of this type is lower than the mortality of colonic resection.

7. Multiple polyps of the colon occasionally require wide resection of portions of the colon, up to and including total proctocolectomy.

8. The association of polyps with mucosal pigmentation represents a syndrome known as Peutz Jeghers disease. Polyps of this type may be present anywhere in the small intestine, colon or rectum and represent hamartomas rather than neoplastic growths. These are benign lesions and may be treated by local excision if they are symptomatic. The incidence of malignancy is negligible.

## DIVERTICULOSIS

### Definition

Diverticulosis represents false outpocketings of the colon without associated inflammation.

### Basic Principles

Diverticulosis is more likely to be associated with massive hemorrhage than diverticulitis. Erosion of underlying vessels can occur and may be the initial presenting complaint of the syndrome. Rarely the bleeding is of sufficient magnitude to warrant emergency colectomy. In most cases, with supportive therapy sufficient time is gained to allow definitive diagnosis.

### Criteria for Diagnosis

1. Repeated episodes of rectal bleeding
2. The presence of massive hemorrhage from the rectum without other lesions present.
3. Barium enema demonstrating diverticula of the colon in the absence of other lesions. Unfortunately, the barium enema examination often fails to delineate the diverticulum which may be bleeding.
4. Inferior or superior mesenteric artery angiography has been successful in demonstrating a leakage of dye into the portion of the colon in which the bleeding diverticulum is located.
5. Sigmoidoscopic examination usually reveals blood coming from above the sigmoidoscope. Rarely are the diverticula visualized.
6. The bleeding is usually short-lived, allowing time for a definitive diagnosis to be made.

### Management

1. On rare occasions massive hemorrhage entails emergency operation. If the bleeding diverticula cannot be easily located, the treatment of choice is a subtotal colectomy with ileoproctostomy.
2. Provide supportive treatment to reestablish adequate blood volume.
3. If the bleeding is mild or if this represents the first episode and barium enema fails to demonstrate significant inflammation or other lesions of the colon, operation may not be indicated. A considerable degree of surgical judgment is necessary in order to select those patients who will benefit from colectomy. If the exact location of the bleeding lesion can be

determined, a partial colectomy may be successful.

4. The presence of persistent deformity of the colon or an area which cannot be clearly differentiated from carcinoma is an indication for operative intervention.

## RECTAL HEMORRHOIDS

### Definition

Rectal hemorrhoids are variceal enlargements of the rectal veins.

### Classification

These venous enlargements are located either within the anus, at the dentate line or immediately above the dentate line within the rectum. These are respectively known as external, mixed or internal hemorrhoids.

### Basic Principles

The etiology of rectal hemorrhoids is not known, although they are occasionally associated with alterations of the venous pressure within the abdomen (i.e., portal cirrhosis). They may be secondary to chronic constipation or excessive straining at the stool. They occur at all ages and frequently are associated with minor rectal bleeding. In every case it is vital to rule out other associated colonic or rectal lesions prior to definitive treatment. The frequent occurrence of hemorrhoids does not mitigate against the concurrent presence of a carcinoma of the colon or rectum.

### Critera for Diagnosis

1. Rectal pain associated with blood-streaking on the toilet tissue or stool
2. Previous history of known hemorrhoids
3. Rectal examination fails in most cases to delineate the hemorrhoidal mass unless thrombosis of the veins has occurred.
4. Sigmoidoscopic or anoscopic examination will confirm the diagnosis.
5. Associated lesions must be ruled out by means of sigmoidoscopy and barium enema.

6. Occasionally the lesions may be seen protruding from the anus (prolapsed hemorrhoids).

### Management

1. Rectal hemorrhoids rarely cause massive gastrointestinal hemorrhage, although on some occasions bleeding may fill the entire colon, giving the impression on sigmoidoscopic examination that the lesion is situated above the sigmoidoscope.
2. Supportive therapy should be directed at reducing the pain and discomfort if the hemorrhoids are thrombosed.
3. Hot sitz baths are extremely helpful in the emergency treatment of prolapsed or thrombosed hemorrhoids associated with bleeding.
4. Emergency excision of hemorrhoids is rarely indicated but can be performed without significant difficulty.
5. Evacuation of a clot from a thrombosed hemorrhoid under local anesthesia will yield immediate specific relief of pain.
6. Nonoperative treatment of hemorrhoids by sclerosing agents has been successful in our experience.
7. Hemorrhoidectomy is to be recommended for most lesions that have been bleeding.

## FISSURE OF THE ANUS (FISSURE IN ANO)

### Definition

A fissure of the anus is a break in the skin of the anus with associated inflammation, occasionally associated with blood-streaking on the toilet paper.

### Basic Principles

Anal fissure is associated with bleeding on rare occasions, except in infants, and is always associated with rectal pain. This is accentuated at the time of bowel movements and may lead to sufficient sphincter spasm to produce constipation and subsequent formation of associated hemorrhoids.

## Criteria for Diagnosis

1. Rectal examination reveals severe rectal pain in a particular quadrant of the anus.

2. Anoscopic examination specifically delineates the lesion.

3. Marked sphincter spasm may prevent adequate rectal examination.

4. In some cases examination may be deferred until local anesthesia can be utilized to provide sphincter relaxation.

## Management

This is rarely a cause of massive hemorrhage. Treatment is directed at symptomatic relief, including the use of sitz baths and suppositories to relieve the associated pain. Rarely, it may be necessary to surgically divide the sphincter in order to allow sufficient relaxation for healing to occur.

# 16. INTESTINAL OBSTRUCTION

*Clarence Dennis,* M.D.

## Definitions

1. *Simple obstruction* is a term applied to obstruction of the lumen of the gut without vascular compromise.

2. *Strangulating obstruction* is obstruction of the lumen of the gut with associated obstruction of the venous or arterial connections of the involved intestine or of both.

3. *Strangling obstruction with necrosis of the gut* refers to the situation in which strangulation has lasted long enough to cause gangrene of the gut. If the vascular compromise is of high degree, this occurs in 3 to 4 hours as a rule. It occurs more quickly in pure venous obstruction than in pure arterial obstruction.

4. *Small bowel obstruction* is that in which the point of obstruction lies between the ileocecal junction and the duodenum.

5. *Large bowel obstruction* is that in which the point of obstruction lies in the colon or rectum. (The large bowel includes the colon and rectum.)

6. *Paralytic* or *adynamic ileus* is a condition in which impairment of function of the muscle of the bowel wall underlies failure of the gut to transport the contents.

7. *Incarcerated hernia* means hernia which is irreducible.

8. *Strangulated hernia* means hernia which compromises the blood supply to the intestine.

9. *Closed-loop obstruction* is one in which a segment of intestine is blocked at two points, thus eliminating the safety valve of removal of increasing content by vomiting.

## Mechanisms of Obstruction

### Small Bowel Obstruction

1. Intestinal adhesions, usually secondary to a previous operation, but occasionally due to an inflammatory process such as a ruptured ulcer, appendicitis or diverticulitis with extension

2. Adhesive bands under which or about which segments of gut may become engaged

3. Hernias, either external or internal. Internal hernia is far less common than external hernia. Internal hernias include paraduodenal (right or left) hernia, hernias through defects in other mesentery (for instance, mesosigmoid) and diaphragmatic hernia. External hernias most likely to produce intestinal obstruction are femoral and inguinal, but ventral and spigelian hernias are also offenders.

4. Herniation through iatrogenic defects, such as incarceration lateral to a colostomy or ileostomy or beneath the jejunal segment after gastrojejunostomy

5. Volvulus of the midgut is seen primarily in the neonatal period and may, if uncorrected, lead within hours to gangrene of essentially the whole jejunum and ileum. This is covered in Chapter 36, Pediatric Surgical Emergencies, as are atresia and stenosis in the newborn.

6. Intussusception of the idiopathic type is seen almost exclusively in the first two years of life, especially in males. Intussusception occurring in later life is nearly always associated with a lesion at the apex of the intussusceptum. This lesion, considered responsible, may be a benign polyp, a malignant polyp or lesion, or just a hypertrophied Peyer's patch.

7. Obturation is obstruction due to entry into the intestine of a body large enough to block passage. The commonest form is gallstone obstruction. In certain areas and seasons, persimmons eaten in excess form solid foreign bodies which may be respon-

sible for obturation. Other bezoars or ingested foreign bodies such as bed springs, spoons, etc., swallowed in demented states, have been seen.

8. Inflammatory disease. In Crohn's disease involving the small bowel, obstruction of greater or lesser degree is commonly observed. Tuberculosis of the gut is now rarely seen in the United States, but it is a definite cause of obstruction in some parts of the world.

9. Primary tumors in the small bowel usually become manifest through obstruction. Tumors which are primary in the stomach, colon, female genitalia or occasionally other organs, all too often become seeded onto or into the peritoneal surfaces and cause small bowel obstruction by secondary involvement.

10. Vascular obstruction without luminal obstruction can occur in mesenteric venous thrombosis, mesenteric arterial occlusion (embolic or degenerative) and in Richter's hernia. In these circumstances, continuing passage of gas is no guarantee against development of gangrene.

### Large Bowel Obstruction

1. Primary carcinoma of the large bowel. Two thirds of these lie in the last 25 cm. of the bowel and can be seen and biopsied through a sigmoidoscope. Eight ninths of obstructing large bowel cancers lie distal to the middle colic artery. Cancer is responsible for two thirds of large bowel obstructions.

2. Diverticulitis of the sigmoid colon is responsible for about one sixth of large bowel obstructions.

3. Volvulus of the sigmoid colon, or less often of the cecum, accounts for most of the remainder.

4. Left inguinal hernia uncommonly leads to incarceration of the sigmoid colon with obstruction.

5. As in the small bowel, secondary cancer occasionally causes large bowel obstruction, usually at the rectosigmoid level.

6. Rare causes of obstruction of the large bowel are congenital bands, inferior mesenteric artery occlusion and segmental vasculitis of the colon.

### Basic Principles

### Small Bowel Obstruction

1. *Small Bowel Muscle Function.* The small bowel is characterized by intrinsic muscular rhythmicity coming in the form of propulsvie contractions every 3 to 10 minutes. After the lumen has been obstructed, fluid and swallowed gas are delivered by the gut far above the point of obstruction to that area of gut just above the obstruction. As dilation of this area just above the obstruction occurs, and the tension on the wall increases as a consequence, the splashing with each peristaltic delivery of more gas and fluid brings a progressively higher musical pitch; at nearly the same moment, the added stretch on the intestinal wall brings a 15- to 60-second cramp of pain. Thus, the hallmark of small bowel obstruction is an audible peristaltic rush of rising pitch and volume over 30 seconds or more, culminating in low tinkling sounds above the musical high C in pitch and finally in an abdominal cramp.

2. *Vomiting and Fluid Loss.* The content emptied into the duodenum by the stomach in normal conditions is approximately isosmolar with the blood, with essential isosmolality being achieved in the duodenum. In the normal adult, the fluids added by salivary glands, stomach, liver, pancreas and duodenum raise the volume which passes the ligament of Treitz to an estimated 8 to 10 liters of fluid per day. The volume of gas varies widely with the gas-swallowing habits of the individuals concerned. The digestive and absorptive processes in passage down the ileum result in sorption of fluid, so that the normal flow through the ileocecal valve is estimated at less than one-half liter per day. For this reason, obstruction at the jejunal level leads to early and very profuse vomiting, with development of severe

dehydration within a day. Obstruction at the cecal end of the ileum, on the other hand, produces slower accumulation of fluid, and vomiting is later to appear and less quickly productive of clinical dehydration. Since application of pressure to the surface of the mucosa appears to accelerate secretion of fluid into the lumen, fluid losses in obstruction may exceed those estimated on the basis of normal exchanges. The deterioration of the hemoglobin waste products from bile poured into the bowel proceeds at such a pace that a period of about 3 days is required for development of vomitus with the appearance and odor of liquid stool. The appearance of such vomitus is an indicator of the duration of obstruction. It is rarely seen in colon obstruction, but it is regularly seen in ileac obstruction of more than 3½ days duration.

3. *Electrolyte Losses.* The electrolyte content of fluid removed from the gut above small bowel obstructions in a series of cases was:

Na+, 132 to 129 mEq./liter
K+, 5.8 to 8.9 mEq./liter
Cl⁻, 104 to 120 mEq./liter

The occasional reduction of levels of these ions observed in the plasma in small bowel obstruction appears to be due to this concentrated loss into the gut, only a portion of which is clinically available for measurement in vomitus or aspirate, the remainder being trapped in the gut.

4. *Distention.* Clinical abdominal distention depends upon the sum total of increase in volume of abdominal content. Jejunal obstruction produces little increase in visceral volume, because the length of gut involved is short and the stomach is quick to be emptied by vomiting. Terminal ileac obstruction usually produces striking distention, because the vast bulk of the small gut becomes overfilled with as yet unvomited gas and fluid.

5. *Obstipation.* After evacuation of the gut distal to the point of obstruction, there is no further passage of stool or gas, and colonic irrigations yield only the slightly soiled fluid instilled.

## Large Bowel Obstruction

1. *The Ileocecal Junction, and Muscle Function of the Large Bowel.* At physiologic pressures, the ileocecal valve normally prevents reflux of contents from the cecum into the ileum. Only after the colon has become distended above a point of obstruction to a mean level well above the normal 6 to 8 cm. of water does reflux occur. (The pressures in colon obstruction have been measured as high as 53 cm. of water.) In two thirds of clinical cases of colon obstruction, there are either no small bowel gas shadows apparent on abdominal scout films or no striking amount of small bowel fluid. In the remainder, there is small bowel distention as striking as that in the colon.

The pattern of contraction of the muscle of the large bowel stands in sharp contrast to that of the ileum, for it consists of mass contractions of great segments of the colon. These come at intervals longer than one-half hour apart, sometimes 12 hours apart, and carry the total content from one side of the colon to the other. Usually any cramps which occur come at long intervals and lack the crescendo peristaltic rush audible in ileac obstruction. Obstruction of the ileocecal junction by cecal cancer presents clinically as low small bowel obstruction. Obstruction of the low right colon may also present in this way, because the volume of the distended colon proximal to it is small enough so that each ileac peristaltic delivery adds stretch to the cecal wall.

The usual competence of the ileocecal valve to prevent reflux permits the ileum to empty into the colon, and vomiting therefore occurs only in an apparently reflex fashion and rarely more than 2 or 3 times in any given patient. Finally, it is rare indeed that the vomitus is fecal in character.

2. Electrolyte and fluid losses are rarely

striking, because most of the fluid of the upper ileum is resorbed. Very little is lost in continuing fashion.

3. Clinical distention is striking and peripheral on the abdominal wall in sigmoid obstruction, because a huge volume of gas and fluid is required to distend the colon above the level of obstruction.

## Criteria for Diagnosis

### Small Bowel Obstruction

1. Colicky pain at intervals of 3 to 10 minutes

2. Colic preceded by crescendo borborygmi of rising pitch, ending in a loud sound above the musical high C

3. Vomiting is invariably present after the first hour or two of symptoms, more profuse in upper obstructions, and usually fecal in character after 3½ days of obstruction.

4. Obstipation (after passage of infra-obstructional content)

5. Distention of the abdomen, more striking in low obstructions than in high obstructions

6. X-ray findings on upright and recumbent films of the abdomen consist of transversely placed segments rising in ladder-like fashion, usually from the left pelvis, with the "ladder" of 3 or more segments crossing the abdomen upward and to the right. There is no gas in the colon (unless incidentally introduced by enemas). Small intestinal gas shadows are normally present in children under 5 years of age.

7. Upper gastrointestinal barium series are not routinely used for establishment of the diagnosis of small bowel obstruction, especially when large bowel obstruction is suspected, since in the latter instance it may make a partial obstruction complete, as well as making it difficult to evacuate the inspissated barium through catheters. Occasionally a small quantity of dilute barium may be instilled through a gastrointestinal tube after the tube has stopped

advancing. This helps to delineate the area of obstruction or differentiate mechanical from adynamic ileus. In most cases of small bowel obstruction, the diagnosis can be made without the use of barium.

### Colonic and Rectal Obstruction Due to Primary Cancer of the Colon

1. History of increasing difficulty in evacuation of the large bowel, often with previous bouts of meteorism relieved by enemas

2. Final failure to pass gas or stool, followed by an increasing pace of abdominal distention over a day or several days. There is a tympanitic percussion note over the course of the colon.

3. Absence of prominent vomiting

4. Abdominal cramps are usually not striking, with an interval between cramps usually of more than one-half hour (unless the lesion is right colonic).

5. X-ray films in the recumbent position show a gas-filled colon from the cecum to the point of the obstructing lesion. This is usually sufficiently precise to permit radiologic localization of the lesion without contrast medium by enema. One third of cases also show ileal distention.

6. The obstructing lesion is within reach of the finger on rectal examination or sigmoidoscopy in two thirds of the cases.

### Colonic Obstruction Due to Volvulus or Diverticulitis

The differential diagnosis may be extremely difficult. In a case of sigmoid volvulus, the abdominal x-ray usually reveals a gigantic gas-filled coffee-bean-like segment which rises from the left lower abdomen and extends to the right diaphragm and all but fills the abdomen. There are only occasionally severe cramps. Diagnosis may be confirmed by a cautious small barium enema and sigmoidoscopy and passage of a rectal tube beyond the end of the sigmoidoscope through the usually obviously twisted bowel. This latter maneuver is not only diagnostic but therapeutic.

Volvulus of the cecum commonly presents as low small bowel obstruction. Recognition of the cecal volvulus as the responsible factor rests upon the radiologic appearance of a huge kidney-shaped gas-filled loop coming from the right lower quadrant into the left upper abdomen, with small bowel distention also present.

Diverticulitis with obstruction is commonly associated with inflammatory responses but may defy identification even with a barium enema.

## Strangulation

This is rare in colon obstructions other than cecal or sigmoid volvulus, but it is all too common in small bowel obstruction. Here, any of the following must dictate the urgent therapy needed for strangulating obstruction:

1. History of abrupt onset (maximal pain reached within 20 minutes of onset)

2. Back pain in addition to abdominal pain

3. Signs of peritoneal irritation (spasm, rebound tenderness)

4. Fever or leukocytosis

5. X-ray demonstration of one or more segments of gas-filled gut in the configuration of a double coffee bean (the result of passage of a loop or loops of intestine under a band)

## Differentiation of Mechanical Obstruction from Paralytic Ileus

In paralytic ileus, the following items are important:

1. The abdomen is usually silent or nearly so.

2. Both large and small bowels appear filled with gas on supine x-ray of the abdomen.

3. X-ray findings in upright films show distended, inverted, U-shaped segments, often outlined by the contained gas. If the patient is maintained 5 minutes in the upright position before a film is taken, continuing peristalsis usually propels some fluid over the top of the inverted U.

Therefore, in the absence of contraction of paralytic ileus the levels are usually identical, whereas in mechanical obstruction the gas-filled levels are uneven.

4. The progress of a small amount of dilute barium instilled into the gastrointestinal tube down to the colon is frequently helpful in differentiating these two types of ileus.

## Lethal Factors

### Small Bowel Obstruction

1. *Acute Dehydration, Electrolyte Loss and Uremia.* In high small bowel obstruction, the massive fluid and electrolyte losses render the patient a fragile candidate for any therapy in advance of correction of these deficits. The common prices of failure to heed this point are acute vascular collapse and sudden death. Uremia results from insufficient fluid in the body to maintain an adequate urine flow. These deficit problems are less severe in obstructions low in the ileum, but even here they are very real.

2. *Acute Shock.* If more than one third of the small intestine is involved in a strangulating process, such as being wrapped about a heavy adhesive band, the easier compression of the venous drainage than of the arterial supply results in huge engorgement and acute loss of circulating blood volume. Death by this mechanism has been observed in 3 hours from onset of symptoms in a patient with acute onset and back pain.

3. *Prolonged Distention.* The mucosal ischemia of prolonged distention permits toxic products from the lumen to pass through the damaged bowel wall and to be absorbed transperitoneally. Two to 3 days of severe distention can be lethal. Free perforation from distention without mesenteric vascular obstruction occurs rarely in dogs but almost never in man.

4. *Strangulation to the Point of Necrosis.* Gangrene of the intestinal wall kills by perforation and peritonitis if the perforation is within the abdomen and by

sepsis of less rapidly overwhelming nature if the involved bowel is entrapped in an external hernia. Survival time can be quadrupled experimentally by administration of broad-spectrum antibiotics at the time of establishment of obstruction.

## Large Bowel Obstruction

1. *Cecal Perforation.* The large diameter and thin anterior wall of the cecum combine to render this the usual site of free perforation in unrelieved colic obstruction. The usual competency of the ileocecal valve converts colon obstruction into a closed-loop obstruction, but even in the presence of an incompetent ileocecal valve, cecal perforation has been observed to occur.

A particularly lethal situation is obstruction of the ascending colon just above the ileocecal valve in the presence of a fully competent valve, for here there is neither clinical distention nor vomiting to give warning, and overwhelming peritonitis from cecal perforation may strike within hours of onset of symptoms.

2. *Strangulation to the Point of Necrosis.* Strangulation has been noted to involve the sigmoid colon in left groin hernias and in volvulus of either the sigmoid colon or the cecum.

### Management

The therapeutic approaches to large bowel and to small bowel obstruction are so different that it is essential to differentiate between them diagnostically. While fluid and electrolyte problems must be evaluated in any emergency situation, the problems are far more serious and the derangements far greater in small bowel obstruction, especially high small bowel obstruction, than is the case in obstruction of the colon. In small bowel obstruction, even the presence of recognized strangulation often cannot dictate proceeding to operative intervention without taking 3 or 4 hours to correct these deficits. In colon obstruction, on the other hand, the urgen-

cy of impending cecal perforation may be handled with surgical intervention within the hour, waiting only for a rapid check on adequacy of electrolytes and fluid. Finally, the incision for small bowel obstruction is usually longitudinal and midabdominal (as the best type for exploration), whereas that for transverse colostomy is transverse across the right upper rectus muscle.

## Small Bowel Obstruction Without Evidence of Strangulation

1. *Nonoperative Decompression of the Gut.* In all patients with intestinal obstruction, bowel decompression should be started as soon as the diagnosis is considered. While decompression alone is rarely indicated for therapy, it may suffice in selected cases such as those in which tube decompression has been used successfully previously, in which obstruction seems incomplete, or in which there may be multiple areas of obstruction secondary to peritoneal metastasis. Operation should not be deferred awaiting the passage of the gastrointestinal tube, but, while preparing the patient for operation, a long tube may be passed down the small bowel to the area of obstruction. The Aloe plastic long sump tube has been most satisfactory.* Suction should be in force during passage of the tubes through the nose and into the stomach in order to handle any vomiting which might be induced by the maneuver. Passage into the stomach is followed by aspiration of the gastric contents, inflation of the balloon with 20 ml. of air, and withdrawal of the tube until it impinges against the esophagogastric junction. The patient is then placed in a forward right lateral decubitus position, and 1 liter of air is quickly instilled into the stomach. The balloon is then emptied, the tube is slowly advanced 18 to 20 cm., and the air is

---

*Dennis, C.: Gastrointestinal sump tube. Surgery, 66:309, 1969. The tube may be ordered from A. S. Aloe Company, 1891 Olive Street, St. Louis, Missouri.

aspirated from the stomach. At this point, the rapid injection of not more than 2 ml. of mercury into the balloon permits both gravity and the mercury-impact-stimulated peristalsis to carry the tube into the duodenum. Thereafter, gravity positioning and slow advancement of the tube permit passage through the duodenum. The balloon should remain deflated until passage through the third portion of the duodenum; thereafter, peristalsis can carry it down the small intestine if the balloon is inflated with 15 ml. of air.

2. *Replacement of Fluids and Electrolytes.* While an initial blood sample is under study for hemoglobin, hematocrit, white blood cell count, blood sugar, electrolytes and crossmatching, Ringer's solution may be added by intravenous infusion. The initial weight of the patient is valuable in calculation. If frank clinical dehydration is present, the assumption is justified that the water lost is equal to 6 to 7 per cent of the body weight. The method of calculation of water and electrolyte deficits is discussed in Chapter 2, Fluid and Electrolyte Problems.

3. Full evaluation of the patient for associated illnesses should be carried out and proper management instituted.

4. *Definitive Correction of Obstruction.* Many cases of adhesive obstruction relent on conservative decompression alone, but it is usually preferable to proceed within 24 hours to explore the abdomen for correction of the adhesions, bands or other lesions responsible. During such interim, the patient must be critically reexamined at least as often as every 2 hours for signs and symptoms of strangulation. If any of these appear, the operation must be performed at once. Exploration is performed through a midline incision, entering the abdomen well away from the scars of previous operations in order to avoid areas of intestinal adhesion to the anterior wall. If decompression has not been fully accomplished by the naso-intestinal sump tube, operative decompression *must* be

done before cutting adhesive bands under which gut has been incarcerated (because the area compressed by the band is commonly necrotic and leaks at once upon section of the band). Passage of the Leonard tube* (or some modification of the Leonard tube) perorally may permit satisfactory emptying of the bowel. If not, aseptic decompression is in order.† In general, relief of adhesive obstruction can be achieved by division of bands and adhesions, but the degree of fibrosis, denudation or dense adhesions may dictate resection. A primary closed (aseptic) anastomosis is essential to maximal success.

Obstruction due to other mechanisms is relieved as indicated by the lesion in question, e.g., removal of an obstructing gallstone by transverse enterotomy (after milking the contents away and securing emptiness of the lumen with gentle Scudder clamps) and aseptic closure of the gut with preplaced silk sutures after the stone has been removed. The linea alba is reapproximated with buried stainless steel wire interrupted sutures, and the wound is washed with 0.2% kanamycin in saline solution before obliteration of the dead space in the subcutaneous fat by mattress sutures through the skin and catching the fascia, and approximation of the skin edges. These mattress sutures are removed at 48 hours.

Suction is continued on the nasointestinal tube postoperatively until good intestinal sounds appear and the patient tolerates 6 hours of tube clamping without discomfort.

---

* Leonard, A.S. et al.: Intestinal decompression: use of a long tube with a coiled spring for relief of distension with enterotomy or enterostomy. Surgery, *49:*440, 1961.

†The full equipment for aseptic decompression should be assembled, sterile, and at hand during any procedure for obstruction. Wangensteen's aseptic decompression is redescribed with other techniques in Dennis, C.: Current procedure in management of obstruction of the small intestine. J.A.M.A., *154:*463, 1954.

## Small Bowel Obstruction with Signs of Strangulation

1. Do not defer operation for the purpose of intestinal intubation, but use the time necessary for partial correction of salt and water losses.

2. Proceed with water and salt estimation and administration as above, but give one half of the estimated needs in 2½ to 3 hours and proceed to operation at that time, slowing the infusion so that the total amount estimated can be administered in approximately 12 hours.

3. At operation, proceed as above, decompressing if there is much distention, and resecting the compromised bowel if there is any question at all of its viability. Primary end-to-end aseptic anastomosis with rotation of one end 180 degrees with respect to the other provides a wide, trouble-free reconstruction.*

4. Proceed to definitive repair of the underlying lesion, e.g., repair of the femoral hernia.

## Right Colonic Obstruction from Carcinoma

1. Decompress as above if there is distention of the small intestine.

2. Proceed with water and salt administration as above.

3. Operative decompression is used if decompression has not yet been achieved, decompressing the right colon through the very terminal ileum in aseptic fashion.

4. Proceed with primary right hemicolectomy.

## Left Colonic and Rectal Obstruction

1. Pass a nasogastric tube.

2. Hydrate as above, noting that dehydration is only relative.

3. All cases of left colon or rectal obstruction should be sigmoidoscoped early. This can safely be performed using a Sims position. If sigmoid volvulus is present, a large amount of gas and liquid feces will pass through the scope. Passage of a No. 40 French long rectal tube will relieve the obstruction long enough to avoid emergency operation and permit preparation of the patient for definitive treatment. Re-x-ray in these cases will demonstrate a decrease in the colonic gas, indicating successful decompression. With rectal or low sigmoid cancer, the visualization of the lesion allows biopsy and definitive diagnosis but does not remove the necessity for emergency colonic decompression. Attempts to pass a tube beyond the lesion should be avoided since this leads to unnecessary delay and is often unsuccessful.

4. Open the abdomen through a right transverse incision across the rectus muscle overlying the transverse colon (position checked by preliminary x-ray of the abdomen with a coin on the umbilicus for measurement).

5. Usually, the distended colon will be filled primarily with gas; this can be removed with a 20-gauge needle on a suction line, tunneling in the substance of the colonic wall for a centimeter in the center of the anterior taenia.

6. After decompression, inspect the cecum cautiously for evidences of perforation or gangrene. If the cecum is intact, proceed with transverse colostomy over a plastic rod, suturing only to the fatty tags. An umbilical tape can be passed about the colon on the distal side of the proposed area of opening the colostomy for later use in occluding around a large Foley catheter to permit meticulous cleansing of the colon before subsequent left hemicolectomy. The colostomy can be opened enough to insert a catheter through a purse-string suture in 24 hours and can usually be opened widely at 3 days. A longitudinal cautery-made incision provides better diversion of the fecal

---

*Dennis, C.: Oblique, aseptic, end-to-end ileac anastomosis, procedure of choice in strangulating small bowel obstruction. Surg., Gynec., Obstet., 77:255, 1943.

stream than a transverse one. If there is question about the viability or intactness of the cecum either preoperatively or at exploration, it should be brought out through a McBurney incision as a cecostomy, with a large catheter in place. In this case, the transverse colostomy may be omitted.

7. The use of a preoperative barium enema is valuable in large bowel obstruction since it may demonstrate the causative lesion. If a carcinoma is present in an area which would necessitate transverse colectomy as a part of the definitive operation (i.e., splenic, flexure or transverse colon carcinoma), decompression by cecostomy is preferred rather than transverse colostomy. This is performed through a right lower quadrant muscle-splitting incision. With careful walling-off of the incision by laparotomy pads, only the disturbed cecum is visible. Decompression through a trocar is accomplished after placement of 2 purse-string non-absorbable sutures. After evacuation of gas and liquid feces by suction, the edges of the cecal incision are grasped with Allis clamps and lifted while a No. 36 to 40 mushroom-tipped catheter with extra side holes is inserted. This tube is brought out through a small lateral stab wound, and the previously placed purse-string sutures are tied as the cecal mucosa is inverted. The sutures are then sewn to the margins of the stab wound incision and the main incision is closed.

## Small Bowel Obstruction Without Evidence of Strangulation

1. Weigh the patient.

2. Send blood to the laboratory for hemoglobin, hematocrit, white blood cell count, differential white blood cell count, sodium, potassium, chloride, total protein, blood sugar and crossmatching (4 units).

3. Gastrointestinal sump tube on continuous (not intermittent) suction. Permit the tube to advance as peristalsis pulls it.

4. Check the temperature, pulse, respiration, blood pressure, urine volume, presence or absence of colic, and function of sump tube every hour.

5. Give intravenous Ringer's solution containing 5% dextrose, 1 liter per hour for 2 hours (in adults), then fluids and electrolytes as reordered (in infants, 20 ml./kg./hour for 2 hours). Add sodium cephalothin, 10 mg./kg., to each hour's allotment the first 2 hours of infusion.

6. Do not give analgesics until the patient is being prepared for the operating room.

7. When the patient is stable, abdominal x-rays are made in 2 positions (i.e., flat and upright or decubitus in a debilitated patient).

8. Prepare the skin from the nipples to the knees anteriorly.

9. Place an indwelling Foley catheter in the bladder with thoroughly sterile bottle-drainage.

10. On call to the operating room, give 50 mg. of Demerol subcutaneously.

# 17. ACUTE INTRA-ABDOMINAL INFLAMMATORY DISEASE

*Bernard Gardner,* M.D.

## Definitions

1. *Acute intra-abdominal inflammatory disease* refers to inflammation of structures within the peritoneal cavity or retroperitoneal area.

2. *Peritonitis* is inflammation of either the visceral or parietal peritoneum.

3. *Visceral pain* is pain caused by stretch of a viscus stimulating the autonomic nervous plexuses in its wall.

4. *Somatic pain* is pain caused by motion of a peritoneum which is the seat of chemical or bacterial inflammation, and it is transmitted by the spinal nerves.

## Basic Principles

1. The first physician consulted by a patient with abdominal pain plays a critical role in determining the subsequent success of treatment.

2. The key question involved is: "Is operation necessary?" Every effort must be directed at finding a prompt answer. This dictates that the physician must:

   A. *Be aware of the possibility* that operation may be necessary

   B. *Obtain early surgical consultation*

   C. *Begin resuscitative measures to prepare* the patient for possible operation

   D. *not* do anything to interfere with the *signs and symptoms* which will be evaluated in any decision to operate

3. Abdominal pain may be either visceral or somatic in origin. *Visceral pain* is caused by sudden stretch or distention of a viscus (e.g., contraction against an obstruction) and is interpreted as crampy or gaseous pain, usually intermittent and referred to the midline of the abdomen. If the viscus involved is derived from the foregut, the crampy pain will be epigastric; midgut pain is periumbilical, and hindgut pain is hypogastric. Most acute intra-abdominal inflammatory diseases requiring operation are preceded by obstruction, and the earliest clinical symptoms and signs will be related to the visceral pain component. This early stage is unaccompanied by any signs of peritonitis and therefore can clearly be distinguished from the later stages. Reflex vomiting occurs with the stimulation of visceral stretch receptors and is easily differentiated from other types of vomiting because it is *unassociated with nausea and is temporally related to the pain.* Examples of intra-abdominal conditions which demonstrate this early visceral phase are appendicitis, cholecystitis (biliary colic), intestinal obstruction, pancreatitis, ureteral stone, common duct stone (choledocholithiasis), etc.

4. *Somatic pain* occurs when fibers located in the *parietal peritoneum* are stimulated by chemical or bacterial inflammation. The pain is constant sharp or aching, depending on its chronicity and amplitude, and is referred to the area of involvement. Any stimulation of the involved peritoneum will produce the pain, so that the patient lies quietly, often with the thighs flexed to relax the peritoneum. Any attempt to palpate the involved area is guarded against by muscular contraction, producing one of the most reliable signs of peritonitis: involuntary guarding. Rebound tenderness is present, as is tenderness to palpation. The peritoneal–intestinal reflex produces immediate cessation of bowel contraction, and therefore the bowel sounds are absent. Localization of the inflammation to specific areas of the peritoneum may be demonstrated by specific maneuvers gauged to stretch the involved areas. Extension of the thigh or the hip produces pain in inflammation of the psoas fascia and adja-

cent peritoneum (psoas sign). Internal rotation of the thigh on the hip produces pain when the obturator fascia is involved (obturator sign).

5. Toxemia secondary to bacterial involvement leads to the rapid development of associated systemic signs and symptoms, such as fever, tachycardia, anorexia, nausea, leukocytosis, etc. Conditions which progress from the early visceral phase to the late somatic phase include appendicitis, cholecystitis, pancreatitis, choledocholithiasis (with cholangitis) and intestinal obstruction (with perforation or gangrene). Some diseases begin with the somatic phase, and these include diverticulitis, perforations of the gastrointestinal tract and ischemic bowel syndromes.

## THE EARLY (VISCERAL) PHASE OF INTRA-ABDOMINAL DISEASE

### Criteria for Diagnosis

1. There is diffuse midabdominal (epigastric, periumbilical or hypogastric) pain, crampy in nature and episodic.

2. Vomiting is not associated with nausea or other systemic signs. The patient may try to eat, in fact, or may retch when the stomach is empty.

3. There are no systemic signs or symptoms such as anorexia, nausea, fever, tachycardia (unless accompanied by hypovolemia), malaise, etc.

4. The onset is acute.

5. Laboratory values confirm the lack of systemic illness. While blood count and erythrocyte sedimentation rate are normal.

6. Physical examination reveals *no signs of parietal peritonitis*.

### Management

1. Call a surgical consultant if you will not operate yourself.

2. Insert a nasogastric tube to avoid aspiration of vomitus and to reduce the volume of swallowed air.

3. Give nothing by mouth to avoid contraction of the involved viscera

(gallbladder) or stimulation of the pancreas and to reduce gastric residual.

4. Start intravenous fluids for maintenance. Since these illnesses are usually acute, we are not contending with a fluid-depleted patient. Exceptions include conditions secondary to underlying malignancy or inflammatory disease or intestinal obstruction with large intraluminal fluid loss.

5. Give no antibiotics or analgesics (*see* below).

6. Obtain the appropriate laboratory tests.

## THE LATE (SOMATIC) PHASE OF INTRA-ABDOMINAL DISEASE

### Criteria for Diagnosis

1. The pain is constant, sharper and localized to the area of involvement.

2. The somatic phase may follow a visceral stage or may develop acutely.

3. It is accompanied by peritoneal signs such as tenderness, rebound tenderness, involuntary guarding, etc. The patient who may have been uncomfortable and moving about during the visceral phase becomes quiet and unwilling to move.

4. Accompanying systemic signs and symptoms develop. The patient appears more ill.

5. Laboratory values reflect systemic disease.

### Conditions Which May Confuse the Diagnosis of Peritonitis

1. Obesity. A thick omentum may lie between the seat of the inflammation and the anterior peritoneum, preventing the abdominal signs of peritonitis from being elicited.

2. Grand multiparity or multiple abdominal operations may denervate the abdominal wall musculature, preventing guarding on palpation and thus misleading the physician.

3. Antibiotics represent the most serious problem, since they may be

successful in treating the bacterial component of peritonitis but not the underlying pathology. For example, in cystic duct obstruction with empyema of the gallbladder, the peritoneal signs of fever and leukocytosis may diminish on appropriate antibiotic treatment while the gallbladder perforates. In patients on antibiotic treatment, on multiple occasions, we have seen the gallbladder or appendix perforate while the abdominal signs were minimal. It is therefore vital to withhold these agents until the over-all plan of treatment is decided by the physician who will have the ultimate responsibility.

4. Analgesics may depress the patient's awareness of painful stimuli, thus leading to difficulty in evaluating the development or progression of signs of peritonitis. They should be withheld until a working diagnosis is firmly established.

## Management

The development of the late phase often signifies impending disaster without early operation. Therefore, prepare the patient for operation.

1. Call a surgeon or prepare to operate.
2. Notify the operating room and the anesthesiologist.
3. Give nothing by mouth.
4. Nasogastric intubation to avoid vomiting.
5. Start intravenous fluids (*see* Chap. 2).
6. White blood count and differential; hematocrit
7. Electrolytes and blood-urea nitrogen
8. Obtain an electrocardiogram as indicated.
9. Crossmatch blood for transfusion, depending on the suspected diagnosis.
10. In any case where the late phase has supervened, delay in operation will lead to increased mortality. The performance of routine x-rays or other examinations should be discouraged unless they may contribute to the diagnosis or are necessary for management of the anesthesia.

11. Antibiotics should be withheld until the decision to operate has been made and *then started preoperatively.* The decision to operate should not be altered by their effects.

The terms early and late phases are used here to alert the responsible physician to the necessity for immediate operation. Early stages of these diseases allow time to make a diagnosis and commence resuscitation. If the late stage (peritonitis) occurs, no unnecessary diagnostic or ritualistic examination should be undertaken, *even if the exact diagnosis is in doubt.* It makes little difference from the patient's point of view if he has an empyema of the gallbladder or a perforated ulcer as long as an early operation is made. Even an incorrect incision is to be preferred to delay of a necessary operation.

# ACUTE APPENDICITIS

## Definition

Acute appendicitis is obstruction of the appendiceal lumen by a mucous plug, fecalith, etc., with supervening bacterial infection and inflammation.

## Basic Principles

1. The differentiation of appendicitis from right-sided pelvic inflammatory disease (PID) may be extremely difficult. PID is not preceded by the visceral phase of midabdominal pain and vomiting, the symptoms usually starting in the right lower quadrant. The point of maximum tenderness is 2 cm. below McBurney's point in ovarian disease, and pelvic examination may clearly demonstrate the ovarian mass or exquisite tenderness on cervical motion.

2. If doubt exists as to the diagnosis, *it is safer to operate.* In general we have found that out of every 8 operations for appendicitis, one is a misdiagnosed PID or a normal appendix. The mortality from appendectomy in such cases has been zero in the past six years of evaluation.

However, delay in operation for acute appendicitis has produced several mortalities during the same period.

3. In cases where the *diagnosis is in doubt,* the patient should be observed while not eating, and on maintenance intravenous fluids. Observation signifies frequent measurements of temperature, white blood count and abdominal and rectal examinations. The natural course of this disease is to progress, so that observation *without antibiotics* will allow the appropriate physical signs to develop, leading to prompt operation. In mild cases of gastroenteritis, etc., the signs and symptoms will resolve within 24 hours. In the rare event of persisting symptoms of mild degree after 24 hours, operation is performed and it is the safest course to follow. The majority of such cases, however, will not have appendicitis as the cause of their symptoms.

## Criteria for Diagnosis

1. *Early Phase*

A. Periumbilical, crampy pain (midgut organ)

B. Vomiting

C. Due to the small size of the appendiceal lumen, the early phase is short-lived and rapidly progresses to the later stages of the disease. The patient may only be aware of transient periumbilical or midabdominal discomfort before localization occurs, but the establishment of this sequence is important in distinguishing the disease from other disorders in the right lower quadrant (i.e., pelvic inflammatory disease).

2. *Late Phase* (6 to 24 hours after onset)

A. The pain in the right lower quadrant is constant.

B. Anorexia, mild fever, leukocytosis, etc., develop.

C. Peritoneal signs develop in the right lower quadrant.

3. The subsequent course of the disease may develop in one of several ways:

A. Free perforation (common in children due to the sparse omentum) → generalized peritonitis → septicemia → death

B. Appendiceal abscess→ septicemia →bowel fistulas→pylephlebitis and liver abscess → death

4. *Unusual Presentations of Appendicitis*

The appendix may be short, stubby, long, thin, etc., and may be anatomically located in the pelvis, overlying the ureter, behind the cecum, alongside of the gallbladder, etc. Therefore, a multitude of signs and symptoms may be indicative of appendicitis. The early visceral phase, however, is usually present, but the later somatic phase may vary considerably, presenting with diarrhea (irritation of a redundant pelvic colon), dysuria (ureteral inflammation); right upper quadrant pain (high-lying paracholecystic appendix) or no anterior wall peritoneal signs (retrocecal appendix).

5. *The Rectal and Pelvic Examination*

When the appendix is located in the pelvis or is retrocecal in origin, peritoneal signs may be limited to the posterior peritoneum. In these cases, the carefully performed rectal examination may clearly demonstrate a difference in pain on palpation to the left or right wall of the rectum. Such differences, when carefully elicited, are highly significant.

## Management

1. The goal of management is early operation—within 2 hours of admission.

2. If the diagnosis after history and physical examination is acute appendicitis:

A. Start intravenous fluids with 5% dextrose in Ringer's lactate at a rate of 2000 ml./24 hours.

B. Give nothing by mouth.

C. Insert a nasogastric tube if the patient is vomiting.

D. Draw blood for white blood count and differential, blood type and hematocrit.

E. In the elderly patient, an ECG may be made.

F. Prepare the abdomen for operation.

G. Take an x-ray of the abdomen and chest.

H. Antibiotics are not used in the stage of early visceral symptoms or localized peritonitis. However, if perforation or abscess formation is suspected:

(1) Start penicillin, 1.2 million units I.M. stat twice daily, and streptomycin, 0.5 gm. I.M. twice daily. The penicillin may be given intravenously if the patient appears septic.

(2) Alternative antibiotics include: kanamycin and cephalothin in combination; nafcillin and ampicillin in combination (not a primary choice for gram-negative sepsis); and chloramphenicol alone.

I. Appendectomy must be performed.

## APPENDICEAL ABSCESS

### Definition

An appendiceal abscess is a localized perforation of the appendix with purulent collection. The remnant of the appendix may not be found at operation.

### Basic Principles

Although early operation is recommended for early, late or perforated appendicitis, under certain specific circumstances we do not operate on a localized appendiceal abscess.

### Criteria for Diagnosis

1. History characteristic of acute appendicitis lasting longer than 72 hours

2. There are no peritoneal signs outside of the right lower quadrant.

### Management

1. Treat the patient with antibiotics and follow the abdominal signs, white blood count and temperature every 2 to 4 hours.

2. If the white blood count and temperature should fall within 12 hours, and the right lower quadrant tenderness

has diminished and no other abdominal signs have developed, this approach may be continued.

3. If the mass has decreased in size and the patient's temperature and white blood count are near normal with 24 to 36 hours, continue observation.

4. If the patient fails to respond as above (5% of patients), operation is carried out at once.

5. This plan of treatment necessitates the performance of interval appendectomy at 6 weeks, since recurrent appendicitis occurs in 20 per cent of these patients between 6 to 12 weeks later.

## ACUTE CHOLECYSTITIS

### Definition

Acute cholecystitis is inflammation of the gallbladder, either chemical or bacterial.

### Basic Principles

1. Cystic duct obstruction is present in 95 per cent of cases, always associated with cholelithiasis. Acute cases not associated with gallbladder stones have common duct pathology (i.e., tumor or stone).

2. *Early Phase: Cystic Duct Obstruction.* With a meal, the gallbladder contracts, producing a midepigastric cramp and vomiting. If there have been recurrent attacks of cholecystitis or long-standing cystic duct obstruction, the pain may be somatic in type (e.g., in the right upper quadrant and sharper). Since the gallbladder is supplied by a branch of the phrenic nerve, pain may be referred to the right scapula, representing the dermatome associated with the C-5, C-6 and C-7 roots.

This stage resolves spontaneously if the stone drops back into the gallbladder, which may then empty. This early stage may occur episodically as attacks of biliary colic without associated infection. There is no fever, peritonitis or abnormal white blood count.

3. If the stone persistently obstructs the cystic duct, the *second phase* of the disease is reached:

The gallbladder is distended and tense

and may become palpable. It is filled with mucus (white bile) secreted by its lining (hydrops), since bile cannot enter through the obstructed cystic duct. Secondary infection may occur, leading to an empyema.

At this stage, peritoneal signs develop, and the patient becomes moderately febrile with an elevated white blood count. The use of antibiotics will produce a gradual decrease in these symptoms and signs, with the appearance of improvement. However, the underlying obstruction is not relieved by antibiotics, and continued mucus secretion and bacterial growth may increase the pressure within the gallbladder, leading to perforation. It is vital to decide if the obstruction is likely to persist or will subside spontaneously, since in the first case operation is indicated. The decision is based on careful observation without the misleading influences of antibiotics or analgesics:

|  | Subsiding Disease | Persistent Obstruction |
|---|---|---|
| Abdominal findings | Decreased | Increased |
| WBC | Decreased | Elevated |
| Temperature | Decreased | Elevated |

With observation every 2 to 4 hours, an early decision can be made as to the need for operation. Once operation has been decided upon, antibiotics may be used as long as the decision to operate is not altered by their effects.

## Criteria for Diagnosis

1. History or previous diagnosis of gallbladder disease or previous hospitalization for right upper quadrant pain
2. Epigastric or right upper quadrant pain, often with radiation to the flank or right shoulder
3. Anorexia
4. Nausea and vomiting
5. Tenderness in the right upper quadrant
6. Rebound tenderness referred to the right upper quadrant

7. Positive Murphy's sign—sudden cessation of inspiration due to pain from the palpating hand thrust deeply into the right upper abdomen just below the costal margin
8. Localized right upper abdominal wall spasm
9. Sensation of a mass in the right upper quadrant
10. Elevated white blood count
11. Elevated sedimentation rate
12. Fever usually over 102° F.
13. Clinical or laboratory evidence of icterus
14. In certain cases, the symptoms may be mild but persistent, or the diagnosis may be in doubt. Under these circumstances, the use of oral cholecystography or intravenous cholangiography is indicated. These studies will often reveal a nonfilling gallbladder. When a cholangiogram demonstrates the common bile duct, failure of the gallbladder to fill is diagnostic of cystic duct obstruction.

## Management

1. Nothing by mouth
2. Nasogastric suction if the patient is vomiting
3. Maintenance intravenous fluid therapy
4. Atropine, 1/150 gr. I.M. every 4 hours, or Pro-Banthine
5. Temperature every 2 hours
6. White blood count every 4 to 6 hours
7. Repeated abdominal examinations
8. No antibiotics or analgesics
9. Chest and abdominal films
10. ECG if indicated
11. Prepare for operation if the patient is getting worse, the symptoms or signs have not subsided in 24 hours or the cholangiogram demonstrates cystic duct obstruction.

## Special Problems Associated with Cholecystitis

1. *Associated jaundice* is a frequent occurrence with acute cholecystitis, but the

serum bilirubin level seldom exceeds 5 mg.%. If the jaundice is deeper, one should suspect a common duct obstruction, with the impending development of cholangitis. This is a serious problem since septicemia quickly follows cholangitis and necessitates emergency common duct drainage for the patient's survival.

2. *Associated pancreatitis* may occur with cholecystitis and may delay operation *unless the patient demonstrates increasing peritoneal signs, fever and leukocytosis.* Under these circumstances, operation is performed promptly and the common duct is explored to rule out the presence of a stone in the ampulla of Vater (and coincidentally to decompress the pancreatic duct in patients with a common channel at the ampulla).

3. *The elderly or very debilitated patient or any patient* in whom general anesthesia is contraindicated (i.e., recent documented myocardial infarction) represents a special problem. Frequently patients with debilitating diseases cannot withstand the ravages of infection and, in our experience, do better with *earlier operation.* However, the procedure may be altered to allow the use of local anesthesia.

In these cases we perform cholecystostomy *under local anesthesia,* being certain to remove the gallbladder stones prior to placement of the cholecystostomy tube. This ensures a patent cystic duct and is important when associated common duct obstruction is present; otherwise, the common duct cannot be decompressed by this operation.

4. *Perforation of the Gallbladder.* The blood supply of the gallbladder is made up of end arteries. The tension on the wall is related to the ratio of the pressure inside to the pressure outside and the *radius* of the viscus. As distention increases, the critical closing pressure of some of the end arteries is exceeded, and patchy areas of gangrene develop, with subsequent leakage of infected contents. This represents a major catastrophe. Ordinarily at least 3 days of persistent obstruction are necessary for perforation to occur, unless there is underlying disease of the small vessels or limited inflow (diabetes and arteriosclerosis). In these cases, the tendency is toward *earlier* operation—with 24 hours.

*Management*

*(1)* Prepare the patient for operation.

*(2)* Nasogastric suction

*(3)* Rapid intravenous hydration

*(4)* Antibiotics: penicillin, 30 million units in intravenous fluid; streptomycin, 1 gm. I.M.

*(5)* Prep the abdomen from the nipple to the knees.

*(6)* Cholecystectomy or tube cholecystostomy

## ACUTE PANCREATITIS

### Definition

Acute pancreatitis is an inflammation, probably chemical or enzymatic, of the pancreas.

### Classification

1. *Acute Edematous Pancreatitis.* This is the most common form of the disease, associated with swelling of the gland, extravasation of pancreatic enzymes and mild retroperitoneal edema. There is no necrosis of the pancreas.

2. *Acute Hemorrhagic Pancreatitis.* There is a release of activated pancreatic enzymes, with the resulting pancreatic and small vessel necrosis. Blood clots, portions of the sloughed pancreas and resulting exudate accumulate in the lesser sac (retroperitoneum). Fluid extravasation tracks toward the left diaphragm and pelvis. The patient appears toxic and prostrate in the severest form. The mortality rate is 20 to 30 per cent.

3. *Acute Recurrent Pancreatitis.* This represents a clinical classification based on recurrent self-limited attacks, and it is often associated with gallbladder disease.

4. *Chronic Pancreatitis.* This represents

the end stage of multiple acute attacks. The pancreas is fibrotic, with dilated ducts and calcifications (parenchymal or ductal). A state of pancreatic insufficiency occurs, with a resulting malabsorption syndrome. The patient loses weight and is in constant pain.

## Basic Principles

A combination of ductal obstruction and pancreatic stimulation will produce pancreatitis experimentally. It has been hypothesized that ductal obstruction in humans occurs secondary to hyperplastic ductal epithelium, common duct stone or spasm of the spincter of Oddi. The last two mechanisms may also produce pancreatitis by reflux of activated bile into the pancreatic duct through a common channel (which is present in two thirds of normal people). In all reported series, there is a high association of the disease with alcoholism or gallbladder disease. In the former case, alcohol acting as a gastric secretagogue promotes duodenal release of secretin, which stimulates the pancreatic secretion. In the latter instance, the gallbladder contains infected bile, which will activate trypsin on reflux into the pancreas. It is therefore advised that cholecystectomy be performed electively in patients with pancreatitis and cholelithiasis.

## Criteria for Diagnosis

1. History of previous similar attacks
2. Recent large alcoholic intake
3. Previous gallbladder disease
4. The pain is bandlike epigastric, radiating to the back, with associated vomiting.
5. The patient may appear prostrate.
6. Tachycardia is a constant finding, often out of proportion to the associated fever and usually unresponsive to fluid replacement.
7. Temperature and white blood count are moderately elevated.
8. The abdomen is soft, since the seat of inflammation is retroperitoneal, but tenderness to deep palpation may be present.
9. When pancreatic ferments enter the peritoneal cavity, signs of peritonitis may develop which mimic perforations of the gastrointestinal tract.
10. Mild jaundice may be present.
11. X-ray findings may be helpful:
    A. Colonic distention to the splenic flexure due to irritation of the sympathetic nerves accompanying the superior mesenteric artery (which underlies the inflamed pancreas)
    B. Left pleural effusion due to direct extension of the retroperitoneal exudate. This may be too small to see on a routine chest plate, so if the diagnosis is suspected, a left lateral decubitus view should be ordered. Left pleural effusion occurs with sufficient frequency to be of important diagnostic value.
    C. Sentinel loop of jejunum or ileum overlying the inflamed pancreas
12. *Laboratory Tests*
    A. The white blood count is mildly elevated in the early phase.
    B. Serum amylase may be normal, slightly or greatly elevated. Our most severe cases have demonstrated only a moderate increase (200 to 400 units) of serum amylase. The elevation may be transient in spite of the persistence of the attack.
    C. Urine amylase values are increased for longer periods of time and may be more valuable for diagnosis later in the course.
    D. There are other enzyme elevations, particularly of pancreatic lipase.
    E. The bilirubin level may be slightly elevated but seldom exceeds 6 mg.%.
    F. The SGOT may be elevated, but values over 400 units invariably imply associated liver necrosis (alcoholic).
    G. Calcium levels may be low (urine Sulkowitch's test negative) due to glucagon release from the inflamed organ. Saponification of fat does not totally account for the low serum calcium levels.
    H. Abdominal paracentesis. When

the diagnosis is in doubt, the collection of peritoneal fluid with amylase values exceeding 2000 units may be helpful. The presence of leukocytes or occasional erythrocytes is nonspecific, whereas bacteria point to a perforation of the gastrointestinal tract. *A negative tap should be ignored.*

## Management

The rationale of treatment is to prevent further stimulation of the gland to secrete enzymes and to correct those deficits which are recognizable.

1. Nothing by mouth
2. Nasogastric suction to avoid presence of acid in the duodenum leading to secretin production
3. Atropine, 1/150 gr. I.M. every 4 hours, to produce a vagolytic effect on gastric and pancreatic secretion
4. Intravenous fluids and colloid to restore oncotic pressure and blood volume and to maintain tissue perfusion. Since the fluid administration may be great, careful control should include monitoring of the central venous pressure and urinary output.
5. Measure temperature every 4 hours and the white blood count daily.
6. If the urine Sulkowitch's test is negative, give calcium gluconate 1 gm. in each 1000 ml. of I.V. fluids.
7. Antibiotics are optional in the routine case or in the early phase, but they should be used when temperature or white blood count elevation persists longer than 3 days.
8. In the routine case, the patient appearing critically ill at first begins to respond within 24 hours by relief of pain. The tachycardia may last 2 to 3 days in spite of adequate fluid replacement. By the third day, the temperature and white blood count have returned to normal. Oral feeding should not be commenced until all pain is gone and the afebrile patient has tolerated 24 hours without nasogastric intubation.

## Complicating Problems

1. *If the Diagnosis is Uncertain*

In some cases, particularly in those cases associated with peritoneal irritation, a differential diagnosis from conditions requiring operation may be difficult. The key points to evaluate will be:

A. Serum amylase values over 600 units

B. Chest x-rays demonstrating left pleural effusion

C. The presence of free air on abdominal upright film or chest x-ray should *rule out* pancreatitis.

D. Abdominal fluid examination

If after thorough evaluation peritonitis cannot be ruled out, it is safer to operate. If cholecystitis is found at operation, it is handled routinely and common duct exploration and drainage are advisable. If only pancreatitis is found with no collection in the lesser sac, the abdomen is closed. With a lesser sac collection, drainage with sump tubes is advised.

2. *If the Patient Remains Febrile*

If by the fourth postadmission day the patient is still running a high fever, then one should suspect the development of a pancreatic abscess. Under these circumstances, the fever will be spiking and the white blood count will be high (occasionally over 30,000/mm.[3]). Antibiotics should be used and a retrogastric mass searched for on a GI series. A high mortality rate can be expected regardless of treatment. If after 5 to 8 days the patient is not responding to this treatment, the temperature is still high, the white blood count is rising and a mass is still evident on x-ray or physical examination, drainage is indicated. There is no wall to the abscess at this stage, so the safest procedure is marsupialization by suture of the lesser omentum to the abdominal wound margins and sump drainage of the lesser sac. If significant bleeding is present, packing of the lesser sac with a head roll for 48 to 72 hours may be helpful. These patients are critically ill and must be monitored frequently and carefully if mortality is to be avoided. On these occasions we do not think of developments on a daily basis, but rather on an hourly basis.

3. *If an Abdominal Mass Develops*

The presence of a mass in a patient with pancreatitis is not an absolute indication for operation. Treatment should include antibiotics because the mass may represent an abscess. Two thirds of these masses will resolve with nonoperative treatment. Indications for operation include a rising white blood count, spiking high temperature and radiographic evidence of enlargement of the mass by serial GI series with a lateral view of the barium-filled stomach. Ten per cent of these masses become infected and need drainage as above, whereas 20 per cent mature and become pseudocysts containing clear, yellow noninfected pancreatic fluid. These may be drained electively by anastomosis to a viscus.

## DIVERTICULITIS

### Definition

Diverticulitis is peridiverticular inflammation, sometimes with perforation and/or abscess formation in a *segment* of the colon.

### Basic Principles

Diverticula of the colon are common in the older age-group, being present in 70 per cent of routine barium studies. They may occur in localized segments of the right or left colon or over the entire colon, but the most common site is the sigmoid colon. They are false diverticula since the outpocketing is not covered by all layers of colon, but the mucosa may be in direct approximation to the serosa. Therefore, with inflammation somatic fibers are almost immediately involved, giving localized pain as the earliest symptom. Irritation of the colon occurs frequently, with the development of diarrhea as an early symptom. The inflamed diverticulum often bleeds, but it rarely bleeds massively enough to repre-

sent a threat to the patient's life. Since the disease involves an intestine containing large numbers of pathogenic bacteria, an abscess will occur unless the diverticulum evacuates itself rapidly into the intestinal lumen. The onset of the disease probably involves obstruction to the neck of the diverticulum with secondary infection. If a segment of colon is involved which is retroperitoneal (i.e., descending colon), the abscess usually burrows along the wall of the colon near the lateral pelvic wall and becomes localized in that area. If the involved segment is intraperitoneal, the abscess may burrow into the mesentery, with walling-off being accomplished by approximation of neighboring small bowel loops or the bladder. With continued inflammation, perforation into these organs may follow, leading to enterocolic or vesicocolonic fistulas. If the small bowel loop fixed to the abscess is kinked upon itself, small bowel obstruction may occur early, presenting with a confusing picture of systemic symptoms (fever, malaise, elevated WBC, localized pain, etc.) preceding the mechanical symptoms (referred midabdominal pain, vomiting, etc.).

On rare occasions, the abscess may perforate freely into the peritoneal cavity, leading to a generalized peritonitis.

### Criteria for Diagnosis

1. The acute attack of right-sided diverticulitis is almost indistinguishable from acute appendicitis and will therefore be treated by early operation.

A. The chief complaint is of localized left lower quadrant abdominal pain, occasionally associated with diarrhea.

B. Previous history of similar episodes, intermittent diarrhea or a proven (x-ray) diagnosis of colonic diverticulitis

C. Occasional blood-streaking on the stool

D. Mild fever (100 to 102° F.)

E. Mild leukocytosis

F. Tenderness in the left lower

quadrant on palpation (localized peritonitis)

G. Occasionally the presence of a mass

This represents the usual mild attack and is treated by systemic antibiotics, nothing by mouth (in case early operation is necessary) and careful observation of the progress of the disease by frequent clinical monitoring (fever, leukocytosis, abdominal examination).

2. In the more advanced cases, the following will be present:

A. Higher fever (102 to 104° F.)

B. Leukocytosis over 15,000/mm.³

C. Peritoneal signs outside the left lower quadrant

D. X-ray examination demonstrating free intraperitoneal air

E. Enlarging mass

F. Evidence of fistulization (pneumaturia, bacteriuria)

## Management of the Early and Self-Limited Phase

1. Nothing by mouth
2. Systemic broad-spectrum antibiotics. Penicillin, 1.2 million units I.M. b.i.d.; streptomycin, 0.5 gm. I.M. b.i.d.
3. Parenteral intravenous maintenance fluids
4. Frequent abdominal examinations
5. Rectal temperatures every 2 to 4 hours
6. Repeat the white blood count every 6 to 8 hours.
7. This nonoperative treatment is maintained as long as there are no abdominal findings outside of the left lower quadrant, the mass and tenderness are improving with each observation, and the fever and white blood count are decreasing.
8. Barium enema examination is delayed as long as peritoneal signs are present. When they diminish, it can be performed for diagnosis. This will avoid leakage of barium from the colon, which represents a serious complication.

## Indications for Operation

1. Continuing, spreading or generalized peritoneal signs
2. Obstruction of the small intestine or colon
3. Failure of the patient to respond to nonoperative management
4. Evidence of vesicocolonic fistula
5. Free intraperitoneal air
6. Leakage of barium outside of the colon

## Choice of Operation

### Primary Resection and Anastomosis

Criteria for anastomosing an unprepared colon include: no proximal colonic obstruction (anastomosis of a dilated proximal colon is dangerous and may lead to leakage); a normal, uninflamed distal segment; no peritoneal inflammation in the area of anastomosis; and ability to resect the involved segment safely. If these criteria are not met, a primary resection without anastomosis or a proximal, diverting colostomy should be performed.

### Primary Resection Without Anastomosis

If the mass is not firmly fixed to the lateral abdominal wall (movable mass), it can usually be resected. This is the preferred treatment since it immediately removes the disease, allowing early recovery of the patient. If safe anastomosis cannot be performed, a proximal-end colostomy is made. The distal segment may be brought to the abdominal wall as a separate mucous fistula or simply closed and returned to the abdominal cavity. A secondary anastomosis can then be performed at a later stage (after 2 weeks to 6 months, depending upon the patient's course and the extent of residual inflammation). This is the preferred treatment in most of our acute cases.

### Proximal Diverting Colostomy

This is the preferred treatment when the mass cannot be removed safely, in the presence of vesciocolonic fistulization, or if carcinoma is suspected. It represents the first stage of a 2- or 3-stage procedure and is the safest procedure in the complicated case. Separate extraperitoneal drainage of the abscess may occasionally be indicated. We cannot stress enough that the colostomy must be truly diverting, since loop colostomies are associated with continued sepsis in many patients, which reflects inadequate treatment.

Proximal-loop colostomy is indicated, however, when the disease is resected and anastomosis is performed below the peritoneal reflection, since the rate of leakage from these anastomoses may reach 30 to 40 per cent in this disease.

Accompanying small bowel obstruction is treated operatively by relieving the obstruction, and the primary disease (diverticulitis) is treated as indicated above (resection and end colostomy if possible).

The major complicating factor is the possible presence of carcinoma. Perforating carcinoma may present with the identical clinical findings as in diverticulitis and may be associated with diverticulosis or diverticulitis. In the latter case, the x-ray diagnosis may be difficult due to associated inflammatory changes in the involved segment. The safest approach is a proximal transverse colon-diverting colostomy so that the definitive resection of the carcinoma is not compromised. A left hemicolectomy can then be performed at a later stage, with removal of the lymph-bearing mesentery *en bloc.*

## ACUTE PERFORATIONS OF THE GASTROINTESTINAL TRACT

### Basic Principles

Gastrointestinal perforation represents an acute surgical condition necessitating early operation. The mortality increases linearly with the delay between perforation and operation, and neither the patient's age nor associated conditions should deter the physician from directing his efforts toward avoiding this delay. Diagnostic procedures should be avoided when the clinical diagnosis is clear but should be performed as emergencies if the diagnosis is only suspected.

Eighty per cent of perforations are gastroduodenal due to ulcer disease, 10 per cent are due to appendicitis, 5 per cent are due to diverticulitis and 5 per cent are due to miscellaneous conditions (i.e., foreign bodies).

### Criteria for Diagnosis

1. Acute onset of abdominal pain without a prodrome. The pain is often generalized, and the patient usually recalls the *exact moment* of onset, which may have the character of a blow to the abdomen.

2. Distinct evidence of peritonitis on examination, which may be localized or generalized. Rapid sealing-off of an ulcer by the overlying liver may limit the findings to the upper abdomen, but this seal is ineffective and delay in operation will often result in continued leakage.

Since the root of the mesentery runs diagonally across the abdomen from left upper quadrant to right lower quadrant, fluid tracking along this course may pool in the right lower quadrant, presenting peritoneal findings similar to appendicitis. Associated upper abdominal tenderness clearly differentiates the two conditions, along with the lack of vomiting and prodromal symptoms in perforation.

3. Temperature and white blood count are usually normal in acute perforations as opposed to acute pancreatitis.

4. The patient refuses to move (peritonitis) and may appear prostrate.

5. Abdominal x-ray films with the patient upright or, more characteristically, a chest x-ray will demonstrate free intraperitoneal air in 60 per cent of cases.

6. An abdominal paracentesis may reveal free gastrointestinal fluid by the presence of mucus or bacteria. *A negative abdominal tap should be ignored.*

7. The use of air or Gastrografin instilled into the stomach under fluoroscopic control has proven useful in some cases to demonstrate the leak. *Barium is contraindicated if perforation is suspected.*

8. With strong clinical suspicion of perforation, operation is carried out. In the presence of acute peritonitis, a condition necessitating operation will usually be discovered.

## Management

1. Operation within 2 hours of admission
2. Nasogastric intubation to reduce further peritoneal contamination
3. Nothing by mouth
4. Resuscitative fluids. Since the onset is usually acute, restoration of blood volume can be accomplished relatively quickly with balanced salt solutions and plasma substitutes.
5. Prepare the abdomen for operation.
6. Obtain x-rays and perform an abdominal tap if the diagnosis is in doubt.
7. In the elderly patient, an ECG and chest films may aid the anesthesiologist in management.
8. Broad-spectrum antibiotics are started at once and continued intraoperatively.

## Choice of Operation

1. The choice of operation, of course, depends upon the nature and site of perforation. In the usual case of gastroduodenal perforation, simple closure of the perforation, reinforced by an omental tag, is performed, and any definitive procedure is delayed. Survival of the patient is of prime importance and treatment of underlying ulcer disease is secondary.

2. We have had occasional complications of an associated posterior ulcer in some patients, and in others the perforation represented the anterior component of a circumferential duodenal ulcer. If there is associated bleeding, or if extensive ulcer disease is suspected, examination at operation is warranted. In many cases, the perforation can be opened further and closed as a pyloroplasty. The performance of a vagotomy then completes the procedure. We have not seen a case of mediastinitis under these circumstances. Primary gastric resection is reserved for special circumstances:

A. Patient under 40 years of age
B. Indication for resection other than perforation (i.e., bleeding, obstruction)
C. Perforation less than 6 hours old
This is done in less than 10 per cent of our cases.

3. Prior to closure of the abdomen, extensive irrigation is carried out with saline containing kanamycin, 1 gm. per liter. At least 6 liters of irrigating fluid are used. Systemic antibiotics are used postoperatively.

## ACUTE REGIONAL ENTERITIS

### Definition

Acute regional enteritis is granulomatous inflammation of segments of the intestinal tract, usually in the distal ileum, but found also in the colon, jejunum, duodenum and stomach.

### Basic Principles

The etiology is unknown. The earliest pathologic changes are submucosal edema of the affected intestine and granulomas in the draining lymph nodes. The bowel becomes thickened and rigid, and mucosal ulceration follows; ulcers are deep and located on the mesenteric border, so that perforations are associated with thickened mesentery, abscesses and fistulae to neighboring loops of bowel, without free intraperitoneal perforations. There is polymorphonuclear and mononuclear cell infiltration in the bowel, with the formation of granulomas.

The bowel appears inflamed, thickened and rigid, with mesenteric fat covering much of its circumference. Abrupt changes to normal-appearing bowel are common, as are skip areas. Any segment of small or large bowel may be involved.

The disease is chronic and recurrent. Any combination of signs and symptoms may occur, from acute peritonitis to mild intermittent diarrhea. Free perforations, however, are rarely seen unless the patient has had treatment with corticosteroids.

## Criteria for Diagnosis

1. History of recurrent abdominal pain and diarrhea, intermittent fever of unknown type, wasting or debility, or previous proven regional enteritis. Occasionally rectal bleeding is evident.

2. Symptoms or signs compatible with intermittent or partial intestinal obstruction (i.e., recurrent crampy pain, vomiting, diarrhea)

3. Symptoms or signs compatible with internal fistulization (i.e., weight loss, sepsis, chronic diarrhea)

4. The acute case may be indistinguishable from acute appendicitis except for an underlying history of chronicity.

5. Abdominal findings may be negative or examination may reveal localized right lower quadrant tenderness. Diffuse peritonitis is absent unless the patient has been on steroid treatment.

6. The white blood count may be normal or elevated.

7. Most accurate diagnoses are made by barium x-ray of the small bowel, which may demonstrate:
   A. Separation of the loops due to thickening of the bowel wall
   B. Partially obstructed loop
   C. Fistulization

Consultation with an experienced radiologist is worthwhile.

## Management

1. The disease is usually treated nonoperatively, using supportive measures, intestinal antibiotics and corticosteroids. In many medical centers, the use of steroids is avoided since effective results have been equivocal and intra-abdominal complications may occur with a reduction in physical findings. Silent perforations may be catastrophic if operation is delayed.

2. Operation is recommended for acute peritonitis, obstruction, fistulization or massive bleeding.
   A. Nothing by mouth
   B. Nasogastric intubation
   C. Maintenance intravenous fluids
   D. Frequent abdominal examinations
   E. Follow the white blood count and temperature.
   F. Obtain electrolyte studies and ECG if necessary.
   G. Chest and abdominal films
   H. Surgical and medical consultation
   I. When the patient's condition is stable, order a GI series with small bowel follow-through.

# ULCERATIVE COLITIS

## Definition

Ulcerative colitis is inflammation of the colon (segmental or total), involving the mucosa primarily.

## Basic Principles

The etiology is unknown. The earliest changes involve the mucosal crypts, with the development of small abscesses. These rupture and lead to mucosal ulceration. Inflammation then involves the submucosa, with resulting polymorphonuclear infiltration followed by scarring. The mucosal ulcers coalesce, producing linear defects. The normal mucosa between the ulcerations gives the appearance of polypoid excrescences (pseudopolyps). Recurrent episodes produce scarring and contraction of the colon, which becomes thickened, rigid and shortened.

The disease may be indolent, chronic, recurrent with frequent acute bouts or, more usually, slowly progressive with persistent diarrhea, weight loss and debility. In long-standing cases, carcinoma occurs with increased frequency. Loss of protein through the stool may be great.

## Criteria for Diagnosis

1. Recurrent or persistent diarrhea, which may contain large amounts of mucus and/or blood
2. Weight loss and debility
3. Fever with the acute phase
4. Abdominal tenderness is usually absent except in cases of impending perforation.
5. The white blood count is normal or slightly elevated.
6. *Sigmoidoscopy* classically reveals rectal involvement, with friable, bleeding mucosa and ulcerations. Biopsy of the rectum will be diagnostic in these cases.
7. *Barium enema* reveals a shortened colon with loss of haustral contractions ("pipe-stem" colon). Mucosal ulcerations or pseudopolyps may be evident. Early mucosal changes and "thumbprinting" may best be diagnosed by a radiologist.

## Management

The acute case may be best treated nonoperatively by steroid enemas or parenteral steroids. Supportive treatment includes restoration of blood volume, maintenance fluids, intestinal antibiotics and low-residue diet.

Bleeding is seldom severe enough to necessitate early operation.

## SPECIAL PROBLEMS ASSOCIATED WITH ULCERATIVE COLITIS

### *Acute Toxic Megacolon*

## Definition

An acute toxic megacolon is acute massive dilation of the colon, associated with high fever, prostration and toxemia.

## Basic Principles

Occasionally the patient with ulcerative colitis may present with a fulminating illness due to acute colonic dilatation, toxemia and prostration. The massively dilated colon is the most striking finding and perforation is imminent. A previous history of steroid administration must make the physician aware of the possibility of "silent" perforation with minimal abdominal findings.

## Criteria for Diagnosis

1. Toxemia, fever, prostration, diarrhea
2. Abdominal distention (occasionally massive)
3. Tenderness indicating impending perforation
4. X-ray evidence of massive colonic dilatation
5. Sigmoidoscopic evidence of acute colitis
6. Elevated white blood count
7. Decreased hematocrit, and serum albumin levels
8. Tachycardia

## Management

In some medical centers, the patient is hydrated, the blood volume is restored by use of albumin and blood, and early operation is performed. The operation may be performed in one or two stages, consisting of colonic resection, ileostomy and a distal-end mucous fistula or oversewing the rectum. Perineal resection of the rectum is the second stage. The results are remarkable, with immediate improvement, reduction in toxemia and fever and early return to normal feeding.

Rarely, if perforation can be ruled out, parenteral steroids are given with supportive treatment, fluids, blood and antibiotics. The risk of perforation may increase with the use of steroids, although some physicians believe the over-all mortality is diminished.

1. Rehydration with saline, albumin, plasma and blood
2. Frequent abdominal examinations for perforation

3. Nothing by mouth

4. Nasogastric suction

5. Monitor the central venous pressure and urine output.

6. If fever and elevated white blood count persist or abdominal tenderness is noted, *early operation* is recommended.

7. If the patient improves over several hours, steroids (prednisone, 20 mg. t.i.d., or cortisone acetate, 50 mg. q.i.d. I.M.) may be used.

## *Complications of Ulcerative Colitis*

### Basic Principles

Long-standing ulcerative colitis may be associated with hepatic damage, arthritis, pyoderma gangrenosum, uveitis, severe hypoproteinemia and carcinoma of the colon.

### Criteria for Diagnosis

1. Careful history and physical examination for changes in the skin, joints or uvea

2. Liver chemistries

3. Barium enema with careful mucosal studies. The diagnosis of early carcinoma is difficult because the mucosal destruction due to the disease masks the earliest changes of colonic cancer.

4. Serum albumin levels are low.

5. Anemia

6. Usually long-standing disease with persistent diarrhea and weight loss

7. Sigmoidoscopy and biopsy

### Management

1. Nonoperative management includes steroids, restoration of blood volume, intestinal antibiotics and low-residue diet.

2. Regression of complications occurs with resection of the disease.

3. Intravenous hyperalimentation is useful in treating hypoalbuminemia and restoring a positive nitrogen balance prior to operation.

4. Definitive operation is indicated in long-standing disease accompanied by:

    A. Debility or chronic weight loss

    B. Persisting diarrhea

    C. Threat of malignancy

    D. Bleeding with persisting anemia

    E. Complications of liver disease, pyoderma and arthritis unresponsive to nonoperative treatment

Operation consists of proctocolectomy and ileostomy.

## ACUTE PELVIC INFLAMMATORY DISEASE

### Definition

Acute pelvic inflammatory disease is inflammation of the pelvic viscera, usually secondary to gonorrheal infection.

### Basic Principles

Pelvic inflammatory disease is included here due to its frequent occurrence and the difficulty in its differentiation from other acute abdominal conditions (e.g., appendicitis). The causative organism is usually gonoccocus (*N. gonorrhea*), which invades the pelvic adnexa after introduction into the vagina. Salpingitis or tubo-ovarian abscess may result, presenting with acute abdominal findings.

### Criteria for Diagnosis

1. History of exposure

2. Pain starting in the lower abdomen without history of shifting

3. Vomiting, absent or late

4. Pelvic examination reveals tenderness on cervical motion to either side; vaginal vault tenderness may be marked. Occasionally the inflamed tube is palpable or an adnexal mass may be felt.

5. Abdominal tenderness is maximal several centimeters inferior to McBurney's point

6. White blood count and temperature is often higher than seen in early acute appendicitis.

7. Erythrocyte sedimentation rate is elevated.

8. Gram stain of vaginal smear may reveal the organism.

## Management

1. Give nothing by mouth until appendicitis is ruled out as unlikely.
2. Observe the patient, with frequent abdominal and pelvic examinations.
3. Repeat the white blood count.
4. If the diagnosis is secure, give procaine penicillin, 600,000 u. I.M. b.i.d.
5. If the diagnosis is in doubt after 6 hours and appendicitis cannot be ruled out, operate.

## RUPTURED ECTOPIC PREGNANCY

### Definition

An ectopic pregnancy is a pregnancy outside the normal intra-uterine location, usually in a salpinx.

### Basic Principles

Ectopic pregnancies with intra-abdominal rupture may lead to catastrophic hemorrhage and death. The earliest signs may be acute abdominal pain.

### Criteria for Diagnosis

1. Carefully elicited history of a missed menstrual period or irregular menses; the possibility of pregnancy
2. Previous pelvic inflammatory disease
3. Vaginal bleeding or staining
4. Tenderness in the adnexa on pelvic examination
5. Anemia or clinical evidence of hypovolemia (i.e., faintness, tachycardia, etc.)

### Management

1. If suspected, a gynecologic consultation should be called for immediate culdoscopy or laparoscopy.
2. Nothing by mouth
3. I.V. fluids
4. Crossmatch 4 units of blood.
5. If an adenexal mass is palpated or hypovolemia and/or shock is evident, immediate operation is indicated.

## PRIMARY PERITONITIS

### Definition

Primary peritonitis is inflammation of the peritoneum without primary intra-abdominal visceral disease.

### Basic Principles

Acute primary peritonitis is uncommon in adults, but it may occur secondary to tuberculous infection or rarely to other organisms. A primary focus may not be clearly evident.

### Criteria for Diagnosis

1. The diagnosis is difficult to make without operation.
2. Diffuse abdominal tenderness
3. High fever, prostration
4. Ascites is common.
5. The white blood count is elevated or normal.
6. Abdominal tap may reveal gram-positive organisms on smear (streptococcus or pneumococcus).

### Management

1. Nonoperative treatment is indicated, but, due to the difficulty of differentiating primary peritonitis from the intraabdominal diseases and its rarity, operation is often performed.
2. Nothing by mouth
3. Nasogastric suction
4. Maintenance I.V. fluids
5. Antibiotics appropriate to cultured organism

## ACUTE TOXIC (ALCOHOLIC) CIRRHOSIS

### Definition

Acute toxic cirrhosis is hepatic necrosis secondary to the intake of toxic amounts of alcohol.

### Basic Principles

Fatty infiltration of the liver and cellular necrosis may follow prolonged large alcoholic intake. Underlying cirrhosis may or may not be evident. The liver is swollen and tender, very soft to the touch and bleeds on mild trauma. Histologic examination in the severe case reveals massive areas of necrosis with few remaining intact liver cells. The mortality rate is high and with operation under general anesthesia rises to 20 per cent.

## Criteria for Diagnosis

1. Recent history of large alcoholic intake
2. Mild abdominal pain
3. Tenderness over the liver
4. Jaundice
5. White blood count occasionally over 25,000/mm.$^3$
6. Liver chemistries may be obstructive in type, with elevated alkaline phosphatase and SGOT.
7. Elevated temperature

8. Abdominal pain, jaundice and fever may be confused with cholangitis.

## Management

1. Nothing by mouth
2. Maintenance I.V. fluids
3. Follow carefully:
   A. Abdominal examination
   B. White blood count
   C. Temperature
4. The obstructive pattern of liver chemistries may be confusing unless accompanied by abnormal cephalin flocculation or a very high SGOT.
5. Avoid operation if possible. If obstructive jaundice with cholangitis cannot be ruled out, then liver biopsy under *local anesthesia* should be done. A simultaneous cholangiogram will delineate any obstruction, and anesthesia can be induced if alcoholic necrosis is not present.

# 18. VASCULAR EMERGENCIES

*Philip N. Sawyer*, M.D.
*Michael R. Golding*, M.D.

Vascular surgical emergencies involve an interruption of normal blood flow to or from an organ, limb or area of the body. If inflow is primarily involved, the ischemic area will not develop edema or swelling. If outflow is blocked, consequent edema will lead to arterial compression and associated ischemia. These factors account for the presenting signs and symptoms of most vascular surgical problems.

## ACUTE ARTERIAL OCCLUSION

### Definition

Acute arterial occlusion is the sudden interruption of arterial inflow to an organ without opportunity for development of collateral circulation.

### Classification

Acute arterial occlusion may be due to:

1. *Embolism.* Material formed in the heart or a vessel is propelled distally, obstructing at a point where the vessel is smaller than the embolus. Emboli may be caused by:

A. Heart disease (either arteriosclerotic or rheumatic) with associated valvular excrescences or thrombi

B. Atrial fibrillation, particularly in patients with rheumatic heart disease and mitral stenosis where left atrial stasis promotes thrombus formation

C. Myocardial infarction with mural thrombus or ventricular aneurysm

D. Subacute bacterial endocarditis

E. Left atrial myxoma

F. Right atrial or systemic venous emboli—"paradoxical" emboli via septal defects

G. Atherosclerotic plaque—either a free-floating fragment or a superimposed recent thrombus on a pre-existing plaque

2. *Thrombosis.* Arterial thrombosis is caused by *in situ* clotting. This is often associated with arteriosclerosis where thrombosis begins on the nidus of the pre-existing atherosclerotic plaque.

3. *Dissecting Aneurysm.* Intramural hemorrhage or dissection in a major artery can produce acute occlusion by narrowing and compressing the lumen. There is often associated thrombus formation.

4. *Low Flow Syndromes.* Low flow syndromes such as those associated with congestive heart failure, hypovolemia, severe dehydration or poor cardiac output can produce thrombosis. Ischemia, however, can occur in these syndromes in spite of vessel patency if the tissue perfusion is inadequate to meet the metabolic demand.

### Basic Principles

1. Establish the cause of the acute blockage of the artery. This can usually be done on the basis of history and physical examination.

A. Without pre-existing signs or symptoms of arterial disease, but with a probable source for an embolus, embolic occlusion is most likely. Under these circumstances, angiography is usually not required.

B. If there is a suggestion of pre-existing arterial disease such as intermittent claudication or other signs or symptoms of chronic arterial insufficiency, aortography is ideally required.

2. *The cardinal principle in the management of acute arterial occlusion is the rapid restoration of pulsatile arterial flow.*

A. If the occlusion is clearly embolic and the extremity is viable, Fogarty catheter embolectomy is indicated.

B. If the occlusion is due to a superimposed thrombosis of a narrowed arteriosclerotic lumen, direct restoration of arterial flow by either endarterectomy or bypass graft is required. Removal of the thrombus alone in cases of arteriosclerotic occlusive disease fails to restore arterial flow, since the conditions that predisposed to the thrombosis remain unchanged.

3. Vasodilators or sympathetic blocks are useless and waste valuable time.

## Criteria for Diagnosis

1. The sudden onset of pain, pallor, coolness, anesthesia and paralysis in a pulseless extremity are the classical signs of acute arterial occlusion. The entire syndrome complex is not necessary for diagnosis. The presence of any one of the signs together with absent peripheral pulses demands consideration of the entity.

2. Acute occlusion to an organ is marked by pain in the region involved, loss of function and bleeding (i.e., acute renal artery occlusion would lead to flank pain, failure of urine formation on the involved side and hematuria).

3. Differentiation between the most common causes of arterial occlusion is important since modes of therapy often vary (*see* Table 18-1).

4. *Dissecting Aneurysms.* Although these are rarely a cause of sudden arterial blockage, absent peripheral pulses with acute chest or back pain in a hypertensive patient who exhibits a shock-like clinical picture suggest the diagnosis. Plain chest or abdominal films may show aortic enlargement, and occasionally a loud bruit may be heard. Confirmation of the diagnosis necessitates aortography when the patient's condition permits.

5. *Venous Gangrene.* This is often sudden, usually occurring in an ill patient, with development of blebs, bullae, cyanosis and edema.

6. *Low Flow.* There is obvious evidence of central pump failure with generalized and symmetrical skin color and temperature changes. Extremity pain is usually not prominent, but cardiac symptoms such as dyspnea, orthopnea, tachypnea and tachycardia are seen.

## Management

### Preoperative Work-up

Preoperative evaluation to determine and correct any systemic deficiency (i.e., anemia, dehydration, acidosis, etc.):

1. Complete blood count, urinalysis, FBS, BUN, SGOT and serum electrolytes (SMA-12) are determined.

2. Electrocardiogram as a baseline and to determine dysrhythmias and/or myocardial infarction

3. Chest x-ray, particularly to rule out

**Table 18-1. Factors Differentiating Between the Most Common Causes
of Arterial Occlusion**

| *Factors Favoring Embolus* | *Factors Favoring Thrombosis* |
|---|---|
| 1. History of heart disease | 1. History suggesting pre-existing arteriosclerotic disease—intermittent claudication, chest pain, night cramps, peripheral skin changes, atrophy, absence of hair, hypertrophy of nails, ulcers or gangrene |
| 2. Arteriosclerotic heart disease or rheumatic heart disease with atrial fibrillation, recent myocardial infarction or ventricular aneurysm | |
| 3. Bounding proximal and absent distal pulse due to lodgement at an arterial bifurcation | 2. History of diabetes, latent diabetes or hyperlipemia |
| 4. Ischemia is severe. | 3. Bruit over the involved artery |
| | 4. Ischemia is moderate because of pre-existing collaterals. |

thoracic aneurysm, cardiomegaly or ventricular aneurysm

4. Cross-table lateral film of the spine and flat film of the abdomen to rule out abdominal aortic aneurysm

5. Place a central venous catheter by cutdown or percutaneously.

6. If the patient is in congestive heart failure or has evidence of low flow, a short period of intense medical therapy is required with use of digitalis and diuretics. If there is central pump failure, any peripheral arterial reconstruction is doomed to failure.

7. Intravenous heparin anticoagulation should be started while preoperative preparations are in progress to prevent proximal and distal propagation of the thrombus. Intermittent intravenous heparin, initially 5,000 units followed by up to 7,500 units every 2 hours as determined by the clotting time, is given.

8. The use of streptokinase and other fibrinolytic agents appears very attractive but has not as yet been added to our routine regimen until further clinical progress in the use of these agents is reported.

9. Angiography is mandatory if there is any question as to the cause of the occlusion. Embolic acute arterial occlusions often *do not* require an angiogram for diagnosis and therapy unless there is a question of other pre-existing chronic arterial disease (Table 18-2).

## Preoperative Orders

1. Keep the patient NPO.
2. Consent and clergy
3. Shave and prep the patient from the neck to the ankle (in case of acute occlusion of the femoral artery).
4. Type and crossmatch 4 units of whole blood.
5. Betadine scrubs to the area from the neck to the ankle
6. Perform a cutdown for central venous pressure monitoring in the contralateral upper extremity, using a No. 210 polyethylene catheter with the catheter

brought out through a separate stab wound below the cutdown incision.

7. Soap suds enema until clear
8. Foley catheter for measurement of hourly urine output

## Operative Management

1. *Anesthesia.* Use general endotracheal anesthesia whenever possible, although local anesthesia may be used for the fragile cardiac patient with a peripheral embolus.

A. A cardiac monitor with a defibrillator should be in the operating room.

B. Cardiac medication available in the operating room should include digitalis, furosemide and Xylocaine.

2. *Prep and Drape*

A. Betadine scrubs and prep

B. Drape the area widely, exposing both groins and abdomen to allow a full-length midline incision for adequate access to the aorta if required.

3. *Operative Technique*

A. *Fogarty Embolectomy*

*(1)* This provides rapid exposure of the artery for proximal and distal control by cutting down over the center of the lowest palpable pulse. Exposure should be adequate and capable of extension should there be a failure to obtain a good "in" or "back" bleeding. At the groin, control the profunda femoral artery with umbilical tapes or atraumatic vascular clamps. Administer systemic heparin prior to applying clamps.

*(2)* Oblique arteriotomy is done with a No. 11 blade.

*(3)* Use an appropriate-size Fogarty arterial embolectomy catheter for removal of the clot. A No. 6 catheter is the usual size needed. The catheter is passed until good forward bleeding and back bleeding are obtained. If there is poor forward bleeding, aortic exploration is indicated. This is done transabdominally. If poor back bleeding is obtained, an arteriogram is done on the operating room table and the run-off is evaluated. If the

## Table 18-2. Complications of Arteriography

| Complication | Treatment |
| --- | --- |
| Extravasation of radiopaque medium | This is usually not important since modern media are rapidly absorbed. |
| Local dissection of the arterial wall or aorta due to partial extrusion of the needle from the aorta | This is also usually not important because the blood pressure will rapidly push the dissected intima and media back against the limiting adventitia. |
| Local destruction of the arterial wall due to catheterization with resulting obstruction | Reconstruction must be considered immediately. The earlier this is done, the more satisfactory it usually is. This usually produces a satisfactory result. |
| Nerve palsy due to local trauma | This usually resolves spontaneously unless the nerve has been cut during dissection relating to exposure of artery or vein. If the nerve palsy is not improving within 24 hours, one must obviously diagnose transection. Repair becomes mandatory. |
| Thrombosis due to wrong positioning of the catheter in the blood vessel | Thrombectomy with reconstruction through a transverse arteriotomy is the treatment. |
| Infection is usually due to a local abscess and may lead to thrombosis of a vessel. | It is immediately imperative that incision and drainage, with reconstruction of the thrombosed vessel if possible, be carried out. This is usually a very serious complication and may lead to loss of the limb. It is mandatory that all attempts possible be made to carry out elective arteriography under sterile conditions for this obvious reason. |
| Allergic reactions | These are very uncommon with modern radiopaque media. However, one must always have Adrenalin, Benadryl, intravenous Nembutal, Isuprel, calcium, etc. in the arteriographic room during these procedures for purposes of therapy in case either shock, acute hyperallergic reaction or cardiac arrest occurs. |
| Excessive radiopaque medium injection given | When more than 150 ml. of even the most highly concentrated radiopaque medium have been injected, it is usually important, if not imperative, to diurese the patient in an attempt to remove the iodinated preparation as rapidly as possible. If by mischance a needle or catheter has been allowed to enter the lumen of a small vessel leading to a single organ rather than one of the main channels during injection, necrosis of the organ may take place. The catheter should be left in place, with immediate injection of 5000 units of heparin, 30 mg. of Benadryl and, if necessary, 0.1 mg. of reserpine to block sympathetic vasomotor tone. |

run-off is inadequate, a bypass graft may be constructed.

*(4)* Closure of the artery is done with double-armed 6-0 Dacron sutures.

*(5)* Meticulous hemostasis is obtained by use of cautery and suture ligatures.

*(6)* If there is any oozing, Hemovac drainage should be instituted prior to closure.

*(7)* Closure to eliminate dead space is accomplished with fine 5-0 silk sutures.

*(8)* Use fine 4-0 interrupted nylon sutures for skin closure.

B. If occlusion is due to a superimposed thrombus on an arteriosclerotic narrowing of the artery, the preoperative angiogram provides the basis for direct reconstruction as follows:

*(1)* Short local segment—gas endarterectomy

*(2)* Long segment—reversed autogenous saphenous vein as a bypass graft

*(a)* The number of vessel run-offs will determine the success of the graft.

*(b)* If no run-off is demonstrated by arteriogram, a limited exploration of the run-off bed is done, exposing the popliteal artery and its divisions (posterior tibial, anterior tibial and peroneal arteries) before deciding as to the feasibility of a direct reconstruction.

## Postoperative Management

1. Keep the patient NPO until he is fully awake, alert and reactive, and there appears to be no need for further operation.

2. Take vital signs every hour.

3. Measure fluid intake and output.

4. Control any coexisting or systemic disease (i.e., diabetes mellitus, etc.)

5. The use of a foot cradle is indicated to avoid undue pressure on the extremity.

6. A cardiac monitor is necessary.

7. Control cardiac rate and rhythm (prevent tachycardia or arrhythmia).

A. Xylocaine, 50 to 100 mg. in a bolus; if arrhythmia is present, a drip of 2 to 4 mg. in I.V.

B. Digitalis as needed if cardiac failure supervenes

C. Volume replacement as indicated by central venous pressure and urine output

D. Prevent peripheral vasoconstriction.

8. Encourage active coughing and deep breathing to prevent pulmonary complications.

9. A serial ECG is needed to diagnose myocardial conduction defects or infarction.

10. Perform blood coagulation studies.

11. Give intravenous heparin intermittently, 3,500 to 7,500 units every 4 hours as indicated by clotting time elevation.

12. Give low-molecular-weight dextran (1 to 2 units per day for 3 days).

13. Peripheral pulses and signs of the arterial circulation should be monitored frequently by:

Color

Temperature

Sensation and motor function

Capillary and venous filling

14. Should a previously present pulse disappear, emergency re-exploration of the vessel is indicated.

15. Perform a fasciotomy or fasciectomy as indicated. If the initial occlusion was long, this should be done at the close of the operation.

## Complications

1. Bleeding

2. Thrombosis

3. Infection

4. Thrombophlebitis with or without pulmonary emboli

5. Late revascularization syndrome Restoration of circulation when ischemic muscle damage has occurred may cause a metabolic acidosis and hyperkalemia with the possibility of renal damage and uremia.

## ACUTE VENOUS OCCLUSION

### Definition

Venous thrombosis is occlusion of one

or more superficial or deep veins by a clot. The difference between thrombophlebitis and phlebothrombosis is artificial, because both can be found pathologically in the same vein. In general, if inflammation is noted with the thrombosis, it is called thrombophlebitis. If the patient is free of pain and inflammation, the entity is termed phlebothrombosis. Edema of the extremity is a sign common to both thrombophlebitis and phlebothrombosis.

## Classification

The clinical presentation varies with the severity of the inflammation and the extent of the veins involved. The natural course of the thrombosis is to propagate centrally, causing more severe symptoms.

1. *Superficial thrombophlebitis* is involvement of only the subcutaneous veins of the extremity.

2. *Deep thrombophlebitis* is involvement of the subfascial veins.

A. Localized to the deep veins of the calf or thigh

B. Extensive to involve the iliofemoral veins

C. Massive involvement of the common iliac veins or higher

3. *Complications of Thrombophlebitis*

A. Massive extension of the thrombosis with venous gangrene

B. The postphlebitic syndrome

C. Pulmonary embolism

## Basic Principles

1. Treatment is aimed at rapid restoration of venous circulation to reduce the risk of massive venous thrombosis and gangrene as well as the development of a postphlebitic leg. Lethal pulmonary emboli must also be prevented.

2. A localized deep thrombophlebitis often begins in the muscular veins of the calf in the deep posterior tibial system. If this process continues, there is a propagation of the thrombus into the iliofemoral system. Thrombosis to the level of the external iliac vein with some inevitable involvement of the collateral venous channels produces the syndrome of phlegmasia alba dolens (milk leg).

If the venous thrombosis is allowed to extend to the common iliac vein, the venous obstruction becomes more extensive, and, as the venous outflow decreases, arterial spasm occurs. Distal arterial pulses may be obscured initially by edema and ultimately by compression and thrombosis. The extremity becomes congested and cyanotic and can progress to gangrene.

3. Massive thrombosis of the entire venous system of the extremity is called phlegmasia cerulea dolens and is associated with ischemic gangrene and massive losses of fluid and electrolytes into the extremity.

A. The process of proximal extension of the thrombus can extend to the renal veins.

B. Renal vein thrombosis is associated with massive proteinuria and may result in irreversible renal failure and death.

## Criteria for Diagnosis

1. *To Establish the Diagnosis of Thrombophlebitis:*

A. Pain in the region of the vein

B. Edema

C. Color change from pale white to cyanosis

D. Homans' sign—deep pain in the calf on active dorsiflexion due to traction on the inflamed vein

E. *Cuff pressure test:* inflate a blood pressure cuff on the calf and note the pressure at which there is onset of pain. If the pain is produced at 40 to 50 mm. Hg or less, thrombophlebitis is probable.

F. Dilatation of the superficial veins

G. Tenderness over the course of the involved vein

2. *Confirmation of Diagnosis*

A. The clinical signs and symptoms as listed above are usually sufficient for diagnosis.

B. When the diagnosis is in doubt,

venograms may be necessary for clarification of the diagnosis. With extensive thrombophlebitis involving iliofemoral thrombosis, venography usually is not necessary. (*See* Table 18-3.)

3. *Diagnosis of Pulmonary Embolism*

A. A high index of suspicion should lead the physician to the diagnosis in a patient with a deep thrombophlebitis or phlebothrombosis with any of the following signs and symptoms.

(1) Undue anxiety

(2) Dyspnea

(3) Tachypnea

(4) Tachycardia

(5) Chest pain

(6) Episodic wheezes, particularly if the wheezes clear on I.V. heparin

(7) Hemoptysis

(8) Sudden cough

(9) Pleural effusion or wedge-shaped density on x-ray

B. ECG, chest x-ray and serum enzymes are necessary to rule out other cardiopulmonary pathology. The ECG may show a right ventricular stain pattern.

C. Confirmation of the diagnosis is essential by:

(1) Lung scan. This is useful as a safe, noninvasive screening procedure, but false positive and false negative studies are reported.

(2) Pulmonary angiogram. This is a definitive and most accurate diagnostic procedure.

**Management**

1. Rapid recognition and establishment of the diagnosis of thromboembolism are necessary so that treatment can be instituted immediately and the risk of complications can be minimized.

A. Bed rest

B. Elevation of the foot of the bed on blocks (8 to 10 inches high)

C. Warm soaks

**Table 18-3. Complications of Venography**

| Complication | Treatment |
|---|---|
| Allergic reaction | Stop the injection; give 30 mg. of Benadryl I.V., along with whatever therapeutic agent is necessary, including 1/2 ml. of 1:5000 Adrenalin. |
| Fainting (loss of consciousness with falling) | The patient should be strapped to the table to prevent this complication of upright venography. |
| Infection of cutdown sites | These should be very carefully cleaned out operatively. Incision and drainage may be necessary to remove fixation sutures, etc. |
| Postinjection thrombosis—thrombophlebitis | Give heparin, 7,500 to 10,000 units I.V., immediately after ruling out extravasation of radiopaque medium in the local areas, which may require specific local therapy. |
| Extravasation of radiopaque medium into the feet. This is more serious here because injection is into a semiclosed space with decreased blood supply. | Give heparin and Benadryl locally. |

D. Intravenous anticoagulation with heparin. Dose is determined by following the Lee-White clotting times to regulate the heparin dose, which averages 7,500 units every 4 hours.

2. If edema fails to resolve rapidly or there is a decrease or absence of the pedal pulses or persistent cyanosis, emergency Fogarty venous thrombectomy may be required.

3. If arterial occlusion is significant, multiple fasciotomies may be necessary to salvage the limb.

4. If there is rapid resolution of edema and decrease of symptoms, a 21-day course of heparin is required to allow for healing of the damaged endothelium.

A. The heparin is tapered after the patient is gradually ambulated. Prior to discharge, the patient is measured for gradient-compression stockings.

B. During the course in the hospital, a work-up to rule out any of the predisposing causes of thrombophlebitis is undertaken:

*(1)* Blood dyscrasias
*(2)* Occult malignancy
*(3)* Collagen diseases

5. If there are suspicions of pulmonary emboli, the diagnosis must be ascertained as above.

A. *Treatment of Pulmonary Emboli*

*(1)* Initial therapy for pulmonary embolization is intravenous heparin. If the patient has a proven pulmonary embolus while on heparin, inferior vena caval (IVC) ligation is indicated. Other indications for IVC ligation are septic emboli and contraindications to anticoagulation.

*(2)* Usually no attempt at the operative removal of pulmonary emboli is required.

*(3)* In the patient without cardiac disease, there will be rapid resolution of the pulmonary emboli. Venous interruption may be necessary to protect the patient from further embolic episodes.

B. *Technique of IVC Ligation*

*(1) Incision*

*(a)* In males the right flank from the tip of the 12th rib to just below the umbilicus—retroperitoneal approach

*(b)* In females or when ligation of the left ovarian vein is mandatory—a full-length midline transabdominal approach

*(2)* Preliminary clamping of the IVC prior to ligation is necessary to test the patient's tolerance for such a major phlebotomy.

*(3)* Ligate immediately distal to the level of the renal veins, with double ligature on the IVC and ovarian vein.

## Postoperative Management

1. Bed rest for 3 weeks
2. Elevation of the extremities
3. I.V. heparin for 3 weeks
4. Gradient-compression stockings

## ARTERIAL ANEURYSM

### Definition

An aneurysm is a pulsatile, expansile, localized dilatation of an artery. True aneurysm contains all the elements of the arterial wall. False aneurysm is usually associated with a disruption of the arterial wall, with the aneurysmal sac being composed of compressed soft tissue and clot.

### Classification

1. Aneurysms may be classified as to location:

A. Thoracic aneurysm
B. Abdominal aortic aneurysm
C. Visceral (splenic, hepatic, renal) aneurysm
D. Peripheral arterial (i.e., popliteal, femoral or carotid artery) aneurysm

2. Pathologic classification as to etiology is possible:

A. Congenital medial defect (i.e., Marfan's disease, Ehlers-Danlos syndrome)
B. Medial degeneration from age, infection or inflammation

*(1)* Poststenotic dilation
*(2)* Mycotic
*(3)* Syphilitic
*(4)* Arteriosclerotic

## Basic Principles

1. *Natural Course and Complications of Aneurysm*

A. Small asymptomatic arteriosclerotic aneurysm, with dilatation of the artery above and below so that the lesion is not clearly delineated, is a benign disease of old age, and the prognosis is more related to the patient's general physical condition and cardiovascular status than to the aneurysm. Therefore, in case of small (less than 5 cm.) symptomless aneurysms in the elderly (over 75 years of age), or frail patient, resection of the aneurysm is debatable and each case must be individualized and the indication for operation ,determined in consultation with an experienced internist.

B. It is the natural course of most aneurysms to progressively enlarge; then any of the following circumstances are ultimately possible:

*(1)* Disruption with exsanguinating hemorrhage, either intraperitoneal or retroperitoneal

*(2)* Peripheral embolism from the content of the aneurysmal sac

*(3)* Pressure symptoms on the gastrointestinal or genitourinary tract, nerve root compression, backache due to vertebral erosion, or iliac vein obstruction with phlebothrombosis

C. Leakage or rupture of an aneurysm and uncontrolled pain due to ischemia or pressure are absolute indications for emergency resection of abdominal aortic aneurysm. A very large aneurysm, rapid enlargement of an existing aneurysm or a pressure effect on other viscera requires urgent resection of the aneurysm.

2. In a ruptured or leaking aneurysm, the following are required:

A. Rapid control of exsanguinating hemorrhage

B. Volume replacement of blood and electrolytes

C. Resection of the aortic aneurysm

D. Restoration of arterial continuity with a Dacron graft

E. Assessment of flow to the colon and both renal arteries prior to closure of the abdomen

3. In dealing with a thrombosed aneurysm, resection or exclusion of the aneurysm with restoration of flow by use of a Dacron graft is required.

4. *Thoracic Aortic Aneurysms.* These are usually seen easily on plain x-rays of the chest. Since the emergency management of a leaking or dissecting aneurysm usually requires cardiopulmonary bypass support which is not generally available on an emergency basis, temporizing management may be accomplished by inducing systemic hypotension to levels between 80 and 90 mm. Hg systolic blood pressure with Arfonad or other vasodilating agents. The patient may then be transferred when stable to appropriate facilities for definitive treatment (*see* Chapter 13, Nontraumatic Cardiac and Thoracic Vascular Emergencies).

5. *Visceral Arterial Aneurysms.* Such aneurysms are generally unsuspected and are incidental findings detected by routine aortography. The treatment will depend on the size of the aneurysm, symptoms and the age of the patient.

6. *Peripheral Arterial Aneurysms.* These are prone to thrombose and thus may present with acute arterial ischemia. Attention is first directed in this instance to restoration of flow, and later the aneurysm may be managed by excision and primary or graft repair.

7. *Abdominal Aortic Aneurysms.* These are the most common aneurysms the surgeon will encounter as an emergency. Many of the principles in the diagnosis and management are equally applicable to the preceding three groups of aneurysms and are discussed below.

## Criteria for Diagnosis

The criteria for diagnosis depend on whether the aortic aneurysm is expanding, has thrombosed or is bleeding and, if bleeding, how rapidly.

1. *Ruptured Aortic Aneurysm*

A. Shock, hypovolemia, syncope,

often confused with myocardial infarction or cerebrovascular accident

B. Pain, severe abdominal and/or back pain

C. Pulsatile, expansile, abdominal mass, with diminution of the other peripheral pulses due to vasoconstriction

D. Duodenal compression due to displacement and angulation of the duodenum across the upper part of the aneurysm

E. True root compression by the aneurysm sac with neurologic deficit

F. Ureteral and bladder compression by the expanding aneurysm

2. *Leaking Abdominal Aneurysm*

A. Abdominal, chest or back pain is very prominent, associated with tenderness and signs of peritoneal irritation. A tender abdominal mass may be palpated.

B. The ECG often suggests myocardial infarction or myocardial ischemia.

3. *Thrombosis of an Abdominal Aortic Aneurysm*

A. Signs of acute peripheral arterial ischemia, usually bilateral

B. Absent femoral pulses

C. Abdominal tenderness and mass, decreased blood pressure, often associated with signs of an ileus and abdominal distention because of mesenteric vascular ischemia due to proximal propagation of the thrombosed aortic aneurysm involving the mesenteric vessels

The presence of an aneurysm with a pulsatile and expansile abdominal mass, a rectal examination to detect the presence of iliac artery aneurysms and a cross-table lateral x-ray of the spine to demonstrate a calcified rim are the requirements for diagnosis.

## Aortography

1. This is not routine because it may be confusing, consume valuable time and occasionally produce a false negative angiographic study.

2. An aortogram can provide valuable information in elective circumstances and may determine management if the aneurysm is associated with peripheral arterial insufficiency or occlusive disease.

3. An angiogram is required:

A. If the diagnosis of aneurysm is uncertain

B. If there is any question of aortic dilatation above the renal arteries

C. If there is an elective aneurysm with coincident occlusive disease of the femoral or popliteal arteries

D. An IVP is useful and may be done rapidly in emergency circumstances to delineate the presence and position of both kidneys.

E. Plain x-ray of the abdomen often shows the partly calcified rim of the border of the aneurysm. The cross-table lateral view of the spine gives more information in delineating the anterior margin of the sac than does the flat film of the abdomen.

## Management

### Preoperative Work-up

1. Complete blood count, urinalysis, BUN, creatine, SGOT, FBS, $Na^+$, $K^+$, $Cl^-$, $CO_2$, VDRL

2. Bleeding work-up (bleeding, clotting and prothrombin time)

3. ECG. Signs of myocardial ischemia are often noted due to hypovolemia, but even in the presence of signs of coronary ischemia, bleeding aortic aneurysms require operation.

4. X-ray studies

A. Chest to rule out thoracic aneurysm

B. Abdomen, cross-table lateral to delineate the aneurysm and to establish the diagnosis

C. IVP to show the position of the kidneys

### Preoperative Orders

1. Keep the patient NPO.

2. Shave and prep the patient from the chin to the midcalves.

3. Betadine scrubs and solution for skin preparation

4. Perform cutdowns in both upper extremities.

5. Record the central venous pressure and maintain it at about 8 to 10 cm. of water.

6. Transfuse the patient to restore blood volume.

A. Plasma and Ringer's lactate initially

B. Blood as soon as it is available

7. Infuse mannitol, 25 to 50 gm., or furosemide, 40 to 80 mg., to protect renal function in the hypotensive patient with a ruptured or leaking aneurysm.

8. Type and crossmatch 10 units of whole blood.

9. Foley catheter

10. A nasogastric tube (No. 18 sump) is inserted after the patient is intubated.

11. If the patient has a history of heart disease and has evidence of left ventricular enlargement or congestive heart failure, rapid digitalization with I.V. digoxin is indicated.

12. Arrhythmias detected on the cardiac monitor should be suppressed with a Xylocaine drip or procainamide.

13. Prophylactic antibiotics, preferably penicillin and tetracycline, are started preoperatively.

## Operative Management

1. *Incision.* The incision is full-length midline to expose the common femoral, superficial femoral and deep femoral arteries in the groin.

2. *Exposure*

A. Mobilize the mesentery and exteriorize the small intestine and right colon.

B. Proximal control below the renal vein is obtained. There is usually a "free" area just below the renal veins where the aorta can be easily and safely encircled.

C. Apply a proximal clamp—Pott's clamp. Start a rapid infusion of blood at this point and continue the infusions until there is a continued diuresis.

D. For distal control, both iliac arteries are encircled with umbilical tape.

E. Resect or excise the aneurysm if possible, oversewing the distal stump of the aneurysm and ligating the lumbar arteries.

F. If resection of the aneurysm is excessively difficult, divide the neck of the aortic aneurysm and leave the back wall and side wall adjacent to the inferior vena cava, particularly if the aneurysm is intimately adherent to the adjacent structures.

G. Ensure hemostasis by suture ligating the lumbar arteries from within the aneurysm sac.

H. *Insertion of the Dacron Graft*

*(1)* Endarterectomize the transected aorta to ensure a suitable adventitia to suture the graft.

*(2)* Continuous No. 000 Dacron suture; end-to-end anastomosis. The distal anastomosis is made in the iliacs or femoral arteries.

*(3)* If there is associated occlusive disease of the iliac arteries, the iliacs are ligated and the graft is carried down to the common femoral arteries, where an end-to-side anastomosis is constructed.

I. Check the renal artery and inferior mesenteric artery as to pulsatile flow.

J. Check the position of the nasogastric tube in the stomach prior to closure.

K. Close the parietal peritoneum over the graft with continuous sutures of 00 chromic catgut.

L. *Closure*

*(1)* Use No. 2 Mersaline or Dacron for a single-layer closure; take large bites for a mass closure.

*(2)* Use No. 0000 silk for closure of the subcutaneous tissue to close dead space.

*(3)* Use No. 0000 nylon interrupted sutures to approximate skin.

## Postoperative Management

1. Take vital signs every 15 minutes.

2. The physician should be called if the blood pressure drops below 100, the pulse rises above 100, the respirations are above 30 or the temperature goes above 102° F.

3. Give nothing by mouth.

4. Maintain the patient in a semi-Fowler position.

5. Turn the patient from side to back to side every 2 hours.

6. Encourage the patient to cough and deep breathe.

7. Give oxygen via nasal catheter at 6 L./minute. If there are any signs of ventilatory insufficiency, the patient should be maintained on a volume-cycled ventilator until blood gases and ventilation as monitored by the Wright spirometer are adequate.

8. Provide endotracheal suction every 2 hours. If copious mucopurulent secretions are aspirated, culture and sensitivity are required for appropriate antibiotic therapy.

9. Attach the nasogastric sump tube to continuous low suction.

10. Irrigate the nasogastric tube with 30 ml. of normal saline every 2 hours.

11. Attach the Foley catheter to straight bottle drainage.

12. Measure urine output every hour.

13. Measure urine specific gravity each shift.

14. Analyze the urine for sugar and acetone every 4 hours without coverage.

15. Monitor fluid intake and output.

16. Cardiac monitor

17. Measure central venous pressure every 2 hours.

18. Hematocrit every 8 hours

19. SMA-12, urinalysis, BUN, creatine and SGOT in A.M.

20. ECG in A.M.

21. Chest x-ray in A.M.

22. I.V. fluids must be adequate to maintain urine output between 50 to 100 ml./hour and central venous pressure at approximately 8 to 10 cm. of water.

23. Give antibiotics prophylactically.

24. Record abdominal girth.

25. Watch for signs of peripheral arterial ischemia—color, temperature, pulses.

## VASCULAR TRAUMA

### Definition

Vascular injury may occur with direct, blunt or penetrating trauma or secondary to laceration by a fractured bone fragment penetrating the arteries and/or veins.

Vascular trauma may cause:

1. *Acute ischemia,* which is the sudden interruption of arterial inflow to an extremity or organ

2. *Pulsating hematoma,* which is due to the complete severance or lateral defect in an artery, with resulting collection of blood and clot compressing soft tissue adjacent to the vessel (also called false aneurysm).

3. *Arteriovenous fistula* which is an abnormal communication between the arterial and venous side of the circulation

4. *False aneurysm* (*See* pulsating hematoma, above.)

### Classification

The classification of vascular trauma may be on the basis of the wounding agent or the damage done.

1. Penetrating trauma may result in any of the following types of injuries which can cause acute ischemia:

   A. Severance

   B. Laceration

   C. Perforation

   D. Spasm

   E. Contusion

   F. Disruption of intima

   G. External compression by hematoma

   H. Intramural hemorrhage

2. Nonpenetrating or blunt trauma may also result in acute ischemia by causing:

   A. Contusion with thrombosis

   B. Intramural hemorrhage

   C. External compression

   D. Disruption of intima

3. Iatrogenic trauma (usually due to transarterial diagnostic procedures) may lead to:

   A. Hematoma

   B. False aneurysm

   C. Hemorrhage

   D. Intimal damage and disruption remote from the puncture site

   E. Thrombosis

   F. Distal embolization

## Basic Principles

1. The aims of therapy in the treatment of vascular injuries are:

    A. Control of hemorrhage

    B. Prevention of secondary or delayed hemorrhage

    C. Preservation of function

    D. Restoration of circulation

2. The patient's life should not be sacrificed in an attempt to save a devascularized or useless extremity. General resuscitation and total evaluation of the patient are required prior to undertaking vascular repair which may be extremely time-consuming and destined to failure in the face of systemic vasoconstriction, central cardiac failure or shock with diminished flow.

3. While not all unrepaired arterial injuries require amputation distally, failure to repair such injuries often results in loss of the extremity. The amputation rate associated with ligation of specific arteries is:

    A. Common femoral artery—81 per cent

    B. Popliteal artery—72 per cent

    C. Anterior and posterior tibial arteries—70 per cent

    D. Superficial femoral artery—55 per cent

    E. Brachial artery (above profunda)—55 per cent

    F. Axillary artery (below profunda)—43 per cent

4. Prompt repair of all arterial injuries will prevent acute ischemia and gangrene, and it will also reduce the incidence of false aneurysms and arteriovenous fistulae. Failure of arterial reconstruction may be due to prolonged ischemia, associated venous clotting, postrepair edema with arterial compression, or technical failure of the reconstruction (anastomotic thrombosis).

5. Failure to recognize an arterial injury may lead to certain delayed complications of vascular trauma.

    A. *Arteriovenous Fistula*

      *(1)* Cardiac failure

      *(2)* Subacute bacterial endocarditis

      *(3)* Distal venous insufficiency

    B. *False Aneurysm* (or pulsating hematoma)

      *(1)* Compression of adjacent structures

      *(2)* Venous distention

      *(3)* An expansile hematoma may avulse nearby arteriolar branches and thereby augment the false aneurysm.

      *(4)* Deep infection

      *(5)* Hemorrhage

## Criteria for Diagnosis

1. Following blunt or penetrating trauma, the appearance of any of the following may indicate peripheral ischemia and vascular trauma:

    A. Pain

    B. Pallor

    C. Paresthesia

    D. Coolness

    E. Pulselessness

    F. Mottled or cyanotic appearance

    G. Prolonged capillary or venous filling

2. The presence of the above physical findings makes angiography mandatory. Prior to the diagnosis of vascular injury, severe shock, with resulting "low flow syndrome," and cold injury must be excluded, because these can also result in decreased temperatures and diminished arterial pulsations without organic vascular injury.

3. The diagnosis of an arteriovenous fistula may be suspected by the presence of a bruit heard over the fistula and the presence of Branham's sign (that is, bradycardia following compression of the fistula). High output failure or distal edema and signs and symptoms of endocarditis are occasionally presenting complaints of an arteriovenous fistula. Pulsating hematoma is suspected on inspection, which discloses a large area of ecchymosis with distal edema and diminished peripheral pulses. The

diagnosis is easily made by palpation of a pulsatile mass.

4. Angiography is necessary to demonstrate the anatomical relationship, the size and position of the fistula or the presence of a false aneurysm.

## Recognition of Vascular Injury

1. Frequently vascular injuries are clear-cut and evident on examination.

2. Usually pulsatile external bleeding does not occur but a subfascial hematoma is developed. This subfascial bleeding makes localization of the injury difficult and confuses the differentiation from traumatic occlusion, temporary spasm or external compression of the vessels.

3. The ischemic extremity is usually cool, pale, mottled or cyanotic, pulseless and somewhat enlarged.

4. The progressive stages of neurologic deficit that follow acute ischemia are:

    A. Hypethesia
    B. Anesthesia
    C. Muscle spasm
    D. Paralysis

5. Prior to the diagnosis of vascular injury, severe shock, low flow and cold injury must be excluded.

6. The presence of a distal pulse does not rule out a proximal arterial injury. A distal pulse may persist through collaterals or through a pulsating hematoma or arteriovenous fistula.

7. Acute ischemia is not the only sequela of arterial injury, since pulsating hematoma and arteriovenous fistula are frequently seen when the arterial wound is not repaired.

8. Angiography is mandatory in all stable patients preoperatively:

    A. No closed vascular injury should be explored without angiography to rule out spasm, external compression or associated distal injury.

    B. To evaluate run-off of the ischemic extremity

    C. To delineate the level of the lesion and dictate the operative approach

## Management

### Initial Treatment: Rapid Resuscitation

1. All patients seen promptly in the emergency room are examined for the presence of:

    A. Shock
    B. Signs of intrathoracic injury
    C. Signs of intra-abdominal injury
    D. Signs of intracranial injury

2. A patent airway is established.

3. A route is established for the rapid infusion of fluids:

    A. At the time an intravenous line is placed, blood is simultaneously drawn for typing and crossmatching, hematocrit and baseline serum chemistries, if necessary.

    B. The selection of the specific extremity to be used for infusion depends upon the presence of central venous or arterial injury.

    C. Central venous pressure monitoring is begun.

4. Sucking wounds of the chest are closed, hemothorax or pneumothorax is evacuated, and closed thoracostomy drainage is instituted.

5. Adequate pleural drainage is mandatory, particularly for the patient who will require general anesthesia.

6. Cardiac injury should be suspected with every chest and upper abdominal wound.

    A. Cardiac tamponade is manifested if there are:

        *(1)* Diminished heart sounds
        *(2)* Pulsus paradoxus
        *(3)* Elevated central venous pressure

    B. Cardiac injury is suspected in a patient who does not respond to the usual therapeutic measures of restoration of cardiac output.

    C. Pericardicentesis is indicated for diagnosis and initial treatment.

7. External hemorrhage is controlled with direct pressure.

8. A Foley catheter is inserted into the bladder to monitor urine output.

9. A nasogastric tube is placed.

10. If shock is not relieved by the above regimen, significant internal injury is likely to be present.

A. In the presence of continued massive bleeding, operation may be an integral part of resuscitation.

B. Emergency operation may be the only chance for salvage of a patient with inferior vena cava, aorta or other major vessel bleeding.

11. If the patient is stable and vascular injury is suspected, angiography with a complementary excretory urogram is extremely important.

In the patient with severe hypotension, delay for angiography may be lethal because it is time-consuming and useless because of the low flow.

## Operative Management

1. The objective is to restore circulation at the earliest possible moment. The time elapsed prior to repair is critical in terms of salvage of tissue.

2. Adequate treatment of soft tissue wounds is required, because these injuries are truly contaminated wounds. Thorough debridement of all devitalized tissue and voluminous wound irrigation are required.

3. Repair of penetrating injury depends on the wounding agent and the nature of the injury.

4. Closed or nonpenetrating injury may cause acute ischemia by disruption of the intima, intramural hemorrhage, contusion with thrombosis and external compression.

5. Ligation of a major vessel is to be avoided.

A. Ligation of a so-called critical artery is associated with a high risk of gangrene or a viable but functionless extremity.

B. Ligation of a major vessel is only a lifesaving procedure which is indicated in the following circumstances:

*(1)* The patient's condition is so precarious that the time required for vascular repair cannot be extended.

*(2)* Infection

*(3)* There is a soft tissue loss so great that coverage cannot be effected after vascular reconstruction (this last indication is questionable since homograft or heterograft skin coverage will afford temporary protection).

## Surgical Technique of Repair

1. Through an anatomical approach, proximal and distal control of the damaged artery is obtained first with tapes or atraumatic vascular clamps.

2. Accurate assessment of vessel damage is carried out. The tendency to underestimate the damage must be avoided.

3. Adequate debridement of the artery is done. The vessel wall is debrided, as is torn adventia, back to normal vessel. This is especially important in wounds from high-velocity missiles.

4. Remove proximal and distal intraluminal thrombus and assess back bleeding. If there is no back bleeding, catheter thrombectomy and irrigation with heparinized lactated Ringer's solution are done (5,000 units of heparin per 500 ml. of Ringer's solution are indicated).

5. Resect 1 cm. on either side of the injury with a sharp scalpel.

6. Mobilize the artery adequately and reanastomose without tension.

A. If mobilization would still result in tension on vascular anastomosis, the imposition of a segment of autogenous vein graft is indicated.

B. If there is no tension, an end-to-end anastomosis using 6-0 Dacron suture can be done.

7. The type of repair construction depends on the nature of the wounding agent as well as the injury.

A. Puncture or laceration of an artery due to a stab wound may only require lateral suture if less than 20 per cent of the wall is involved and lateral suture will not compromise the lumen.

B. Resection and reanastomosis are required for all gunshot wounds and all blunt trauma to major vessels.

C. Thrombosis of an injured vessel without loss of continuity cannot be treated with thrombectomy alone. Resection and anastomosis of the involved segment are required for a successful revascularization.

8. Simultaneous injury of an associated vein requires repair, complete hemostasis and interposition of viable tissue between the repaired artery and vein to diminish the chance of the development of an arteriovenous fistula.

9. If associated osseous injury can be stabilized adequately by internal fixation, it should be done because it will simplify subsequent extremity management.

10. Cover the arterial repair with healthy soft tissue.

11. Close the skin over a dry wound without drainage.

## Postoperative Management

1. Edema, particularly after prolonged ischemia and/or extensive venous injury, must be minimized.

A. Early fasciotomy may be required to control edema and muscle-damaging compression. Incipient ischemic muscle contracture may be prevented by complete fasciotomy or fasciectomy.

B. Elevation of the injured extremity is useful in enhancing the rapid resolution of edema.

2. The use of heparin postoperatively is controversial.

A. It increases the risk of hematoma and infection postoperatively.

B. Heparin treatment will not salvage a poor reconstruction.

C. It does not affect platelet thrombosis.

D. Heparin is definitely indicated when extensive venous ligations are required for hemostasis and there is the risk of venous insufficiency, or if there is associated venous thrombosis.

3. Antibiotics and tetanus prophylaxis are utilized.

4. Splint or use a bivalved cast to immobilize the extremity when an associated fracture must be stabilized.

A. A splint may be needed if flexion is required to prevent tension on the anastomosis.

B. In civilian life, internal fixation of fractures, when possible, may prevent the disruption of the anastomosis and facilitate the postoperative care.

5. Maintain the part at rest until soft tissue healing is progressing satisfactorily prior to any exercise.

## Treatment of Complications of Missed Arterial Injury

### Pulsating Hematoma (False Aneurysm)

1. Operation is indicated as soon as the diagnosis is established and confirmed by adequate angiography and the patient is stable and free of infection.

A. Since there is no hope for spontaneous cure, unnecessary delay makes operative repair more difficult. A pulsating hematoma tends to expand and shear off vascular branches which augment the false aneurysm.

B. With the increase in size of the false aneurysm there is edema of the skin which predisposes to infection.

2. Operative management includes:

A. Generous exposure to obtain proximal and distal control of the involved vessel

B. Leaving the skin over the false aneurysm intact until control is obtained

C. Sharp dissection which is less traumatic and avoids hemorrhage

D. After this control is obtained, evacuation of the hematoma and creation of a dry field

E. Resection or repair of the artery according to the nature of the injury, wounding agent and the involved vessel

### Arteriovenous Fistula

1. The indication for operation is the

same as above for pulsating hematoma except with added urgency because of the risk of cardiovascular disorders (i.e., congestive heart failure and endocarditis).

2. *Operation*

A. Obtain proximal and distal control of the vessel at a distance through a normal and easily accessible field.

B. Identify the fistula and its branches.

C. Repair the fistula with resection of the artery and its branches and suture repair of the vein.

D. Absolute hemostasis is required to prevent infection or recurrence of the fistula.

E. Interposition of viable tissue between the reconstructed artery and sutured vein is very useful to prevent recurrence.

## FROSTBITE

### Definition

Frostbite is thermal injury due to excessive supercooling with intracellular ice-crystal formation.

### Basic Principles

It is important to realize that the gangrenous (necrotic) changes observed occur from an external source and do not involve a primary deficiency in blood flow. Therefore, they do not indicate irreversible tissue loss in the area. However, gas formation and crepitation in the tissues with severe infection, if secondary to frostbite, may necessitate amputation.

### Criteria for Diagnosis

#### Signs and Symptoms

Classically a patient arrives in the emergency room complaining of having fallen asleep in the cold or of other long exposure, with frozen, usually thawed, swollen, blistered, erythematous, distal limbs and toes. The lesions may be quadralateral.

The classical changes in the fingers and toes plus the history of long exposure to cold usually make diagnosis easy. Most frequently the patient has thawed the tissues before entering the hospital. They enter because of extreme pain produced by frostbite.

### Management

1. If frozen, thaw the part at ambient room temperature between 70 to 80° F. with only air warming. Occasionally a low-velocity fan may be helpful.

2. Daily cool pHisoHex soaks and debridement keep the local tissues clean.

3. Immediate regional sympathectomy, if not contraindicated by other systemic disease, is very useful in terms of increasing the blood supply to the damaged tissues, limiting tissue loss, decreasing edema and increasing the speed of healing.

4. Following this, local debridement is frequently all that is necessary.

# 19. INFLAMMATORY CONDITIONS OF THE HEAD AND NECK

*David H. Harshaw,* M.D.

Although there are many types of inflammatory conditions affecting the head and neck region, only a limited number of them become acute emergencies. There are also some noninflammatory conditions which can resemble the inflammatory conditions by the swelling they produce. These too have been included in the following discussion.

## ACUTE BACTERIAL INFECTIONS

### ERYSIPELAS AND STREPTOCOCCAL INFECTIONS

#### Definition

These are acute cellulitic streptococcal infections, usually of the face, with progressive and expanding erythema.

#### Basic Principles

In this era of antibiotics, the one danger with streptococcal infections of the face is when the infections are present near the angular vein adjacent to the ala nasi. Involvement of this vein can lead to cavernous sinus thrombosis. The clinical picture of impending cavernous sinus thrombosis is periorbital edema, proptosis and increasing lethargy.

#### Criteria for Diagnosis

Erysipelas is characterized by:
1. A marked progressive erythema expanding outward from where the infection began
2. The boundary between the involved and uninvolved tissues is shown by a sharp end of the erythema.
3. The erythema can progress to involve the entire face.
4. There is high fever, swelling and systemic toxicity but little if any abscess formation.

#### Management

1. Streptococcal infections should be treated with penicillin or Keflin, which are capable of rapidly destroying the organisms.
2. For severe erysipelas infections, ampicillin or Keflin, 1 to 2 gm. every 4 hours by intravenous push, should be used in the adult.
3. Involvement of the angular vein with possible cavernous sinus thrombosis is treated by heparinization of the patient simultaneously with intravenous penicillin. The heparinization should be continued for about 1 week after subsidence of all symptoms.
4. Moist warm soaks can be applied to the area involved.
5. Once the fever and erythema begin to subside, oral antibiotics can be used.

### ACUTE PAROTITIS

#### Definition

Acute parotitis is an inflammatory infection of the parotid gland.

#### Basic Principles

The offending organism in acute parotitis when occurring in children is usually a staphylococcus, whereas in the adult the offending organism varies. The infection in the child can occur without any antecedent cause; however, in most adult cases, an initiating cause can be found. One should look for recent dental work, tooth abscesses or an infection in the upper face. Patients with dehydration, prolonged nasogastric suction and poor oral hygiene are prone to parotitis. Salivary duct obstruction rarely causes acute bacterial parotitis. Often the parotitis is a lymphadenitis of the nodes within the gland.

## Criteria for Diagnosis

The gland is hot, swollen and exquisitely tender. The onset is sudden and abscess formation is rare.

## Management

1. Acute parotitis is best treated in children with a penicillinase-resistant penicillin (250 mg. I.V. of nafcillin every 4 to 6 hours). When the inflammation subsides, 100 mg. of nafcillin are given orally every 6 hours for 10 days.

2. Warm soaks are applied to the area and the gland is checked for fluctuation.

3. If such an area presents, it is aspirated and a culture and sensitivity are done. It is better to frequently aspirate an abscess rather than to open and drain it, for fear of cutting a facial nerve branch.

4. Acute parotitis in the adult is not as often due to staphylococci as it is in children. A predisposing cause, such as a dental infection, should be searched for and treated.

5. The parotid infection in the adult is treated with soaks, a penicillinase-resistant penicillin and a gram-negative antibiotic such as streptomycin.

6. If the infection continues in the adult, a short course of radiation therapy to the gland will stop its secretion and usually will allow the antibiotic to bring the infection under control.

7. If the patient is dehydrated and has poor oral hygiene, this must be corrected.

## LUDWIG'S ANGINA

### Definition

Ludwig's angina is a closed-space infection of the mouth and throat.

### Basic Principles

The cellulitis or abscess is deep to the mylohyoid muscles and encircles the submaxillary gland, extending into the base of the tongue. It can progress to muscle and nerve necrosis, as well as producing pharyngeal and supraglottic airway obstruction. In most cases the offending organism is streptococcal.

## Criteria for Diagnosis

1. Brawny edema of the upper neck
2. Oral cavity swelling
3. Fever and leukocytosis

## Management

1. Ludwig's angina should be treated by covering the patient with a broad-spectrum antibiotic such as ampicillin.

2. Under general anesthesia and endotracheal intubation, the submaxillary triangles on both sides are incised with a semicircular transverse upper neck incision. The incision is kept just above the hyoid bone to avoid the marginal branch of the facial nerve which runs about 1 cm. below the mandible.

3. The platysma muscle is incised and the fascia over the submaxillary gland is exposed and incised. Upon entering the submaxillary triangle, the tissue around the submaxillary gland is bluntly dissected and the space deep to the gland entered, thus allowing the abscess to drain. Care should be taken to avoid injury to the hypoglossal and lingual nerves.

4. The abscess cavity is irrigated, and drains which allow further irrigation are left in place.

5. In order to drain the abscess and expose it properly, the mylohyoid muscle may have to be divided.

## ACUTE TONSILLITIS

### Definition

Acute tonsillitis is an acute infection of the tonsil.

### Basic Principles

Acute tonsillitis can be a painful and partially obstructing enlargement of the tonsils, with many small abscess foci. It has the danger of progressing to peritonsillar abscess, retropharyngeal abscess or parapharyngeal abscess. The causative organism may be streptococcal, in which case the tissues deep to the tonsil are swollen. If an abscess forms during the progression of the tonsillitis, it forms between the tonsillar capsule and the superior constrictor muscle and can displace the tonsil and soft palate forward and medially. Trismus can develop, swallowing becomes difficult and aspiration can occur. This abscess is called a peritonsillar abscess. The retropharyngeal abscess is usually a disease of young children and it is secondary to retropharyngeal lymphadenitis. In the retropharyngeal abscess, there is a collection between the constrictor muscles and the prevertebral fascia.

### Criteria for Diagnosis

1. In acute tonsillitis, there is fever and leukocytosis. The tonsil is enlarged, inflamed, and may have multiple focal abscesses on the surface or may be covered with a thick exudate.

2. The peritonsillar abscess presents as a swelling in the region of the tonsillar fossa, displacing the tonsil, the tonsillar pillars and the soft palate.

3. The retropharyngeal abscess presents as a forward displacement of the entire posterior pharyngeal wall. This will give:

A. Stridor and swallowing difficulty

B. A soft, boggy area at the back of the throat through which the vertebral bodies cannot be felt

C. The child tends to hyperextend his neck in order to swallow and relieve pain. The position the child assumes may resemble meningitis.

### Management

1. Acute tonsillitis is usually treated with broad-spectrum antibiotics and hydration, allowing the inflammation to subside.

2. If there are many small abscess foci in the tonsil, a tonsillectomy should be done after the acute infection has subsided.

3. A peritonsillar abscess, because of its tendency to obstruct the pharynx, should be drained by a semicircular incision in the posterior tonsillar pillar.

4. A parapharyngeal abscess is drained through the neck by an incision in the neck at the angle of the jaw and carried down to the level of the carotid bifurcation. At this point, the parapharyngeal space can be entered and drained.

5. A retropharyngeal abscess is drained through the constrictor muscles. Care must be taken in draining a peritonsillar or retropharyngeal abscess to prevent aspiration of the abscess contents, especially in children.

6. If the child can be anesthetized, it is safer to drain these abscesses under endotracheal anesthesia to prevent aspiration.

7. The fever in the child should be brought under control prior to anesthesia, and he should be covered with ampicillin pre- and post-operatively.

## ACUTE THYROIDITIS

### Definition

Acute thyroiditis is an acute bacterial inflammation of the thyroid gland.

### Basic Principles

In acute thyroiditis, the danger is tracheal compression since the infection is a closed-space-type infection.

### Criteria for Diagnosis

1. Acute thyroiditis presents as a diffuse, exquisitely painful swelling in the thyroid region. It is accompanied by fever and leukocytosis.

2. Early in the disease, the swollen gland is recognized.

3. Late edema in the surrounding tissues makes outlining of the thyroid difficult.

4. The causative organism is usually streptococcal, although sometimes staphylococcic abscess can occur.

5. Abscess formation should always be looked for and drained.

### Management

1. Acute thyroiditis is best treated with

antibiotics, usually a penicillinase-resistant penicillin.

2. If an abscess is present, it can be aspirated, and if purulence is obtained, it can be drained.

3. The swelling of the gland may be such that there is impending tracheal obstruction.

4. Stridor and difficulty in clearing pulmonary secretions are indications for a tracheotomy.

5. A tracheotomy in the face of acute thyroiditis is difficult and should be done in the operating room with an endotracheal tube inserted prior to commencing the procedure. The gland is enlarged and hyperemic, overlies the trachea, makes the trachea seem to move posterior and the normal fascial planes are obscured. The patient should be hyperextended and a low vertical incision should be made in the neck to get adequate exposure of the trachea.

## SUPPURATIVE SINUSITIS

### Definition

Suppurative sinusitis is an acute suppurative inflammation of one of the paranasal sinuses.

### Basic Principles

Mild cases are often self-limited with antibiotic coverage, whereas severe cases necessitate drainage to avoid complications such as venous thrombosis, osteomyelitis or meningitis.

### Criteria for Diagnosis

1. Suppurative sinusitis presents with a diffuse swelling of the area over the sinus and is accompanied by an unrelenting headache of the upper side of the face.

2. There is fever and tenderness over the sinus, which is usually the maxillary sinus.

3. It can be diagnosed by an anteroposterior film of the face showing an opacified sinus.

### Management

1. Suppurative sinusitis is treated by draining the sinus.

2. For a maxillary sinus, a Caldwell-Luc approach gives excellent drainage and leaves no visible scar. It is made by incising the mucosa of the upper gingival labial sulcus. The incision should be high in the sulcus and lateral to the canine tooth. This avoids injury to the roots of the upper teeth. The mucosa is freed from over the maxillary bone with a periosteal elevator. It is freed almost up to the inferior orbital rim, with care being taken not to injure the inferior orbital nerve. An opening about the size of the index finger is made in the maxilla with an osteotome. The opening is widened with a rongeur. A culture is obtained, the sinus is extensively irrigated and a Penrose drain is inserted. The sinus is then irrigated for the next several days postoperatively until the infection has subsided. At this point the drain can be removed.

3. The patient should also be covered with the appropriate antibiotic.

4. An antral trocar can be used to widen the natural opening into the maxillary sinus beneath the middle turbinate. This can be done under local anesthesia, but the nasal cavity must be well anesthetized. Swelling of the nasal tissue may make it difficult to adequately do an antrotomy, and for this reason and because the drainage is small, an antrotomy is usually inadequate to drain a suppurative maxillary sinus. A Caldwell-Luc operation is a preferred procedure.

## NONSPECIFIC INFLAMMATIONS
### CERVICAL LYMPHADENITIS

### Definition

Cervical lymphadenitis is an inflammation of the cervical lymph nodes.

### Basic Principles

Cervical lymphadenitis is an infected lymph node secondary to infection in the oral cavity or oral pharynx. In older patients, oropharyngeal cancer should be ruled out.

## Criteria for Diagnosis

1. It can present as a massive swelling of the neck with either brawny induration or fluctuation.

2. The mass is usually located along the main lymphatic routes.

3. The subdigastric nodes or those adjacent to them along the upper jugular vein are generally involved.

4. The oral cavity and pharynx should be carefully inspected in the older-aged patient. The infected node may be an infected, necrotic, metastatic lymph node from oropharyngeal cancer.

## Management

Cervical lymphadenitis, if presenting as a matted mass of hard inflamed or fluctuant nodes, should be managed as follows:

1. Soaks and antibiotics until the inflammation subsides

2. Fluctuation in the mass is drained and cultured, and, if possible, a piece of the abscess wall is submitted to pathologic examination.

3. Careful inspection of the oral cavity, oropharynx, hypopharynx, nasopharynx and larynx is needed to rule out neoplasm.

4. One month after inflammation has subsided, if the node or mass is still present and no primary neoplasm has been found, an open lymph node biopsy is done with frozen section.

5. If the frozen section is positive:

A. The upper neck node shows:

*(1) Squamous Carcinoma.* Then a radical neck dissection, followed by postoperative radiotherapy to the areas most suspect for occult primaries, is done.

*(2) Adenocarcinoma.* Then a radical neck dissection is done. The salivary glands and sites below the clavicle are watched for development of the primary.

*(3) Lymphoma.* Then an intact lymph node is submitted and the patient is treated appropriately. Lymphomas rarely get inflamed.

B. *Supraclavicular Nodes*

If the first presenting node is a supraclavicular node, it usually will arise from a primary below the clavicle and an open biopsy is done alone. Although the site of the primary is still searched for, any treatment is palliative.

## NONINFLAMMATORY NON-NEOPLASTIC SWELLINGS

### SALIVARY GLAND OBSTRUCTION

## Definition

Salivary gland obstruction is obstruction of the parotid or submaxillary duct, usually due to stones.

## Basic Principles

Salivary gland obstruction is of two types, nonspecific and that due to calculi. Calculi mostly occur in the submaxillary gland duct and can readily be palpated in the floor of the mouth. Upon removing the stones, the swelling rapidly subsides. In the nonspecific type, a sialogram will show a distorted but unobstructed duct. Any hard mass within the gland should be considered a tumor until proven otherwise.

## Criteria for Diagnosis

1. Boggy, indurated nontender salivary gland

2. Sialographic demonstration of obstruction or distortion of the duct system

3. Palpation of a stone

4. Open biopsy of the gland or mass

## Management

1. *Submaxillary Gland.* This is the gland most commonly obstructed, and the calculus can vary from the size of a poppy seed to a bean. The small calculi are usually able to work their way out of Wharton's duct. The larger calculi require incision over the duct to remove the stone and then marsupialization of the opening. If the calculi are recurrent, a removal of the submaxillary gland should be done.

2. *Parotid Gland.* Calculus obstruction is extremely rare and the stone is difficult to palpate. A sialogram should be done to

demonstrate the obstruction of Stensen's duct. Local procedures to the duct are usually ineffective, and, if the calculus fails to pass, a superficial parotidectomy should be done.

## CHRONIC PAROTITIS

### Definition

Chronic parotitis is a nonspecific or viral inflammation of the parotid gland.

### Basic Principles

Chronic parotitis can be due to nonspecific causes and rarely is it due to a stone in Stensen's duct. The enlargement can be due to an enlarged node within the gland which may be a lymphoma or a metastatic node. This will usually present as a well-outlined mass and should be treated as a tumor. Mumps can occur in the adult and may be unilateral. Mumps is usually accompanied by an elevated amylase.

### Criteria for Diagnosis

1. Nontender enlarged gland
2. Swelling aggravated by stimulation, especially citrus fruits and alcohol
3. High serum amylase
4. Fever if due to a viremia

### Management

1. *Gustatory Swelling.* If the enlargement of the gland is aggravated by eating, sectioning Jacobson's nerve in the ear may partially relieve the swelling by interfering with the reflex arc of salivary secretion.

2. A hard mass located within a diffusely enlarged gland is always suspect as tumor. A sialogram may disclose a distorted duct. A superficial parotidectomy should be done to rule out a possible tumor.

3. If the gland is diffusely enlarged and the enlargement occurs in recurrent episodes, usually the cause is nonspecific. Pathologic examination shows chronic sialadenitis and a sialogram is not helpful in diagnosing the cause. There is usually no pain with this enlargement and treatment is cosmetic. Treatment is a superficial parotidectomy.

## THYROIDITIS

### Definition

Thyroiditis is a nonbacterial inflammation of the thyroid.

### Basic Principles

Thyroiditis may be of the acute viral type (De Quervain's thyroiditis). This is characterized by a somewhat tender, swollen gland with little inflammation. It can occasionally produce tracheal compression. Hashimoto's thyroiditis is an autoimmune disease and is self-limited.

### Criteria for Diagnosis

1. Enlargement of the thyroid which may be asymmetrical
2. The gland may be mildly tender or sometimes acutely tender as with the viral type. Pain may be referred to the side of the face or teeth.
3. Despite the swelling and tenderness, there are few signs of systemic toxicity as with acute thyroiditis.
4. The patient may be hypothyroid in the Hashimoto's type.
5. In the acute stage, the following tests may be helpful in distinguishing these two types of thyroiditis:

|               | PBI      | RAI Uptake |
|---------------|----------|------------|
| De Quervain's | Elevated | Decreased  |
| Hashimoto's   | Normal   | Elevated   |

### Management

1. De Quervain's thyroiditis, although painful, is self-limited and rarely will produce enough swelling to interfere with respiration.

2. Hashimoto's thyroiditis can produce enough swelling and pressure to constrict the trachea. These patients may become hypothyroid later; therefore, removing any thyroid is contraindicated unless carcinoma is suspected. Dividing the isthmus of the thyroid will usually relieve the constricting type of obstruction, and this should be done before resorting to a tracheotomy.

## LARYNGEAL EDEMA

### Definition

Laryngeal edema is swelling of the vocal cords due to edema.

### Basic Principles

Laryngeal obstruction has two causes: (1) *extrinsic,* due to compression from a retro- or parapharyngeal abscess, mediastinal adenitis and cervical adenitis; (2) *intrinsic,* due to obstruction from diphtheria, exanthema (measles, pertussis) and laryngotracheobronchitis. A laryngeal cyst or papilloma of small size can become obstructing with a superimposed laryngitis. Laryngeal edema is manifested by stridor in the infant and young child. Because of the small and easily compressible airway it can quickly develop into an emergent situation, whereas in the adult it rarely progresses to actual airway obstruction.

### Criteria for Diagnosis

1. Stridor
2. Hoarseness
3. History of acute allergic reaction, drug toxicity, or previous similar episode

### Management

1. *Laryngotracheobronchitis.* This is a nonspecific inflammation, usually of a viral origin, and occurs in infants and children. It can become an emergency and can involve just the larynx or the entire tracheobronchial tree. Treatment is mainly observation and supportive care since the disease is self-limited.

   A. Antibiotics are used to prevent secondary pneumonia.

   B. A throat swab for culture and Gram's stain are done first.

   C. A high-humidity (90%), cool oxygen tent or croupette is used. This is to create a moist atmosphere to loosen secretions and to aid the child in expelling them.

   D. Careful observation of the child

for progressing anoxia or $CO_2$ retention is done. Blood gases before and during treatment are more accurate than clinical impressions.

   E. *Endotracheal Intubation by an Orotracheal or Nasotracheal Airway.* Prior to intubation, the child should be sedated and the mouth sprayed with 1% tetracaine. Laryngeal intubation, if kept in for over 24 hours, is highly prone to damage the vocal cords and leads to glottic stricture at a later date.

   If the tube cannot be removed in 24 hours, a tracheotomy must be done. After removing an endotracheal tube, the child must be watched for recurring obstruction.

   F. Tracheotomy does allow better removal of secretions and application of positive-pressure breathing. However, the tracheal opening can become the site of a stricture. A child is more difficult to extubate than an adult even after the cause for the tracheotomy has been resolved. It may take several months before the child can tolerate removal of the tube once he has become dependent upon it.

2. *Diphtherial Laryngitis.* In the past this was a frequent cause of death in children with diphtheria. This fact is mentioned here to keep it in mind, especially in a child who has not had DPT immunization. A rapidly progressing laryngitis in a toxic child may be the first clinical sign. Laryngoscopic visualization of the larynx should further make one suspect diphtherial laryngitis. The larynx is covered with a heavy exudate, while the usual tracheobronchitis has a swollen larynx with a clear mucous secretion. Tracheotomy, antibiotics and antitoxin are administered as well as DPT.

3. *Acute Allergic Laryngeal Edema*

   A. Dexamethasone, 1 gm. by I.V. push .

   B. Adrenalin (1:100,000), 1 ml. I.V.

   C. Antihistamines (i.e., Benadryl, 50 mg. I.M.)

   D. Calcium gluconate, 1 gm. slowly (5 minutes) I.V.

E. Intubation is usually impossible and an emergency tracheotomy is required if the patient is not responding and stridor is progressing.

## MANAGEMENT OF A TRACHEOTOMY

This is one of the simplest of operative procedures and yet, if conducted wrong, done under unfavorable conditions or in a difficult patient, it can become a surgical nightmare.

### Indications for a Tracheotomy

1. *General Indications*

A. Progressive airway obstruction at the level of the larynx. This is manifested by a croupy cough, stridor and progressive hoarseness. Anoxia initially manifests itself in restlessness, use of accessory respiratory muscles, then later by apathy and cyanosis.

B. Airway access to allow the use of a pressure or volume ventilator. Although an endotracheal tube can be used, it has certain inherent problems.

C. Airway access to remove secretions, frequently in paralytic conditions, brain injury, atelectasis and comatose state

2. *Specific Indications*

A. Congenital malformations of the larynx

B. Post thoracic surgery

C. Post neurosurgery

D. Post head and neck surgery

E. Inflammatory obstruction of the larynx and trachea, intrinsic inflammation as in laryngotracheobronchitis, extrinsic inflammation as in thyroiditis

F. Neoplasms

(1) Laryngeal or supraglottic cancer

(2) Vocal cord cysts and papilloma

G. Trauma

(1) To the larynx or head and neck region

(2) Burns to the pharynx and airway

H. Foreign body in the airway

## Type of Patient for a Tracheotomy

The attitude, approach and conduct of the surgeon should be conditioned by the type of patient who is to have the tracheotomy.

1. *Body Habitus.* A patient with a short, fat or thick neck is much more difficult to properly position for tracheal exposure than one with a long, thin, supple neck. Likewise, an elderly patient with kyphosis, in whom the cervical contents have partially sunk into the thoracic inlet and migrated posteriorly, presents a difficult trachea to approach.

2. *Age.* In addition to his kyphosis and emphysema, which makes the trachea more difficult to expose, the elderly patient is hard to position, he cannot extend his head and his cardiorespiratory situation may not allow a supine position, periods of anoxia, or any undue excitement. His blood vessels are more fragile and, if he has an element of congestive failure, there will be more bleeding from dilated veins.

The child and infant are, in general, uncooperative for such a procedure and are best sedated and/or intubated prior to the procedure.

3. *Disease States Necessitating the Tracheotomy*

A. Impending airway obstruction may require a rapid and dexterous procedure, and, if it would seem that the patient is going to be difficult, endotracheal intubation prior to tracheotomy may be wise.

B. Any inflammation or edema of the neck will increase the difficulty of dissection.

C. An overlying or enlarged thyroid gland may make a direct approach to the trachea impossible without a formal dissection of the thyroid to raise it off the trachea.

D. Emphysema or cardiovascular disease may distort the anatomy, increase the venous engorgement or produce a very unstable patient (arrhythmias secondary to anoxia).

## Conduct of Procedure

1. *Bedside or Operating Room.* Unless the surgeon does not think he has the time, a tracheotomy in a child or in the group of patients which present with intrinsic difficulties as enumerated above should be done in the operating room where the facilities are at their best.

2. Endotracheal intubation should be at least attempted in those patients who have impending obstruction or who present with certain physical and medical problems making a tracheotomy more difficult. This converts a harried and stormy procedure into a more tranquil one both for the patient and the surgeon.

3. *Anesthesia.* An anesthesiologist should be present. If an endotracheal tube has been passed, oxygen and anesthetic gases can be delivered in order to quiet the patient. If the patient's condition is too precarious for general anesthesia, oxygen and assisted ventilation can be given. If the case is done at the bedside, it is good to have some means to assist in ventilating the patient and the equipment ready for endotracheal intubation if necessary.

4. *Assistants.* Whether at the bedside or in the operating room the surgeon and his assistants should be gowned and gloved (there may not be time to scrub). He should have at least one assistant and, in a difficult type of patient, two assistants. If done in the operating room, a scrub nurse and circulating nurse should be present. If at the bedside, there should be someone to run errands.

5. *Intravenous Fluid and Monitoring.* If time permits, whether the patient is an adult or child, an intravenous line should be present and working. In the poor-risk patient, a line which allows central venous pressure monitoring is preferable. Again, a poor-risk patient should have his blood pressure, pulse and electrocardiogram monitored during the procedure. In a truly emergency procedure, this cannot be done, but most tracheotomies allow enough time for this monitoring.

6. *Who Does the Procedure?* Often on a surgical service this procedure is relegated to the intern or an inexperienced resident as a good opportunity to do some surgery and gain experience. He is often poorly supervised and assisted, and it is not uncommon that something that could have been prevented, if in the proper hands, occurs. The poor-risk and difficult patient should not only be done under optimum conditions but by a thoroughly experienced surgeon or resident. The intern and inexperienced resident should do this procedure on relatively good-risk patients and then under good supervision until they have obtained a certain degree of technical skill.

## Anatomy

The site of the tracheotomy is that part of the trachea between the cricoid cartilage and the suprasternal notch. Normally there are 5 to 8 semicartilaginous tracheal rings in this interval. The trachea is a midline structure, but in certain disease states it can be deviated to one side, such as after a pneumonectomy or with an enlarged compressing thyroid lobe. This should be noted prior to the operation. Behind the trachea lies the cervical esophagus separated by a distinct fascial plane. The esophagus is only tightly adherent at the cricoid level. The normal thyroid extends from the cricoid cartilage to about the fifth or sixth tracheal ring, which places the lower pole of the thyroid about 2 to 3 cm. above the clavicle. The isthmus of the thyroid, which is variable in width, usually covers the third and fourth tracheal rings and frequently sends a pyramidal lobe up over the cricoid and thyroid cartilage. The thyroid is invested in a thin capsule, which is separate from the fascia which encircles the trachea. This allows separation of the lower thyroid from the trachea. The trachea and thyroid are covered with two layers of strap muscles, the sternothyroid and the more superficial sternohyoid. These are fused in the midline in a relatively avascular plane.

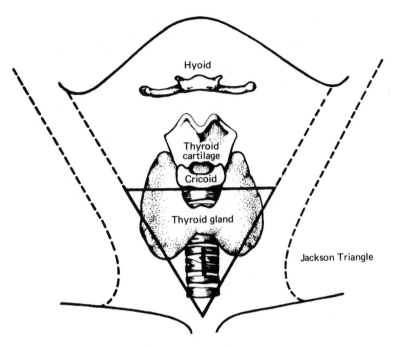

Fig. 19-1.

The sheaths of these muscles proceed laterally, fusing with the deep cervical fascia which forms the carotid sheath surrounding the carotid artery, jugular vein and vagus nerve. High in the neck at about the level of the cricoid cartilage, the omohyoid muscle crosses the carotid sheath superficially. The sternal head of the sternocleidomastoid muscle is lateral to the carotid sheath at the level of the thyroid cartilage and crosses and covers it as it converges to insert at the suprasternal notch. Jackson's triangle is that space bounded by the anterior edges of the converging sternocleidomastoid muscles and the cricoid cartilage, with its apex at the sternal notch. This is the region where a tracheotomy is done. The strap muscles are overlain with the superficial cervical fascia and the platysma muscle. Anterior superficial jugular veins may lie in this fascial plane in a vertical direction, and supraclavicular superficial jugular veins

proceed in this plane in a transverse direction to empty into the jugular vein beneath the sternocleidomastoid muscle. A patient with congestive failure may have these veins significantly enlarged. The thyroid gland is supplied by an inferior thyroid artery which approaches the thyroid from behind the gland and arborizes at about the level of the first to third rings. It lies lateral to the trachea. The superior thyroid artery enters the upper pole of the gland, usually above the level of the cricoid. A rare thyroid ima artery approaches the isthmus of the gland along the anterior surface of the trachea. In addition to the vein which accompanies each artery, an inconstant middle thyroid vein approaches the gland laterally. The recurrent laryngeal nerve ascends in the tracheo-esophageal groove along the posterior wall of the trachea, crosses beneath the inferior thyroid artery and enters the larynx at the junction of the inferior horn of the thyroid cartilage with the cricoid. Thus the lower tracheal fifth to eighth rings are covered with no vital structures, and the only interfering vascular structures may be the anterior and supraclavicular superficial jugular veins and the rare thyroid artery. The upper trachea is covered with the thyroid isthmus and pyramidal lobe, which can be divided between clamps. They are relatively avascular. The cricoid cartilage is the only complete cartilaginous ring in the airway. The tracheal rings extend about two thirds around the trachea and are absent posteriorly. The wall of the trachea and the posterior fascia are quite strong in the adult and can give good support posteriorly. In the child this is not true and care should be taken not to extend an incision too far laterally. The blood supply to the trachea comes primarily from behind the trachea.

## Instruments

The following list of instruments is what an adequate tracheotomy tray should include:

1. *Knife Blades:* 2 handles with 2 No. 11 and No. 15 blades

2. *Retractors:* 2 skin hooks (plastic); No. 4 Senn retractors; No. 4 Army-Navy retractors, 2 small Deaver retractors; No. 3 tracheal hooks

3. *Hemostats:* 10 curved mosquito hemostats; 4 Mixter or right angle clamps; 4 Carmault or Kelly clamps; 2 Kocher clamps; 4 tonsil clamps

4. *Scissors:* 2 Metzenbaum surgical scissors; 1 Mayo scissors; 1 nurse's scissors

5. *Forceps:* 2 Ochsner 8-inch needle holders; No. 2 De Bakey vascular forceps; 2 toothed forceps; 1 Trousseau tracheal dilator

6. *Suction and Catheters:* No. 1 tonsil suction tip; No. 1 Frazier suction tip; 2 20

ml. syringes with No. 20, 22 and 25 needles; 4 rubber Robinson catheters, sizes No. 12, No. 14, No. 16 and No. 18 French

7. *Needles and Suture:* Intestinal needles (regular eye), $T_3$, $T_6$, and $T_{12}$ (3 of each); 3 atraumatic swedged needles, $T_5$ with 3-0 silk; 1 pack of 2-0 silk; 1 pack of 3-0 silk; 1 pack of 3-0 chromic gut (for ties); 1 pack of atraumatic swedged needles $T_5$ with chromic gut; 1 pack of 0 Tevdek sutures

8. *Other Items:* 2 medicine cups, 1 preparation cup; 1 ring forceps; 20 4" x 8" sponges; 10 regular sponges; 1 kidney basin; 1 jar of ¼-inch iodoform gauze; 8 towels, 6 towel clips, 2 large drapes, 1 small drape with exposure opening, suction tubing

The most critical instruments are De Bakey tissue forceps, Senn retractors, Army-Navy retractors and tracheal hooks along with suction. If the operation is done in the operating room, an electro-coagulation apparatus is useful but not necessary. If the operation is done at the bedside, 2 gooseneck lamps or a portable overhead light is absolutely necessary. A portable headlamp is also helpful at the bedside.

## Tracheotomy Tubes

The approximate size of the patient's trachea is estimated from either his size or, in a child, from his age. The average adult male should take a No. 9 or larger and the average adult female should take a No. 7 or larger. The surgeon should also decide prior to doing the tracheotomy whether he will need a cuffed tube to prevent aspiration of saliva or vomitus or for positive-pressure ventilation. He should also estimate how long the patient is going to require the tracheotomy and how long the cuff needs to be inflated. He should also consider whether the patient may receive anesthesia after the tracheotomy and, if so, use a tube with a cuff and an extension to the cannula which will fit the anesthesia equipment or ventilator.

1. *Metal Tubes*

A. *For Adults.* Inner and outer cannulae with inserting trocar. The cuff does not come with these tubes and must be placed on the tube by the surgeon. To get a cuff which will not slip off, use a cuff one size smaller than the tube. The adult sizes range from No. 6 to No. 11.

B. *For Children.* No cuff is necessary with infants and small children because the tube usually is fairly snug in the trachea. If a respirator is to be used for the child, in order to get this snug fit, use a tube one size larger than the recommended size.

| *Age* | *Size of Tube* |
|---|---|
| Newborn | No. 00 |
| 6 months | No. 00–0 |
| 12 months | No. 0 |
| 18 months | No. 0–1 |
| 2 years | No. 1 |
| 3 years | No. 1–2 |
| 4 years | No. 2 |
| 5–7 years | No. 2–3 |
| 8–12 years | No. 3–4 |

An extension-type of inner cannula (often called a Lyons tube) is desirable if the tube is to be connected to a respirator.

2. *Plastic Tubes*

A. The Portex tube is a thick, Tygon plastic tube whose smallest outer diameter is No. 6. Its inner diameter is considerably less than the corresponding metal tube, including its inner cannula. This tube has no inner cannula or trocar for insertion. Its advantage lies in its cuff, which is incorporated into the tube and will not come off. The balloon on the cuff can be preset to 30 ml. capacity by annealing it in hot water. Then when it is placed in the trachea at say 5 to 10 ml. inflation, it exerts a minimal degree of pressure on the tracheal wall, causing less wall necrosis than a corresponding rubber balloon. A proper adapter must be found to fit it to a respirator.

These tubes have a considerable degree of friction between themselves and the tracheal wall. They are difficult to in-sert into a trachea and it is quite easy to tear the tracheal opening while inserting this tube. This difficulty in insertion and its small inner diameter to outer diameter are its chief disadvantages.

B. *Sheiley Tube.* This is a thin-walled, acrylic plastic tube with an inner and outer cannula and a preattached cuff. It can be reused and has a surface which impairs the adherence of secretion to its walls. The attachment of the tube to the face plate is swivelled so that the tube can accommodate itself to the tracheal angle with the face plate flush against the neck. It has an extension on the locking inner cannula, allowing easy attachment to the respirator. Its chief disadvantages are its limited number of sizes and its nonannealing cuff.

## Operation

1. *Position of the Patient*

A. Hyperextend the neck, allowing it to fall posteriorly by placing a rolled-up towel between the scapular blades.

B. The shoulders should be pulled caudad and allowed to fall posteriorly.

C. If the operation cannot be done with the patient supine, it can be done with the patient in a high semi-Fowler's position; but again, the neck should be hyperextended as much as possible. This will pull the trachea up from the thorax and bring it anteriorly.

2. *Skin Incision*

A. *Vertical Midline Incision.* In a difficult patient with a short neck and indistinct landmarks, a vertical incision will allow better access to the proper site in the trachea for entry. It should begin 1 cm. above the sternal notch and extend upward for 2 cm. It can be extended in either direction. Its disadvantage is that it leaves a noticeable scar.

B. *Horizontal Incision.* This incision, if made properly, leaves little in the way of a scar, which is easy to revise if necessary. However, it requires precise positioning. It should, in the normal neck, be positioned about 2 cm. above the notch with the head hyperextended and should be about 3 cm. long.

### 3. *Tracheal Opening*

A. *Position on the Trachea.* A high tracheal opening (rings 2 to 4) is recommended if a laryngectomy is to be done at a later date for cancer, if a later revision of the tracheal opening is to be done, or if the patient is elderly and kyphotic.

A low tracheal opening (rings 5 to 7) is recommended if other surgery is to be done in the neck and one hopes to prevent contamination of the other incision by the tracheotomy. The lower incision and lower tracheal opening give a better cosmetic result and this is the usual tracheotomy

done in young people. It may, however, be associated with severe bleeding if the tube erodes into the innominate vein by continued pressure.

B. *Tracheal Incision*

*(1)* Vertical

*(2)* Vertical with a window

*(3)* Transverse with removal of ring(s)

*(4)* Transverse with a ring flap sutured to the skin

*(5)* Transverse (between rings)

Types 2 and 3 are preferred in children; they extend upward a distance of 2 rings and horizontally about one fourth to one third of the circumference. Type 4 is used in adults; the flap provides a good

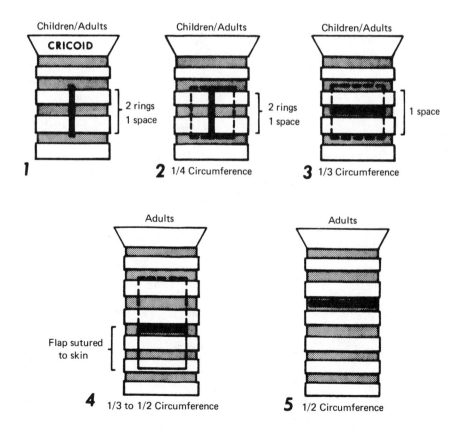

Fig. 19-2.

tracheal tract and can be released when need for the tracheotomy is over, closing the defect in the trachea. It can only be done in patients with a thin neck. Type 5 is used only in adults, and, on removing the tracheal tube, it closes with a minimum of scar. The most important aspect of inserting the tracheal cannula is to do it with as little trauma as possible to the tracheal wall.

C. *Retention Sutures.* Sutures of 0 Tevdek are inserted around the intact rings above and below the tracheal opening. These are untied and left long. They provide ready access to the trachea if the cannula should be dislodged before a mature tracheotomy tract has formed.

4. *Procedure.* If the patient is not intubated, local anesthetic, usually 1% Xylocaine, is infiltrated into the skin at the selected site of incision. This is done with a No. 25 needle until a good wheal is obtained, then using the No. 22 needle for the deeper tissues. This usually takes 5 to 10 ml. of local anesthetic. The more anesthetic that is injected, the more the tissues are distorted. The incision is made through the skin and skin hooks are used to pull back the skin. The incision is deepened and the rake ends of the Senn retractors are now used. The platysma muscle is identified and divided and the strap muscles are exposed. Any large veins crossing the exposure field are divided and ligated. The trachea is palpated, the midline determined and the sheath over the strap muscle is vertically incised. The Army-Navy retractors are now inserted as the muscle fibers of the strap muscle are bluntly separated. These retractors, if used properly, will completely retract these muscles. If the thyroid overlies the trachea, it can be palpated and the fascia over it wiped away. A 2-0 silk suture is placed in the thyroid gland in a figure-of-eight fashion. This can be pulled upon to elevate the gland off the trachea and allow it to be sharply dissected free. The tissue on either side of the trachea is bluntly dissected free and the long ends of

the Army-Navy retractors (or in a very deep neck, the small Deaver retractors) are inserted on either side of the trachea, thus exposing over half its circumference. The fascia overlying the trachea is wiped free with a sponge, and a small amount of Xylocaine is injected into the lumen. The selected type of opening is made and then the tracheal hooks are inserted into the upper and lower rings. The two retention sutures of 0 Tevdek are inserted with a T-6 needle. The lumen of the trachea is aspirated with a Robinson catheter and, while pulling on the tracheal hooks, which widens the opening, the proper-size tracheal cannula is inserted. The hooks are carefully removed so as not to tear the cuff, the trocar is removed, and the inner cannula is inserted. Any hemostats in the skin are now tied, and any residual ooze of blood from the wound can be stopped with iodoform packing. The face plate can be sewn to the skin but usually the ½-inch umbilical tape attached to the plate is sufficient. It is tied snugly around the neck with a square knot. The tube is now aspirated and the cuff is inflated if it needs to be. The opening in the skin should not be sewn tight around the tube or packed too tight because there must be a wide enough route to allow air to escape and avoid subcutaneous emphysema.

## Complications of Tracheotomy

1. *Hemorrhage*

A. During the procedure, this is usually from a superficial thyroid vessel or a superficial jugular vein. Adequate exposure, identification of these vessels and ligation will usually prevent it from occurring. If it should occur, digital pressure stops it; the blood is aspirated and the bleeding vessel is identified and ligated. Mass suture ligature into the paratracheal tissue is useless. Bleeding from an inflamed thyroid can be controlled with a figure-of-eight suture ligature. Bleeding from the tracheal wall is best treated with electrocautery.

B. Delayed hemorrhage (several hours later) is usually from the same vessels as in A or from the tracheal wall. Packing the tracheotomy incision with ¼-inch iodoform gauze may control it. These vessels were missed at the time of surgery and for some reason did not bleed; then coughing or clot lysis allowed them to bleed. If the bleeding recurs after packing, the patient is taken back to the operating room and the bleeding vessel is searched for.

2. *Air Embolism.* This usually occurs from an open superficial jugular vein which is greatly dilated. The patient generally has some degree of heart failure in order to dilate these veins, enabling them to aspirate sufficient air. The patient quickly becomes shocky and an audible chest murmur is heard. This can be treated by quickly packing the wound or closing the vessel and turning the patient on his left side.

3. *Subcutaneous Emphysema and Mediastinal Emphysema.* This may be caused by either too extensive dissection into surrounding tissues or too tight closure of the tracheotomy site. It can be treated by opening the wound and allowing air to escape through the neck.

4. *Damage to Vocal Cords.* This is caused by inserting the tracheotomy too close to the subglottic region.

5. *Damage to the Recurrent Nerve.* This is caused by missing the midline and extensively dissecting the paratracheal tissues.

6. *Damage to the Trachea.* This is usually from traumatic cannulation, either from poor exposure or from inserting a cannula too large for the tracheal opening. A very high tracheotomy can cause osteochondritis of the cricoid. The result of either is tracheal stricture. In a child, too great traction of the trachea or too lateral an incision can lead to partial transection of the trachea, which again develops into stricture despite attempts at immediate repair.

7. *Perforation of the Esophagus.* This is usually due to an incision through both walls of the trachea. This may provide a route for a later fistula. It is treated by operative exposure of the esophagus and immediate closure of the perforation.

8. *Erosion of the Trachea.* This is due to an ill-fitting and improperly angled tracheotomy tube. Anterior impingement can lead to penetration into a great vessel, usually the innominate vein, with fatal hemorrhage. A posterior erosion into the esophagus leads to fistula and continuous aspiration pneumonia. The repair of this usually requires several thoracic procedures, isolating the esophagus and then reconstructing it.

9. *Stricture.* Any damage to the trachea or loss of blood supply can lead to a stricture. A large opening in the trachea when it closes over will have at least a relative degree of stricture.

10. *Aspiration.* The tracheotomy may interfere with swallowing in some patients and they tend to aspirate through the glottis. A cuffed tube can help prevent this. A bleeding vessel in the tracheal wall can lead to aspiration of blood. Some of these vessels can be quite persistent and require operative exposure and coagulation.

11. *Slipping Off of the Cuff with Resulting Airway Obstruction*

12. *Insertion of the Tube Down a Main Stem Bronchus with Occlusion of the Other Bronchus.* This usually occurs in infants where too long a tracheotomy tube was used.

13. *Dislodgment of the Tracheotomy Tube by Swelling of the Neck.* This gives a partial obstruction. A longer tracheotomy tube or anode-type endotracheal tube is the solution.

14. *Pneumothorax.* This can occur in the kyphotic emphysematous patient where the pleural apex enters the neck.

15. *Infection.* This is rare due to easy drainage afforded by the tracheotomy incision.

## Postoperative Care

1. *Humidification.* A nebulizer (preferably ultrasonic) on the respirator or a tracheotomy cover equipped with high-humidity oxygen or cold-steam mist will protect the trachea from drying out and will allow easier removal of secretions. During the first several days after a tracheotomy, humidification is essential until the patient adjusts to the tracheotomy.

2. *Aspiration*

A. Five ml. of saline and Mucomyst (acetylcysteine) are injected down the trachea at least every 4 to 6 hours or more if secretions are thick and heavy.

B. Soft rubber catheters (No. 14 or No. 16 adult) are used for aspiration. Between aspirations, the catheters are soaked in benzalkonium chloride for 30 minutes. The catheters are cleansed with peroxide and saline after use and before soaking. After soaking, the catheters should be rinsed in saline before being inserted into the trachea.

C. For the first 2 weeks, in face of no respiratory infection, a culture and sensitivity should be done every 3 days.

D. Aspiration is done as often as necessary to remove secretions. It should be done with a gloved hand. The need for frequent aspiration becomes less as the patient adjusts to his tracheotomy.

3. *Cuff deflation* for 5 to 15 minutes should be done every 6 hours if the patient can tolerate being off his respirator that long.

4. *Change* and clean the inner cannula every 8 hours.

5. *No antibiotics* should be used unless there is a compelling reason for them. A tracheotomy alone is not a reason for antibiotics.

6. *Self-instruction.* If the patient appears to require the tracheotomy for a considerable time and he is able to care for himself, he should be taught to care for his tracheotomy as soon as possible.

7. *The tracheotomy tube* should be changed after a good tract has been formed. This is usually 3 to 5 days after the tracheotomy was done. It is then changed every 3 days thereafter.

8. *Extubation*

A. In the adult, the opening in the tracheotomy tube is gradually closed, at first during the day and then during the night, by progressively inserting a half cork or three quarters cork and finally completely corking the opening. If the patient can tolerate corking for 24 hours, the cannula is removed and the opening in the neck is covered with a bandage.

B. In the child, the tracheotomy tube itself is progressively changed to a smaller tube. Eventually the tube is corked, and, when the child can tolerate corking for 24 hours, the tracheotomy tube is removed.

9. *Precautions*

A. Anteroposterior and lateral films of the chest are done to check for air dissection, mediastinal bleeding, midline position of the tracheotomy tube and to see if the position of the tube does not impinge on the anterior or posterior tracheal wall. This lateral film is especially important if the tube can not be easily changed or aspirated. It may be dislodged within the wound or against the wall.

B. Retention sutures aid in locating the tracheal opening if the tracheotomy tube comes out before a tract has formed.

C. Do not force reinsertion of the tube. If it will not go easily, get a tracheotomy set and insert the tube under direct exposure.

## CRICOTHYROIDOTOMY

This is a temporary opening into the trachea between the cricoid and thyroid cartilage. It is usually done under extremely emergent conditions and should always be followed by formal tracheotomy at a lower level. A cannula left at this site for any extended period of time leads to vocal cord damage and cartilage necrosis. There are trocars available that can accomplish this rapidly after making a small skin incision. It is only feasible in a neck which is thin enough to discern the anatomy.

# 20. ACUTE CRANIOCEREBRAL INJURIES

*Albert W. Cook,* M.D

## Definition

Acute craniocerebral injury is a series of pathophysiologic events that occurs following contact trauma to the head. The nature and extent of these changes are determined by:

1. The site and severity of the injury to the head

2. The character of the injury (i.e., whether the head is fixed or moving)

3. The nature of the injurious force (broad or focal force)

4. The presence and severity of other injuries in terms of their effect on the circulatory, respiratory and autonomic systems

## State of Consciousness

The state of consciousness is defined in standard, though arbitrary, terms.

1. *Alert:* The patient is considered to be alert when he is completely aware of his surroundings, is oriented to time and place, is not confused and reacts appropriately to verbal and painful stimuli.

2. *Drowsy:* The patient is reactive to verbal and painful stimuli but falls asleep easily when not disturbed.

3. *Stupor.* This can be graded depending upon the degree and promptness of response to pain. There is no response to verbal stimuli.

4. *Coma.* This exists when there is no response to verbal and painful stimuli.

## Factors Determining the Operative or Nonoperative Management

The most important element in therapeutic assessment is the neurologic examination, especially the state of consciousness, neuro-ophthalmologic signs and general and other focal signs such as increasing hemiparesis. All neurologic signs must be interpreted in terms of the general condition of the patient. Marked systemic hypotension or pulmonary insufficiency, when associated with a craniocerebral injury, may exaggerate or produce abnormal neurologic signs, occasionally suggesting brain stem dysfunction. Therefore, documentation of systemic and metabolic disorders associated with head injury is necessary.

## Metabolic, Respiratory and Circulatory Changes in Intracranial Dynamics

After head injury, patients with traumatic brain lesions often have a primary intracerebral metabolic acidosis, leading to a compensatory hyperventilation. If this persists and is marked, ventilatory assistance may be necessary. Although oxygen desaturation of the arterial blood may be present, changes in the arterial $pCO_2$ are more important. Increased $pCO_2$ stimulates respiration and decreased $pCO_2$ depresses it. Cerebral blood flow responds to intracerebral pH, so that with increased $pCO_2$, dilation and increased flow occur in normal cerebral blood vessels but there may be decreased flow to diseased areas. Increased blood flow to diseased areas may be accomplished by reducing the arterial $pCO_2$. With ventilatory assistance, it may be necessary to reduce arterial $pCO_2$ to 25 mm. Hg before any change in intracerebral pH occurs. In addition, changes in $pCO_2$ are rapidly reflected in the cerebrospinal fluid, whereas changes in bicarbonate are not, leading to a discrepancy between the acid–base changes in the peripheral blood and cerebrospinal fluid.

Of importance is the fact that increased intracranial pressure may tend to vasoparalysis with vascular dilation. Therefore, management of increasing intracranial pressure becomes mandatory. The manner in which these abnormalities may be handled can be tabulated in a general manner by considering the general nonoperative management of the patient with acute craniocerebral injuries.

## Nonoperative Management of Patients with Head Injury

In addition to the general observations that are necessary in the patient with craniocerebral injury, basic management principles are as follows.

### General Care

1. The unconscious patient should be maintained in a flat position, or possibly with the head elevated 15 to 30 degrees, on his side and turned every 2 hours day and night.

2. Temperature should be maintained within normal limits with cold ice sponging and preferably a hypothermic mattress.

3. Movement of all uninjured joints should be carried out through a normal range once or twice a day.

4. Emergency endotracheal intubation should be performed, but this must be considered temporary. If the patient remains unconscious for any long period of time, a tracheostomy should be accomplished.

5. Control of arterial hypotension and prophylactic antibiotics are useful, as well as Levin-tube feeding and urinary catheters.

6. Steroid therapy (i.e., Solu-Medrol, 240 mg. daily) is appropriate.

7. Controlled respiration, if facilities are available, may be helpful.

### Suggested Standard Orders

1. Depending upon circumstances, temperatures should be recorded as frequently as necessary to maintain normothermic conditions, usually every 2 hours and later every 4 hours.

2. Record the blood pressure and pulse, initially every 15 minutes until stable, then every hour and then every 2 hours, etc.

3. Respiratory rate and rhythm are noted early and recorded with blood pressure and pulse rate.

4. Respirator and tracheostomy setups should be available at the bedside.

5. Steroids (Solu-Medrol) are given, 40 mg. every 4 hours.

6. Intravenous fluids, including colloids, are administered as necessary. In general, the amount of 1500 to 2000 ml. daily is adequate. Insensible fluid loss may be large, and fluid balance should be managed as in any injured patient.

7. Blood count, hematocrit and, if possible, blood volume should be obtained, although acute head injury is usually not associated with blood volume alterations.

8. Obtain a urinalysis and monitor urine output.

9. Blood-urea nitrogen, sodium, potassium and chloride determinations are made, and potassium supplements should be added to the intravenous fluid as necessary to replace losses.

10. Multivitamins are administered.

11. An electrocardiogram is recorded.

12. Daily repeated arterial blood gases ($pO_2$ and $pCO_2$) and pH and, where possible, cerebrospinal fluid $pO_2$ and pH are obtained.

13. Give Dilantin Sodium, 1½ gr. t.i.d.

14. For the agitated patient, various drugs may be used, such as phenobarbital, ½ gr. t.i.d., chlorpromazine, 75 mg. every 4 hours, or Valium, 10 mg. every 4 hours.

15. Obtain an echoencephalogram.

16. Take x-rays of the skull and cervical spine.

17. A spinal puncture is indicated if special reason exists.

18. Under ideal circumstances, monitoring of intracranial pressure by intraventricular catheter or intracranial sensor is helpful in the severely injured patient. With evidence of rising pressure,

drugs such as mannitol should be added to the therapeutic regimen.

19. Arteriography is done when indicated, as discussed under Intracranial Hematoma, page 272.

20. Special attention should be directed to the possible presence of alcoholism or narcotic addiction in patients with severe head injury. These states may cloud the clinical picture and, if unrecognized, may result in misdirected treatment and death. In both instances, neurologic signs may be altered and there may be systemic signs of uncontrollable failing circulation. In addicts, the addition of methadone to the therapeutic regimen may be necessary.

21. The patient with severe systemic and cardiorespiratory problems should have monitoring of central venous pressure and even pulmonary artery pressure in addition to monitoring of intracranial pressure. Death due to head injuries is often associated with a so-called "shock lung."

22. Provide general neurologic observation as detailed below.

## Clinical Observation

In the injured patient, general consideration should be directed to the nature, character and time of the injury, and particularly to the state of consciousness of the patient at the time of injury. This last has to be evaluated in terms of the adequacy of the reporter and any progressive changes which may have occurred since injury. The classical signs of intracranial hematoma, which include the presence of a relatively lucid interval, enlargement of the pupils and contralateral hemiparesis (tentorial herniation), may be uncertain guides for the localization of the hematoma. Very often a hematoma may occur without a lucid interval, and the hemiparesis may be on either the opposite or the ipsilateral side. Lateralizing signs or other signs of transtentorial herniation may occur in the absence of a blood clot. For this reason, additional diagnostic procedures other than clinical observation are often

necessary and will be discussed subsequently.

The following items are of major importance in evaluating a patient with altered consciousness following craniocerebral injury, since stupor or coma may be present in a patient with injury to the head but with the primary cause being an underlying disease. An example is a patient with a primary cerebrovascular accident who, following the ictus, falls and injures his scalp, skull, etc. The signs of injury to the scalp and skull may lead one to incorrectly diagnose a primary head injury. Attention to the following details, however, will help in differentiating the cause of altered consciousness and therefore lead to appropriate therapy.

1. *Nature of the Alteration in the State of Consciousness.* Ominous signs are ones associated with progressive deterioration in the state of consciousness toward coma. Observation of other signs will help to evaluate the cause of the progressive deterioration.

2. *Nature of the Change in Respiration.* Various types of abnormal respiratory patterns in patients with head injuries in stupor are related according to their head injury, the presence of associated disease and changes in acid–base balance. Differential diagnosis of abnormal respiratory function will be aided by a determination of any respiratory or metabolic acid–base disturbances.

3. *Nature of Changes in the Pupils.* The reactivity of the pupils to light, establishment of the presence or absence of nystagmus, and other induced eye movements provide essential information in the differential diagnosis of the patient in stupor or coma. Caloric stimulation and head movement are excellent means to obtain information regarding the pathways serving these functions in the brain stem.

4. *Changes in Ocular Movements and Disorders of Motor Function.* Varying degrees of hemiparesis are significant in indicating an advancing process, and states

such as decerebrate rigidity specifically indicate brain stem dysfunction. The reader is referred to more detailed neurologic texts for further description about the specificity of these neurologic tests.

## Special Diagnostic Procedures

### Electroencephalogram

1. *Definition.* The EEG reflects the electrical pattern of the cortex and deep structures of the brain. It may be changed by dysfunction of cortical neurons, by interruption of connections between the brain stem and the cortex and by alterations of diencephalic and brain stem structures.

2. *Use and Interpretation*

A. A normal EEG in an unresponsive patient may indicate either a lower brain stem disturbance or a functional state.

B. The EEG in patients with intracranial hematomas characteristically exhibits low-voltage slowing or a dampened effect on the side of the lesion, although these changes are not always pathognomonic. Occasionally they may occur in cerebral contusion-laceration without significant subdural masses.

C. EEG changes may persist for weeks after evacuation of subdural collections.

### Cerebral Arteriography

1. *Definition.* Cerebral arteriography is visualization of the cerebral vasculature by injection of contrast material into the carotid arteries.

2. *Use and Interpretation*

A. Contrast visualization of the intracranial vascular system is an effective and reliable means of diagnosing cranial hematoma. Surface lesions such as epidural and subdural hemorrhage classically produce vessel displacement, although the anterior cerebral artery may not be displaced even by large collections in the epidural space.

B. In bilateral subdural hematoma, midline structures may appear fixed in the midline, but displacement of the surface brain vessels from the inner table of the skull may indicate the correct diagnosis.

### Brain Scanning

1. *Definition.* Brain scanning is isotope-uptake visualization of brain substance following the injection of technetium-99.

2. *Use and Interpretation.* Brain scanning has been helpful in identifying surface hematomas and is also used serially to follow the course of bilateral fronto-temporal contusion.

### Air Encephalography (Ventriculography)

1. *Definition.* Air encephalography is radiographic visualization of the ventricular system by injection of air into the system as a contrast medium.

2. *Use and Interpretation.* Air encephalography is used less frequently in acute head injury. It may show a shift of intracranial structures and ventricular dilation in post-traumatic hydrocephalus. This latter phenomenon may require a shunt procedure to promote recovery from acute craniocerebral injury.

## Clinical Features Leading to Operation

After the initial clinical assessment and appropriate treatment to correct extracranial abnormalities such as abnormal respiratory and metabolic changes, attention can be directed to the possible presence of an intracranial clot. This is likely to be present in a patient whose clinical state deteriorates after a period of improvement or who fails to show continued improvement over a period of several days. Under these circumstances, arteriography is indicated. Although acute arteriography may be normal early in the phase of a craniocerebral injury, a repeated study, possibly in conjunction with ventriculography, may demonstrate that the failure to improve was due to the presence of a clot. The shift of the ventricular system may remain for weeks after evacuation of an intracranial clot and may not necessarily require further operation. The patient's clinical state, unclouded by respiratory or metabolic changes, in association with the observed radiographic findings dictates the subsequent management.

In general, patients with head injuries should follow a pattern of improvement or regression related to the length of time since injury. Lack of such improvement should lead one to suspect the presence of an intracranial hematoma or multiple intracranial clots. If a clot has been evacuated and improvement does not occur, another intracranial clot should be suspected, either epidural, subdural or intracerebral, or in another position in the cranial cavity. For such cases, all available methods of diagnosis should be used. The failure to find a hematoma by multiple burr holes does not exclude the presence of an epidural hematoma. If an epidural clot or subdural hemorrhage is not found at operation and progressive clinical deterioration occurs, arteriography and, if necessary, air ventriculography should be employed so that the presence of a clot can be unequivocally excluded.

Although there are classical signs of intracranial clots in different compartments of the head, those who await these classical situations will often be dismayed by an unexpected death from undiagnosed clots or operation may be delayed until mortality and morbidity are high. Preferably, intracranial clots should be identified before severe signs of brain stem dysfunction appear. Some of the essential clinical features associated with various types of clots are recorded below.

## INJURIES TO THE SCALP

### Lacerations

The scalp is highly vascularized and has a tendency to separate when hit by a flat or blunt object. At times it may be necessary to search diligently for a laceration of the scalp which is hidden by matted and dirt-laden hair. The area of laceration should be carefully recorded and may be important in the future evaluation of intracranial alterations. Since the scalp is extremely vascular, some lacerations may cause arterial hypotension and tachycardia due to hemorrhage. Lacerations may be simple, multiple, jagged, linear, curvilinear, small or large. There may be partial or complete avulsion. The proper care of these wounds is best executed in a hospital rather than on the street or in an ambulance, and should include the following:

1. Shaving should be done with a sharp razor and should always be directed away from the laceration.

2. Complete debridement of the wound should be performed, with removal of macerated edges of scalp by sharp-knife dissection, washing away all debrided tissue.

3. Before closure of the laceration, the underlying skull should be palpated with a sterile gloved finger in an effort to find osseous injury. X-ray examination of the skull is not a substitute for this maneuver.

4. The wound is closed with through-and-through fine silk sutures, which are tied tightly enough to control hemorrhage but without strangulation of tissues.

5. Sutures are not buried and antibiotics are not applied topically. With palpation in the open scalp laceration, the presence of a ridge due to hemorrhage in or under the periosteum may suggest a depressed fracture. Here the combination of palpation and x-ray often resolves the situation. More complicated or larger lacerations of the scalp should be repaired in the operating room and may require transposition of flaps of scalp, followed by skin grafting.

### Electrical Burns

1. Electrical burns of the scalp often involve the entire thickness of scalp, periosteum and outer surface of the skull.

2. When first seen, the extent of destruction is difficult to estimate.

3. Careful cleansing of the wound

should be carried out and systemic antibiotic therapy instituted.

4. Sequestration of the underlying bone is awaited before consideration of closure of the defect.

5. Early closure of these wounds is contraindicated since subsequent sequestration appearing beneath the closed wound will lead to infection.

6. As in any wound, appropriate use of tetanus toxoid or tetanus immune globulin should be made.

## INJURIES TO THE SKULL

Fractures of the skull may be simple or compound, linear, depressed or penetrating, and may involve the vault and/or the base.

### Linear Fractures

When subjected to an external force, the skull shortens in one direction and lengthens in another. The fracture line is usually in the direction of the shortest meridian. With an associated scalp laceration, there is danger of entrapment of dirt and other foreign material. The position of the fracture line within the skull assumes special significance if it is in direct relationship to vascular grooves, the posterior fossa or major neurosinus, which may lead to a laceration of one of these major structures with intracranial hemorrhage. The position of the fracture may also indicate the mechanism of brain injury; for example, an occipital fracture may be associated with intracranial shearing forces, leading to frontal and temporal contusion-laceration.

1. The simple linear fracture of the skull demonstrated by x-ray requires no specific treatment.

2. When there is an extension of the fracture into the paranasal sinuses or the middle ear, systemic antibiotics have supplanted operation.

3. Simple comminuted depressed fractures of the vault of the skull may require operative correction for a better cosmetic result or if there is associated cerebral dysfunction.

4. Surgical elevation of a cranial depression is emergent when there is severe neurologic deficit and occasionally when an underlying epidural or intracerebral hematoma is responsible for the cerebral disorder.

5. Open fractures should be promptly debrided in the operating room.

6. Depending upon the degree of wound contamination, the comminuted fracture pieces may be used to restore bony alignment at surgery or discarded with delayed repair of the skull defect. With minimal contamination, a simple prosthesis of a suitable material may be used at the time of debridement. If the dura has been lacerated, the implicated area is then excised, all macerated tissue removed and the dura closed unless the defect is too large. With proper treatment of an open fracture of the vault, post-traumatic abscess and meningitis rarely occur. Such infections more commonly follow open fractures at the base of the skull, but intracranial infections of all types are infrequent with the early use of antibiotics.

## CRANIAL NERVE INJURIES

Although all dysfunctions of the cranial nerves are important, the following are emphasized:

### First Cranial Nerve

In severe craniocerebral injury, particularly when associated with shearing forces in the skull, some unilateral or bilateral impairment of smell may be noted. This is secondary to tears of the filaments in the olfactory nerve or hemorrhage about the olfactory bulb and may be permanent. There is no specific treatment.

### Second Cranial Nerve

The optic nerve may be injured in a great variety of ways following a craniocerebral trauma. Often in these acute injuries there is little spontaneous return of vision.

Mechanisms of injury include:

1. A fracture line extending through the orbit or optic foramina with fragments of bone compromising the nerve. This is an indication for operation only if the vision is grossly impaired but not completely lost, but, although the nerve may be freed of all compression, manipulation of the optic nerve after acute injury is dangerous and may result in permanent blindness. The presence of a bony spicule compressing the nerve at the optic foramen, demonstrated by x-ray, may be followed by complete functional recovery without operation. The decision for emergency operation is difficult and can only be made by an experienced neurosurgeon.

2. Perineural hemorrhage in and/or about the orbit

3. Compression of the nerve by hemorrhage within the sella turcica. This may be associated with loss of pituitary function. Usually the etiology is a fracture extending to the base of the sella. Clinical features include alteration of the visual fields or total blindness. On occasion, operation has been followed by minimal return of vision, but, in those cases, resolution may have occurred spontaneously without operation.

### Third Cranial Nerve

Embarrassment of the oculomotor nerve frequently occurs in combination with intracranial hematoma and tentorial herniation. Dysfunction may persist with total ophthalmoplegia except for the structures that are served by the fourth and sixth nerves. Late recovery may ensue. Treatment for a third-nerve lesion is directed at the underlying pathology producing the difficulty.

### Fourth Cranial Nerve

Dysfunction of the trochlear nerve is hard to detect and does not warrant specific treatment acutely.

### Fifth Cranial Nerve

Trigeminal nerve palsy is often temporary and there is no specific treatment.

### Sixth Cranial Nerve

Occasionally trauma involves the abducent nerve, but this is rare and does not require surgery in the early phases after the injury.

### Seventh Cranial Nerve

The facial nerve is frequently involved and associated with a compound fracture at the base of the skull in the middle ear:

1. Facial palsy occurring immediately after injury should have a guarded prognosis about recovery, although recovery often occurs. Although the underlying pathology is a structural alteration within the nerve, patients who have an electromyographic indication of complete functional loss may require decompression of the facial nerve within the facial canal.

2. When the facial palsy appears within 4 to 6 days after injury, there usually is complete or incomplete spontaneous recovery. These patients are treated with antibiotics and followed with serial electromyograms to observe their progress. Steroids may be used to reduce swelling within the canal and promote recovery.

3. When the peripheral facial palsy appears 10 to 14 days following a compound fracture at the base of the skull, it is usually inflammatory in origin and associated with an unpleasant odoriferous discharge from the ar. Treatment is with antibiotics. The use of prophylactic antibiotics has almost completely eliminated this clinical entity.

### Eighth Cranial Nerve

With any craniocerebral injury, either or both the cochlear and vestibular divisions of the acoustic nerve may be impaired. A conductive hearing deficit associated with hemorrhage into the middle ear can be diagnosed by careful examination and may necessitate decompression. Patients with compound basilar skull fractures through the petrous bone and middle ear often have a bloody or spinal fluid discharge from the ear, which ceases spontaneously. No attempt should be made to plug the ear.

Varying degrees of sensory neural conductive hearing loss may remain as permanent residuals after slow, graded recovery. Injury to the vestibular portion of the eighth nerve can be due to hemorrhage in the labyrinth, producing horizontal nystagmus only on gaze to one side. Associated vomiting, particularly on movement of the head, may occur. Differentiation from a posterior fossa lesion, such as a hematoma, is important but may be difficult. Chronic disorders due to vestibular dysfunction may occur but do not affect acute management.

## Ninth, Tenth, Eleventh and Twelfth Cranial Nerves

Injuries to glossopharyngeal, vagal, spinal accessory and hypoglossal nerves are of importance in indicating a focal site of injury, but they do not require treatment.

## INTRACRANIAL HEMATOMA

### Epidural Hematoma

This hemorrhage may result from a tear of the middle meningeal arteries and/or veins, or from a laceration of a dural sinus.

1. The identification of a fracture line crossing the site of the meningeal vessels or a sinus alerts the physician to the possible presence of an epidural clot.

2. Huge epidural clots, particularly those situated in the frontal fossa, may occur without fracture of the skull.

3. The classical syndrome of epidural hemorrhage consists of a head injury with or without change in consciousness, relative improvement (lucid interval) and then depression of the conscious state to stupor, with unilateral pupillary dilation followed by contralateral hemiparesis. This may be rapidly followed by dilation of the other pupil, decerebrate rigidity, ineffectual respiratory function, slow pulse or rising blood pressure.

4. Early diagnosis is essential.

5. Mortality is related primarily to the immediate preoperative clinical state, and, due to the rapid development of dysfunction, emergency treatment is vital.

## Acute Subdural Hematoma

This hemorrhage results from a laceration of the bridging veins or from a contusion-laceration of the brain.

1. Tentorial herniation may develop rapidly, and extraordinary efforts must be directed at early diagnosis and complete evacuation of the clot as well as control of intracerebral swelling and cardio-respiratory abnormalities, if survival is to be obtained.

2. In the stable patient, nonoperative management followed by delayed evacuation of the clot will lead to lower mortality.

## Intracerebral Hemorrhage

Intracerebral hemorrhage may be focal or coalescing in association with contusion-laceration of the brain, and it may be associated with other hematomas. Intracerebral hematoma and focal contusion-lacerations may simulate other hematomas by producing the signs of tentorial herniation. In general, from the surgical standpoint, most clots should be evacuated through a suitable dural flap.

## Hematoma in the Posterior Fossa

Hemorrhage in the posterior fossa deserves special consideration, since a relatively small amount of blood can have devastating effects by embarrassment of the hind brain. Usually the clots are unilateral, but epidural clots may be bilateral, particularly if bleeding is from a transverse sinus.

1. The syndrome of a posterior fossa clot occurs with contact trauma to the posterior part of the head and is often associated with occipital fracture.

2. It is characterized by a relative lucid interval, or at least a temporary plateau in the clinical course, further drowsiness and stupor, slow, irregular and even sighing respiration and slow pulse rate.

3. The striking feature is the respiratory dysfunction.

4. If a relatively alert patient with obvious respiratory change not due to thoracic or lung injury demonstrates nystagmus, emergency exploratory burr holes over the posterior fossa should be carried out. Death may occur in less than 45 minutes in such patients.

5. Even though rapid decisions are necessary, it is mandatory to consider other potential causes of the syndrome, such as traumatic labyrinthitis. In this case, horizontal nystagmus usually occurs only on gaze to one side and respiration is not disturbed. In both instances, vomiting and drowsiness may be present.

6. If uncertainty still exists, exploratory burr holes should be made and arteriography employed. The fact remains that death is still more common than survival in patients with hematoma in the posterior fossa.

## ACUTE CRANIOCEREBRAL INJURIES IN CHILDREN

### Introduction

Children with head injuries behave differently from adults. The plasticity of the skull, yielding suture lines, consistency of the brain and absence of a significant subdural space in children account for some of these differences. Intracranial hematomas and frontotemporal contusions are not as frequent in children as in adults with comparable injuries. In addition, the craniocerebral structures of children tolerate injury better, with lower mortality rates than adults, unless there is pre-existing cerebral disease such as hydrocephalus, which predisposes to more disastrous effects.

### Diagnosis

The diagnosis of intracranial hematoma in a child is difficult because the usual clinical manifestations do not have the same significance as in adults. In addition

to the fact that neurologic signs may be more insidious in their development, several clinical syndromes in children require emphasis.

1. Following head trauma, a child may exhibit the classical picture of intracranial hematoma and then suddenly recover. Classically, after head injury with or without loss of consciousness, a distinct lucid interval is followed by drowsiness, confusion or even light stupor. Babinski's sign may be present bilaterally, as well as hemiparesis and inequality of pupils. After a variable period of time, progression of the abnormal signs ceases and the child awakens and recovers. Other neurologic signs may endure for several days. In general, the cause of this common syndrome is thought to be related to focal cerebral edema, and of importance is the fact that the recovery occurs rapidly and no intracranial clot is present. However, persistent stupor and a falling or low hemoglobin indicate the presence of intracranial hematoma, necessitating arteriography, exploratory trephination or other appropriate treatment.

2. Convulsive seizures followed by postictal stupor commonly occur in children after head injury, and this may be difficult to differentiate from the depression of consciousness occurring with a progressive intracranial lesion.

3. Very large hematomas may exist acutely after injury, with only a few abnormal clinical signs. A change in behavior, for example, undue cooperativeness instead of the usual resistance and crying on examination may be significant. The child is reasonably cooperative during the examination but, when not disturbed, will tend to fall to sleep or tilt over in his mother's arms, or may simply lie down to sleep, which may be the onset of stupor. The diagnostic use of arteriography may disclose large clots before stupor supervenes, thereby reducing the mortality.

4. Epidural hematomas in children may progress to intracranial decompensation

rapidly or over a period of up to 14 days. Prolonged observation is therefore indicated.

5. Acute subdural hematomas may occur in infancy, associated with long bone fractures or other prenatal injury. Characteristically these children demonstrate rapid deterioration, consisting of:

A. Systemic hypotension and shock (from blood loss in the head)

B. Bulging fontanelle

C. Massive retinal hemorrhage and edema

D. Stupor and failing respiration with cyanosis

E. Decerebration

## Management

1. Urgent evacuation of the clot (which is often bilateral) is necessary if life is to be preserved. Simultaneously, blood replacement is necessary to treat the shock. Treatment in the presence of an open fontanelle consists of simply introducing a needle into the subdural space and aspiration of blood. Frequently aspiration is unnecessary because the blood will spurt out under considerable pressure. When the fontanelles are closed, trephination is required.

2. The nonoperative treatment of head injuries in children is similar to that previously outlined for adults. Particular attention should be directed toward control of abnormal respiratory function. In our experience, the occasional use of barbiturates in conjunction with other supportive treatment has helped provide more normal respiratory function.

# 21. NONTRAUMATIC NEUROSURGICAL EMERGENCIES

*Robert R. Sparacio,* M.D.

## BRAIN ABSCESS

### Definition

A brain abscess is any collection of liquid pus and/or necrotic suppuration, with or without encapsulation, located within brain tissues.

### Classification

1. *Single Abscess*

A. *Acute.* These produce *rapidly advancing* signs and symptoms of *localized* cerebral, cerebellar and/or brain stem dysfunction (e.g., focal seizures, hemiparesis, aphasia, visual field defects, cranial nerve palsies), together with depressed states of consciousness.

B. *Chronic.* These produce similar but *slowly progressive* signs and symptoms.

2. *Multiple Abscesses*

A. *Acute.* These produce *rapidly advancing* signs and symptoms of *generalized* cerebral, cerebellar and/or brain stem dysfunction (e.g., grand mal seizures, confusion, disorientation, personality changes, ataxias), together with depressed states of consciousness.

B. *Chronic.* These produce similar but *slowly progressive* signs and symptoms.

### Basic Principles

1. Single acute abscesses are usually direct extensions of bacterial infection from an extracranial site (e.g., from an otitis media to a temporal lobe; from a mastoiditis to a cerebellar hemisphere; from a frontal sinusitis to a frontal lobe; from a contaminated puncture wound or open fracture of the skull to any contiguous brain area). The connecting link is either a local osteomyelitis or infected,

thrombosed veins. The pathogenic bacteria are most frequently *Staphylococcus aureus,* less frequently strains of *Streptococci* and *Pneumococci,* and on rarer occasions *E. coli, H. influenzae, Proteus vulgaris, Salmonellae,* etc.

2. The single chronic abscesses arise from larger areas of necrotic suppuration developing in the course of prolonged secondary central nervous system infection by tuberculosis, fungi or parasitic organisms. They may be found anywhere in the brain but tend to favor more basal locations. The most common fungus pathogenic to the central nervous system is *Cryptococcus neoformans* (Torula). On rare occasions, other types occur, including *Actinomyces, Coccidiodes, Nocardia, Blastomyces, Mucor* and *Candida albicans,* but these tend more to produce a meningitis or cerebritis rather than abscesses. Central nervous system fungal infection is most often secondary to an independent, pre-existing disease process such as diabetes mellitus or lymphoma, or to radiation therapy or prolonged corticosteroid therapy. Granulomatous infestations of the central nervous system by parasites are uncommon in the United States but frequent elsewhere, particularly in Latin America and the Orient. The major pathogenic organisms are *Echinococcus* and *Cysticercus.* Very rarely, helminthiasis (*Schistosoma japonicum, Paragonimi westermani*) and amebiasis cause brain abscess; malaria, toxoplasmosis and trypanosomiasis produce diffuse lesions of microscopic caliber.

3. The multiple abscesses (acute and chronic) occur as a diffuse dissemination of microabscesses within brain tissues, predominantly within the cerebral hemispheres. They originate in the lungs

(pneumonia, lung abscess, bronchiectasis), in the valvular or congenital septal vegetations of subacute bacterial endocarditis, in pelvic suppurative disease and in foci of osteomyelitis. The microabscesses are more densely distributed in areas supplied by the middle cerebral artery circulation and characteristically have small arterioles as nuclei.

4. All types of brain abscesses incite and coexist with brain swelling (edema), often of marked degree, which in itself is significantly disruptive of cerebral activity.

5. All types of brain abscesses may cause hydrocephalus of varying intensity, the signs and symptoms of which (nausea, vomiting, headache, papilledema) may then be added to, or superimposed on, those evoked by the suppurative lesions and brain swelling. In the acute forms, the hydrocephalus is usually obstructive (noncommunicating) in type. Hydrocephalus may remain as a permanent residuum after the central nervous system infection is controlled.

6. Abscesses or granulomas situated within the brain stem are ordinarily not approachable by operation.

7. Meningitis does not usually cause a brain abscess, but it may coexist with an abscess if pus from an infected brain area finds its way into the subarachnoid space.

8. A brain abscess may suddenly rupture into the ventricular system, causing a marked ventriculitis and profound neurologic dysfunction, leading rapidly to death.

9. Metastatic abscesses are an increasingly frequent complication of heroin addiction and other drug abuses, because of unsterile injection techniques.

10. Subdural abscesses or empyema are rare, resemble the clinical picture of solitary brain (parenchymal) abscess and are treated in the same way.

## Criteria for Diagnosis

1. Headache, dizziness, depressed state of consciousness

2. Presence of progressive neurologic abnormalities, especially focalizing manifestations

3. Presence of an extracranial site of infection (e.g., otitis media, sinusitis, pulmonary infection, etc.) and/or a history of preceding infection

4. Grand mal or focal convulsions (over 50% of cases)

5. Persistent low-grade fever

6. Mild nuchal rigidity, positive Kernig's sign

7. Increased sedimentation rate and mildly increased white blood cell count in peripheral blood

8. Normal or near-normal cerebrospinal fluid content (total protein and cell count may be slightly elevated), together with increased cerebrospinal fluid pressure

These criteria in combination strongly suggest intracranial abscess, particularly of the more acute type. Chronic abscesses are very difficult to diagnose and often behave like, and are mistaken for, brain tumors. An extracranial site of infection (e.g., pulmonary tuberculosis) may be the only differentiating clue.

## Management

### Preoperative

1. Careful examination of the patient for possible sources of infection and for localizing neurologic signs

2. X-rays of the skull and chest

3. Complete blood count, sedimentation rate, urinalysis, blood sugar, serology, blood-urea nitrogen and sputum analyses (if obtainable)

4. Lumbar puncture to determine cerebrospinal fluid pressure, total protein (and gamma globulin), glucose, chlorides and cell count. Serology and India ink preparations for *Cryptococcus,* as well as smears and culture of cerebrospinal fluid for routine bacteria, AFB and fungi, are advisable.

*Caution:* if papilledema is present, lumbar puncture should be deferred until other diagnostic procedures are done and until a consultant neurologist or neurosurgeon is present.

5. Brachial (R) *and* carotid (L) arteriography should be performed. With a large solitary abscess, major shifts of the larger cerebral blood vessels by a nonstaining mass will usually be visualized.

6. PEG or ventriculography may be required if cerebral arteriograms are not diagnostic.

7. Brain scans and EEG are helpful diagnostic adjuncts, but they should be done only if they do not significantly delay the primary work-up.

8. If no mass lesion is found, but the clinical picture is that of intracranial infection (i.e., cerebritis), with or without accompanying meningitis, antibiotic therapy should be instituted and continued indefinitely or until both the intracranial infection and its extracranial source are eradicated.

## Operative

If a mass lesion is detected, proper treatment consists in the following:

1. I.V. antibiotics (by catheter) in high dosage. An infusion of 10 million units of aqueous penicillin in 1000 ml. of 5% glucose in water is begun and given every 8 hours, unless cultures of the pus obtained indicate other specific antibiotics.

Suspected tuberculous infections demand intensive therapy with streptomycin, 1 gm./day, isoniazid (INH), 300 to 600 mg./day, p-aminosalicylic acid (P.A.S.), 4 gm. t.i.d., or ethambutol, 400 mg. t.i.d., and pyridoxine, 100 mg./day.

Torula infections require therapy with amphotericin B. The initial I.V. dose (given over a period of 2 to 6 hours, diluted in 500 to 1000 ml. of 5% glucose in water) is 1 mg. on the first day, with gradual increments daily to a total (optimal) dose of from 1.0 to 1.5 mg./kg. Dosage is adjusted so that the blood-urea nitrogen remains less than 50 mg./100 ml. and serum creatinine remains less than 3.0 mg./100 ml.

2. Immediate burr holes over the abscess site. The abscess is punctured with a ventricular cannula and drained. Irrigations with antibiotic solutions may be done.

3. If the patient's condition is satisfactory and the abscess is encapsulated, craniotomy is performed immediately and the entire abscess is removed. In more critical circumstances (e.g., if the patient is moribund), this procedure may be delayed until the patient's condition improves.

## Postoperative

1. Continue antibiotic therapy until both the intracranial infection *and* the extracranial source are eliminated. Antituberculous and antifungal therapy may be required for months or years.

2. Give anticonvulsants. Dilantin, 100 mg. every 6 hours and/or phenobarbital, 30 to 60 mg. every hour, may be required to control seizure activity.

3. Maintain an adequate airway, utilizing a prophylactic tracheotomy if necessary.

4. Keep the patient's temperature at normal or subnormal levels with aspirin, alcohol spongings and an ice mattress.

5. Turn the patient from side to side every 2 hours.

6. Keep the patient's head elevated 30 degrees.

7. Periodic infusions of mannitol may be used to help control brain swelling.

8. Record and regulate fluid intake and output (indwelling Foley catheter is necessary).

9. Maintain adequate nutrition.

10. If hydrocephalus develops, a shunt may be required.

# SPONTANEOUS SUBARACHNOID HEMORRHAGE

## Definition

Spontaneous subarachnoid hemorrhage (SSH) refers to nontraumatic, active bleeding or extravasation of blood into the subarachnoid space of the central nervous system.

## Causes

1. Intracranial aneurysm
2. Hypertensive, arteriosclerotic cerebrovascular disease
3. Arteriovenous malformations
4. Intracranial tumors, primary and secondary
5. Blood dyscrasias

## Basic Principles

1. SSH has an estimated incidence in the United States of 16 cases per 100,000 population per year, 50 per cent of which (or approximately 16,000 cases) are caused by ruptured intracranial aneurysm. Sex distribution is about equal, but age is an important relative indicator of the probable etiology of SSH: arteriovenous malformations are a frequent cause in adolescents and younger adults; aneurysms predominate in the 40- to 60-year-old age-group; and hypertensive, arteriosclerotic vascular disease and tumors are common causes in the elderly. Blood dyscrasias occur in all age-groups.

2. Approximately 90 per cent of patients with symptomatic intracranial aneurysms present with SSH, and about 40 per cent of these will die from the initial hemorrhage. Unruptured symptomatic aneurysms give rise to unilateral ocular pain and/or palsy and headache. Multiple aneurysms occur in about 15 per cent of symptomatic cases. The true incidence of intracranial aneurysm is unknown because asymptomatic aneurysms are a not uncommon finding at autopsy, and postmortem examinations are not mandatory in this country except in criminal or other legal situations. Recurrent bleeding from a ruptured aneurysm usually occurs between the first and second week after the first bleeding episode, and it carries an estimated risk of death which is twice that of the initial hemorrhage.

3. The clinical state of the patient who survives the initial hemorrhage is a reflection of the intensity of disturbance of his cerebral metabolism and is the major determinant of his further management. SSH produces profound alterations in cerebral blood flow, nutrition and oxygenation, often associated with pronounced vasospasm and brain swelling. The mechanisms involved are poorly understood but may be roughly correlated with the degree of observed functional disability: patients who are awake, communicative and show minimal neurologic deficit soon after the original bleeding episode may be inferred to have considerably less derangement of cerebral metabolism than those patients who are stuporous or comatose. Patients in the former category should be investigated early, the cause of the hemorrhage clarified and appropriate therapy, including any necessary operation, carried out. Patients who are more seriously ill should be given general supportive treatment and allowed to improve their clinical state, in particular their level of consciousness, before undergoing diagnostic tests such as cerebral arteriography. Any patient in this category who is suspected of harboring an intracerebral or subdural clot should have immediate angiographic evaluation.

4. SSH may give rise to communicating hydrocephalus, acute or chronic. The acute form may develop within hours after the initial hemorrhage or within the first few days, may cause rapid deterioration in the patient's clinical state, and may erroneously be interpreted as a rebleeding episode or as massive cerebral edema. Definitive diagnosis depends on cerebral arteriography.

5. SSH which occurs during pregnancy has the same prognosis, referable to cause, as in the nonpregnant state. Consequently, cerebral arteriography and any necessary surgical procedures should be carried out as if the patient were not pregnant.

6. Untreated hypertension may predispose to initial aneurysmal rupture,

and it probably hastens recurrent bleeding episodes. In addition, hypertensive patients who undergo aneurysmal surgery have greater morbidity and mortality than those who are normotensive.

7. Aneurysms customarily arise at the branching of major cerebral arteries. Principal sites include the internal carotid, middle cerebral, anterior communicating, anterior cerebral, posterior communicating and basilar arteries. Less common sites are the origins of the anterior choroidal, pericallosal and ophthalmic arteries.

8. Three major types of aneurysm are recognized:

A. Saccular or "berry" (over 90%)

B. Fusiform

C. Intracavernous

Giant aneurysms which present clinically as an expanding intracranial mass, without SSH, are usually of arteriosclerotic origin (fusiform).

9. When dealing with multiple aneurysms, arteriographic evidence of which aneurysm has bled includes:

A. Large size

B. Presence of lobulations in the aneurysm

C. Presence of an intracerebral hematoma adjacent to the aneurysm

D. Spasm of the feeding vessel to the aneurysm

10. Arteriovenous malformations are composed of interconnected, tortuous, thin-walled venous channels fed by one or more major arterial branches. They frequently cause convulsions and may act as an expanding mass. A distinct bruit over the lesion may sometimes be present. In many instances the SSH they produce is less severe than SSH arising from other sources, possibly attesting to a venous origin. Adequate visualization of all feeding arteries is essential for proper surgical evaluation.

11. Brain scans and EEG's may be helpful in localizing arteriovenous malformations or tumors, but they are of little value in localizing aneurysms, except where an intracerebral or subdural clot may be present.

12. SSH caused by hypertensive, arteriosclerotic cerebrovascular disease is usually associated with intracerebral hematoma. Mortality is high with or without surgical evacuation of the clot, especially if the clot's location is "nuclear," i.e., in the deeply situated nuclear masses (thalamus basal ganglia, internal capsule). Rupture into the lateral ventricles and secondary brain stem hemorrhages are common.

13. SSH occasionally originates within cerebral neoplastic tissue. At times it may be the initial presenting sign, and it may be associated with a large intracerebral hematoma which obscures the underlying tumor. It is more likely to occur in highly malignant neoplasms (e.g., glioblastoma multiforme).

14. Blood dyscrasias such as leukemia, thrombocytopenic purpura and aplastic anemia may cause SSH, but more characteristically these give rise to small, multiple parenchymal hemorrhages, implicating supratentorial and infratentorial structures.

## Criteria for Diagnosis

SSH is characterized by the sudden onset of most or all of the following:

1. Headache, usually severe and generalized

2. Depressed state of consciousness, ranging from drowsiness to deep coma

3. Nausea, vomiting, photophobia

4. Signs of meningeal irritation (e.g., nuchal rigidity, positive Kernig's and Brudzinski's signs). At times, severe pain in the neck or lower back is present.

5. Convulsions, focal or generalized

6. Focal neurologic manifestations (e.g., unilateral oculomotor cranial nerve palsy, hemiplegia, aphasia)

7. Bloody cerebrospinal fluid, with xanthochromic supernate on centrifuga-

tion. On occasion, xanthochromia without gross blood will be found.

## Management

### Preoperative

1. Strict bed rest. If no surgically correctable lesion is discovered on subsequent investigations, or if the patient's general physical condition does not permit operation, or if proposed operation is refused, bed rest is continued for a minimum of 3 to 4 weeks.

2. An unobstructed airway must be maintained at all times, utilizing a prophylactic tracheotomy if necessary. Poor respiratory exchange contributing to cerebral hypoxia, increased intracranial venous and cerebrospinal fluid pressure and further brain swelling is incompatible with survival.

3. Body temperature should be maintained at normal or slightly subnormal levels with aspirin, alcohol spongings, ice packs and/or an ice mattress.

4. Fluid intake and output must be precisely recorded. An indwelling Foley catheter is required. Fluid intake should not exceed 2000 ml./day since some SSH patients may develop inappropriate excessive antidiuretic hormone secretion and retain water. I.V. fluids are administered in the more acute phase of illness and in cases in which oral intake is either impossible or inadvisable.

5. Reduction of cerebral edema, especially in more seriously ill patients, may be achieved by:

A. Mannitol, 25% solution, in doses of 1 to 2 gm./kg. of body weight, administered intravenously over 30 to 60 minutes every 6 hours.

B. Lyophilized urea, 30% solution, in 5 to 10% glucose, in doses of 1.0 to 1.5 gm./kg. of body weight, administered intravenously over 30 to 60 minutes every 6 hours.

C. Glyceryl, in doses of 0.5 gm./kg. of body weight, administered orally or by nasogastric tube every 4 hours

6. Dexamethasone (Decadron), 4 mg. I.M. or I.V. stat and 2 mg. every 6 hours I.M., or methylprednisolone (Solu-Medrol), 40 mg. I.M. or I.V. stat and 40 mg. I.M. every 4 hours. Use cautiously or not at all in patients with a history of peptic ulcer, gastrointestinal bleeding or severe diabetes.

7. Dilantin, 100 mg. I.M. or orally q.i.d.

8. Phenobarbital, 30 to 60 mg. I.M. q.i.d., for restlessness and/or to help control seizures

9. Reduction of hypertension:

A. If blood pressure is 160 to 180 mm. systolic, reduce by 25 per cent.

B. If blood pressure is over 180 mm. systolic, reduce by at least 30 per cent.

Reserpine (Serpasil) is the most effective single drug, but methyldopa (Aldomet), chlorothiazide (Diuril), furosemide (Lasix), and others are also used singly or in combination, depending on response.

### Operative

1. *Aneurysm*

Operation for aneurysm is a *prophylactic procedure,* i.e., it is designed to prevent recurrent bleeding. It is ideally performed at the earliest time after arteriographic detection consistent with an acceptable clinical state in the patient. If a second hemorrhage has already occurred and the patient survives, an *immediate* attempt should be made to repair the aneurysm.

Proper facilities (operating microscope, hypothermic blanket, volume respirators, monitoring equipment, etc.) as well as trained O.R. personnel should be available to deal with the particular needs attendant to intracranial aneurysmal surgery.

Hyperventilation and continuous cerebrospinal fluid drainage (to reduce intracranial bulk) and hypothermia (to reduce metabolic needs of cerebral tissues) may be employed according to the discretion of the individual surgeon.

Techniques to deal with the aneurysm are of two basic types: (1) direct attack on the aneurysm itself, and (2) reduction or elimination of its blood supply.

A. *Methods Used to Obliterate the Aneurysm Directly*

*(1)* Clipping or ligating the neck of the aneurysm (most successful and most widely used)

*(2)* Wrapping with muscle, fascia or gauze

*(3)* Coating with layers of polymerized plastic adhesives

*(4)* Production of thrombosis by injection of horsehairs

*(5)* Production of thrombosis by direct insertion of an electrode

*(6)* Production of thrombosis by stereotaxic injection of an iron suspension, held in place by a magnet

B. *Methods Used to Reduce or Eliminate the Blood Supply to the Aneurysm*

*(1)* Clipping the parent vessel intracranially, including "trapping" procedures

*(2)* Carotid ligation in the neck

C. Carotid ligation in the neck may be employed for aneurysms of the internal carotid system either alone or as part of a multistaged attack on a single aneurysm, or as part of a combined treatment for multiple aneurysms. Ligation may be done in several ways:

*(1)* Partial (at least 80%) ligation of the common carotid artery, followed in 4 or 5 days by complete ligation of the internal carotid artery

*(2)* Partial ligation of the common carotid artery, followed in 4 or 5 days by complete ligation of the external carotid artery

*(3)* Total occlusion of the common carotid artery done *gradually* over a period of a few days, utilizing a Selverstone clamp which has been placed around the artery

*(4)* Similar *gradual* total occlusion of the internal carotid artery

D. Sudden or rapid *total* occlusions of the common carotid or internal carotid arteries are poorly tolerated and should not be done.

2. *Arteriovenous Malformation*

A. Surgical excision of the arteriovenous malformations is performed to:

*(1)* Prevent recurrent bleeding

*(2)* Remove a compressive mass (the malformation itself, an intracerebral hematoma, or both)

*(3)* Halt shunting of blood away from normal brain tissues

*(4)* Help reduce or eliminate convulsions

B. Surgical excision is *not* performed in the following situations:

*(1)* The malformation is located in an inaccessible area (e.g., brain stem structures)

*(2)* Removal would result in serious neurologic deficits (e.g., lesions in motor areas, the speech area on the left, the region of the angular gyrus).

C. Operable lesions must be removed *totally*. Ligation of feeding arteries alone, or with subtotal removal, is inadequate treatment and should be avoided.

3. *Hypertensive, Arteriosclerotic Cerebrovascular Disease*

Craniotomy is advisable for evacuation of *large* intracerebral and intracerebellar hematomas. (Early surgical intervention is especially critical in cerebellar hemorrhage, before pontine-medullary decompensation occurs.) Morbidity is high even with surgery because of the destruction rendered to brain tissues by the clot before evacuation. Prognosis is more favorable when the excised hematoma is located laterally in the subcortical white matter and has not precipitated secondary brain stem hemorrhages.

4. *Tumors*

Surgical evacuation of a coexisting intracerebral clot usually accompanies excision of the neoplasm. All spontaneous intracerebral hematomas which are treated by operation should have biopsies of the wall of the clot cavity if no tumor or other etiologic source is evident.

5. *Blood Dyscrasias*

Surgical intervention is necessary only in rare instances when a large intracerebral hematoma occurs in an operably favorable position.

## Postoperative

1. General postoperative care is essentially the same as outlined under Brain Abscess, page 227, without the high-dose antibiotics.

2. High-dose steroids are gradually reduced over a 7- to 10-day period and then discontinued.

3. Antihypertensive therapy is continued indefinitely.

4. Ambulation should not proceed too rapidly, allowing for a "settling period" for injured brain tissues.

# HYDROCEPHALUS

## Definition

Hydrocephalus refers to the retention and accumulation of cerebrospinal fluid, usually under increased pressure, within the ventricles and subarachnoid space of the brain, resulting in ventricular enlargement and variable degrees of internal compression of brain tissues.

## Classification

1. *Obstructive Hydrocephalus* (noncommunicating). This is due to blockage or obstruction of the flow of cerebrospinal fluid in the ventricular system from within or from without, so that the cerebrospinal fluid is unable to enter the subarachnoid space.

2. *Communicating Hydrocephalus.* This is due to defective absorption of cerebrospinal fluid which enters the subarachnoid space.

Both communicating and noncommunicating hydrocephalus may develop acutely, within hours, or chronically, over months or years.

## Causes of Hydrocephalus

1. *Neoplastic.* Intra-axial tumors involving the third or fourth ventricles, aqueductal region and posterior fossa are primary offenders.

2. *Postinflammatory.* This may be caused by subarachnoid hemorrhage from any traumatic or nontraumatic source, including birth injuries.

3. *Postinfection.* This may be due to any type of bacterial, fungal or parasitic meningitis and/or cerebritis, as well as some instances of viral encephalitis.

4. *Congenital.* Possible causes are lesions of the aqueduct of Sylvius, including atresia, stenosis, gliosis and septal membranes;, Arnold-Chiari malformations; obstruction of the foramina of Luschka and Magendie (Dandy-Walker syndrome); vascular malformations.

## Basic Principles

1. The cerebrospinal fluid is continuously formed as a clear dialysate by the choroid plexuses of the lateral, third and fourth ventricles. From its points of origin in the ventricles, it flows in one direction out of the foramina of Luschka and Magendie into the basal cisterns and the subarachnoid space around the spinal cord, then over the surfaces of the cerebral and cerebellar hemispheres to the major midline venous sinuses. The cerebrospinal fluid is absorbed principally through the walls of capillaries of the pia-arachnoid covering the brain surface and through the arachnoid villi of the venous sinuses, although some fluid escapes through perineural lymphatic channels. The normal adult ventricular and subarachnoid spaces contain approximately 100 to 150 ml. of cerebrospinal fluid. Any disease process which causes impaired cerebrospinal fluid flow or absorption produces hydrocephalus.

2. Clinical manifestations of hydrocephalus differ with the age of the patient. In infants and young children, in whom the cranial bones are not yet firmly fused, ventricular dilatation is apt to be accompanied by:

A. Enlargement of the head at a rapid rate

B. Bulging fontanelles

C. Separated sutures (Macewen's "cracked-pot" tympany may be elicited).

D. Engorgement of scalp veins

E. Downward displacement of the eyes ("setting-sun" sign)

F. Prominent forehead with a small face

G. Variable neurologic deficits, depending on the efficacy of natural compensation to elevated intracranial pressure

3. In older children, adolescents and adults, in whom fusion of the cranial bones is more complete and the cranial vault is unyielding, increasing intraventricular pressure is transmitted more fully to the brain itself, with a strong tendency to herniation through natural openings (e.g., the tentorial notch and the foramen magnum). Ventricular enlargement is accompanied by:

A. Constant headache

B. Nausea and vomiting

C. Papilledema

D. If the hydrocephalus is not relieved, tentorial and/or foraminal herniation will occur, followed by functional failure of brain stem structures and death.

4. A chronic hydrocephalus which took months or years to develop may reach a level of maximum accommodation by intracranial tissues and, suddenly, upon little or no provocation, precipitate an acute crisis requiring immediate ventricular decompression.

5. Rapid decompression of ventricular pressure, while restoring brain function to a more normal level, on some occasions may cause a tearing of meningeal vessels or bridging veins, giving rise to epidural or subdural hemorrhage which must be evacuated by craniotomy.

6. In older patients, a normal pressure hydrocephalus may occur, associated with progressive dementia, bradykinesia and mild ataxic gait, all of which may successfully respond to a shunting procedure.

## Management

1. *Ventricular Drainage*

A. This method is used whenever *immediate* decompression is vital (e.g., in case of rapidly progressive tentorial herniation).

B. It is also used as an adjunct to posterior fossa and other cranial surgery, in order to:

   (1) Relieve compression and herniation of brain tissues

   (2) Aid in reducing venous bleeding

   (3) Help provide better exposure

C. Drainage is accomplished by introduction of a metal or rubber cannula into the lateral ventricle through a burr hole.

D. Prophylactic antibiotics are given if drainage is continued for hours or days.

2. *Direct Removal of Cause of Obstruction*

Whenever possible, blockage to cerebrospinal fluid flow should be removed (e.g., excision of posterior fossa neoplasms, cysts or vascular malformations; excision of third ventricular cysts or tumors; suboccipital and upper cervical decompression of Arnold-Chiari malformation; perforation of congenital aqueductal membrane, etc.).

3. *Shunting Procedures*

A. Shunts provide the only adequate treatment for communicating hydrocephalus and those types of noncommunicating hydrocephalus in which the obstruction cannot be removed directly. All shunts employ the principle of diversion of cerebrospinal fluid from a lateral ventricle into either the venous system, visceral cavity or an organ.

B. The ventriculo-atrial shunt is by far the most successful and most widely used type of shunt. Several kinds with specialized one-way valves (Pudenz, Holter, Hakim) are available.

*Types of Shunts:*

   (1) Ventriculo-atrial

   (2) Ventriculo-peritoneal

   (3) Ventriculo-cisternal (Torkildsen)

*(4)* Ventriculo-sinus    (superior sagittal or transverse sinus)

*(5)* Ventriculo-pleural

*(6)* Ventriculo-ureteral

*(7)* Ventriculo-fallopian

*(8)* Arachnoidal (lumbar)-ureteral

*(9)* Ventriculostomy of the third ventricle

C. Shunts which use the ureter require removal of the ipsilateral kidney. Ureteral and fallopian shunts produce problems of fluid and electrolyte balance, because the cerebrospinal fluid merely exits from the body and is not passed over a reabsorbing surface. Shunts frequently cease to function properly and must be replaced if the cause of hydrocephalus is still operative. Special care must be exercised when installing a shunting apparatus (strict aseptic technique, antibiotics, etc.) or else serious infection (e.g., meningitis, subacute bacterial endocarditis, peritonitis, etc.) might develop. If infection of any kind does occur, the shunting apparatus should be completely removed, and it should be replaced only after the infection has been adequately controlled with antibiotic therapy.

## INTRACRANIAL NEOPLASMS WITH ACUTE SIGNS

Intracranial neoplasms classically evolve as slowly growing masses, and they produce signs and symptoms of subtle onset and gradually progressive intensity which are reflections of this indolent process. However, tumors of any type, whether malignant or benign, may signal their presence rather precipitously on occasion, demanding rapidly corrective medical treatment and/or operation. They may do so in several ways: (1) by producing an obstructive hydrocephalus; (2) by creating marked cerebral edema (metastatic tumors are notorious in this respect); (3) by causing a subarachnoid hemorrhage, with or without an intracerebral hematoma; (4) by inducing an intravascular occlusion in a major brain

arterial system; (5) by provoking severe epileptic states, including status epilepticus; (6) by masquerading as a different disease (e.g., demyelinating disease or essential hypertension), until brain stem decompensation occurs. Iatrogenic etiologies, such as cerebral herniations occurring during pneumoencephalography, also must be included.

The only effective containment against such circumstances is a clinical awareness or alertness on the part of the physician, and even then, any of the described events may take place without advance warning. Proper therapy mandates excision of the tumor whenever possible, with adjunctive cobalt radiotherapy and/or chemotherapy whenever indicated. Prior to, and together with, such surgery, any complication must be treated: hydrocephalus should be decompressed, cerebral edema reduced, convulsions stopped, hypertension controlled, etc. Otherwise an already high morbidity and mortality will be increased.

## SPINAL EPIDURAL ABSCESS

### Definition

A spinal epidural abscess is any collection of liquid pus and/or necrotic suppuration located within the extradural space of the spinal canal.

### Classification

1. *Acute Abscess.* This abscess is characterized by abrupt onset and rapid progression of spinal cord compression and neurologic dysfunction below the level of the lesion. It is caused by pyogenic bacteria, primarily *Staphylococcus aureus,* but including various strains of *Streptococci, Pneumococci, E. coli,* etc.

2. *Chronic Abscess.* This is characterized by slow onset and less rapid progression of spinal cord compression. It is caused almost exclusively by tubercle bacillus.

### Basic Principles

1. Pyogenic spinal epidural abscesses arise from contaminated wound per-

forations (including lumbar puncture), surgical wound infections, extensions from local skin infections (carbuncles, furuncles), vertebral osteomyelitis, and from remote infected areas (e.g., from visceral abscess via bacteremia). Any spinal level may be affected.

2. Tuberculous granulomas and abscesses have a constant predilection for the thoracic spine, but they may be encountered anywhere along the spinal axis. The intervertebral disk space is first affected, with progressive destruction of the contiguous vertebral bodies. The granulomatous mass with centralized necrosis and caseation gradually enlarges in all directions, eventually encroaching upon the spinal canal and its neural contents, as well as producing a clearly definable posterior mediastinal mass. In younger people in particular, this process may occur at multiple levels. At times, no true abscess will form, and the bony lesions on x-ray may resemble osteomyelitis of nontuberculous origin or even carcinomatous metastases.

3. Abscesses and/or granulomas of any etiology produce their neurologic disturbances by:

A. Direct compression of neural structures (spinal cord, nerve roots)

B. Vasculitis and thrombosis of the blood supply to neural structures

4. Tuberculous granulomas may also have a certain "toxic" effect on neural metabolism. Collapse of weakened vertebrae with posterior buckling and outright dislocation may occur, particularly in the cervical area, with further embarrassment of neural function. The transverse myelitis and malacia which take place may not be reversible, and permanent neurologic deficits may remain.

5. Paraplegias resulting from pyogenic abscesses may differ clinically in their behavior from similar paraplegias resulting from tuberculous disease. The former tend to be permanent if not treated by operation within 2 to 6 hours, while the latter may recede and recur and fluctuate in intensity for many days, especially when under proper antibiotic and chemotherapeutic treatment. The exact reason is unknown but is probably a reflection of local changes in edema and vasculitis of the inflammatory mass adjacent to neural structures.

## Criteria for Diagnosis
### Acute Abscess

1. Pain in the back, usually sharply localized to one or two vertebrae
2. Radicular pains, secondary to nerve root inflammation
3. Fever, malaise, headache, signs of meningeal irritation
4. Paraparesis or paraplegia below the level of the spinal lesion. In cervical abscesses, quadriparesis and respiratory disturbances may occur.
5. Paresthesias and objective sensory disturbances below the level of the spinal lesion
6. Sphincteric disturbances below the level of the spinal lesion
7. Presence of an infected area near to (e.g., vertebral osteomyelitis, puncture wound) or remote from the spinal lesion (e.g., pulmonary abscess)
8. History of preceding infection
9. Any age-group may be affected.

### Chronic Abscess

The findings are the same as in the acute type, but also include:
1. Anorexia and weight loss
2. Slower evolution of neurologic signs and symptoms is the rule, but occasionally it may be rapid.
3. X-ray picture of Pott's vertebral spondylitis with paraspinal abscess
4. Presence of pulmonary tuberculosis
5. Preponderance in young adults

## Management
### General

1. Careful examination of the patient for possible sources of infection and for es-

tablishing the clinical level of the spinal lesion(s)

2. X-rays of the spine and chest

3. Complete blood count, urinalysis, blood-urea nitrogen, blood sugar, serology

4. Work-up for tuberculosis (in suspected granulomas), including PPD skin test, sputum examinations, gastric analyses, etc.

5. Myelography. A complete extradural block at the level of the spinal lesion is demonstrable in most cases.

## Acute Pyogenic Abscess

1. Immediate laminectomy and drainage of the abscess. The dura is *never* opened at the time of operation, so that potentially fatal meningitis may be prevented.

2. Intravenous antibiotic therapy in high dose is carried out coincident with operation. Ten million units of aqueous penicillin every 8 hours are given until cultures specify the nature of the infecting organism and other more appropriate antibiotics may be given.

3. Antibiotic therapy is continued for 2 to 4 weeks or until all signs of infection have disappeared.

4. Any coexisting metabolic disorder which might enhance the infective process, such as diabetes mellitus, anemia or hypoproteinemia, should be vigorously controlled.

5. Ambulation of the patient may begin 7 to 10 days postoperatively in uncomplicated cases.

## Chronic Tuberculous Granuloma and/or Abscess

The keynote of therapy embraces a constellation of factors, namely: elimination of pus and all necrotic, granulomatous material; protection of neural function; reconstruction of bony vertebral defects; and control of pulmonary infection. Although variations in modes of application occur, most methods utilize the following principles:

1. *Neural Aspect*

A. If a patient presents with progressing spinal cord dysfunction but is not yet paraplegic and has never been under treatment, therapy consists in complete bed rest, streptomycin, 1 gm./day I.M., isoniazid (INH), 300 to 600 mg./day, p-aminosalicylic acid (P.A.S.), 4 gm. t.i.d., or ethambutol, 400 mg. t.i.d., pyridoxine, 100 mg./day, and general supportive measures (e.g., adequate nutrition, proper ventilation, etc.).

B. If such a patient already has a complete paraplegia when first seen, decompressive laminectomy should be performed, in addition to rest and antituberculous medications.

C. If a patient presents with progressing spinal cord dysfunction *despite* adequate therapy with rest and antituberculous medications, decompressive laminectomy should be performed.

D. Advanced cervical spinal lesions, with or without dislocation, should be treated with traction with Crutchfield tongs (or other skeletal traction) prior to any operation. Traction should be maintained until sufficient healing has taken place with or without fusion of the bony vertebral lesion.

E. Whenever decompressive laminectomy is performed, the dura must *never* be opened, to prevent a potentially fatal tuberculous meningitis.

2. *Vertebral (Bony, "Structural") Aspect*

Since the granulomatous destruction of the vertebral bodies and the anteriorly located paraspinal abscess are not affected by decompressive laminectomy, further surgical therapy may be necessary

A. Exposure of the posterior mediastinum via thoracotomy, or, in the cervical area, exposure of the retropharyngeal or retro-esophageal space (The odontoid area is best exposed through the back of the mouth.)

B. Drainage of the abscess, and excision of all necrotic and granulomatous tissues

C. Vertebral body fusion at all necessary levels, using pieces of ribs as struts. High cervical (odontoid) levels are best fused posteriorly.

3. Ambulation after fusion may begin in 4 to 6 months.

4. Antituberculous medication is continued for a minimum of one year but, depending on clinical and x-ray evaluation, may be required for several years. In the later recovery phase, this may be limited to combinations of the oral antituberculous agents.

5. Physiotherapy during bed confinement and during early ambulation is essential to proper recovery.

6. Stringent care of bowel and bladder function must be instituted early and maintained throughout the course of illness.

## SPINAL EPIDURAL METASTASES

### Definition

Spinal epidural metastases means the spread of malignant neoplastic growths from a primary source to the extradural space of the spinal canal.

### Classification

1. *Direct Metastases.* This refers to uninterrupted extensions of the neoplasm into the spinal extradural space from a contiguous primary source, usually posterior mediastinal or retroperitoneal. Common types include lymphosarcoma, Hodgkin's granuloma, reticulum cell sarcoma, neuroblastoma and multiple myeloma.

2. *Indirect Metastases.* This refers to extensions of the neoplasm into the spinal extradural space from a remote primary source by way of the blood stream. Common types include carcinomas arising in the lung (most frequent), breast, gastrointestinal tract, prostate, kidney and thyroid.

### Basic Principles

1. Extradural tumors in the cervical and thoracic areas produce weakness in the limbs and trunk, associated with "cord" signs (e.g., hyperreflexia, early spasticity, bilateral Babinski's toe sign); in the lumbar region, such weakness is accompanied by "cauda equina" signs (e.g., hyporeflexia or areflexia, flaccidity, depressed or absent plantar reflexes and no Babinski's toe signs); and at the thoracolumbar junction (where the spinal cord ends and the cauda equina begins—the conus region), the weakness is associated with mixed signs, with early loss of bladder control and with a tendency for "cord" signs to predominate. In addition, in this area "saddle" patterns of sensory loss may be detected prior to more total sensory catastrophe.

2. Any vertebral level may be affected by a metastatic neoplasm, whether direct or indirect, but the indirect types favor the thoracic spine.

3. Although some degree of spinal pain may be present for several weeks prior to the onset of neurologic signs, the spinal neurologic deficits are apt to proceed swiftly to totality once they begin. The time interval may be as short as one hour, but it often takes from several hours to a few days. The reason for this is related to the mechanism of spinal cord and/or cauda equina dysfunction, namely: (1) direct compression by the mass, and (2) interruption of the vascular supply to neural structures. With operation, the chances of recovery of functional loss are most specifically determined by the metabolic derangement in the neural structures immediately preceding decompression. A compressed infarcted spinal cord is not likely to recover much, if at all. Clinically total deficits (e.g., anesthesia, complete paraplegia in the limbs) are consistently associated with infarctions of the spinal cord and are usually irreversible, particularly if present for longer than 4 to 6 hours. Therefore, the principal guiding factors to successful treatment are: (1) early diagnosis and (2) decompressive laminectomy *before complete paraplegia occurs.*

## Criteria for Diagnosis

1. Pain and palpable tenderness in the spine, precisely localizable to one or two vertebrae

2. Rapid onset and progression of neurologic abnormalities below the level of spinal pain, including:

  A. Paraparesis proceeding to paraplegia in the lower extremities. In cervical lesions, quadriplegia may ensue.

  B. Sphincteric disturbances, with varying degrees of loss of bladder and bowel control

  C. Subjective sensory disturbances (paresthesias) (e.g., numbness, tingling, pins-and-needles sensations and coldness in the trunk and limbs)

  D. Objective sensory disturbances, ranging from mild bilateral hypalgesia to pin-prick to complete anesthesia, either up to the level of the bony vertebral lesion or to one to three dermatome levels below the bony vertebral lesion

3. X-ray evidence of destruction of vertebral bone (e.g., pedicle erosion) at the site of spinal pain and tenderness

4. Presence of complete extradural block on myelography

5. Presence of known malignant neoplasm elsewhere in the body

## Management

Since time is crucial to preservation of neural function, all work-up and tests should be done without delay, prior to emergency operation.

### Preoperative

1. Adequate history and careful physical examination to determine the existence and location of the primary neoplasm, as well as to pinpoint the level of the spinal lesion

2. Keep the patient NPO

3. Complete blood count, urinalysis, blood-urea nitrogen, blood sugar, ECG. More detailed blood studies, such as serology, acid and alkaline phosphatase, calcium, phosphorus, serum electro-phoresis, etc., often provide important diagnostic information and may be drawn preoperatively, but they should not cause delay in myelography or surgery.

4. X-rays of the chest and spine, with special attention to areas of pain and palpable vertebral tenderness

5. Myelography. The level of complete epidural block defines the lower border of the tumor. An opaque marker or scratch on the skin at this point can be a useful guide at surgery. Cisternal myelography may be required if the lesion is located in the lower lumbar area.

### Operative

Immediate decompressive laminectomy and excision of the tumor are performed. The dura is not opened at the time of operation.

### Postoperative

1. Postoperative orders may include:

  A. Keep the patient NPO until fully reactive; then fluids are added to the diet as tolerated.

  B. Take vital signs every 15 minutes until stable and then every 2 hours.

  C. Foley catheter in bladder

  D. Monitor fluid intake and output.

  E. Talwin, 30 mg. I.M. every 4 hours, or Demerol, 50 to 75 mg. I.M. every 4 hours p.r.n., for pain

  F. Prophylactic antibiotics (optional)

  G. Nembutal, 100 mg. I.M. at bedtime

  H. Keep the patient on his side; do not lay him flat.

  I. Turn the patient from side to side in a "log-rolling" manner every 2 hours.

  J. Complete blood count and hematocrit 12 to 24 hours after operation

  K. I.V. fluids are continued only until the patient takes sufficient nutrition orally.

2. If the primary neoplasm is not evident, an adequate search for it must be conducted. The histologic features of the neoplastic tissue excised at laminectomy may identify the source of the mass or at

least narrow the possibilities. Special studies such as IVP, barium enemas, etc. are best performed after the patient has been allowed a short period of time to recuperate from operation. When found, the primary tumor should undergo appropriate treatment.

3. Cobalt radiation therapy should be given to the area of spinal malignancy, since laminectomy ordinarily does not permit total excision of the tumor. Cobalt radiotherapy should *not* be given as a *substitute* for operation except in those instances in which:

A. The patient's general physical condition precludes the performance of a major operation (e.g., acute myocardial infarction).

B. *Complete* paraplegia and sensory anesthesia have been present for a prolonged period of time (i.e., over several days or weeks).

C. The patient refuses surgery.

4. Hormonal therapy and/or removal of the gonads (surgically or by radiation) may be a useful adjunct in some types of malignancies (e.g., cancer of the breast, prostatic cancer).

5. Chemotherapy may be employed in certain situations where multiple lesions are present in addition to the spinal metastasis.

6. Physiotherapy during early convalescence and beyond is necessary to ensure maximal recovery of limb function.

7. Measures to maintain optimal bladder and bowel function must be instituted early and applied throughout the course of illness.

## "MASSIVE" LUMBAR DISK HERNIATION

### Definition

"Massive" lumbar disk herniation refers to a large rupture of a lumbar disk dorsally into the spinal canal, usually with extrusion of the nucleus pulposus, causing severe extradural compression of the cauda equina.

### Classification

This type of herniation occurs only as an *acute* disease.

### Basic Principles

1. "Massive" lumbar disk herniation is uncommon, but not rare, and presupposes anatomical failures which are exceptional in disk disease. Disk herniations are usually posterolateral protrusions of soft nucleus pulposus under a thinned-out, weakened fibrocartilaginous capsule (annulus fibrosus), which exert pressure on the nearest exiting nerve root. On occasion, actual rupture of a localized area of the fibrocartilage occurs, with extrusion of the softer nuclear core material. In the average protruded or extruded disk, unilateral direction and relatively discrete nerve root compression tend to remain constant because of two factors: (1) the weakness in the annulus is localized, and (2) the midline posterior longitudinal ligament persistently remains strong and unyielding. In massive herniations, both of these factors appear to be altered (i.e., the fibrocartilaginous capsule of the disk is more diffusely affected, and the posterior longitudinal ligament apparently is defective and gives way). The result is disastrous: even a trivial traumatic event or motion may precipitate an acute, marked, dorsally directed herniation or rupture of the disk, with compression of *all* adjacent cauda equina roots within the dural sac. The severe neurologic deficits which result may remain permanently unless operative intervention to relieve the compression is performed promptly, within a few hours after onset. Myelography should always be done prior to operation to clearly define the level of the herniation.

2. Preceding the onset of massive herniation, signs and symptoms referable to the lower back may be conspicuously absent, but not infrequently a history of

prolonged, intermittent minor back pain or discomfort may be elicited.

3. At times, upon herniation, a dissociation of degrees of motor impairment may be seen (e.g., a very mild paraparesis will coexist with total urinary and fecal incontinence).

## Criteria for Diagnosis

Typically, there is a sudden or rapid onset of:

1. Pain in the lower back (lumbosacral region), radiating into both sciatic nerve distribution areas. The intensity of the pain may range from a mild to a marked degree, but often it is exacerbated by straining, coughing, sneezing, etc.

2. Paraplegia or paraparesis in the lower extremities, associated with depressed or absent deep tendon reflexes, flaccidity and no Babinski's toe sign

3. Sensory diminution or loss (all modalities) in the lower extremities, up to complete anesthesia

4. Paresthesias (numbness, coldness, pins-and-needles sensations) in the lower extremities prior to advanced sensory depression

5. Loss of control of bladder and bowel function

6. On plain x-rays, narrowed intervertebral disk space (lumbar), with *no* evidence of destruction of bone or of soft tissue masses

7. On myelography, a complete block *at the level of the interspace* where the disk herniation took place

## Management

1. Preoperative work-up, urgently executed, and immediate postoperative orders are the same as outlined under Spinal Epidural Metastases, page 288.

2. *Operative.* Immediate decompressive laminectomy and excision of the disk are performed. If the disk material cannot be excised extradurally, the dura is opened and a transdural approach is used to remove the herniation.

# CLOSURE DEFECTS: SPINA BIFIDA AND CRANIUM BIFIDUM

## Definitions

1. *Spina bifida* is a defect of the spinal column caused by a failure of closure of the bony vertebral spinal canal in embryonic life.

2. *Cranium bifidum* is a midline defect involving failure of closure of cranial bones. The encephalocele which results is a herniation of the cranial dural sac, with or without neural tissue content.

## Classification

1. *Spina Bifida Occulta.* This is a vertebral bony defect (absence of spinous process, maldevelopment of laminae, nonfusion of laminae, rachischisis) without herniation of intraspinal elements.

2. *Meningocele.* This is a vertebral bony defect associated with herniation of the spinal dural sac which contains no neural tissue.

3. *Meningomyelocele.* This is a vertebral bony defect associated with herniation of the spinal dural sac which contains neural tissue (spinal cord, nerve roots, cauda equina).

## Basic Principles

1. Spina bifida bony fusion (mesodermal) defects and any associated maldevelopments of cutaneous (somatic ectodermal) and neural (neuroectodermal) tissues take place before the third month of embryonic life, although the actual herniations develop progressively throughout intra-uterine life. These congenital abnormalities may occur anywhere along the spinal axis, but they favor the lumbosacral area. The cranial defects favor the suboccipital region. A history of maternal trauma, infection or metabolic disorder during the first trimester of pregnancy is usually absent, and little or no familial tendency is present.

2. Spina bifida occulta is most often an incidental x-ray finding, since the vast ma-

jority of cases are asymptomatic. A small group may exhibit neurologic disabilities at any age, due to intraspinous fibrous adhesions or stalks, lipomas, bony spicules or malformations of neural structures.

3. Meningoceles and encephaloceles which contain no neural tissues produce no neurologic disturbances. Meningomyeloceles and encephaloceles which contain neural tissues are associated with a variety of neurologic deficits, including paraplegias, bladder and bowel incontinence, loss of anal reflex and marked sensory loss below the level of the lesion.

4. Spina bifida defects of all types are commonly accompanied by overlying cutaneous abnormalities (e.g., abnormal hair, dimpling of the skin, fat deposits or lipomas, telangiectases). Herniations may be covered by a thick layer of skin, or by a very thin layer or no skin at all. Hernations often have a broad, sessile base, but may be pedunculated.

5. Hydrocephalus may coexist with closure defects at birth, or it may develop when the defect is surgically repaired. Other congenital defects (e.g., clubfoot, heart disease, cleft palate, hip dislocations, etc.) may also be present.

6. The danger of bacterial contamination possibly fatal meningitis is great in meningocele and meningomyelocele, even though no spinal fluid leak occurs. This is especially true when the defect has scanty or no skin covering; therefore, prophylactic antibiotics are advisable in such cases. When a cerebrospinal fluid leak does occur, a meningitis may follow quickly, within a 24-hour period, even with antibiotic therapy.

## Criteria for Diagnosis

The presence in a newborn infant of a protruding mass anywhere along the spinal axis (or midline cranial area), with or without neurologic abnormalities, associated with a bony vertebral defect, is sufficient for diagnosis.

## Management

1. Spina bifida occulta which is asymptomatic requires no specific treatment.

2. Spina bifida occulta associated with progressing neurologic disability requires myelography, followed by laminectomy and removal of fibrous stalks and lipomas, and lysis of adhesions.

3. Meningoceles and encephaloceles should be repaired surgically soon after birth, within the first few weeks of life, if technically feasible. The purposes of surgery are (1) to remove a disfiguring mass and (2) to prevent infection. Some herniations which are not amenable to early repair may become operable at a later date, when the defect has become relatively smaller in relation to increased body size and the surrounding skin has toughened. Whenever a cerebrospinal fluid leak occurs, *immediate* surgical repair is indicated.

4. Meningomyelocele repair is performed if *both* of the following two conditions exist:

A. Only *partial* neurologic disability is present, and the possibility of functional recovery exists.

B. Hydrocephalus is either absent or arrested.

5. Meningomyelocele repair is not performed if *either* of the following two conditions is present (even if a cerebrospinal fluid leak exists):

A. Advanced neurologic defects, namely, total paraplegia and bladder and bowel incontinence

B. Progressive hydrocephalus

6. Hydrocephalus which develops after surgical repair of a meningocele, encephalocele or symptomatic spina bifida occulta defect should be treated with a shunt.

## SPONTANEOUS SPINAL EPIDURAL HEMATOMA

### Definition

Spontaneous spinal epidural hematoma

refers to nontraumatic bleeding or extravasation of blood into the spinal epidural space.

## Classification

It occurs primarily as an *acute* disease.

## Basic Principles

1. Spontaneous spinal epidural hematoma is a relatively rare disease, less than 60 surgically treated cases having been reported in the medical literature in the past 100 years. It often is clinically indistinguishable from a number of other diseases which affect spinal neural structures rapidly (e.g., metastatic tumors, massive disk herniation, occlusions of the abdominal aorta with spinal cord dysfunction, transverse myelitis of vascular, inflammatory or demyelinating origin, Guillain-Barré's syndrome, etc.). Definitive diagnosis is possible only after surgical exposure.

2. The majority of cases of spinal epidural hemorrhage lack a demonstrable causative factor. In a few cases, arteriovenous malformations have been tentatively identified; similarly, at times blood dyscrasias and excessive anticoagulant therapy have been implicated. Tumors practically never give rise to such bleeding. Rupture of epidural veins, which are thinwalled, numerous, extensively anastomotic and responsive to sudden changes in pressure and blood flow induced by increased abdominal pressure, has been causally indicted, especially since most of the reported cases have had some kind of physical strain (coughing, sneezing, vomiting, bending) just prior to the onset of symptoms. In general, prognosis is good if the hematoma is removed before neurologic deficits become complete.

## Criteria for Diagnosis

1. Sudden onset of focal pain anywhere along the spinal axis, usually accompanied by a radicular component
2. Evidence of spinal cord or cauda equina compression below the level of the lesion:
   A. Paraplegia or paraparesis
   B. Sphincteric disturbances
   C. Paresthesias and objective sensory loss (all modalities)
3. Complete extradural block on myelography
4. Normal plain x-rays of the spine

## Management

1. Preoperative work-up, urgently executed, and immediate postoperative orders are the same as outlined under Spinal Epidural Metastases, page 00.
2. *Operative.* Immediate decompressive laminectomy and removal of the epidural clot are performed.

# 22. FRACTURE DISLOCATIONS OF THE SPINE WITH NEUROLOGIC INVOLVEMENT

*Albert W. Cook,* M.D.

## Introduction

1. Fracture dislocations of the spine with neurologic involvement will be considered under the following headings:

    A. Upper cervical spine
    B. Lower cervical spine
    C. Thoracic spine
    D. Lumbar spine

The structures to be considered in each of these areas are bony, cartilaginous, ligamentous, vascular and neural (i.e., nerve roots and spinal cord). Different complicating features arise, depending on the level of the spinal axis, the type of injury and the structures involved, all of which determine the type of treatment and the prognosis. Injuries to the bone are considered elsewhere but influence the choice of treatment. The goals of treatment of patients with neurologic involvement are: (1) preservation of remaining neurologic function and (2) maximum reversal of any dysfunction of nerve roots and spinal cord. These considerations take precedence over all else, including restoration of bony alignment. Satisfactory bony alignment is desirable but not at the expense of neurologic deficits. Manipulation of a fracture dislocation of the cervical spine may lead to an irreversible neurologic injury when none existed previously.

2, *Reversibility of Neurologic Damage.* Spinal roots, particularly ventral roots, have a greater potential for recovery than the spinal cord since they are peripheral nerves and exhibit better regenerative powers and more resistance to injury. Delay in treatment of spinal cord injury potentiates irreversibility. The site of damage significantly influences the choice of treatment and the prognosis. In addition, the general condition of the patient, including associated diseases and other in-

juries, may greatly influence the degree of neurologic dysfunction. For example, cervical cord injury with respiratory embarrassment in an emphysematous patient may reduce the arterial blood oxygenation enough to affect both the prognosis of the local spinal cord lesion as well as the patient's survival. Pre-existing bony abnormalities (i.e., cervical spondylosis) may exaggerate or predispose to serious spinal cord damage. There is great variability in the size of the spinal canal at different levels, in different sexes and at different ages. A combination of a congenitally small canal and an acquired bony abnormality may produce a serious neurologic deficit after a relatively minor injury.

## Basic Principles

### Spinal Cord

Fracture dislocations of the cervical spine, thoracic spine and lumbar spine may be associated with complete or partial spinal cord injury. In the lumbar area the nerve roots of the cauda equina may be disturbed while in the cervical spine there may be a significant combination of root and spinal cord injury. The most common fracture dislocations are in the cervical and lumbar area because of the great mobility, and partial lesions are encountered more frequently here than in the thoracic spine.

(1) Complete anatomical or physiologic transection of the cord at first results in the state of spinal shock. This consists primarily of the abolition of all types of activity below the level of the lesion. (2) After this has passed, various stages of reflex spinal activity appear. (3) Babinski's sign may appear. (4) The bladder and rectum empty automatically. (5) In general, in varying degrees, there is a general increase of autonomic activity below the level of the le-

sion, such as penile erection, sweating, evacuation of the bladder and rectum, general flexion movements and increases in blood pressure due to vasoconstriction. (6) In association with vasoconstriction and a rise in blood pressure, there is a reflex response from the sino-atrial nodes resulting in changes above the level of the lesion, namely, vasodilation of the skin, headache, etc. (7) Various inflammatory changes such as cystopyelonephritis can occur rapidly. (8) Rapid decalcification of bone and metastatic calcification occur. The duration of this period of hyperactivity is variable and depends upon the type of injury that the cord has sustained. (9) Ultimately, all reflex activity may disappear when the spinal reflex centers below the level of the lesion become functionless or indeed may persist in their dysfunction from the time of injury. Under these circumstances, reflexes may never appear or, having once appeared, may disappear. Finally, all reflexes may be abolished and the muscles show marked wasting. Even the automatic activity of the bladder and rectum may disappear so that urine and feces are either retained or there may be continued dripping of urine and frequent incontinence. (10) The skin becomes dry, scaly, cold and mottled. (11) Very rapidly, too, there may be bed sores in which there is atrophy of the skin, subcutaneous and deep tissue and muscle, and even the bone becomes involved and destroyed. There is little tendency to heal. It is of considerable importance to recognize the significance of this type of disturbance in autonomic activity in terms of treatment. Specifically, although it is of great importance to monitor the skin from the standpoint of pressure sores, which undoubtedly are initiated by prolonged pressure in any one area, it is the intrinsic neurologic disturbance in the skin itself which rapidly leads to this deterioration, even at times without known local pressure, although the sores invariably appear over obvious places of continued trauma. (12) So too with the gastrointestinal tract. Soon after injury there may be dilation of the stomach and also lack of all type of peristaltic activity of the intestines. This not only has to be monitored, but consideration should be given to the function of the intestinal tract as regards its absorptive capacity. In spinal injuries in man, the absorptive capacity of the upper gastrointestinal tract is altered as regards various nutritional elements. This has bearing on the general nutrition of the patient and his treatment.

## FRACTURE DISLOCATION OF THE UPPER CERVICAL (ATLANTOAXIAL) SPINE

### Definition

A fracture dislocation of the upper cervical spine is any fracture with or without displacement of the occipital atlas and axis articulation.

### Basic Principles

1. The degree of neurologic dysfunction associated with fracture dislocation at this level depends almost entirely on the integrity of the odontoid process.

2. Fracture dislocation in this area should be suspected in any patient with craniocervical or simple cranial trauma.

3. X-ray examination, including laminagrams, is necessary for diagnosis.

4. All cases of anteroposterior dislocation of the atlas and axis can be classified as follows:

    A. Those caused by incompetence of the odontoid

    B. Those caused by incompetence of the transverse atlantoid ligament

5. A fresh fracture of the odontoid may be difficult to distinguish from a congenitally separated odontoid even with a history of trauma. In the latter there are often other congenital anomalies and the line of separation is not irregular.

6. Once fracture of the odontoid has occurred, there may be immediate spinal cord dysfunction or, because of an unstable articulation, repeated cord trauma may occur over many years.

## Criteria for Diagnosis

1. The diagnosis of atlantoaxial dislocation and odontoid fracture is made with a frequency commensurate with the suspicion of the examiner.

2. Detailed scrutiny of appropriate roentgenograms, including laminagrams, is necessary. Important points in evaluating the x-rays are as follow:

A. The atlanto-odontoid interval in adults is usually less than 2.5 mm. and there is no movement of C-1 or C-2 with flexion of the head. In children there will be movement and the interval may be 4 to 5 mm.

B. When odontoid fracture produces anterior dislocation with an intact transverse atlantoid ligament, the atlanto-odontoid interval may be normal. Here measurements of the anteroposterior diameter of the spinal canal is necessary.

C. If the antero-posterior diameter of the spinal canal behind the dens is less than 19 mm., abnormal neurologic signs can be anticipated.

## Management

1. Treatment of the atlantoaxial dislocation depends on:

A. The etiology of the dislocation

B. Whether the dislocation is reducible or nonreducible

C. The presence or absence of neurologic findings

2. Because of the distinct possibility of nonunion in fracture dislocations with fractures of the odontoid, delayed neurologic injury may occur.

3. Operation is indicated whether or not neurologic complications are present.

4. In the presence of neurologic complications after acute injury, treatment with skeletal traction is indicated until the acute effects of trauma have subsided.

A. Crutchfield tongs are used to reduce the dislocation, followed by operation and posterior fusion as soon as the patient's condition permits.

(1) In the application of Crutchfield tongs, the patient is placed in a supine position.

(2) The scalp is shaved and prepared in an appropriate fashion in an area extending across the head at the level of the ears.

(3) The tongs are placed in this line, with the center of the tong in the midline of the head. Indentations are made in the scalp by the projecting points as markers for incisions.

(4) After procainization of the scalp in the area of marked points, a stab incision is made and the periosteum is freed.

(5) With the drill designed for this procedure, an opening is made in the skull down to the depth of the guard on the bit of the drill.

(6) The points of the tongs are then inserted into these openings. The tongs are then cocked and tightened, and 4 to 6 lbs. of weight are applied.

B. When the dislocation is not reducible in the presence of neurologic signs, immediate treatment to relieve cord compression and achieve stabilization is indicated.

C. Since operative risk is high with postdecompressive procedures, an anterior approach through the mouth permits removal of the odontoid process and anterior decompression.

D. Posterior fusion can be done before or at a later date. Alternatively, fusion of the lateral masses transorally at the time of the removal of the odontoid may be indicated.

E. In some patients, simple skeletal traction followed by immobilization with a collar has produced favorable results without operation.

5. Persistent instability at this level of the craniospinal axis may lead to serious neurologic damage. Simple unroofing (laminectomy) posteriorly may be disastrous if no consideration is given to the lack of stabilizing influence of the lateral joints and the disruption of the odontoid joints in the fracture dislocation; therefore,

after this procedure stabilization is necessary.

## LOWER CERVICAL SPINE FRACTURE DISLOCATION

### Definition

Lower cervical spine fracture dislocation is any fracture with or without displacement involving cervical vertebrae 3 to 7.

### Basic Principles

1. Injury to the cervical spine may result in damage to the bony, cartilaginous, ligamentous and neural structures. Skeletal injury affects the vertebral body, facets or posterior elements, singly or in combination.

2. Persistent dislocation may not be easily reduced, and, if reduction is accomplished, instability may lead to recurrent dislocation.

3. Dislocation may be followed by spontaneous reduction.

### Factors Influencing Neurologic Injury

The mechanism of injury includes hyperflexion, hyperextension or compression.

1. With hyperflexion, the anterior cord is pressed against the ventral wall of the spinal canal and the cord is stretched. Occasionally the pia may be ruptured or the cord trapped between the bony structures.

2. In hyperextension injuries, the spinal cord is pinched between the upper vertebral body and the lower vertebral arch.

3. With compressive forces, there is fracture of the vertebral body.

4. Pre-existing disease or anomalies contribute to the degree of nerve injury.

5. The normal diameter of the spinal canal is 12 to 20 mm., and variations affect the severity of nerve injury.

6. Additional factors which affect spinal cord injury include: (1) hemorrhage (extrinsic and intrinsic); (2) compression by a herniated disk, ligaments or bone; and (3) stretching, swelling and vascular insufficiency.

### Criteria for Diagnosis

Specific treatment depends on the type of neurologic syndrome: complete or incomplete spinal cord dysfunction. The latter category includes the central cord syndrome, anterior cord syndrome, posterior cord syndrome, Brown-Séquard syndrome and various other admixtures of partial lesions.

1. *Complete cervical cord lesions* are associated with thoracic muscle paralysis and a complete loss of sensation, motor function and reflexes below the lesion. Occasionally the complete cord lesion reverts into an incomplete cord lesion within hours. The presence of a slow flexor plantar reflex with a short interval between the stimulus and the response (Gordon Holmes toe reflex) or priapism indicates a poor prognosis for recovery, particularly if there is no improvement within the first twenty-four hours.

2. *With posterior cord contusion* the symptoms are mostly sensory and always disappear within several days to a week. This is also the case in spinal concussion.

3. *The anterior cervical cord syndrome* is characterized by a total paralysis below the level of the lesion, with serious impairment of sensation and urinary retention. The senses of touch and position are largely preserved. This syndrome occurs as the result of compression of the anterior part of the spinal cord by either a vertebral body or a protruding intervetebral disk. It is commonly seen in hyperflexion injuries. If myelography shows a block, decompressive laminectomy or interbody fusion is considered.

4. A *central cervical cord injury* is diagnosed by disproportionate involvement of the upper limbs compared to the lower limbs, representing a syndrome called diplegia brachialis, and may manifest various degrees of severity. Laminectomy is contraindicated.

5. A *modified Brown-Séquard* syndrome is exhibited by an asymmetrical paresis of the lower extremities, with

analgesia on the side opposite to the paretic side.

6. Other subtotal cord lesions include those in which there is total paralysis with retained sensation or those with minimal movement of the toes and nearly total absence of sensation.

7. In the Brown-Séquard syndrome and in most cases of the central cord syndrome the prognosis is reasonably good, while with the anterior cervical cord syndrome and some other subtotal lesions the prognosis is generally unfavorable.

8. Root lesions can be observed as isolated entities or in conjunction with spinal cord dysfunction. They can be diagnosed by neurologic examination and include symptoms of radicular-type pain.

9. Spinal puncture combined with the Queckenstedt maneuver may suggest the need for myelography. Although a block may disappear spontaneously, its demonstration may relate the type of bony injury to the type of neurologic dysfunction.

## Management

1. The treatment of the patient with spinal injury can be directed to the focal lesion or its effects.

A. Operative treatment consists of: (1) decompressive laminectomy, open reduction of the fracture dislocation and relief of compression by bone, hematoma or disk; (2) anterior interbody exploration and fusion.

B. Nonoperative treatment consists of various forms of immobilization of the site of injury and traction.

(1) Skeletal traction is preferred if this is to be maintained over a long period.

(a) In the application of Crutchfield tongs, the patient is placed in a supine position.

(b) The scalp is shaved and prepared in an appropriate fashion in an area extending across the head at the level of the ears.

(c) The tongs are placed in this line, with the center of the tong in the midline of the head. Indentations are made in the scalp by the projecting points as markers for incisions.

(d) After procainization of the scalp in the area of the marked points, a stab incision is made and the periosteum is freed.

(e) With the drill designed for this procedure, an opening is made in the skull down to the depth of the guard on the bit of the drill.

(f) The points of the tongs are then inserted into these openings. The tongs are then cocked and tightened, and 4 to 6 lbs. of weight are applied.

(2) The indications for cervical skeletal traction are as follow:

(a) Any sign by radiograph or neurologic examination of dysfunction relative to the cervical area

(b) When either bony injury or neurologic damage is suspected, particularly since spontaneous reduction of a dislocation may not be evident on x-ray

(c) Early reduction is vital if neurologic function is to be restored. The use of muscle relaxants, Demerol or general anesthesia may aid the application of traction, but care is necessary to avoid aggravation of neurologic damage.

(d) If reduction is accomplished, traction is maintained for 2 to 6 weeks and, depending upon the general condition of the patient, change in neurologic signs, improvement, stability or progression, operative stabilization of the spinal canal can be considered. Anterior interbody fusion can shorten the period of traction and confinement to bed, allowing earlier ambulation.

(e) If reduction is not accomplished, posterior operation (laminectomy) is indicated for open reduction. Once again, the timing of these procedures is guided by the interval since injury, the type of abnormal neurologic syndrome and the general condition of the patient, particularly the state of ventilatory function.

(f) Timing is important to

produce maximum restoration of function and to avoid further damage. If there is progressive deterioration in neurologic signs, myelogram and operative intervention should be seriously entertained.

2. *Summary of Orders for Patients with Acute Spinal Cord Injury*

A. *Initial Evaluation*

*(1)* Immobilization of the injured part in a suitable manner, usually with sandbags

*(2)* Appropriate radiographs of the cervical spine, thoracic spine or lumbar spine

*(3)* Record of neurologic deficit

B. *Systemic Features*

*(1)* Blood pressure, pulse and respiration are recorded every fifteen minutes, every thirty minutes and every hour, and the intervals increase when there is stability.

*(2)* Measurements of tidal volume with a spirometer

*(3)* Arterial $pCO_2$ and $pO_2$, as often as necessary

*(4)* Tracheostomy set and respirator made available

*(5)* Intravenous fluid, as indicated

*(6)* Indwelling catheter, preferably tidal drainage

*(7)* Decompression of stomach if appropriate

*(8)* Circular bed, Stryker frame or special mattress, depending upon other forms of treatment to be employed

*(9)* Frequent turning, as often as every two hours

*(10)* Padding of pressure points

*(11)* Urinary antisepsis with drugs such as Gantrisin

*(12)* Irrigation of the catheter three times a day

In general, the nutritional status of the patient should be maintained in as normal a fashion as possible, preferably by use of the gastrointestinal tract. Alternatively, intravenous therapy should be used. If this is prolonged, hyperalimentation should be considered. Antibiotics should be given. In our experience the use of steroids to reduce spinal cord swelling is not warranted routinely.

## THORACIC SPINE FRACTURE DISLOCATIONS

### Basic Principles

Many of the principles of management of neurologic dysfunction in the thoracic area are similar to those in the cervical area. Since the thoracic spinal canal is smaller compared to the diameter of its contents, complete lesions are more common. Systemic complications include urinary sepsis, bed sores and respiratory embarrassment which results from local thoracic injury, as well as respiratory muscle paralysis.

### Management

After four to six hours of complete paralysis, operation is of little value unless local hypothermia has been instituted. With partial lesions, however, decompressive laminectomy may be useful.

## LUMBAR SPINE FRACTURE DISLOCATIONS

### Basic Principles

Injuries of the lumbar spine produce different effects since the lumbar spinal canal is larger and contains ventral and dorsal roots along with the conus medullaris. Partial lesions are the rule, and varying degrees of spontaneous recovery occur even with significant fracture dislocations.

### Management

Progressive partial lesions and complete lesions affecting special segments should be subjected to early operation. Urinary bladder and bowel dysfunction may be improved by early or even late decompression is some cases, since the cauda equina has a greater potential for recovery than the cord.

## SPECIAL PROBLEMS IN SPINAL CORD INJURY

### RESPIRATORY DISORDERS ACCOMPANYING TRAUMATIC CERVICAL CORD LESIONS

#### Basic Principles

Patients with major injury to the spinal cord demonstrate several types of respiratory disturbances.

1. With injury above the level of the thorax, there will be paralysis of the thoracic muscles, and only diaphragmatic action may maintain ventilatory activity.

2. In patients with a high cervical cord lesion, the voluntary control of respiration may be impaired so that during sleep grave difficulties may occur.

3. Cervical cord injuries are often associated with injuries which may lead to aspiration of blood or other foreign material. With thoracic muscle paralysis, ventilatory volume is reduced to one half to two thirds of normal values. In addition to this, the volume is further diminished by paradoxical respiration as may occur with extensive thoracic injury.

#### Criteria for Diagnosis

1. In general, 500 ml. of vital capacity is sufficient to maintain arterial oxygenation, but these patients cannot exhale forcibly or cough. It is therefore extremely important to establish normal ventilatory function early and to persistently re-evaluate it daily.

2. Two simple instruments which help are a spirometer with a recording graph or a Wright's spirometer.

3. When the arterial $pCO_2$ is measured, these data indicate the necessity for tracheostomy.

#### Management

1. Hypercapnia may lead to stupor or mental confusion and predisposes to cardiac irregularity when stimulation is applied to the upper air passage. A combination of hypercapnia and acidosis may indicate the need for tracheostomy.

2. One of the most serious complications that may occur soon after injury is aspiration from a dilated stomach. Gastric intubation or gastrostomy are measures taken to avoid this complication.

### BLADDER DYSFUNCTION IN SPINAL INJURY

#### Basic Principles

Bladder infections are common in patients with spinal cord injury. Reflex control may be delayed from weeks to a year due to overdistention of the bladder following inadequate drainage or in patients who exhibit severe flexor spasms. In our experience, an early return of reflex activity occurs when extensor reflexes can be elicited early, as occurs in incomplete lesions. In complete lesions of the cervical spinal cord with return of reflex bladder activity, the bladder contractions are initially weak and poorly sustained. Gradually the amount of urine which is evacuated increases and consequently there is a decrease in the frequency of reflex contractions.

#### Criteria for Diagnosis

1. The typical reflex bladder finally evacuates most of its contents at a capacity of 300 to 400 ml., indicating that the activity of the reflex center is not necessarily high. This is a so-called normal reflex bladder.

2. The spastic reflex bladder is characterized by frequent discharges of small quantities of urine at irregular intervals at a capacity of less than 100 ml. and is also observed in the presence of bladder infection.

3. With complete lesions in the spinal cord there is the uninhibited neurogenic bladder. It is characterized by urgency of micturition with loss of sensation of bladder filling and sometimes associated with precipitate micturition with little residual urine.

## Management

1. Fluid intake is forced to produce a regular urinary output.

2. At the end of each period of one hour, the catheter is opened and the patient is submitted to micturition reflex by massage of the abdomen or Crede's maneuver. If no leakage occurs, the interval is increased gradually to three hours.

3. The catheter is then removed and the same regimen is used without a catheter.

4. When early catheterization is instituted and bladder infection is prevented by careful management, supported by oral administration of antiseptics, the non-irritated bladder may carry a normal quantity of urine before reflex discharge occurs.

5. One of the most effective methods for encouraging automaticity in cord bladders and avoiding infection is the use of tidal drainage. This sytem automatically permits filling and evacuation of the bladder, but it can lead to overdistention of the bladder if not applied correctly. For this reason, repeated catheterizations are suggested by some urologists as superior.

# 23. FRACTURES AND DISLOCATIONS OF THE SPINE WITHOUT NEUROLOGIC INVOLVEMENT

*Leroy S. Lavine*, M.D.

## Introduction

Spinal injuries are common, and they are not limited predominantly to industrial accidents as is often supposed. Fractures may be sustained in sports such as football, diving, polo, and the like; in the home from slipping and landing heavily in a "sit-down" position or from falling from a ladder or chair, the impact on a hard surface causing the spine to suddenly flex or "jackknife"; or in traffic or highway accidents, many of which may seem trivial.

## CERVICAL SPINE

### FRACTURES OF THE ATLAS

#### Basic Principles

The atlas may be fractured by a vertical force acting through the skull, the bony ring formed by the anterior arch and the posterior arch of the atlas being forced open by the occipital condyles. Displacement is seldom severe, and, more often than not, the spinal cord escapes serious injury.

#### Criteria for Diagnosis

1. History of trauma involving a vertical force acting through the skull
2. Spasm and tenderness of the paracervical musculature with tenderness involving the upper cervical spine
3. X-ray examination which discloses the fracture

#### Management

1. In the absence of injury to the spinal cord, it is sufficient to support the injured region for three months by a plaster or plastic collar.
2. Prior to the application of the collar, the patient should be placed in head-halter traction with 5 pounds of weight until

definitive evidence of neurologic involvement is absent.

### FRACTURE OF THE BASE OF THE ODONTOID WITHOUT DISPLACEMENT OF THE AXIS OR ATLAS

#### Basic Principles

The mechanism of injury can be direct trauma to the area or a sudden flexion-extension injury.

#### Criteria for Diagnosis

1. History of injury to the cervical spine
2. Severe pain associated with spasm and tenderness of the cervical spine
3. Marked limitation of motion
4. Careful neurologic examination which reveals the absence of any neurologic findings
5. X-ray examination, which includes an open-mouth view, lateral views in extension and flexion, and oblique views, reveals the fracture without displacement.

#### Management

1. Immediate splinting of the cervical spine and skull in the position of the deformity without attempts at correcting the deformity until a diagnosis has been made
2. After the diagnosis has been made, immediate application of skull-tong traction
3. The patient should be carefully evaluated for possible development of neurologic findings.
4. After the patient is symptom-free, immobilization should be continued with a Minerva-type plaster or plastic jacket.

### FRACTURES OF THE BASE OF THE ODONTOID WITH SUBLUXATION OF THE ATLAS OR AXIS

#### Basic Principles

The mechanism of injury is similar to

that described for fractures without displacement. The normal atlantoaxial joint depends for its stability upon the snug fit of the anterior arch and the transverse ligament of the atlas over the odontoid process of the axis. This stability may be lost if the transverse ligament is defective or if the dens is fractured. Forward displacement of the atlas on the axis is much more common than backward displacement. Forward displacement of the atlas from inflammatory softening of the transverse ligament is well recognized in cases of infection of the throat or neck.

### Criteria for Diagnosis

1. History of trauma to the cervical spine
2. Severe spasm, pain and tenderness of the cervical spine
3. Limitation of motion
4. Clinically, the patient is often seen supporting his head in his hand.
5. *Radiographic diagnosis* reveals the fracture of the base of the odontoid process with displacement. Occasionally tomographic and cineradiographic examination may be required to make the diagnosis.

### Management

Treatment is similar to that outlined previously for fractures without displacement. However, immobilization in skull-tong traction should be continued for 8 to 10 weeks. Immobilization in a plaster-type Minerva jacket should be maintained for 3 to 6 months. At the end of this time, cineradiography should be employed to determine if stability of the atlantoaxial joint is present. If the joint is unstable, spinal fusion should be carried out.

### WEDGE COMPRESSION FRACTURES OF THE CERVICAL VERTEBRAE

### Basic Principles

The injury is caused by a flexion force. The posterior ligaments are intact so that the spine is stable and neurologic involve-

ment is not seen. If the posterior ligaments are not intact, transection of the spinal cord may ensue.

### Criteria for Diagnosis

1. Local pain over the site of compression
2. Prominent spinous process on palpation
3. Tenderness on percussion
4. Painful limitation of cervical motion
5. X-ray discloses the compression fracture.

### Management

1. Head-halter traction (5 pounds) until acute symptoms subside
2. A plastic or plaster collar should be worn for 10 to 12 weeks.

### SUBLUXATION OF ONE CERVICAL VERTEBRA ON ANOTHER

### Basic Principles

The direction of the displacement depends on whether the injury is either a flexion or extension injury.

### Criteria for Diagnosis

1. History of injury to the cervical spine with mechanism of injury
2. Local pain and spasm, with tenderness over the site of subluxation
3. A "step-off" may be palpable over the level of the subluxation.
4. X-ray diagnosis discloses the subluxation of one vertebra on another.

### Management

1. Immediate application of skull-tong traction to reduce the subluxation. If the subluxation recurs after reduction, this is indicative of an unstable spine. Spinal fusion is indicated.
2. The skull-tong traction should be maintained for 8 to 10 weeks and then immobilization should be continued in a plaster- or plastic-type jacket for 3 to 6 months. Cineradiography may then be employed to determine the stability of the

spine. If the spine is found to be unstable, fusion may be indicated.

## FRACTURES OF THE SPINOUS PROCESSES

### Basic Principles

These fractures usually follow trauma involving violent muscular contractions. The types of fractures produced are avulsion-type fractures.

### Criteria for Diagnosis

1. Local spasm, tenderness and pain
2. X-ray examination reveals the fracture.

### Management

Treatment consists of immobilization in a collar until acute symptoms have subsided.

## DORSOLUMBAR SPINE

## WEDGE COMPRESSION FRACTURE OF A VERTEBRAL BODY WITHOUT NEUROLOGIC INVOLVEMENT

### Basic Principles

The mechanism of injury may be due to:
1. A severe flexion force which may crush the cancellous bone of one or more vertebral bodies. The compression is always most marked at the front of the vertebral body, which consequently becomes wedge-shaped. The posterior ligaments are intact, so the fracture is stable.
2. Fall from a height
3. Compression from a pathologic process involving the vertebral body (e.g., senile osteoporosis and tumor metastasis).

### Criteria for Diagnosis

1. Severe pain localized to the area of the vertebral body, associated with muscle spasm
2. Paralytic ileus and urinary retention may be associated with compression fractures.
3. Radiographic confirmation of the diagnosis

### Management

1. Bed rest on a hard surface until the pain has subsided
2. Analgesics to control pain
3. If paralytic ileus is present, nasogastric suction may become necessary.
4. Stool softeners while on bed rest (e.g., Colace)
5. Mobilization with an external support when acute pain has subsided. For dorsal spine fractures, a Knight Taylor or Jewett hyperextension brace may be utilized. For lumbar spine compression fractures, a Knight spinal brace or high lumbosacral corset may be ordered.

## FRACTURES OF THE TRANSVERSE PROCESSES

### Basic Principles

These fractures are usually associated with a fall from a height and other vertebral fractures. Torsion injuries to the spine may also produce fractures of the transverse processes.

### Criteria for Diagnosis

1. Localized pain and tenderness, with associated muscle spasm
2. Radiographic confirmation of the diagnosis

### Management

1. Rest until the acute symptoms have subsided
2. Analgesics for pain
3. Mobilization with a corset when acute symptoms have subsided

## FRACTURE OF THE SACRUM

### Basic Principles

The mechanism of injury is usually associated with a fall on the buttocks.

### Criteria for Diagnosis

1. Localized pain and tenderness
2. Radiographic confirmation of the diagnosis

## Management

1. Bed rest until acute symptoms have subsided. A firm mattress is necessary.
2. Analgesics for pain
3. Sacral corset if chronic pain persists

## FRACTURES OF THE COCCYX

### Basic Principles

A fracture of the coccyx is usually caused by a direct fall. The coccyx may or may not be displaced.

### Criteria for Diagnosis

1. Localized pain and tenderness in the coccygeal area which may radiate to the rectum or low back area
2. Rectal examination discloses tenderness on palpation
3. Radiographic examination for confirmation

## Management

1. Bed rest if warranted by severe pain
2. Analgesics for pain
3. Sitz baths
4. Stool softeners if bowel movement is painful
5. Occasionally, a sacro-iliac support may be needed.
6. If pain persists, occasionally excision of the coccyx is warranted.

# 24. ACUTE INFECTIONS AND INJURIES OF BONES AND JOINTS

*Irving Lustrin*, M.D.
*Walter H. Rubins*, M.D.

## ACUTE PYOGENIC OSTEOMYELITIS

### Definition

Acute pyogenic osteomyelitis is an inflammatory or infectious process of bone, of sudden onset, caused by pyogenic organisms settling from the blood stream; therefore, it is the local manifestation of bacteremia.

### Classification

1. *Acute Pyogenic Osteomyelitis in the Infant* (under one year of age). The epiphyseal vessels are still open; infections involving the metaphysis will usually involve the adjacent joint space and the epiphyseal side of the plate.

2. *Acute Pyogenic Osteomyelitis in Childhood.* Most common metaphyseal vessels are the last ramifications of the nutrient artery which eventually reach a large system of sinusoidal veins and venous lakes. This is an ideal medium for the development of infection secondary to an infected embolus because of the specialized anatomy. The metaphysis of long bones is the most common site, usually around the knee.

3. *Acute Pyogenic Osteomyelitis in the Adult.* This is rare and is usually localized to short bones (e.g., the spine). If it is localized to long bones, the site is usually the diaphysis.

### Basic Principles

1. Since acute pyogenic osteomyelitis is usually spread from a pre-existing focus by way of the blood stream, there is a transient and intermittent bacteremia. The capillaries, end arteries and venous lakes of the metaphysis are usually the site of the septic thrombi which lead to septic infarction. An inflammatory process then commences with hyperemia, edema and infiltration with polymorphonuclear leukocytes. Proteolytic enzymes are produced, yielding further necrosis of ischemic tissue which culminates in abscess formation. Under sufficient pressure, the abscess spreads inward toward the medullary canal and outwardly along the vascular channels to form a subperiosteal abscess. The purulent exudate also follows Haversian and cortical Volkmann's canals to enter the subperiosteal space. If allowed to progress, the pus will strip the entire periosteum. This purulent exudate thus bathes both the medullary canal and the subperiosteal space, producing necrosis of the entire shaft. Occasionally the disease process may spread further to involve the adjacent joint space, producing septic arthritis, or may metastasize to other sites.

2. Although pre-existing infection elsewhere in the body is the common precursor, it is well known that bacteria are often present in bone in a dormant state. Minor trauma may excite activity of the infection organism, producing osteomyelitis.

Clinical infection, therefore, is a result of host factors and infecting organisms. An individual with lowered host resistance thus is more susceptible to predisposing clinical infection.

3. The object of treatment of this disease is to abort the pathologic process prior to the development of the fulminant picture described previously. If treatment is commenced early enough with effective antibiotic therapy, subsequent complications should be minimal. Therefore, if this condition enters into the differential diagnosis, treatment should be instituted immediately. If another entity is later found to be responsible, very little is lost. If one waits to prove the diagnosis by x-ray or other

means, a golden opportunity has been missed.

4. Acute pyogenic osteomyelitis should be suspected in any patient with sepsis, local pain and tenderness at the end of a long bone. Antibiotic therapy should be instituted and continued as long as required. Aborting the process and preventing the onset of x-ray changes should be considered successful treatment rather than "overtreatment" of a minor condition.

## Criteria for Diagnosis

1. *General Signs*
   A. The child appears acutely ill, with signs of sepsis, malaise, general weakness, headaches, chills and fever.
   B. Site of previous infection
2. *Local Signs*
   A. Discomfort and eventually severe pain at the end of a long bone
   B. Splinting of the extremity and protective muscle spasm
   C. Refusal to bear weight
   D. Swelling and erythema over the involved area
   E. Sympathetic effusion in the adjacent joint
   F. Aspiration of pus from the area
3. *Laboratory Diagnosis*
   A. Elevated white blood count with a polymorphonuclear shift to the left
   B. Elevated erythrocyte sedimentation rate (ESR). This test is most important and is used both for diagnosis and to follow the effects of treatment.
   C. Anemia
4. *Radiographic Findings*
   A. Bone changes are relatively late in this disease. Treatment should be commenced long before they are seen.
   B. Early changes can be identified with good technique. In 2 to 3 days, the deep soft tissues adjacent to the area involved will show blurring of the muscle planes and swelling of the deep layers.
   C. Several days later, haziness or mottling of the metaphysis may be seen, and in 7 to 10 days, the typical findings of bone destruction, periosteal elevation and sequestration will be seen.

5. *Etiologic Organisms.* Approximately 95 per cent of all infections will involve coagulase-positive *Staphylococcus aureus*. In infants, there is an increased incidence of *Haemophilus influenzae*. Other rare organisms are *Escherichia coli* and *Pneumococcus sp.* Sickle cell disease is a special problem, with *Salmonella sp.* commonly as the infecting organism.

## Differential Diagnosis

1. Rheumatic fever has a slower onset; there is usually more than one site involved, with less bone and more joint tenderness.
2. Cellulitis
3. Pyogenic arthritis
4. Ewing's sarcoma, osteogenic sarcoma, tuberculosis

## Management

If the diagnosis is suspected:
1. Admit the patient to the hospital.
2. Complete blood count, erythrocyte sedimentation rate and blood cultures are drawn.
3. If possible, locally aspirate the involved area with a large bore needle. If purulent material is obtained, an immediate Gram's stain should be done and the material sent for culture and sensitivity.
4. *General Supportive Measures*
   A. If the patient is lethargic, dehydrated or appears ill, intravenous fluids should be given.
   B. If septicemia is present, anemia may be present and requires blood replacement.
   C. The limb should be placed at rest either in a plaster shell or in traction.
   D. Analgesics and good supportive nursing care
5. *Antibiotic Therapy*
   A. Since the most common causative organism is *Staphylococcus aureus,* the best antibiotic is still penicillin. With an increasing incidence of penicillin-resistant

organisms, it has been our practice to add a penicillinase-resistant antibiotic; at present we are using methicillin. When the cultures and drug sensitivities are returned in 24 to 48 hours, the drugs are changed according to this additional information

B. The intravenous route is used initially and changed to the intramuscular or oral route as clinical conditions dictate. If the patient is allergic to penicillin, other appropriate bactericidal antibiotics should be used.

C. Our usual regimen is:

*Intravenous:*

*(1)* Penicillin, 10 to 20 million units, half sodium, half potassium, every 8 to 12 hours for the average adult. The same dosage is used for a child.

*(2)* Methicillin or oxacillin, 1 gm. every 6 hours as the adult dosage; 100 mg./kg./day or higher for a child

D. Treatment is continued until all acute signs have subsided and the patient is responding well, which is usually after about 2 weeks.

E. Drug therapy is then changed to lower doses intramuscularly.

F. Prior to discharge, the patient is placed on an oral antibiotic regimen, usually only one—penicillin or dicloxacillin, which is continued for 8 to 10 weeks.

G. The patient is followed by x-ray and appropriate laboratory tests. The sedimentation rate is extremely valuable as a simple aid in assessing subsidence of infection.

6. *Local Measures*

A. When treatment is started as soon as the diagnosis is suspected, further local therapy may be unnecessary.

B. If there is continued or further swelling at the site, repeat aspiration should be performed.

C. Operative decompression is mandatory if the above is not successful; this usually consists of decompressing the medullary canal by opening a window in the involved area.

D. Drip and suction with local antibiotic irrigation should be utilized if open decompression is required.

## Prognosis

Local bone destruction, sequestrum formation, distant seeding and disturbances of the growth plate are complications encountered if the disease process is allowed to progress or treatment is not adequate. With proper early therapy, these severe complications which were seen in previous years are rarely encountered.

# ACUTE PYOGENIC ARTHRITIS

## Definition

Acute pyogenic arthritis is an acute infectious process of a synovial joint. The most common joints involved are the hip and the knee. Other joints less commonly involved are the elbow, ankle and shoulder.

## Etiology

The joint may become infected by:

1. Hematogenous spread from a distant focus

2. Direct or lymphatic spread from a nearby focus, such as osteomyelitis

3. Inoculation via a penetrating wound, with or without a foreign body

4. In infants, femoral puncture is a common cause of hip joint involvement.

## Basic Principles

1. In the early stages, the synovial membrane is involved; it becomes hyperemic, edematous and thickened and produces an increased amount of fluid. There is local infiltration with inflammatory cells. The synovial fluid is at first serous, thin and watery. If allowed to progress, the fluid becomes frankly purulent, with rapid destruction of articular cartilage by proteolytic enzymes. These enzymes are released from the polymorphonuclear leukocytes which are destroyed. This process, if allowed to progress, culminates in fibrous and bony ankylosis.

2. It should be emphasized that the diagnosis of a septic joint must be considered in the examination of every swollen joint. If this diagnosis is suspected, treatment should be instituted until a definitive diagnosis is made. Only prompt vigorous and active treatment will prevent joint destruction. Pyogenic arthritis of the hip in infants and children warrants special emphasis because of difficulty in diagnosis and the catastrophic results of delayed treatment.

3. The commonest causative organism, as in acute osteomyelitis, is *Staphylococcus aureus*. In infants, *Haemophilus influenzae* and hemolytic streptococcus are commonly seen. Other rare organisms are pneumococcus, gonococcus and *Escherichia coli.*

## Criteria for Diagnosis

1. General weakness, malaise, fever and chills

2. Gradually increasing joint swelling and pain

3. Inability to bear weight and painful joint motion

4. Physical examination discloses a swollen, erythematous joint with marked limitation of motion. The joint is held in a position in which the capsule is most lax. The hip assumes an attitude of flexion, abduction and external rotation.

5. Joint aspiration discloses infected fluid.

6. *Laboratory Diagnosis*

A. The white blood cell count is elevated with a shift to the left (usually 14,-000 to 18,000/mm.$^3$).

B. The erythrocyte sedimentation rate is elevated.

C. One may encounter a falling hemoglobin and hematocrit with prolonged sepsis.

D. *Nature of Synovial Fluid*

*(1)* The fluid does not necessarily manifest as a frankly purulent exudate. Early in the process, the fluid is cloudy, thin and less viscous than normal joint fluid. If allowed to progress, the fluid becomes thickened and purulent.

*(2)* Microscopic examination discloses a marked increase in acute inflammatory cells. Gram's stain may identify the etiologic organism.

*(3)* The lowered viscosity is easily determined by a marked diminution in the mucin clot formation.

*(4)* There is a marked increase in synovial fluid protein with a decrease in fluid sugar content. Simultaneous blood sugar glucose and joint fluid glucose disclose a differential of 20 to 30 mg.

7. *Radiographic Findings.* The most common radiographic finding is distention of the joint capsule with fluid. There may be associated soft tissue swelling and osteoporosis of the bone. In cases of septic arthritis of the hip joint, one finds separation of the joint surfaces with lateral and superior displacement of the fat lines and, frequently, frank subluxation or dislocation of the hip.

## Differential Diagnosis

1. Synovitis. In this condition there is usually a low-grade fever. The white blood cell count and erythrocyte sedimentation rate are normal and the joint fluid does not disclose many of the findings previously enumerated. The general systemic symptoms of a seriously ill patient are usually not present.

2. Rheumatic fever

3. Sympathetic effusion

4. Hemarthrosis

5. Acute inflammatory conditions such as gout, acute rheumatoid arthritis, acute osteomyelitis and tuberculosis

## Management

### Systemic

1. Intravenous fluids with antibiotics as discussed above under Acute Pyogenic Osteomyelitis

2. Blood replacement if a septic hemolytic anemia is present

## Local

1. Cast or traction immobilization of the joint
2. Aspiration decompression of the joint should be performed every 8 hours for 36 hours. If the general systemic symptoms subside and the volume of the joint aspirations markedly lessens, this is the treatment of choice. Aspiration should be continued until 3 negative aspirations are obtained. If the fluid becomes purulent and the volume increases despite aspirations, immediate incision and drainage should be performed.
3. Pyogenic arthritis of the hip joint presents a special problem. The major blood supply to the head of the femur transverses the capsule of the hip joint. With increasing distention there is obliteration of the blood supply with a superimposed aseptic necrosis upon an already infected head. Rapid destruction of the head of the femur ensues. It is imperative that accurate early diagnosis is made and treatment instituted. Immediate surgical decompression of the joint is mandatory. This is combined with drip-and-suction technique. There is no place for repeated aspiration in the treatment of septic arthritis of the hip joint. Traction of the extremity is extremely important because of the inherent danger of dislocation of the hip.
4. Septic arthritis of the shoulder joint should be treated similarly to the above.

## Complications

1. Joint fibrosis and ankylosis
2. Dislocation
3. Osteomyelitis
4. Growth plate disturbances

## OSTEOMYELITIS (CHRONIC)

### Definitions

1. *Chronic osteomyelitis,* an infection of bone of long duration, is characterized by numerous sinus tracts, sequestra (necrotic bone) and often repeated skin breakdown.

2. *Brodie's abscess* is a localized form of chronic osteomyelitis; it has a sharply delineated focus of infection, usually present only in one bone. This abscess is most often seen in the tibia. It may be from 1 to 4 cm. in diameter. Its wall is lined by chronic inflammatory granulation tissue, and, around its periphery, the spongy bone is likely to present areas of sclerosis.

### Basic Principles

The two commonest causes of chronic osteomyelitis are:
1. Transition from acute osteomyelitis cases that are either diagnosed late, when there is already bone necrosis, treated with insufficient intensity or for too short a time and thus recur, or cases which progress to the chronic stage no matter how well they are treated. This may be due to the virulence of the organism or lack of resistance of the patient.
2. Infection of bone following open fractures. The fractures may have been open primarily or may have been opened for surgical intervention.

### Criteria for Diagnosis

The diagnosis is usually self-evident if there are:
1. Draining sinuses
2. Repeated episodes of swelling
3. Discomfort over the involved bone
4. Evidence of sequestra on x-ray

### Differential Diagnosis

When the diagnosis is not clear, the following conditions must be considered:
1. Ewing's sarcoma
2. Osteogenic sarcoma
3. Osteoid-osteoma
4. Tuberculosis

### Management

The patient is no longer acutely ill; the treatment is aimed toward obliteration of a localized disease process, including eradication of sinuses and cavities, removal of necrotic bone and sequestra and achieving adequate skin coverage where necessary.

1. Appropriate cultures are taken and long-term antibiotic treatment is instituted. It should be noted, however, that antibiotics do not penetrate these usually poorly vascularized areas and the primary treatment is surgical.

2. Sinus tracts should be identified, often with the use of sinograms. Cavities and sequestra are identified, often with tomograms.

3. *Surgical Management*

A. Surgery consists of:

(1) Complete removal of all dead bone

(2) Eradication of infected cavities

(3) Excision of sinus tracts

B. If the bone is weakened, it must be protected by casting.

C. Usually this surgery is followed by drip and suction. Two or three polyethylene catheters are inserted into the operative site.

D. If sensitivities are available, appropriate antibiotics are placed in the normal saline irrigating fluid.

E. Do not use glucose because this promotes the growth of bacteria.

F. Suction is applied to keep the surrounding area comparatively dry.

G. This is continued until all cultures are negative on at least two occasions or until there is no further drainage.

4. The treatment of this phase of osteomyelitis is difficult and tedious and should not be undertaken lightly. Multiple procedures are often required.

### Prognosis

1. Recurrences are common.

2. Growth disturbances may occur. Infection may either stimulate or arrest growth in young patients with open epiphysis.

3. Deformities may result.

4. Amyloidosis is seen in a significant number of patients with osteomyelitis of long duration.

5. Carcinoma in sinus tracts has been reported.

6. Amputation of a limb is occasionally required if all treatment fails or if the complication noted above occurs.

## TENDINITIS AND BURSITIS

### Definition

Tendinitis and bursitis are non-infectious inflammatory processes involving tendons and bursae, with or without an accompanying calcium deposit.

## THE SHOULDER

### Basic Principles

1. The subacromial (subdeltoid) bursa lies between the deltoid muscle and rotator cuff and inferior to the acromion process. Bursitis usually occurs in young and middle-age people.

2. The bicipital tendon lies in the bicipital groove between the greater and lesser tuberosities.

*Subacromial Bursitis*

### Criteria for Diagnosis

Patients with acute subacromial bursitis present with:

1. Pain

2. Swelling

3. Marked limitation of shoulder motion

4. Physical examination discloses joint tenderness over the subacromial bursa and marked limitation of active and passive shoulder motion.

5. X-ray examination usually discloses a large calcific deposit over the greater tuberosity. The absence of such a deposit does not rule out the diagnosis of subacromial bursitis. The calcium deposits are found initially in the supraspinatus tendon and work their way to the surface, eventually rupturing into the bursa. While the deposit is under tension within the tendon, it irritates the overlying bursa, which exhibits a reddened, congested appearance in the area immediately overlying the deposit.

## Differential Diagnosis

1. Tears of the rotator cuff can be differentiated from acute subacromial bursitis by the injection of a local anesthetic. In tears of the rotator cuff, the first 20 degrees of shoulder abduction cannot be initiated despite the local anesthetic. In subacromial bursitis, the first 20 degrees of shoulder abduction are present after local infiltration of the supraspinatus tendon.

2. Septic arthritis of the shoulder joint and of the bursa

3. Metastasis to the upper end of the humerus

4. Cervical spondylosis with radiculitis

5. Arthritis of the acromioclavicular joint

6. Fractures of the greater tuberosity of the humerus

## Management

1. The limb should be placed at rest in a sling or Velpeau dressing until the acute symptoms have subsided. Prolonged immobilization is contraindicated, since adhesive capsulitis (frozen shoulder) rapidly develops.

2. Ice packs should be applied to the shoulder, and all forms of heat should be avoided.

3. Local infiltration of the bursa with 10 to 20 ml. of 1% Xylocaine solution and 1 to 2 ml. (10 to 20 mg.) of intra-articular hydrocortisone frequently affords immediate relief. We feel that the bursa should be punctured with a large bore needle in multiple areas.

4. Anti-inflammatory drugs, such as phenylbutazone (100 mg. q.i.d. after meals for 5 days), or oral steroids (prednisone, 5 to 40 mg. daily for 3 days and then gradual reduction over a 10-day period) are a helpful adjunct to therapy.

### *Bicipital Tendinitis*

## Basic Principles

Tenosynovitis of the biceps tendon is usally produced by trauma to the shoulder in the area of the bicipital groove or by calcific deposits in this area.

## Criteria for Diagnosis

The patient presents with:
1. Pain in the shoulder
2. Restriction of motion
3. Swelling and point tenderness over the long head of the biceps in the bicipital groove
4. Resistance to flexion and supination of the elbow reproduces the pain.

## Management

1. Temporary immobilization
2. Ice packs
3. Local infiltration into the bicipital groove and shoulder joint as described above with local anesthetic and steroid
4. Systemic anti-inflammatory drugs (as for bursitis of the shoulder)

# THE ELBOW

### *Lateral Epicondylitis of the Humerus (Tennis Elbow)*

## Basic Principles

The extensor muscles originate from the lateral epicondyle of the humerus and fan out to form the large extensor mass on the dorsolateral aspect of the forearm. The usual lesion is a partial rupture of the origin of the extensor muscles, with a secondary traumatic periostitis over the lateral epicondyle.

## Criteria for Diagnosis

1. Pain on the lateral aspect of the elbow and over the extensor surfaces of the forearm

2. Swelling and point tenderness over the lateral epicondyle of the humerus

3. Frequent complaints of pain with dorsiflexion of the wrist; inability to carry heavy objects

## Management

1. Temporary immobilization
2. Ice packs

3. Local infiltration with 10 ml. of 1% Xylocaine and 1 to 2 ml. (10 to 20 mg.) of hydrocortisone

4. Anti-inflammatory drugs are frequently helpful.

5. Surgical treatment is rarely indicated.

### *Medial Epicondylitis*

## Basic Principles

The flexor muscle mass originates from the medial epicondyle of the humerus and forms a large mass on the anterior aspect of the forearm. The lesion is usually produced by a partial tear of the flexor tendon as it originates on the medial epicondyle. There is a secondary traumatic periostitis.

## Criteria for Diagnosis

1. Pain over the medial epicondyle
2. Point tenderness over the medial epicondyle
3. Pain on forced flexion of the wrist against resistance

## Management

1. Immobilization for a short time
2. Ice packs to the involved area
3. Infiltration of the medial epicondyle with 10 ml. of 1% Xylocaine and 1 to 2 ml. (10 to 20 mg.) of hydrocortisone
4. Anti-inflammatory drugs are prescribed as an adjunct

## WRIST AND HAND

### *Acute Tenosynovitis*

## Basic Principles

The flexor carpi ulnaris tendon is laterally situated at the wrist and inserts into the pisiform. Calcium deposits within the tendon sheath frequently cause an irritative tenosynovitis.

## Criteria for Diagnosis

1. Local pain
2. Swelling
3. Limitation of wrist motion
4. Marked tenderness over the flexor carpi ulnaris tendon

## Management

1. Plaster or splint immobilization
2. Systemic anti-inflammatory drugs
3. Local infiltration with 10 ml. of 1% Xylocaine and 1 to 2 ml. of hydrocortisone is frequently helpful.

### *Stenosing Tenosynovitis*

## De Quervain's Disease

### Basic Principles

This is a chronic inflammatory process of the tendons of the abductor pollicis longus and extensor pollicis brevis, as they overlie the radial styloid process.

### Criteria for Diagnosis

1. Pain
2. Swelling
3. Tenderness over the radial styloid
4. A positive Finkelstein's test (severe pain over the radial styloid process with thumb flexion and sharp ulnar deviation of the wrist)

## Trigger Thumb and Trigger Finger

### Basic Principles

Stenosing tenosynovitis of the flexor pollicis longus at the level of the head of the first metacarpal impinges upon full tendon excursion and produces "locking" of the interphalangeal joint of the thumb. A similar process involving the flexor tendon sheaths of the other fingers (most commonly the ring finger) produces locking of the distal and proximal interphalangeal joint.

### Criteria for Diagnosis

1. Pain
2. A palpable nodule is easily felt at the distal palmar crease of the hand.
3. Tenderness is localized to the area of the nodule.
4. Locking of the distal joint

### Management

1. Local infiltration of 1 to 2 ml. (10 to

20 mg.) of hydrocortisone under local anesthesia

2. If conservative measures fail, operation is warranted, which consists of incision of the fibrous tendon sheath of the involved tendons distal to the nodule (*see* Chap. 32).

## HIP JOINT
### *Trochanteric Bursitis*

**Basic Principles**

There are two trochanteric bursae, the superficial and the deep. The deep trochanteric bursa is located behind the greater trochanter and in front of the tendinous portion of the gluteus maximus muscle. The superficial bursa is located between the greater trochanter and the skin and subcutaneous tissue.

**Criteria for Diagnosis**

1. Pain
2. Swelling
3. Tenderness over the greater trochanter. The pain may radiate to the back of the thigh, and motion of the hip joint causes discomfort.

Differential Diagnosis

1. Septic arthritis of the hip joint
2. Herniated disk
3. Osteomyelitis of the upper end of the femur
4. Tuberculous bursitis

**Management**

1. Ice packs to the hip
2. Rest
3. Anti-inflammatory medication
4. Infiltration of the area with 10 ml. of 1% Xylocaine and 2 to 3 ml. (20 to 30 mg.) of hydrocortisone
5. Analgesics for pain

### *Iliopsoas Bursitis*

**Basic Principles**

The iliopsoas bursa is located between the iliopsoas muscle and the iliopectineal eminence on the anterior surface of the hip joint capsule.

**Criteria for Diagnosis**

1. The patient presents with tenderness at about the middle of the inguinal ligament.
2. Pain, caused by pressure on the femoral nerve, may radiate down the front of the leg.

Differential Diagnosis

1. Femoral hernia
2. Iliopsoas abscess
3. Synovitis of the hip joint
4. Infectious arthritis of the hip

**Management**

Similar to that of trochanteric bursitis, above

## KNEE JOINT
### *Pes Anserine Bursitis*

**Basic Principles**

This bursa lies posterior to the tendinous insertions of the sartorius, gracilis and semitendinous tendons, on the anteromedial surface of the tibia. The bursa is directly anterior to the insertion of the medial collateral ligament.

**Criteria for Diagnosis**

1. Localized pain
2. Localized swelling
3. Tenderness over the bursa on the upper anteromedial surface of the tibia
4. Ambulation is painful and there is a pronounced limp.

**Management**

1. Immobilization with a Jordan splint if disability is severe
2. Ice packs
3. Anti-inflammatory medication such as phenylbutazone or prednisone
4. Infiltration of the area with 10 ml. of 1% Xylocaine and 1 to 2 ml. (10 to 20 mg.) of hydrocortisone

## ANKLE AND FOOT

### *Achilles Bursitis and Tendinitis*

#### Basic Principles

The retrocalcaneal bursa lies between the calcaneous and the Achilles tendon. Irritation from a tight shoe sometimes causes the formation of a bursa between the Achilles tendon and the skin (the superficial calcaneal bursa).

#### Criteria for Diagnosis

1. Pain on motion
2. Local tenderness
3. Differentiation between bursitis and tendinitis cannot be made and is unimportant in treatment.

#### Management

1. Limited activities
2. Heel lift (¼ inch)
3. Phenylbutazone, 100 mg. q.i.d. after meals for 5 days
4. If severe, inject locally with 10 ml. of 1% Xylocaine and 1 to 2 ml. (10 to 20 mg.) of intra-articular hydrocortisone.

### *Posterior Tibial Tendinitis*

#### Basic Principles

Posterior tibial tendinitis is an inflammation of the posterior tibial tendon which runs along the posteromedial aspect of the ankle, behind the medial malleolus, and inserts mainly into the tarsal navicular.

#### Criteria for Diagnosis

1. Severe tenderness along the course of the tendon
2. Pain on ambulation, often referred to the arch of the foot

#### Management

1. Immobilize the foot and ankle with strapping or an Ace bandage.
2. Ice packs to the area
3. Anti-inflammatory medication, either phenylbutazone, 100 mg. q.i.d. after meals for 5 days, or prednisone, 40 mg.

day for 3 days, and gradually reduce the dosage over a 10-day period.

### *Calcium Deposits in the Foot*

#### Criteria for Diagnosis

1. Pain and tenderness along the outer border of the foot in the area of the cuboid
2. X-rays show a calcific deposit in the area involved.

#### Management

1. Ice packs to the area
2. Injection of 10 ml. of 1% Xylocaine and 1 to 2 ml. (10 to 20 mg.) of intra-articular hydrocortisone
3. Phenylbutazone, 100 mg. q.i.d. after meals for 5 days

## TENDON AND MUSCLE RUPTURES

### Definition

Tendon and muscle ruptures are complete, or almost complete, tears of tendon or muscle fibers.

### Basic Principles

In general, a violent, forceful contraction of a muscle with resistance to the contraction will produce a rupture of its tendon or of the muscle itself.

With increasing age (usually over 40 years) there is a physiologic tendon degeneration, so that a less than violent contraction may produce tendon rupture. The most common sites for tendon and muscle rupture are:

1. Achilles tendon
2. Plantaris tendon
3. Medial head of the gastrocnemius muscle
4. Quadriceps tendon
5. Patellar tendon
6. Biceps tendon or muscle belly
7. Rotator cuff of the shoulder

## RUPTURE OF THE ACHILLES TENDON

### Basic Principles

The site of rupture is:
1. The musculotendinous junction—

usually seen in individuals under the age of 40

2. In and around the tendon insertion into the os calcis—usually seen in individuals over the age of 40

## Criteria for Diagnosis

1. History of injury
2. Gait abnormality. There is a lack of push-off and an inability to stand on the toes of the affected side.
3. A palpable gap is present at the site of the rupture.
4. The Thompson test discloses a lack of function of the Achilles tendon. The Thompson test is performed with the patient in the prone position and the knee flexed to 90 degrees. Squeezing the gastrocnemius-soleus muscle in the calf will not produce plantar flexion of the foot when the rupture is complete.

## Management

1. Treatment consists primarily of surgical repair of the ruptured tendon.
2. Cast immobilization with the ankle in equinus and the knee flexed has recently been described but has not been employed by us.

## RUPTURE OF THE PLANTARIS TENDON AND THE MEDIAL HEAD OF THE GASTROCNEMIUS TENDON

## Criteria for Diagnosis

1. History of a sudden onset of pain in the calf with the sensation of "being kicked in the calf or struck by a bullet"
2. Tenderness and ecchymosis at the musculotendinous junction
3. The Thompson test discloses full function of the Achilles tendon.

## Management

1. Heel lift on the affected side
2. Ice packs for the first 36 to 48 hours, followed by warm compresses
3. Crutches if ambulation is very painful, either for partial or complete non-weight-bearing

4. Occasionally strapping the ankle in equinus will relieve the pain.
5. Analgesics for pain

## RUPTURE OF THE QUADRICEPS TENDON AND THE PATELLAR TENDON

### Basic Principles

The site of rupture may be above or below the patella.

1. *Suprapatellar.* This is a rupture of the tendon as it inserts into the superior pole of the patella. This type of rupture is usually seen in individuals in the third and fourth decade of life.
2. *Infrapatellar Tendon*

A. Rupture at the inferior pole of the patella is seen in individuals over 40 years of age.

B. Avulsion of the tibial tubercle with the patellar tendon is seen in teen-agers.

### Criteria for Diagnosis

1. History of injury
2. Pain, swelling and ecchymosis in the region of the rupture
3. Inability to extend the knee or maintain the passively extended knee
4. Palpable gap in the region of the rupture
5. Occasionally electric stimulation of the quadriceps muscle can be used when one cannot determine whether the inability to extend the knee is due to severe pain or to a rupture of the quadriceps mechanism.

### Management

1. If full extension of the knee is present, a cylinder walking cast in extension is applied for 6 weeks.
2. Lack of, or inability to maintain, full extension requires surgical repair of the tendon.

## RUPTURE OF THE BICEPS TENDON OR MUSCLE BELLY

### Basic Principles

The site of rupture is usually found in:

1. The long head of the biceps throughout its course
2. The muscle belly
3. The tendinous insertion into the radial tuberosity at the elbow

## Criteria for Diagnosis

1. History of injury
2. Pain and swelling in the area of the rupture
3. Inability to flex and supinate the elbow against mild resistance
4. Abnormal bulge of the biceps in the arm

## Management

1. Sling and swathe immobilization
2. Analgesics for pain
3. Early motion when the patient is free of pain
4. Surgical intervention is usually unnecessary.

## RUPTURE OF THE ROTATOR CUFF OF THE SHOULDER

### Basic Principles

Rupture of the shoulder rotator cuff is usually seen in individuals over the age of 40 years.

### Criteria for Diagnosis

1. History of injury
2. Pain
3. Swelling
4. Tenderness over the lateral aspect of the shoulder
5. The first 20 degrees of abduction of the shoulder cannot be initiated against light resistance.

### Management

1. Immobilization until the pain subsides
2. Early active exercises when pain-free
3. Abduction cast and surgical intervention are rarely indicated, since results with conservative therapy are usually satisfactory.

## SLIPPED CAPITAL FEMORAL EPIPHYSIS

### Definition

A slipped capital femoral epiphysis is displacement of the upper femoral epiphysis from the neck of the femur.

### Basic Principles

Slipped capital femoral epiphysis is most often seen in children between the ages of 10 and 16 years of age. The condition is more common in males and is bilateral in 40 per cent of cases. It is frequently seen in:
1. Very tall, thin children, undergoing a rapid growth phase
2. The Fröhlich type, with underdeveloped sexual characteristics

The etiology is unknown; however, various theories implicate rapid growth, minor trauma and endocrine factors.

### Criteria for Diagnosis

1. Gradual onset of fatigue after walking, pain and stiffness about the knee and hip and a visible limp
2. Spiralling. Flexion of the hip makes the hip assume an attitude of rotation.
3. Knee pain may be the one and only presenting symptom. *Any child in the age-group of 10 to 16 presenting with knee pain should be examined for a slipped epiphysis.*
4. X-rays. Early slipping can be recognized in the lateral x-ray before it becomes apparent in the anteroposterior view. When further slipping has taken place, it becomes apparent in the anteroposterior view. The head is usually displaced posteriorly, medially and inferiorly. The epiphyseal plate is widened (epiphysiolysis) and may show evidence of cartilage necrosis by narrowing of the joint space.

### Differential Diagnosis

1. Fracture about the hip and pelvis
2. Synovitis and septic arthritis of the hip joint

3. Late-appearing septic arthritis of the hip joint

4. Rheumatoid arthritis of the hip

5. Tuberculosis of the hip

6. Avulsion of the iliopsoas tendon

## Management

1. Immediate treatment after diagnosis (or suspected diagnosis) consists of complete bed rest with Buck's extension traction with 5 pounds of weight.

2. The patient should then undergo immediate surgical treatment (usually pinning *in situ*).

3. We do not feel that treatment with cast immobilization is indicated.

## JOINT INJURIES

### Definitions

1. *Internal Derangement.* This is a term commonly used to describe affections of the knee (although it may be applied to other joints), most often traumatic in origin, which are the result of lesions of the semilunar cartilages, joint surfaces, ligaments or synovial membranes.

2. *Strain.* This refers to a stretching of the ligament without interruption of its fibers.

3. *Sprain.* A sprain is an interruption of the fibers of a ligament which is an incomplete tear. A tear is complete interruption of the ligament fibers.

4. *Avulsion of Attachment.* This is the detachment with or without a piece of bone of the ligament from its origin or insertion.

5. *Hemarthrosis.* This is the accumulation of blood within a joint.

### INJURIES OF THE KNEE JOINT

#### Basic Principles

1. Major injuries of the knee joint may involve the medial collateral ligament, lateral collateral ligament and/or cruciate ligaments or menisci. Displacements and tears of the semilunar cartilages or menisci constitute by far the most frequent cause of internal derangement of the knee joint. The medial cartilage is injured about eight times as frequently as the lateral cartilage; the reason for this is:

A. The medial cartilage is larger and bifurcated at its anterior pole.

B. The mechanism of injury which causes injury to the medial cartilage is far more common than that which affects the lateral cartilage.

C. The medial meniscus, by being attached firmly to the deep posterior fibers of the medial collateral ligament, is more likely to be split than the more mobile lateral meniscus.

2. Tears of the lateral meniscus are difficult to diagnose, since true locking rarely occurs. Curiously, tears of the lateral meniscus often cause symptoms that seem to indicate that the medial meniscus is torn, because pain and tenderness are often present on the medial side of the joint next to the patellar tendon.

3. The functional anatomy is:

A. *Medial Collateral Ligament.* The ligament is composed of 2 layers. The superficial layer originates on the femoral condyle, 2 inches superior to the medial joint line, and inserts on the tibia deep into the pes anserine bursa. The deep layer is shorter than the superficial ligament and is anchored to the margin of the medial meniscus; thus it stabilizes the medial meniscus and keeps it from becoming trapped between the femur and tibia during motion. The medial collateral ligament prevents valgus and rotatory instability of the knee joint.

B. *Fibular (Lateral) Collateral Ligament.* This ligament originates on the lateral femoral condyle, 2 inches above the lateral joint line, and inserts on the fibular head. It functions in preventing varus instability and also plays a role in rotatory stability.

C. *Anterior Cruciate Ligament.* This ligament originates on the lateral femoral condyle in the area of the intercondylar notch and inserts on the anterior tibial spine, thus taking an oblique course and inserting anterior and medial to its origin. Its major function is to prevent rotatory and anterior displacement of the tibia on the femur.

D. *Posterior Cruciate Ligament.* This ligament originates on the medial condyle in the areas of the intercondylar notch and inserts on the posterior spine. Its major function is to prevent rotatory and posterior instability of the tibia on the femur.

E. Semilunar cartilages are 2 crescentic plates of fibrocartilage which are placed on the condylar surface of the tibia. They are triangular in cross section, the wide base facing externally, the apex directed internally. Each meniscus has 2 horns which are attached to the intercondylar area of the tibia. The lateral semilunar cartilage is larger in breadth than the medial meniscus and forms an almost complete circle, the horns attaching adjacent to each other. The anterior horn is attached to the tibia just in front of the intercondylar eminence, partly beneath the anterior cruciate ligament. The posterior horn is attached directly to the posterior intercondylar eminence. The medial meniscus is semicircular and its anterior horn attaches in front of the anterior cruciate ligament. The larger posterior horn is fixed to the intercondylar area in front of the posterior cruciate and behind the posterior horn of the lateral meniscus. The outer aspect of the meniscus is attached to the posterior deep fibers of the medial collateral ligament.

4. It must be emphasized that all of the structures that stabilize the knee are important and interrelated. Therefore, proper function depends upon the normal function of the muscles and tendons, the cruciate ligaments, the collateral ligaments, the capsule and the menisci. The articular surface must be smooth and congruous. The muscles, quadriceps, hamstrings and gastrocnemius and the tendons that cross the knee are active stabilizers of the joint, so that tone and

strength must be maintained. The mechanism of injury in these structures in general is:

A. *Medial Collateral Ligament.* A valgus force applied to the lateral or posterolateral side of the knee, with the foot firmly fixed to the ground, will produce injury to the medial structures of the knee, including the medial collateral ligament, medial capsule, medial meniscus, anterior cruciate ligament and posteromedial capsule.

B. *Lateral Collateral Ligament.* A varus force applied to the medial side of the knee produces injury to the lateral collateral ligament, lateral capsule, lateral meniscus, and biceps femoris tendon and may even injure the peroneal nerve.

C. *Cruciate Ligaments.* Isolated cruciate ligament injuries are rare. They are usually associated with injuries to the other stabilizing structures of the knee. The most common combination consists of injury to the medial collateral ligament, medial meniscus and anterior cruciate ligament, frequently called "O'Donohue's Triad."

D. *Menisci.* The meniscus is torn by a rotational force incurred while the joint is partially flexed. During vigorous internal rotation of the femur on the tibia with the knee in flexion, the femur tends to force the medial meniscus posteriorly and toward the center of the joint. When the joint is suddenly extended, a longitudinal tear results, producing the classical "bucket-handle" tear. Transverse and oblique tears may also result. The meniscus may also be torn at its peripheral attachment. Vigorous external rotation of the femur on the tibia with the knee in partial flexion may injure the lateral meniscus. Because of its mobility and structure, the lateral meniscus is not susceptible to bucket-handle tears; the lateral meniscus frequently sustains incomplete transverse tears.

5. Any force exerted against the knee that exceeds the passive stabilizing element will strain the ligaments or incompletely

rupture or avulse the attachments of one or more of the major ligaments.

## Criteria for Diagnosis

1. History of injury, especially the type of injuring force

2. Physical examination of the knee joint must be carried out in a logical and systematic manner. The entire physical examination of the knee, including stress x-ray examination, may require local anesthesia to be properly carried out.

   A. *Inspection.* Determine if a visible effusion is present and whether the knee assumes an unnatural position.

   B. *Palpation.* The origins and insertions of the medial and lateral collateral ligaments must be palpated for tenderness. The medial and lateral joint lines should be palpated for areas of tenderness.

   C. *Stress Examination of the Knee*

   *(1)* A valgus stress (attempted bending of the leg laterally) to the knee joint with the knee held in 20 degrees of flexion will disclose instability of the medial collateral ligament and medial capsule.

   *(2)* A varus stress (attempted bending of the leg medially) of the knee joint with the knee held in 20 degrees of flexion will disclose instability of the lateral collateral ligament.

   *(3)* Tests for rupture of the anterior and posterior cruciate ligaments are made with the knee flexed to 90 degrees. If the anterior cruciate ligament is ruptured, the tibia can be forced to move anteriorly on the femur (anterior drawer sign). If the posterior ligament is ruptured, the tibia can be forced to move posteriorly on the femur.

3. *X-ray Diagnosis*

   A. X-ray examination in the anteroposterior plane, with a varus or valgus stress in 20 degrees of flexion, will disclose instability of the collateral ligaments of the knee with their associated capsule.

   B. When there is varus or valgus instability of the knee, roentgenograms should always be made to detect any fracture that might cause or exaggerate it. Frequently, varus instability in elderly people is caused by both fracture of the lateral tibial condyle and rupture of the medial collateral ligament.

   C. Arthrography, especially double contrast studies, is invaluable for diagnosis of ligament and cartilage disruptions that are doubtful clinically.

4. *Internal Derangement.* The syndrome caused by tears of the menisci alone may be divided into two groups, depending on whether locking of the knee is present or absent.

   A. A locked knee is one in which there is the inability to extend the knee, classically produced by a bucket-handle tear of the medial meniscus. The patient presents with:

   *(1)* History of rotational injury to the knee

   *(2)* Walking with the affected knee flexed and limping

   *(3)* Effusion with inability to extend the knee joint

   *(4)* Marked tenderness over the medial joint line with a positive McMurray and Apley test

   The McMurray sign is elicited by flexing the knee beyond 90 degrees and externally rotating the leg as far as possible; then the knee is slowly extended. As the femur passes over the tear in the meniscus, a click may be heard or felt. The lateral meniscus is checked by internally rotating the leg as far as possible and slowly extending the knee. This click, produced by the McMurray test, is caused by a posterior peripheral tear of the meniscus.

   The Apley (grinding) test is performed with the patient prone. The knee is flexed to 90 degrees and the thigh is fixed against the examining table. The foot and leg are then pulled upward to distract the joint and are then rotated to place rotational strain upon the ligaments: if the ligaments are torn, this part of the test is painful. Next, with the knee in the same position, the foot and leg are pressed downward and rotated as the joint is slowly flexed and extended. If a meniscus is torn, this part of the test is painful.

(5) The differential diagnosis of the locked knee includes:

(a) Protective muscle spasm. The hamstrings may be in spasm. This will not allow full extension of the knee.

(b) Knee joint effusion and hemarthrosis

(c) Loose bodies, including osteochondritit dessicans fragments

(d) Diseases involving the synovial membrane such as synovial chondromatosis

(e) Foreign bodies

(f) Tumors—intraarticular

B. When locking is absent, the diagnosis is more difficult.

(1) Complaint of a sensation of "giving way," usually noticed on rotary movement of the knee and often associated with a feeling of subluxation or instability of the joint

(2) There is often a difficulty in walking up and down stairs.

(3) Physical examination shows:

(a) Effusion in the joint

(b) Quadriceps atrophy

(c) Tenderness over the affected joint line

(d) Positive McMurray sign

## Management

1. *Strain*

A. Strains of the ligaments of the knee, depending upon the severity, should be treated with either:

(1) A Jordan extension splint

(2) A cylinder walking cast

B. A large hemarthrosis, which is frequently associated with trauma to the knee, should be aspirated under aseptic technique (using a large bore needle with local 1% Xylocaine).

2. *Sprain plus Ligamentous Avulsion*

A. A mild sprain with less than 10 degrees of varus or valgus instability should be treated conservatively with plaster immobilization.

B. A severe sprain or ligamentous avulsion with more than 10 degrees of instability is best treated by early operative intervention.

3. *Hemarthrosis*

A. Small accumulations of blood should be treated conservatively with ice packs initially and splinting, but not with aspiration.

B. Large accumulations of blood, which distend the joint, should be treated by aspiration with a large bore needle and a compressive dressing. An attempt should then be made to make a definitive diagnosis.

4. *Internal Derangement*

A. Locked Knee

(1) Patients with a locked knee and effusion should first be treated conservatively.

(a) The effusion should be aspirated with a large bore needle under aseptic technique.

(b) The extremity should be placed in Buck's extension traction with 5 pounds of weight.

(c) If the knee extends fully within 72 hours, a cylinder cast is applied for 4 to 6 weeks.

(d) If after 72 hours the knee remains locked, operation is indicated.

(2) With a recurrent history of locking, operation is the treatment of choice.

B. *Knee in Which Locking Is Absent*

(1) These patients are usually treated conservatively.

(2) Aspiration of any effusion that may be present

(3) Progressive resistive quadriceps exercises

(4) If symptoms and disability persist, arthrography of the knee is indicated, with arthrotomy if injury is found.

## INJURIES OF THE ANKLE JOINT

### Basic Principles

A torn ankle ligament is a serious injury,

reducing ankle stability to the same precarious state as that of a man with a broken stirrup astride a galloping horse. The ligaments most commonly injured are the laterally placed anterior talofibular, posterior talofibular, calcaneofibular and the medially situated deltoid ligament.

## Anatomy

1. The medial (deltoid) ligament is large and strong, investing the medial malleolus on three sides as it blends with the tibial periosteum. Distal to the malleolus, it spreads fan-like to insert diffusely into the talus, navicular and calcaneus.

2. The lateral ligament is weaker and more subject to injury. It is comprised of the three main fasciculi, originating jointly at the lateral malleolus and inserting separately into the talus and calcaneus.

## Mechanism of Injury

Any ligament about the ankle may be torn by a force which exerts traction in the direction of its fibers. When the ligament is strong, a fragment of bone is avulsed from the point of attachment of the ligament.

## Criteria for Diagnosis

1. *Injury to the Deltoid*
   A. History of forceful eversion
   B. Pain on the medial side of the ankle
   C. Swelling about the medial side of the ankle
   D. Marked tenderness directly below the medial malleolus

E. Physical examination may disclose instability of the joint with eversion stress.
F. X-ray examination may show soft tissue swelling or an avulsed fragment of bone. Stress films may show rocking of the talus laterally.

2. *Injury to the Lateral Ligaments*
   A. History of inversion injury over the lateral ankle joint
   B. Swelling
   C. Tenderness below the lateral malleolus, especially anterolaterally
   D. Difficulty in ambulation
   E. Ecchymosis may be present over the dorsolateral aspect of the ankle, foot and over the os calcis.
   F. X-ray examination may disclose marked soft tissue swelling or an avulsed fragment of bone. In complete tears, stress views may disclose subluxation of the talus medially in the ankle mortise. Comparison views of the unaffected ankle should be obtained to rule out individual variation and generalized ligamentous laxity.

## Management

1. Strains and incomplete tears of the ligaments may be treated conservatively by means of taping or cast immobilization.
2. Complete ruptures, in which the ankle mortise is intact or can be reduced, may be treated with plaster immobilization for 4 to 6 weeks.
3. Operation is indicated in those cases in which there is subluxation of the talus in the ankle mortise which cannot be reduced.

# 25. EXTREMITY FRACTURES

*Horace Herbsman,* M.D.
*Gerald W. Shaftan,* M.D.
*Manfreds Munters,* M.D.

## Introduction

A detailed discussion of the management of each type and variety of fracture is obviously beyond the scope of this book. Since fractures, however, represent such a large proportion of the common emergencies seen both in the adult and pediatric age-groups, this chapter will attempt to outline broad principles of management of all fractures, as well as the specific details of diagnosis and treatment of the common fractures and dislocations.

## Definitions

1. *Fracture.* This is a disruption of cortical continuity of a bone which may be complete or incomplete. An incomplete fracture does not extend across the entire bone.

2. *Closed (Simple) Fracture.* This is a fracture with no wound extending from the skin surface to the fracture site.

3. *Open (Compound) Fracture.* This is a fracture with a skin wound communicating with the fracture site or in close proximity to it.

4. *Comminuted Fracture.* This refers to a fracture with more than one fracture line, producing more than two fragments.

5. *Pathologic Fracture.* This refers to a fracture through an area of abnormal bone.

6. *Dislocation.* This is the displacement of the articular surface of one of the bones of the joint from the other.

7. *Subluxation.* This is an incomplete dislocation, in which the articular surfaces remain in partial contact.

8. *Displacement.* This refers to the shifting of normal anatomical alignment at a fracture or dislocation site. Unless otherwise stated, displacements are described as distal change to proximal fragment normality.

9. *Axial Displacement.* This is the displacement of fracture fragments perpendicular to the long axis of the bone.

10. *Rotary Displacement.* This refers to rotation of the distal fracture fragment relative to the proximal fragment around the long axis of the bone.

11. *Angular Displacement.* This refers to angulation of the fracture fragments from the normal long axis of the bone (*see* Varus and Valgus, below).

12. *Adduction.* This is the act of bringing the extremity toward the midline.

13. *Abduction.* This is the act of drawing the extremity away from the midline.

14. *Varus.* This is a deformity in which the distal extremity is toward the midline, when the proximal portion of the extremity is in normal anatomical position.

15. *Valgus.* This is a deformity in which the distal extremity is away from the midline, when the proximal part is in normal anatomical position.

## Criteria for Diagnosis

1. *History.* Fractures are produced by direct or indirect force. A tibial fracture resulting from a blow by an automobile bumper is an example of a fracture produced by direct force. Indirect force usually produces a fracture at a more distant site, such as a femoral shaft fracture resulting from a sudden body twist with the foot fixed. The history of the method of injury will often give clues to the type of fracture present. Fractures in pathologic bone frequently will be produced by minimal trauma.

2. *Clinical Signs and Symptoms of Fracture*

A. *Pain and Tenderness.* Local soft tissue injury with associated swelling and hemorrhage produces pain and tenderness at the fracture site. Any movement of the extremity will aggravate the pain by causing displacement of the bone fragments and increased local muscle spasm. If the fracture involves a joint, pain may be severe due to bleeding into the joint under tension.

B. *Swelling and Ecchymosis.* Local swelling is rapid in onset after fracture, due to hemorrhage and edema of the soft tissues surrounding the bone. Swelling may be severe enough to produce local skin blisters. Hemorrhage from the fracture will produce varying degrees of ecchymosis. The rapidity with which ecchymosis appears is dependent on the proximity of the bone to the skin surface and the extent of hemorrhage. Delayed ecchymosis may appear at an area distant from the fracture, indicating seepage along tissue planes.

C. *Deformity and Loss of Function.* Severe fractures may present obvious gross deformity and loss of normal function. Less severe fractures, especially those without displacement, will present little deformity other than the local swelling, and loss of function may be minimal. Palpation of the fracture area occasionally may detect loss of bony contour. *False point of motion* may be present due to the fracture, but this should never be tested for intentionally because of the danger of compounding and injury to major vessels and nerves.

D. *Crepitus.* Grating (crepitus) of the bony fragment ends on each other sometimes is present but should never be elicited intentionally because in producing the grating additional bony and soft tissue injury occurs.

E. *Axial Compression and Osteophony.* Compression or percussion in the long axis of the fractured bone will often result in pain at the fracture site. If a stethoscope is applied on one side of the fracture and the other side is percussed, a sound diminished in pitch and intensity will be heard compared to the same sound transmitted through an intact bone. This phenomenon is known as osteophony and occasionally can be helpful in the clinical evaluation of an extremity fracture. It is invaluable as a screening technique for mass casualties and in the unconscious patient. The upper extremities are evaluated by listening over the manubrium while the radial styloids are percussed. For the lower extremity, major fractures will be found by auscultation over the pubis while each medial malleolus is thumped.

3. *Associated Injuries.* Always check for other fractures since the severity of an obvious fracture may obscure a lesser one, either local or distant. Injury to major vessels in the fracture area will produce changes in the circulation distal to the injury, such as pallor, coldness and loss of pulses. Injury to major nerves in the fracture area will produce sensory and motor changes in the involved extremity. Always examine for and record all nerve, vascular and bony injury *before* any treatment is instituted to avoid implicating the therapy in any subsequently discovered problem.

4. *X-Ray.* Accurate diagnosis requires x-rays of the injured part. Anteroposterior and lateral films are the minimum acceptable study, and occasionally oblique or special views may be necessary. Without two-plane radiography, a fracture can easily be missed. In children, comparison views of the uninjured side also will help in fracture assessment. Poor-quality films or inadequate views are worse than no x-rays at all.

## Management

### Emergency Management

1. Control external hemorrhage.
2. Evaluate the patient for associated injuries.
3. Cover all open wounds with a clean dressing.
4. Splint all injured extremities before attempting transportation of the patient to

a hospital. Splints are meant to immobilize the part, not to reduce the fracture. Always include the joints above and below the suspected fracture in the immobilization.

## Definitive Management

1. The aim of fracture treatment is early reduction of the fracture, followed by immobilization until healing is sufficient to allow resumption of function.

2. Reduction should be performed as soon as possible after injury without waiting for swelling to subside.

3. Muscular relaxation is essential for proper reduction and usually only can be obtained by regional or general anesthesia.

4. The bone fragment that can be controlled is manipulated into alignment with the fragment that cannot be controlled. The reduction is usually carried out by reversing the forces which originally produced the fracture, but using gentle, purposeful movements.

5. Certain fractures may be treated by minimal immobilization while others will not even be effectively managed by closed means and will require open reduction and internal fixation.

6. The methods of fracture management are as follow:

A. *Minimal Immobilization.* Fractures which will heal satisfactorily without prolonged immobilization can be treated by minimal immobilization, thereby allowing earlier functional use of the injured part. Impacted humeral neck fractures and nondisplaced radial head fractures are examples of this category.

B. *Closed Reduction and Casting*

(1) This is the commonest and most desirable method of fracture management for displaced fractures. If the position of the fracture fragments is adequate without reduction but protection of the injured part is necessary, cast immobilization is provided without further manipulation.

(2) Closed reduction is performed by applying slow, steady, manual traction in the long axis of the extremity to dis-

engage the fragments and then manipulating them into proper anatomical relationship.

(3) If reduction of a displaced fracture results in a stable position of the fracture fragments, cast immobilization, including the joints above and below the fracture, will be sufficient to maintain position during the healing period.

(4) Although closed reduction and casting involve no risk of infection, careful attention must be paid to the extremity during the immediate postcasting period to ensure that the cast is not too tight. If circulatory embarrassment becomes obvious, manifested by pain, pallor, paresthesias and absent or diminished pulses, the cast and padding must be split and opened immediately.

(5) Maintenance of reduction also must be checked immediately postcasting and frequently thereafter by repeated x-ray examinations until early callus has appeared.

(6) Muscles should be exercised within the cast by isometric exercises to maintain as much muscular tone as possible.

C. *Continuous Traction*

(1) Continuous traction is a method of maintaining reduction in those fractures where comminution or obliquity of the fracture line would make maintenance of reduction difficult in a cast. It is also useful in restoring length in an overriding fracture where muscle spasm cannot be overcome by a single manipulation. Occasionally, soft tissue injury is too extensive to permit immediate casting and continuous traction is chosen as an alternative method. Continuous traction is maintained by either skin or skeletal traction.

(2) Skin traction is applied to an extremity distal to a fracture by the use of adhesive strips or moleskin plaster.

(a) Bony prominences under the adhesive strips are padded.

(b) A circular bandage is used to

secure the adhesive strips, and the lower ends of the strips are attached to a weight device.

(c) In Buck's extension, traction for the lower extremity is applied over a pulley at the end of the bed.

(d) With Russell's traction, a sling under the knee is incorporated into a pulley system with Buck's traction, providing a resultant of forces (described on p. 353, Fractures of the Shaft of the Femur).

(e) Skin traction is satisfactory for prolonged periods of time in the young, but the skin of the elderly is too fragile to tolerate skin traction and will develop blisters and ulcerations. In these cases, skeletal traction is used.

(3) Skeletal traction is more direct, with the force being applied to the distal bone fragment or to an adjacent bone.

(a) A small-caliber wire (Kirschner wire) or pin (Steinmann pin) is drilled into the bone under strict aseptic conditions using local anesthesia.

(b) A traction bow is then attached and connected to a weight system.

(c) If the extremity itself is suspended by a counterbalanced weight system, the traction is termed continuous balanced traction.

D. *External Skeletal Fixation.* Certain fractures, such as oblique fractures of the tibia, lend themselves to treatment by external skeletal fixation. After reduction, the reduced position is difficult to maintain in plaster due to the obliquity of the fracture line. Continuous sketetal traction relies on counter traction by the weight of the body, but with external skeletal fixation a wire or pin is placed proximal as well as distal to the fracture. Manual traction is then used to effect reduction and the extremity is casted, incorporating the pins into the cast. The pins are removed when callus formation is visible on x-ray and loss of position is no longer probable.

E. *Open Reduction and Internal Fixation.* Open reduction is operative ex-

posure of the fracture site and manually put back in place the fragments in proper anatomical position. Usually the reduced position is held by internal fixation with "hardware" such as screws, plates or intramedullary nails. This method of fracture management is resorted to only if closed methods are not applicable, since opening the fracture site risks the complication of infection. With some fractures, such as femoral shaft fractures, the use of the open method is a matter of choice on the part of the surgeon, but with others, such as displaced patellar fractures, where closed methods are unsuitable, open reduction is a treatment of necessity. The use of internal fixation allows early mobilization of joints and decreases the period of functional disability.

7. *Open Fractures.* The primary objective of open fracture management is prompt and thorough wound treatment in order to avoid or minimize subsequent wound infection.

A. As soon as possible after injury, the patient should be taken to the operating room.

B. Systemic antibiotics and tetanus immunization are administered as soon after injury as possible.

C. The extremity is cleansed and draped. All devitalized tissue and foreign matter should be debrided from the wound. The wound is extended as necessary to uncover all damaged deeper structures.

D. Thoroughly irrigate the wound with several liters of warm saline solution, containing 1 gram of kanamycin per liter.

E. Small crushed bone fragments should be removed and discarded. Major fragments should be cleansed but retained.

F. The fracture fragments are reduced by direct manipulation. If external methods of immobilization will maintain reduction, no internal fixation is used. Internal fixation is avoided wherever possible, because in the presence of a contaminated wound, any foreign body implant is undesirable. If maintenance of reduction *requires* internal fixation, it is better to risk the use of buried metal than to have the fragments move, producing further tissue damage and a better milieu for infection.

G. The wound is closed primarily if the delay from injury to debridement is less than 6 hours, contamination is minimal, soft tissue damage is mild and there is no tension on the wound closure. If these conditions are not present, the wound is packed open. If the wound is clean after five days, delayed primary closure can be attempted. If infection is present, healing by secondary intention should be permitted.

## FRACTURES AND DISLOCATIONS OF THE UPPER EXTREMITY

### SHOULDER GIRDLE INJURIES

*Sternoclavicular Dislocations*

**Basic Principles**

Sternoclavicular dislocations are classified according to the displacement of the medial end of the clavicle and may be anterior or, much less commonly, posterior, depending upon the mechanism of injury. The anterior displacement is usually due to a medially directed force on the point of the shoulders; posterior dislocation is secondary to a direct blow to the medial half of the clavicle. The need for management in anterior dislocations is primarily for adequate cosmesis; in posterior dislocations, reduction may be necessitated because of compression of structures in the thoracic inlet.

**Criteria for Diagnosis**

1. History of injury, and pain and tenderness at the sternoclavicular junction
2. Evident deformity of the sternoclavicular joint, with either prominence of the medial end of the clavicle in anterior dislocations or of the lateral border of the manubrium in posterior dislocations

3. Oblique x-rays are required, usually in multiple views, to determine the degree of dislocation and the precise location of the clavicular head.
4. In posterior dislocations of the clavicle, particular attention must be paid to the presence of the brachial and carotid pulse on the side of the dislocation and the presence of brachial plexus palsies.

**Management**

1. Closed reduction under general anesthesia with complete muscle relaxation may be accomplished in anterior dislocations with relative ease.
2. Posterior dislocations may also occasionally be reduced closed by bracing the shoulders, using sandbags to elevate the upper dorsal spine from the table.
3. If these maneuvers are successful, reduction can frequently be maintained with a standard or modified figure-of-eight bandage or a clavicular splint to maintain the shoulders in a brace position.
4. Open reduction should be reserved for cosmetically unacceptable anterior dislocations which fail closed reduction or posterior dislocations which produce thoracic outlet symptomatology. The maintenance of the reduction is accomplished with heavy Kirschner wires through the sternoclavicular joint.

*Caution:* the ends of the wires must be bent over into a hook, because medial migration of the wires into the mediastinum is not a rare complication even with threaded wires.

*Clavicular Fractures*

**Basic Principles**

This common injury, usually occurring in the mid third of the clavicle, is frequently seen following comparatively mild trauma in children. Typically, the lateral fragment is displaced medially and inferiorly while the medial fragment is pulled superiorly through the sternocleidomastoid attachment. Because of the proximity of the subclavian vessels and trunk of the brachial plexus, distal vascular and nerve continuity must be checked. Large hematomas in the area should suggest the possibility of subclavian vessel injury. Pneumothorax also may be a concomitant finding.

### Criteria for Diagnosis

1. History of injury, usually a fall on the outstretched hand or a direct blow to the clavicle

2. Clinical signs of fracture

3. Pain on forward or backward motion of the shoulder as well as on abduction of the arm

### Management

1. Closed management is usually undertaken without anesthesia, except for sedation or injection of the fracture hematoma with 1% Xylocaine solution.

2. Reduction is accomplished in most instances by forcing the shoulders backward (braced position), usually against the knee of the operator which is placed against the upper dorsal spine.

3. Reduction is maintained either by a standard figure-of-eight bandage wrapped snugly over padding in the axilla, with the use of commercially available clavicular splints with Velcro straps, or by a simple technique using stockinette, which has proved most useful in our experience, especially in children (Fig. 25-1).

In the technique using stockinette, a 6-foot length of 2- or 3-inch stockinette is stuffed, sausage-like, with cast padding material from both ends, leaving about 1 inch unpadded in the center. This is draped over both shoulders and the unpadded center is brought through the large lap ring. (The use of the new disposable lap rings is more comfortable for the patient and will endear the surgeon to the operating room supervisor.) The stuffed ends are then brought over the shoulder, under the axilla, under the lap ring, and through the unpadded center portion of the stockinette. Excess padding may then be removed and extra stockinette length cut off. At this point the fracture is reduced

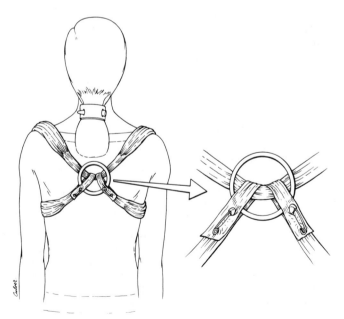

Fig. 25-1. A modified stockinette figure-of-eight bandage using a lap ring (*see* text).

by bracing the shoulders, and the two ends of stockinette are pulled down toward their respective axilla until the braced position is maintained. The stockinette edges are then pinned to each other, usually using two safety pins on each side for security. The parent or spouse is shown how to remove the safety pins from each side alternately, tighten up on the modified figure-of-eight dressing and re-pin the dressing to maintain the brace. This permits the constant snugging of a figure-of-eight bandage which, in our experience, no matter of what material it is made, rapidly loosens and ceases to provide immobilization.

4. Following the application of the figure-of-eight bandage, modified bandage or splint, the pulse must be checked with the arms at the side. If the pulse disappears when the arms are lowered to the side, the bandage must be loosened.

5. The patient or parent should be cautioned that evidence of swelling, blue discoloration or loss of sensation is cause to loosen or cut away the bandage entirely. It is better to have an unreduced fracture than a Volkmann's paralysis.

6. X-rays should be taken immediately after the application of the immobilizing bandage to ascertain that length has been restored to the clavicle. Axial reduction is of lesser importance because the fracture will heal even with 100 per cent displacement. The closer the approximation of the fragment, however, the smaller will be the residual callus which even in children usually will not remodel.

7. Repeat x-rays should be taken at one week and the immobilizing bandage should be checked at that time for adequacy.

8. Immobilization should be maintained until the fracture is clinically healed, that is, when it is no longer painful to the touch and the palpable callus is not tender. In general, this is after 2 to 3 weeks in a child, and 4 to 6 weeks in the adult.

9. After the healing is confirmed radiographically, active range-of-motion exercises may be begun to provide full shoulder abduction and forward flexion.

*Acromioclavicular Separation*

## Definitions

1. *Acromioclavicular Subluxation.* This is a tear of the acromioclavicular ligaments with an incomplete tear of the coracoclavicular ligaments, providing for separation at the acromioclavicular joint without widening of the coracoclavicular space.

2. *Acromioclavicular Dislocation.* This is a complete tear of both the acromioclavicular and coracoclavicular ligaments, permitting an upward dislocation of the entire clavicle with widening of the coracoclavicular space.

## Basic Principles

This injury is commonly seen in contact sports and is due to severe direct trauma on the shoulder forcing it downward. The downward motion of the clavicle is arrested by the first rib, and continued downward motion of the scapula and humerus produces initially a tear of the acromioclavicular ligaments and, with continued force, a complete rupture of the coracoclavicular ligaments.

## Criteria for Diagnosis

1. There is a history of direct injury to the shoulder as in a football blocking attempt.

2. There is prominence of the distal end of the clavicle, with tenderness over the acromioclavicular joint, and evident motion at the acromioclavicular joint on depressing the clavicle.

3. The patient has loss of voluntary use of the shoulder because of pain.

4. A plain upright chest x-ray, with the film placed in a horizontal position to visualize both clavicles, may be diagnostic. Stress films, that is, with the patient carrying weights (a 1-liter infusion bottle will suffice) in both hands, will provide suf-

ficient downward traction to differentiate between a simple subluxation and a complete dislocation.

## Management

1. Acromioclavicular subluxations or ligamentous strains are adequately treated with supportive slings such as a well-padded Jones bandage. An arm sling should be added to the supportive dressing.

2. Immobilization need not be carried out for more than 2 weeks, or until the patient is free of pain. Active motion at that time will prevent shoulder stiffness and eliminate many of the postinjury complications.

3. Complete acute separation may also be treated with this type of closed immobilization. In our experience, such management neither maintains permanent reduction, obviates the residual deformity, nor prevents postinjury symptomatology. Open reduction is required for good anatomical and functional results.

4. *Open Reduction*
    A. Our usual method of repair is restoration of the coracoclavicular ligament with an adjacent ligamentous structure, such as a coracohumeral ligament, and maintenance of the acromioclavicular reduction with temporary joint transfixion wires.

    B. Following open reduction, the shoulder girdle should be immobilized for 2 to 3 weeks in a modified Velpeau dressing, followed by pendulum exercises in a sling for an additional 3 weeks.

    C. At 6 weeks the wires are removed, and full active use of the shoulder is permitted after 8 weeks.

5. *Caution:* Even in patients with perfect closed or open reductions as well as those in whom reduction was never accomplished, late acromioclavicular arthritis may necessitate excision of the distal end of the clavicle at that time.

*Fractures of the Scapula*

## Basic Principles

A wide variety of scapula fractures may be seen. These are invariably due to severe direct trauma to the posterior thorax and, because of this, frequently will have associated soft tissue as well as intrathoracic injuries. Isolated fractures of the glenoid are occasionally seen following direct trauma to the shoulder.

## Criteria for Diagnosis

1. History of direct posterior shoulder injury

2. Clinical signs of fracture in the region of the scapulae. The patient also voluntarily splints his shoulder as in acromioclavicular separation.

3. Anteroposterior views of both scapulae as well as oblique views to delineate the scapula spine and the glenoid may be necessary to completely evaluate the type of fracture.

## Management

1. Since the scapula is entirely surrounded by muscle, displacement of the body of the scapula is rare. For that reason, conservative management using a supportive sling suffices until local pain and tenderness subside.

2. This usually occurs from 2 to 3 weeks, and active motion is encouraged at that time.

3. Open reduction is only of value in scapula fractures when they involve the acromial process, which may become displaced into the shoulder joint, or in transglenoid fractures. When the former obtains, the displaced acromial process fragments should be excised. Likewise, a smooth, congruous, articular surface of the glenoid may be obtained by open wiring.

*Dislocations of the Shoulder*

## Definition

Dislocation of the shoulder is an injury producing displacement of the humeral head out of its normal congruous relation to the glenoid cavity.

## Classification

1. *Anterior Dislocation.* The usual

anterior dislocation is a subcoracoid dislocation. The rarer subglenoid dislocation (luxatio erecta) is distinguished by a locking of the limb in the position of full abduction.

2. *Posterior Dislocation.* This is frequently associated with impression fracture of the humeral head.

3. *Recurrent Anterior Dislocations*

## Basic Principles

Anterior dislocations account for approximately 95 per cent of all glenohumeral dislocations. They are frequently associated with avulsion fractures of the greater tuberosity or tears of the supraspinatus tendon (rotator cuff). The avulsion fracture will generally return to anatomical position following reduction. When this does not happen, or when an injury of the rotator cuff is diagnosed when motion is started after immobilization, surgical repair is indicated.

The sooner the reduction is accomplished following the dislocation, the simpler will be the task of reduction. Within 24 hours, most reductions can be accomplished with sedation alone. General anesthesia with muscle relaxation is usually required for later attempts at reduction. Since the dislocating humeral head may injure axillary structures, the distal vascular and neurologic status of the arm, forearm and hand must be assessed *prior* to reduction.

Chronic recurrent anterior dislocations always have a history of a previous dislocation which was inadequately immobilized at the first occurrence.

## Criteria for Diagnosis

### Anterior Dislocation

1. There is a history of either a fall backward on the outstretched arm or a forcible external rotation injury with the arm abducted. In patients with recurrent dislocations, trauma may be minimal, such as reaching over the head for a book.

2. *Physical Signs*

A. There is pain and tenderness in the

affected shoulder, and the symmetry of the shoulders is disturbed, with loss of the normal rounding of the shoulder joint.

B. Occasionally a prominence will be seen inferiorly in the region of the coracoid process, especially in thin individuals.

C. Palpation will disclose an empty glenoid, with the head of the humerus palpated in the subcoracoid position.

D. The patient is unable to fully abduct his arm across his chest.

3. Anteroposterior, oblique and transthoracic lateral examinations should disclose the dislocated humeral head.

### Posterior Dislocation

1. The injury force will be a direct backward blow over the shoulder or, more usually, a violent internal rotation movement.

2. *Physical Signs*

A. The glenoid fossa is empty and the humeral head cannot be palpated anteriorly although it may be felt in the axilla.

B. External rotation is markedly limited, and the arm is generally held in an attitude of adduction and internal rotation.

3. X-ray in the ordinary anteroposterior view is often deceptive because the humeral head appears to lie in proximity to the glenoid. An oblique view will disclose the posterior dislocation, but an axillary view is necessary to diagnose the impression fracture of the humeral head which is a frequent concomitant injury.

## Management

### Anterior Dislocation

1. The simplest technique which will accomplish the reduction is the best treatment.

2. Criteria for relocation either spontaneously or by manipulation are: (1) immediate relief of pain in the affected shoulder; (2) normal contour of the affected shoulder as contrasted to the opposite side; (3) ability to internally rotate and abduct the shoulder.

*Warning:* do not attempt a full range of

motion of the shoulder, especially external rotation; otherwise, redislocation may occur.

3. Adequate sedation should be given. In our experience, intravenous muscle relaxants are ineffective.

4. *Methods of Reduction*

A. The simplest technique is that of Milch, in which the patient lies in a prone position on a firm surface, such as a stretcher, with the dislocated extremity hanging downward with 10 or 15 lbs. of weight attached to the wrist and forearm by adhesive tape. If after one-half hour in this position the shoulder does not spontaneously reduce, the surgeon, sitting on the floor, may exert continued traction downward with manual manipulation of the palpable head of the humerus to effect relocation.

B. The classical or Hippocratic maneuver (which differ in that the latter uses the unshod foot of the surgeon in the patient's axilla both for counter traction and for manipulation of the humeral head) depends on sustained traction on the outstretched and slightly abducted arm until the patient's muscle relaxation is sufficient to allow the humeral head to ride over the glenoid rim and relocate into the glenoid fossa. It requires continuous steady traction and tenacity. Slight rocking of the extremity in abduction and adduction during the maintained traction occasionally will assist in reducing the humeral head.

*Special Note:* it must be emphasized that the traction must be steadily maintained, and as the surgeon tires, so does the patient's musculature. Therefore, if steady traction is maintained for an additional five minutes after the time that the surgeon feels he no longer can exert traction, he will effect reduction.

C. The Kocher maneuver, unlike the Milch supine or classical technique, depends on leverage rather than traction alone to reduce a dislocation. As such it should be used with care and with experience, because fracture of the humeral

shaft can occur during manipulation. With the patient supine, the dislocated arm is held with the elbow flexed and steady traction is applied while the humerus is externally rotated. The externally rotated arm is then adducted and flexed at the shoulder with the elbow approaching the midline of the anterior chest. These maneuvers should nally rotated until the forearm lies against the anterior chest. These manuevers should be done slowly and smoothly without any sudden movement, and only moderate force should' be applied.

5. Clinical reduction should always be confirmed with postreduction x-rays.

6. *Immobilization.* The reduction is maintained by preventing abduction and external rotation. This can be accomplished with a standard Velpeau dressing, or with a sling which supports the elbow and forearm and a swathe around the body *and* sling preventing abduction and external rotation. The latter has the advantage of being simpler to apply and cooler than the standard Velpeau.

A third immobilizing bandage, which we favor, is the stockinette Velpeau described by Gilcrist (Fig. 25-2) which accomplishes all of the objectives of immobilization of the anterior dislocated shoulder with one single length of stockinette. It is cool, easy to keep clean and adaptable even in patients with large pendulous breasts.

7. *Duration of Immobilization.* For the elderly, a short period of immobilization for 10 to 14 days, with resumption of pendulum exercises in a sling, will lead to a satisfactory result. In the younger individual, immobilization should be maintained for a minimum period of 3 weeks to allow capsular healing.

8. Associated neurologic injuries are treated conservatively, with most falling in the realm of neurapraxias with uneventful subsequent recoveries. Vascular injuries require direct surgical repair.

9. Fracture of the greater tuberosity associated with anterior shoulder dislocations usually does not require opera-

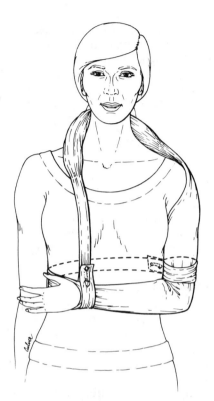

Fig. 25-2. A modified stockinette Velpeau bandage after Gilchrist's technique (Gilchrist, D. K.: A stockinette Velpeau for immobilization of the shoulder girdle. J. Bone & Joint Surg., *49A*:750, 1967)

tion, because after reduction it invariably will be almost perfectly reduced. If the tuberosity fragment does not lie in satisfactory position after shoulder relocation, open fixation is indicated.

## Posterior Dislocation

1. Posterior dislocation of the shoulder should be treated only under general anesthesia.

2. With complete relaxation, traction is exerted on the flexed elbow and the arm is slowly externally rotated while pressure is applied posteriorly to the dislocated humeral head.

3. Immobilization does not need to be done in the "football pass" position with the arm abducted at 90 degrees and externally rotated, but may be accomplished in sling and swathe or modified Velpeau dressing, as noted above.

4. Old dislocations or dislocations associated with impression fractures of the humeral head will require open reduction.

## Recurrent Anterior Dislocation

These dislocations should be reduced as soon as possible. Definitive treatment, however, almost invariably will require a surgical reconstructive procedure.

### *Rotator Cuff Injuries of the Shoulder*

## Definition

A rotator cuff injury of the shoulder is a tear of the musculotendinous insertion of the shoulder abductors, either primarily traumatic or through a degenerated and attenuated region, characterized by the inability to initiate abduction.

## Basic Principles

These injuries are frequently seen in the elderly individual and are associated with sudden trauma such as a fall on the shoulder or strenuous exertion. In younger patients, rotator cuff injuries are only seen after severe abduction-type trauma. The lesions are often overlooked or misdiagnosed because x-rays fail to reveal any bony injury.

## Criteria for Diagnosis

1. History of severe injury to the shoulder in the middle-aged or elderly patient

2. Localized pain in the subacromial area of the shoulder

3. Inability to abduct the arm against resistance

4. Occasionally, a defect may be palpated overlying the greater tuberosity, but in acute cases this is often obscured by swelling.

5. Local injection of 1% Xylocaine into the area of acute tenderness will, with relief of pain, permit motion of the shoulder.

Passive abduction to 90 degrees at the scapulohumeral joint will be maintained by deltoid pull even though active abduction was not possible.

6. Contrast arthrography of the shoulder joint will demonstrate a tear in the anterior and lateral capsule.

## Management

1. Incomplete tears, that is, when the pain is relieved by local anesthetic injection and abduction is possible, will respond to treatment with a sling and analgesics.

2. Similarly, minor complete tears which respond favorably to local anesthetic injection with the return of range of motion may also be treated with analgesics and sling immobilization together with local heat. After 10 to 14 days, pendulum exercises may be begun and active range-of-motion exercises started after 3 weeks.

3. Major tears of the rotator cuff should be surgically repaired as soon as they are diagnosed. There is little advantage in delaying operative correction.

*Fractures of the Neck of the Humerus*

## Definitions

1. *Surgical Neck.* The surgical neck of the humerus is the usual site of fracture of the upper end of the humerus and lies at the proximal end of the shaft just below the greater and lesser tuberosities.

2. *Anatomical Neck.* The anatomical neck of the humerus is an area just proximal to the greater and lesser tuberosities and distal to the articular surface of the humeral head which is a site of attachment of the capsule of the shoulder joint.

## Basic Principles

There is a wide variety of types of this common injury which usually is seen in the region of the surgical neck of the humerus, varying from a simple impacted fracture to the four-fragment fractures in which the head, shaft and both tuberosities are separated.

Fractures of the anatomical neck of the humerus are comparatively rare and are generally impacted with minimal displacement. Fracture lines occasionally will extend into the humeral head, in which case operative reduction to obtain a smooth articular surface is mandatory.

## Criteria for Diagnosis

1. History of trauma to the shoulder or to the outstretched arm

2. Clinical signs of fracture in the region of the shoulder

3. A minimum of two-plane radiography to delineate the type, degree of comminution and displacement of the fracture.

## Management

1. In cases of impaction of the anatomical neck of the humerus, immobilization with the sling and swathe or modified Velpeau bandage will suffice. Pendulum exercises may be begun within the first week.

2. Impacted fractures of the surgical neck of the humerus, even with moderate displacement, should also be treated by immobilization with early active gravity exercises.

3. With marked displacement of the fracture fragments, closed reduction under anesthesia may be attempted. If this is successful, immobilization of the humerus in a sling and swathe or Velpeau-type dressing, often with an axillary pad, will be effective in maintaining the reduction. The use of the abduction shoulder spica or the Magnuson splint, in our experience, seems to afford no better maintenance of reduction than the sling and swathe.

4. If the fragments cannot be maintained in alignment in the elderly patient, prolonged immobilization will give a less satisfactory result than marked deformity, so that in these patients one must be prepared to accept deformity or chance open reduction in order to minimize immobilization time.

5. Open reduction is mandatory when markedly displaced fractures, or markedly comminuted fractures, cannot be maintained in satisfactory alignment by closed means, especially in the younger individual. If open reduction has produced a satisfactorily stable internal fixation, the initial immobilization in a sling and swathe is discontinued within one week, and pendulum exercises in a sling are begun for the shoulder and active exercises out of the sling are begun for the wrist and elbow..

6. Fracture of the humeral neck with dislocation of the humeral head presents a therapeutic nightmare.

A. Occasionally closed reduction under general anesthesia with total muscular relaxation will permit manual manipulation of the humeral head and reduction of the dislocation while traction is maintained on the arm and forearm. If this is successful, the management of the fracture is the same as for a simple fracture of the neck of the humerus.

B. If manual reduction cannot be accomplished, open reduction is mandatory as an urgent surgical procedure under the same anesthetic used for the attempt at closed reduction. Once open reduction of the dislocation has been accomplished, if the fracture fragments lie in satisfactory anatomical alignment, internal fixation is not mandatory since immobilization should continue anyhow for at least three weeks prior to the institution of pendulum exercises.

*Fractures of the Humeral Shaft*

## Definition

Fractures of the humeral shaft are fractures of the diaphysis of the humerus extending from the neck of the humerus distally to the supracondylar area above the elbow.

## Basic Principles

Fractures of the shaft of the humerus are deceptively difficult because of the high incidence of delayed union and nonunion, malunion with rotary and angular deformity, and injury, both immediate and late secondary to callus compression, of the radial nerve. To evaluate the latter, it is essential that extension of the wrist and/or fingers at the metacarpophalangeal joints be checked repetitively before and after manipulation and during postoperative cast checks and follow-up.

Because of the necessity to immobilize the shoulder, elbow and frequently the wrist, joint stiffness, even with good anatomical reduction and healing, may end with a poor functional result.

## Criteria for Diagnosis

1. History of direct or twisting trauma to the arm
2. Signs and symptoms of fracture of the arm
3. Anteroposterior and lateral x-ray examination of the entire humerus

## Management

1. Closed treatment is preferable if satisfactory axial and rotary alignment can be maintained. In fractures with minimal displacement, immobilization against the thorax with a Velpeau dressing or a sling and swathe may provide for adequate treatment.

2. If overriding is not severe, axial alignment may be obtained and maintained by wrapping the arm snugly in an immobilizing dressing, incorporating 3 or 4 gutter splints to provide stability. Instead of gutter splints, the use of 2 sugar tongs plasters of 2- or 3-inch width, with one sugar tong arching proximally over the shoulder down to the elbow and the other arching over the bent elbow and wrapped with stretch bandage, provides some flexibility in correcting angular deformity. Support of the wrist with a "collar-and-cuff" arrangement will complete the immobilization.

3. The use of the hanging cast (a long arm cast going from the distal palmar crease to the level of the fracture site, fre-

quently with a 1- or 2-pound weight incorporated at the level of the elbow) may provide reduction for spiral or oblique fractures which override because of muscle pull. In the hanging cast, anterior or posterior angulation is corrected by shortening or lengthening the rope, fastening the loop incorporated in the wrist of the cast to a padded collar. The hanging cast requires a cooperative patient who is willing to sleep in a sitting or semi-sitting position for at least the first few weeks.

4. *Open Reduction of Humeral Shaft Fractures*

    A. Indications for open reduction are:

        *(1)* Rotary or angular deformities that cannot be corrected by closed means

        *(2)* Open fractures

        *(3)* Mid or lower third humeral fractures associated with radial nerve injury

    B. The use of compression screws and compression plates has proved superior in our experience to the loosely fitting intramedullary rod.

5. Although nonunion is not rare in humeral shaft fractures, most of these fractures heal sufficiently within 6 to 8 weeks so that the immobilization can be discontinued and active joint motion can be begun.

6. Occasionally when other injuries mandate bed rest, especially in the multiply injured patient, reduction and maintenance of immobilization may be carried out with skeletal olecranon traction in overhead Zeno fashion (Fig. 25-3). (*See* Supracondylar Fracture of the Humerus, p. 339.)

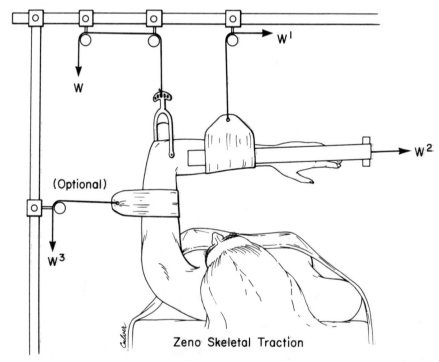

Fig. 25-3. Zeno skeletal traction. Primary traction (W) is applied through a Kirschner wire through the olecranon. The forearm is supported by a sling (W¹) and the direction of forearm rotation is controlled by forearm skin traction (W²). Counter traction with an arm sling (W³) may be necessary for supracondylar fractures.

## ELBOW INJURIES

*Supracondylar Fractures of the Humerus*

### Classification

1. *Extension Type.* This type of fracture is produced by a fall on the extended elbow, with the fracture fragment displaced posteriorly and the fracture line running from posterior proximally down to anterior distally. This comprises over 98 per cent of the supracondylar fractures.

2. *Flexion Type.* This type of fracture is produced by a fall on the flexed elbow, with the distal fragment displaced anteriorly and the fracture line running from anterior proximally to posterior distally.

### Basic Principles

These fractures, which are most common in children, are frequently associated with significant soft tissue damage. The restoration of anatomical alignment and the prevention of valgus, varus or rotational displacement of the distal fragment are necessary for a good functional result. If axial alignment is proper, anterior or posterior displacement, especially in children, will have less functional significance. The firm encircling superficial fascial covering of the elbow joint anteriorly permits little room for hemorrhage or swelling. Compression of the vascular structures passing under the fascial envelope, especially when the fracture fragments remain displaced, may lead to Volkmann's ischemic paralysis (*see* Chapter 31). The prevention of this tragedy depends upon early fracture reduction and careful observation, with emergency fasciotomy for release of antecubital compression if there is diminution or absence of pulse, power of the fingers or loss of voluntary motion or sensation.

### Criteria for Diagnosis

1. History of a fall on the outstretched arm or elbow
2. Signs and symptoms of fracture

3. Thorough evaluation of the presence of the distal radial *and* ulnar pulses and sensation and motor function in the hand
4. Anteroposterior and lateral films of the lower humerus. *Note:* it is essential for adequate evaluation that there be a true lateral view of the distal humerus, not an oblique view. An anteroposterior film of the distal humerus may be difficult to obtain in an elbow that is splinted in a right-angle position but this also is needed for fracture assessment.

### Management

#### Extension-Type Fractures

1. In undisplaced fractures, immobilization with a posterior molded plaster with the elbow at greater than 90 degrees of flexion will suffice. The posterior mold is held in place by stretch gauze above and below the elbow, excluding the antecubital space and with a window at the wrist for palpation of the pulse.

2. In displaced fractures, closed reduction is always performed under general anesthesia.

   A. With complete muscle relaxation, counter traction is exerted both cephalad and posteriorly on the arm at the level of the axilla.

   B. Traction is exerted on the forearm and the forearm is flexed while being pulled forward and the distal humeral fragment manipulated into position with the thumbs.

   C. Elbow flexion should be at as acute an angle as swelling will permit.

   D. The forearm is then forcibly pronated to lock the reduced fragments into position.

   E. Temporary immobilization to permit anteroposterior and lateral x-rays to check reduction can be accomplished with the use of a figure-of-eight bandage between the arm and forearm (Moorehead dressing).

   F. If reduction is adequate and the radial and ulnar pulses are present, a posterior molded plaster, as described above, is substituted for the Moorehead dressing.

G. If the pulse is absent, the elbow is extended 5 degrees beyond that point at which the pulse returns and immobilized either with a Moorehead dressing or posterior molded plaster.

H. X-rays must be taken after the application of the definitive immobilization.

I. If the immobilization is at an angle greater than 90 degrees, it is probable that the reduction will not be stable; therefore, progressively increase the angle of flexion each day as the swelling decreases until an acute angle of 65 to 45 degrees is reached.

J. Check radiographs must be done during this period and before discharge of the patient from the hospital to assure the maintenance of the reduction.

K. *Caution:* the severe crippling of Volkmann's paralysis demands that the nurses during hospitalization, and the parents or patient after hospital discharge, be aware that any loss of pulse, numbness of the hand or fingers, pallor, coldness or inability to move the fingers is a surgical emergency demanding the immediate release of the immobilization and extension until circulation and function return. *The loss of fracture reduction and malunion can be corrected subsequently; Volkmann's ischemic necrosis is a permanent disability.*

3. When swelling prevents the reduction of the fracture fragments without loss of radial pulse, the use of Dunlop-type traction frequently will permit maintenance of fracture position until the swelling subsides.

A. Dunlop traction (Fig. 25-4) is accomplished through adhesive traction

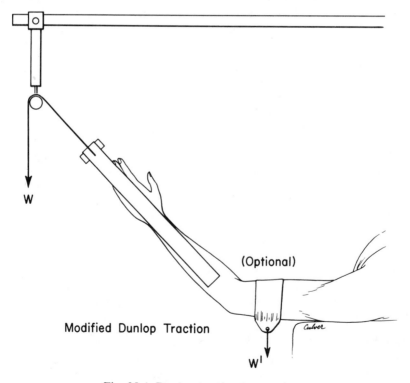

Modified Dunlop Traction

W

(Optional)

W¹

Fig. 25-4. Dunlop traction (*see* text).

applied to the forearm to the level of the wrist, with the traction force applied through a side frame so that the elbow is kept at about 135 degrees of extension.

B. Occasionally the use of a sling over the proximal arm, with a weight providing counter traction downward on the proximal fragment, is necessary to maintain reduction. It is advantageous if the use of this proximal counter traction be deferred until substantial swelling of the antecubital area has subsided so that the sling will not add to proximal venous obstruction.

C. If reduction in Dunlop's traction is satisfactory, it should be maintained for 10 to 21 days, at which time elbow flexion and a posterior molded plaster can be used to continue the immobilization.

4. Severe swelling requires the use of Zeno-type traction (Fig. 25-3).

A. The pull is directed overhead through a Kirschner wire inserted into the olecranon.

B. In this type of traction, the body weight acts as counter traction.

C. A sling is added over the forearm to support the forearm and maintain the proper angle at the elbow while adhesive traction applied to the forearm and directed laterally adjusts the rotation of the distal fragment relative to the proximal arm.

D. Occasionally a counter traction sling on the arm may be required as in the Dunlop's traction, with lateral pull on the proximal humerus to effect reduction of the fracture fragment. This sling, however, should not be used until there has been marked subsidence of swelling, as in the Dunlop's traction.

5. Open reduction, especially in children, is rarely necessary. Most supracondylar fractures can be adequately managed by closed manipulation or traction. However, the failure to achieve proper anatomical alignment or the inability of the patient to tolerate prolonged bed rest may make open reduction the treatment of choice.

A. Percutaneous pinning under image intensification can obviate the need for traction and markedly reduce the incidence of Volkmann's paralysis.

B. Another advantage of stable internal fixation is the ability to begin elbow and shoulder motion early with the diminution of late joint stiffness.

C. Internal fixation with crossed intramedullary pins or posteriorly applied plates and screws usually provides a very satisfactory means of fixation.

## Flexion-Type Fractures

Theoretically, flexion-type supracondylar fractures may be stabilized by reduction and maintenance of the elbow in extension. From a practical viewpoint, this is difficult. If after reduction moderate extension will not maintain reduction, Zeno traction or open reduction is preferable.

### *Single Condylar and T or Y Fractures*

### Basic Principles

It is essential that the congruity of the distal condylar surfaces be restored to minimize traumatic arthritis. Additionally, it is helpful if relatively stable immobilization is obtained so that early motion can reduce postfracture joint stiffness.

### Criteria for Diagnosis

As above for Supracondylar Fractures of the Humerus.

### Management

1. Closed reduction of single condylar fractures in adults and T or Y fractures may be attempted; with marked displacement they are rarely successful.

2. Zeno traction may be effective when open reduction is contraindicated.

3. Single condylar fractures in children and fractures in adults that cannot be accurately reduced closed require open reduction with transcondylar fixation as well as fixation to the proximal shaft if there is a T or Y component. Postoperative

motion should be started within 3 weeks to provide optimal return of joint function.

4. As with ordinary supracondylar fractures, Volkmann's ischemic paralysis must be anticipated in order to prevent this crippling disability.

*Epicondylar Fractures*

## Basic Principles

Fractures of the lateral epicondyle are rare. Fractures of the medial epicondyle are more commonly seen due to avulsion injury produced by sudden extension of the flexed wrist and fingers pulling off the insertion of the volar flexor muscles.

## Criteria for Diagnosis

1. History of a fall on the hand with the wrist in neutral position and the elbow flexed
2. Signs and symptoms of fracture at the ulnar side of the elbow
3. Anteroposterior and lateral views of both elbows to ensure that the apparent fracture line is not an ununited epiphysis

## Management

1. Undisplaced epicondylar fractures require protection with a posterior molded plaster for approximately 3 weeks.
2. If the medial epicondyle is minimally displaced (still above the joint line), similar conservative treatment will suffice.
3. Epicondylar fractures at the joint level or with the fragment in the joint, as well as those with ulnar nerve sensory and motor deficits, require open reduction and fixation of the fracture fragment. Transposition of the ulnar nerve anterior to the medial epicondyle is sometimes advisable if there is a fracture line running through the ulnar nerve groove posterior to the medial epicondyle. After open reduction, motion may be begun in from 10 to 21 days, depending upon security of fixation.

*Elbow Dislocations*

## Basic Principles

Dislocations of the radius and ulna on the humerus are always posterior except when there is an associated fracture of the olecranon, which will permit anterior, medial or lateral displacement of the distal fragment. Reduction of the dislocation should be accomplished as soon as possible. Evaluation of the distal extremity following reduction must be done for evidence of median, ulnar or radial nerve damage.

## Criteria for Diagnosis

1. History of a fall on the hand with the elbow extended or slightly flexed
2. Signs and symptoms of fracture. A characteristic deformity with the olecranon usually palpable posteriorly will be seen if there is not massive swelling about the elbow.
3. Anteroposterior and true lateral views of the elbow are necessary, not only to confirm the dislocation, but to evaluate the presence of associated fractures (radial head, coronoid process of the ulna, medial epicondyle of the humerus).

## Management

1. Closed reduction under general anesthesia is accomplished by applying traction to the flexed forearm while counter traction is maintained on the humerus and it is pulled posteriorly. If relaxation is complete, this can be accomplished with ease and the dislocation reduced almost without recognizing the relocation.
2. *Caution:* attempts at levering the humerus back into the olecranon concavity without adequate relaxation can produce fracture of the coronoid process or of the radial head where none existed before reduction.
3. If reduction is assured, a posterior molded plaster may be applied before postreduction x-rays are obtained. A true lateral film is mandatory. If there is a question of reduction, x-rays may be taken before the plaster is applied but they must be repeated after the application of immobilization.

4. Immobilization in the posterior molded plaster should be with the elbow flexed at least 90 degrees if swelling permits. (*See* Supracondylar Fractures of the Humerus, above.) If this cannot be accomplished initially, the posterior mold must be replaced repeatedly until the patient can maintain the radial pulse with at least 90 degrees of flexion of the elbow.

5. Repeat x-rays must be taken after each change of plaster.

6. Immobilization is continued for 3 weeks, with active motion of the shoulder, wrist and fingers during this time. A "collar-and-cuff" support is preferable to the use of the sling.

7. After 3 weeks the immobilization may be discontinued and gentle active motion encouraged.

8. Anterior, medial and lateral dislocations of the elbow are always associated with humeral or olecranon fractures and usually require open reduction for restoration of a congruous elbow joint.

### *Fractures of the Olecranon*

## Basic Principles

Olecranon fractures are a common injury resulting from either a sudden pull on the triceps tendon or direct trauma such as a fall on the point of the elbow. The fracture may vary from a simple small avulsion fragment to a comminuted fracture essentially involving the whole ulnar articular surface. As a principle of management, treatment is directed toward restoring the triceps' integrity and a smooth congruous joint for the trochlear of the humerus.

## Criteria for Diagnosis

1. Fall on the hand with the elbow semiflexed or direct trauma to the olecranon

2. Signs and symptoms of fracture about the posterior elbow

3. Anteroposterior and true lateral views of the elbow joint to ascertain the extent of injury and the presence of associated fractures

## Management

1. Essentially undisplaced olecranon fractures not involving a major portion of the articular surface of the olecranon may be treated by immobilization with a posterior molded plaster with the elbow at 90-degree flexion.

2. Displaced simple olecranon fractures or slightly separated fractures involving the major articular surface require open reduction and fixation. This is most easily accomplished using two parallel intramedullary Kirschner wires and a figure-of-eight posterior tension wire after the technique of the ASIF group.

3. Alternately, small avulsion fragments which will not affect the stability of the elbow joint may be excised with direct bone-to-tendon reconstruction, using wire sutures.

4. Markedly comminuted olecranon fractures represent a therapeutic jigsaw puzzle that is frequently best handled by interfragmentary fixation and the use of a posterior plate.

5. Open reduction is protected with a posterior molded plaster with the elbow at 90 degrees of flexion for 10 to 21 days.

6. At the end of this time, depending upon the type of repair and the security of fixation, active nonresistive motion may be begun.

### *Fractures of the Radial Head*

## Basic Principles

Fractures of the radial head are quite common following injury to the elbow or a fall on the outstretched hand. Three degrees of severity are distinguished: (1) *first degree,* a fracture of the head or neck of the radius, which is essentially undisplaced; (2) *second degree,* a fracture of the head of the radius with comminution and displacement of the fracture fragments which do not, under adequate anesthesia, block elbow flexion or extension or wrist pronation or supination; (3) *third degree,* comminuted and displaced fractures of the radial head in which the fragments of the radial head block elbow function.

Since the principle of management of these fractures is the restoration of full pronation and supination, as well as flexion and extension of the elbow, in general the first two classes of fracture will respond well to early active motion without operation.

## Criteria for Diagnosis

1. History of a fall on the hand with the elbow extended, with or without concomitant dislocation of the elbow

2. Signs and symptoms of fracture about the elbow, especially on pronation and supination

3. Anteroposterior and lateral views of the elbow and proximal forearm. Anteroposterior views of the radial head with the hand both in pronation and supination will often be required to see small rim fractures.

## Management

1. In first- and second-degree fractures, immobilization of the elbow in a well-fitting cloth sling is usually sufficient to permit early pronation and supination and flexion, as pain permits.

2. At the end of 7 to 10 days, the patient should be encouraged to remove the arm from the sling and begin extension as well as flexion exercises. The sling may be discarded after 21 days.

3. When the radial head fracture is associated with elbow dislocation, a posterior molded plaster with 90 degrees of elbow flexion is needed for 3 weeks before flexion–extension may be started. Pronation–supination exercises should be encouraged during this time.

4. Immediate operative excision of the radial head should be done whenever there are fragments blocking elbow motion or when there are associated fractures of the lateral condyle or of the proximal articular surface of the olecranon. Following excision of the radial head, sling immobilization with early active motion is essential.

# FRACTURES OF THE FOREARM
*Fractures of the Shaft of the Radius and Ulna*

## Basic Principles

Rotary as well as axial alignment is essential in the reduction of injuries to both bones of the forearm. Because of the powerful rotators of these bones, particularly the supinators, the following are essential for rotary realignment: (1) in fractures of the proximal one third of the radius or of both bones, the reduction must be maintained in supination; (2) for fractures of the mid third of these bones, a mid position between pronation and supination will provide proper alignment; (3) in the distal third, full pronation usually will give the most satisfactory anatomical alignment.

Angular deformity will similarly impair function by preventing rotation of the radius around the ulna.

Cross union is a complication rarely seen except following open fractures or open reduction. It is this complication that "must give us pause," and "makes us rather bear those ills we have than flee to others that we know not of." Were it not for the fear of cross union, open reduction with its simplicity and ability for early return of function would be the treatment of choice for many, if not most, forearm shaft fractures.

## Criteria for Diagnosis

1. History of forearm injury, usually direct trauma. Occasionally forced pronation or supination will produce spiral fractures of one or both bones.

2. Signs and symptoms of fracture in the forearm

3. Anteroposterior and lateral x-rays of the forearm, including the elbow and the wrist for complete delineation of any associated fracture or dislocation

## Management

1. Undisplaced fractures of one or both

forearm bones should be studiously treated *without* manipulation by simple immobilization in a snug, well-fitted, long arm plaster cast extending distally to the metacarpophalangeal crease of the palm and molded into the palm to prevent pronation and supination.

2. Displaced fractures must be treated under general anesthesia or a regional block anesthesia which produces complete relaxation of the forearm musculature. Such relaxation will permit distraction of the fracture fragments to obtain at least partial end-on apposition. Frequently, if one bone is reduced it can be used as a fulcrum on which the other bone may be levered into position, with rotation controlled by pronating or supinating the distal wrist as noted above.

3. Postreduction films after the application of immobilization must confirm the maintenance of the reduction, and check radiographs should be done at 48 and 96 hours, especially if swelling was present at the time of initial cast application.

4. The extremity should be elevated, preferably from an I.V. pole, for the first 24 hours postreduction. Splitting of the cast should *only* be done if swelling of the hand does not remit after 6 hours of adequate elevation, because loss of reduction is a frequent concomitant of loosened external immobilization.

5. If closed reduction is inadequate after at least two attempts under satisfactory muscle-relaxant anesthesia, open reduction and internal fixation are indicated. We prefer compression plate fixation for at least one of the two bones because it permits early functional rehabilitation.

6. Following open reduction, immobilization in the long arm plaster frequently is necessary for 10 to 28 days, depending upon the stability of the fixation. The external immobilization should be discarded as soon as it is prudent to permit exercise of the elbow, wrist and rotary joints of the forearm.

## Monteggia and Galeazzi Fracture Dislocations

### Definitions

1. *Monteggia Fracture Dislocation.* This is a fracture of the ulna with a dislocation of the intact proximal radius out of the elbow joint. Forward dislocation of the radial head is the common injury, while posterior dislocation is often referred to as a "reverse Monteggia."

2. *Galeazzi Fracture Dislocation.* This is a fracture of the shaft of the radius, with disruption of the distal radial-ulnar joint and subluxation of the distal ulna.

### Basic Principles

Both of these fractures are due to direct force. The true extent of the injury often is not suspected because the elbow and/or wrist is not included in the original film, and closed reduction of the fracture of the radius or the ulna usually will not suffice to maintain the dislocation.

### Criteria for Diagnosis

1. Direct injury to one aspect of the forearm (cf., "parry fracture")
2. Signs and symptoms of fracture of the forearm and pain in the elbow or wrist respectively
3. Anteroposterior and true lateral views of the forearm. Separate lateral views of the elbow or wrist may be required for a more accurate appraisal of the dislocation.

### Management

1. Closed reduction occasionally is effective in the treatment of the anterior Monteggia fracture in children. If the reduction is satisfactory with complete reduction of the radial head against the capitellum, immobilization in mid pronation–supination in a long arm cast will yield a satisfactory result.

2. Most adult Monteggia fractures, especially the posterior type, require open reduction of the dislocated radial head,

repair of the orbicular ligament and compression plating of the ulnar fracture.

3. In all Galeazzi fractures, open reduction with compression plating of the radial fracture is mandatory. This will stabilize the subluxation-dislocation of the distal ulna and usually obviates the necessity for ligamentous repair at the distal joint.

4. Both fractures, following open reduction, require immobilization in a long arm plaster cast for 3 to 6 weeks, depending upon the stability of the internal fixation.

### *Fractures of the Distal Radius— Colles' Fracture*

### Definition

Colles' fracture is a fracture through the cancellous portion of the distal radius, with the distal fragment commonly exhibiting:
1. Dorsal displacement
2. Dorsal angulation
3. Impaction and radial shortening (hence radial deviation of the hand).

There may be an associated fracture of the ulnar styloid.

### Basic Principles

These fractures are more common in the elderly and result from a fall on the outstretched hand. In the child, a similar fall results in a fracture of the distal radius, not through the cancellous portion of the bone, or a fracture through the distal radial epiphysis.

The normal anatomical relationships of the wrist on lateral x-ray projection show a volar tilt of the distal articular surface of 10 to 15 degrees. On anteroposterior projection, the distal radius will have normal median facing of 27 degrees or a radial-ulnar styloid angle of approximately 15 degrees. In the normal wrist, therefore, the radial styloid should be 1 cm. distal to the ulnar styloid.

Radial length is the most important deformity to be corrected, followed by dorsal displacement and then dorsal angulation. While tremendous stress is often placed by the novice in restoring the volar tilt of the articular radial face, late disability results from pain due to the stretch of the radial-ulnar triangular ligament. Shortening of the radius, therefore, should be corrected in all but the extremely elderly patient.

### Criteria for Diagnosis

1. History of a fall on the outstretched dorsiflexed hand
2. Signs and symptoms of fracture with the characteristic silver fork deformity (*Note:* since this name is of European origin, it refers to a fork placed with the tines down and the hump of the fork up.)
3. X-rays of the wrist and the forearm in anteroposterior and lateral projections. Since injuries of the carpal bones are also seen with this history of injury, good visualization of the wrist is imperative.

### Management

1. An undisplaced Colles' fracture needs immobilization in a long arm plaster cast or in a snug-fitting sugar tongs plaster for 4 to 6 weeks. The sugar tongs plaster is especially favored because it: (1) permits slight expansion with swelling; (2) enables the snugging of the immobilizing bandage with reduction in swelling; (3) allows some motion at the elbow, while preventing pronation and supination; and (4) is easy to remove without fear of injuring aged skin.

2. Displaced and comminuted fractures require closed reduction under adequate anesthesia.

A. General anesthesia or regional block anesthesia permits the best attempt at reduction because the forearm musculature is completely relaxed and traction reduction of the fragments is possible

B. The injection of local anesthetic into the fracture hematoma will obviate local pain and will suffice for minor fracture displacements that require manipulation. However, distraction of the fracture fragment is difficult because of forearm muscular spasm.

C. The use of a narcotic and Valium intravenously has occasionally been effective but is potentially dangerous and still does not provide the total muscular relaxation needed for difficult reductions.

3. After adequate relaxation and anesthesia are obtained, traction is applied to the hand, especially to the thumb, with counter traction to the arm above the flexed elbow. Frequently, the fragments must be disimpacted so that the deformity may be increased even though this produces additional bony injury. With adequate traction, the disimpacted fragments may then be pressed into axial alignment and proper angular facing. Ulnar deviation should restore radial length.

4. If radial shortening is prominent, immobilization must be carried out with the wrist in neutral position and forcibly ulnar deviated. If shortening is not a major component of the fracture, volar flexion of the wrist in mid-deviation may serve to maintain the volar angulation of the articular surface.

The surgeon must choose the deformity that he most wishes to correct, since the combination of volar flexion and ulnar deviation serves to correct neither of the above deformities, since it relaxes all tension on the ligaments and tendons which otherwise would maintain the fragment in desired position.

Successful maintenance of the fracture reduction depends upon a snug-fitting forearm plaster cast with minimal or no padding, well molded around the carpus and base of the metacarpals and into the palm. The cast must obviate pronation or supination either by completion as a long arm cast or by a U-shaped extension around the elbow, but it must not prevent full 90-degree flexion at the metacarpophalangeal joints by extending beyond the distal palmar crease.

5. Postreduction x-rays must be taken after the plaster immobilization has been completed, after 48 hours and weekly at one, two and three weeks.

6. In elderly patients, rigid immobilization is discontinued after three weeks in favor of a volar plaster splint that is removed periodically by the patient for exercise of the wrist and hand and then replaced for protection of the early healing fracture.

7. Most of the patients will tolerate 6 to 8 weeks of immobilization until solid union of the distal fracture has been accomplished. In those patients in whom forced volar flexion of the wrist was used to maintain the fracture fragments initially, the cast should be changed at three weeks and the wrist brought to a more neutral position.

8. Open reduction and internal fixation have been of little value in our experience because of the marked comminution of the cancellous bone and the small size of the distal fragment to be transfixed.

9. The use of a Kirschner wire for skeletal traction, placed either through the distal portion of the thumb metacarpal or through the necks of the second and third metacarpals, may be advantageous in maintaining radial length, especially in a markedly swollen wrist. This traction initially can be dynamically balanced with weights overhead and later (sometimes after manipulation while in traction with analgesia) incorporated in a long arm plaster cast maintaining the reduction achieved. Again, immobilization should continue for 6 to 8 weeks, although the Kirschner wire usually can be removed at the end of 4 weeks.

*Fractures of the Distal Radius—*
*Smith's Fracture*

## Definition

A Smith's fracture is a fracture of the radius through its cancellous portion with volar displacement of the distal fragment.

## Basic Principles

This fracture is essentially the opposite of a Colles' fracture and results from a fall on the volar flexed hand. Frequently there is disruption of the articular surface of the distal radius.

## Criteria for Diagnosis

1. History of a fall on the volar flexed hand
2. Signs and symptoms of fracture about the wrist
3. Anteroposterior and lateral x-rays of the wrist

## Management

1. Closed reduction is usually successful in reducing the fracture fragments, especially if satisfactory muscle relaxation has been accomplished by general or regional block anesthesia.
2. The technique of reduction involves initial increase in volar flexion deformity, followed by dorsiflexion with immobilization of the wrist in the dorsiflexed "cock-up" position.
3. Occasionally these fractures are unstable and open reduction has been recommended but, as noted above, is difficult to accomplish.
4. Immobilization time is 6 to 8 weeks but may be shortened to 3 weeks in the elderly, as noted with the Colles' fracture, above.
5. Active use of the fingers and elevation of the injured extremity at night are advantageous in reducing the postfracture morbidity.

### FRACTURES OF THE CARPUS AND HAND

*See* Chapter 31.

## FRACTURES AND DISLOCATIONS OF THE PELVIS AND LOWER EXTREMITY

### PELVIC FRACTURES

## Definition

The pelvic ring is a rigid structure composed of the two innominate bones connected anteriorly by the symphysis pubis and posteriorly by the sacrum. The expansive aspect of each half of the pelvis, the ilium, is connected to the sacrum at the sacro-iliac joint. The inferoposterior portion of the pelvis (ischium) and the inferoanterior portion (pubis) comprise the remainder of each half of the pelvic ring. All three bones on each side contribute to the formation of the acetabulum, which houses the head of the femur. The inferior and superior rami of the pubis surround the obturator foramen on each side.

## Basic Principles

Pelvic fractures are usually sustained by application of a violent force, such as occurs in automobile accidents and falls from a height. If the basic integrity of the pelvic ring is undisturbed, as in isolated fractures of a ramus or iliac wing, the stability of the pelvis remains intact. Fractures through both the anterior and posterior portions of the pelvic ring allow the pelvis to open like a clam shell. In addition, proximal displacement of the fractured hemipelvis produces shortening of the involved lower limb.

Visceral injuries are frequent with pelvic fractures and must be suspected. Injuries to the bladder and urethra are common but other intra-abdominal organs also may be affected. Retroperitoneal hemorrhage from disruption of major vessels is an occasional serious complication.

## Criteria for Diagnosis

### Clinical

1. Initial diagnostic studies should be aimed at determining the extent of pelvic fractures and the presence of any associated visceral injuries.
2. Integrity of the pelvic ring can be tested by compression of the pelvis between one hand of the examiner anteriorly over the symphysis pubis and the other hand behind the sacrum. Additionally, compression of the iliac ala between both hands and attempt at separation of the innominate bones by lateral pressure on the pelvic rim will help to

assess pubic or sacro-iliac separations. In the absence of pain with these three maneuvers, pelvic fracture is unlikely.

## Laboratory

Urine must be examined for the presence of blood. If necessary, catheterize the patient. If bloody urine is present, a cystourethrogram is indicated to rule out bladder perforation.

## X-ray

1. X-ray of the pelvis in one plane (anteroposterior) is sufficient to identify most fractures of clinical significance.
2. Acetabular fractures, associated with hip dislocation, may require several views for accurate detection.

## Management

1. Attention is directed primarily in the immediate postinjury period to any visceral injuries associated with the pelvic fracture.
2. Following this, most undisplaced pelvic fractures are treated by bed rest for 2 to 3 weeks, followed by progressive ambulation on crutches until full weight bearing is achieved at 6 weeks.
3. Displaced fractures resulting from fractures through both rami on one side and either an ipsilateral sacro-iliac dislocation or an ipsilateral fracture of the wing of the ilium should be reduced initially. Displacement will be either medial or lateral, as well as superior.

   A. Reduction of lateral displacement can be accomplished by a pelvic sling which compresses the "open clam shell" back to normal position. Reduction can sometimes also be effected by placing the patient on the uninjured side, using the weight of the body to compress the pelvis back into position.

   B. Superior displacement is treated initially by strong skeletal traction through the distal femur or tibial tubercle of the injured side. If after 12 hours reduction has not been accomplished, manipulative closed reduction under anesthesia is indicated,

followed by maintenance of reduction with skeletal traction.

C. Medial displacement requires manipulative reduction under anesthesia, followed by traction, either skin or skeletal, for maintenance of reduction, and bed rest in the supine position.

D. Combinations of traction and pelvic sling may be necessary for superiorly and laterally displaced fractures.

E. After reduction, 6 weeks of immobilization are necessary before ambulation can be instituted.

## DISLOCATIONS OF THE HIP

### Basic Principles

Dislocations of the hip may be posterior, anterior or central.

1. Posterior dislocations are the most common and usually result from a strong force exerted on the flexed thigh, as for example when the crossed knee hits the dashboard in an automobile collision. The femoral head comes to rest above and posterior to the acetabulum. Frequently, a portion of the posterior lip of the acetabulum is fractured as the head is forced posteriorly.
2. Anterior dislocations are rare and usually result from a posterior blow on an abducted and externally rotated thigh. The femoral head is forced through the anterior capsule and comes to rest in the obturator foramen.
3. Central dislocation is the result of a severe force applied to the greater trochanter or the abducted thigh, driving the femoral head through the acetabulum into the pelvis.

### Criteria for Diagnosis

#### Clinical

1. The leg with a posteriorly dislocated hip usually appears flexed, adducted and internally rotated. In most cases the femoral head is sitting above the acetabulum, and the extremity is shortened. The knee on the affected side is usually resting on the opposite thigh.

2. With the anteriorly dislocated hip, the lower extremity usually appears extended, abducted and externally rotated. Since the femoral head is resting on the obturator foramen which is below the level of the acetabulum, the leg appears lengthened.

3. The centrally dislocated hip produces leg shortening due to superomedial migration of the femoral head through the fractured acetabulum. The extremity is usually extended in midrotation position.

### X-ray

1. While the dislocated extremity usually assumes a characteristic position following injury, definitive diagnosis can only be established by adequate x-rays.

2. Two-plane radiography is essential, since occasionally a dislocated femoral head will appear in normal position on anteroposterior view.

3. Fractures of the posterior lip of the acetabulum also may be difficult to identify on routine two-plane x-rays. When a fracture of the posterior lip is suspected, repeat films must be taken after relocation of the head. At that time, with the patient prone and the uninvolved hip elevated 30 degrees off the table, posteroanterior x-rays taken directly over the involved hip will show the posterior acetabular lip adequately.

4. Fracture of the femoral head may complicate posterior dislocation of the hip and may appear on x-ray as a fragment in the acetabulum. This must be differentiated from an acetabular fracture by the views described above.

### Management

Manipulative reduction should be performed under general or spinal anesthesia whenever possible. Analgesics and sedation usually will not suffice and forceful manipulation without adequate muscle relaxation may result in further injury.

### Specific Techniques

1. *Posterior Dislocation*

  A. *Preferred Method*

    *(1)* The patient lies supine on a padded floor or low operating table.

    *(2)* An assistant applies counter traction by downward pressure on the anterior superior spines of the pelvis.

    *(3)* Flex the knee and thigh to 90 degrees and exert strong steady traction upward on the knee until the femoral head is felt to snap back into the acetabulum.

  B. *Bigelow Method*

    *(1)* The patient lies supine.

    *(2)* Flex the knee and thigh to 90 degrees, grasp the flexed knee and abduct it over the abdomen.

    *(3)* Circumduct the thigh laterally while applying traction.

    *(4)* Externally rotate and extend the thigh to bring the head into the acetabulum.

    *(5)* While this method has been advocated for many decades, it is a hazardous one, since improper or excessive manipulation can result in fracture of the femoral shaft or neck.

  C. *Stimson Method*

    *(1)* The patient lies prone on the operating table with his thighs flexed at the hip, and hanging over the end of the table.

    *(2)* The affected knee is brought to a right angle and steady pressure is exerted downward on the flexed knee until the head clicks into the acetabulum.

2. *Anterior Dislocation*

  A. *Preferred Method*

    *(1)* The patient lies supine on a padded floor or low operating table.

    *(2)* An assistant applies counter traction by downward pressure on the anterior superior spines of the pelvis.

    *(3)* Flex the knee and thigh to 90 degrees, allowing the femoral head to slide posterior to the acetabulum; this converts the anterior dislocation into a posterior one.

    *(4)* Exert strong steady traction upward on the knee until the femoral head is felt to snap into the acetabulum.

  B. *Alternate Method*

    *(1)* A modified Bigelow maneuver

may be used by flexing the knee and thigh, circumducting the thigh medially and then internally rotating and extending the thigh.

(2) The hazards which exist for the Bigelow maneuver in posterior dislocations apply here as well.

3. *Central Dislocations*

A. If displacement of the femoral head is minimal and the major portion of the femoral head rests under the weight-bearing dome of the acetabulum, maintenance of position by balanced skeletal traction through the distal femur and tibial tubercle is sufficient (*See* Fractures of the Shaft of the Femur).

B. If central displacement of the femoral head is marked, reduction may be achieved by skeletal traction or manipulation under general anesthesia. A hook screw (Green screw) is inserted into the greater trochanter in addition to the Kirschner wire in the distal femur or tibial tubercle. Traction is then applied laterally as well as distally to effect reduction.

C. Open reduction is rarely indicated since the medially fractured wall of the acetabulum. even if not anatomically restored, will scar sufficiently to prevent redisplacement.

D. In those rare instances where the superior dome of the acetabulum is severely fractured, open reduction may be attempted to restore a weight-bearing surface.

E. After 8 weeks of skeletal traction, crutch walking is begun. Full weight bearing on the affected extremity is not resumed until 12 weeks after injury, and subsequent periodic x-rays are necessary to detect avascular necrosis of the femoral head.

## Postreduction Care

1. Following reduction of anterior and posterior dislocations, the patient is kept on bed rest with the affected extremity in Buck's extension for 3 weeks.

2. Crutch walking without weight on the involved side is then begun and con-tinued for 6 weeks, with active exercises of the hip and knee joints during this time.

3. Following resumption of full weight bearing, periodic x-rays of the hip at 3-month intervals are necessary for two years to check for the possible late complication of avascular necrosis of the femoral head.

## Associated Injuries

1. If a fracture of the posterior acetabular lip has been noted, postreduction films are necessary to confirm proper repositioning of the fracture fragment. When a large fragment remains unreduced or appears unstable, open reduction and internal fixation are indicated.

2. Fractures of the femoral head complicating posterior dislocation may result in a small fragment of femoral head within the joint cavity. If this fragment interferes with complete reduction of the dislocated head, or if it is lodged between the femoral head and acetabulum in a weight-bearing area, it has to be removed by operative intervention.

## Complications

1. Injury to the sciatic nerve may complicate posterior dislocation of the femoral head, making motor and sensory evaluations of the extremity mandatory in all cases.

2. Central dislocation may result in injury to the obturator or femoral nerves.

3. Vascular injury is uncommon in these cases.

4. Late aseptic necrosis of the femoral head should be anticipated.

## FRACTURES OF THE HIP (PROXIMAL FEMUR)

### Basic Principles

Fractures of the hip usually occur in the elderly, following a fall on the involved side.

The fracture line may fall within the joint capsule (intracapsular) at three common sites: (1) below the femoral head (subcapital); (2) through the midneck region;

or (3) at the base of the neck. There may be varying degrees of separation of the fragments. If the neck is driven into the head at the fracture site and rigidly locked in this position, the fracture is said to be impacted. Impacted fractures can occur in valgus and varus position, but unimpacted fractures usually assume a varus deformity. A stable impacted fracture is usually in valgus position without anterior or posterior tipping. All intracapsular fractures result in local vascular disruption since the blood supply to the femoral head is primarily through intramedullary and reflected capsular vessels. The closer the fracture line is to the femoral head, the greater is the severity of vascular disruption. The high incidence of nonunion and avascular necrosis following intracapsular fractures is believed to be related to this loss of blood supply.

Extracapsular fractures usually occur between the greater and lesser trochanters (intertrochanteric) or just below the lesser trochanter (subtrochanteric). Vascular deprivation of the fragments is minimal at these locations, making nonunion and avascular necrosis rare in extracapsular fractures.

## Criteria for Diagnosis

1. History of a fall
2. Clinical evaluation
    A. Pain in the hip area is the most prominent symptom of a hip fracture.
    B. The patient usually is unable to lift the involved extremity, unless the fracture is impacted.
    C. Impacted fractures, especially if in the valgus position, will display little deformity, and diagnosis will only be possible by x-ray.
    D. Displaced neck fractures and extracapsular fractures usually present a typical picture of shortening and external rotation of the injured extremity.
3. X-ray: in all cases, anteroposterior and lateral x-rays are necessary for diagnosis.

## Management

1. As in all fractures, initial emergency treatment in a suspected hip fracture requires splinting and immobilization of the involved extremity, which can be accomplished with the aid of a Thomas splint, allowing traction and counter traction to be applied during transportation to the hospital.
2. Once x-rays have been obtained, the Thomas splint, with its hazardous ankle hitch, can be replaced by Buck's skin traction.
3. In the elderly, the skin of the lower extremity may not tolerate skin traction, and in those patients bed rest without traction usually suffices while awaiting operation.
4. Since most patients with hip fractures are in the older age-groups, they present with many complicating problems in addition to the fracture. We believe that a 24- to 48-hour delay, while associated problems are evaluated and treated, is preferable to immediate operation with minimal preparation. Cardiac, pulmonary and renal status should be well investigated before undertaking operation.

### Specific Management

1. *Impacted Neck Fractures*
    A. Well-impacted neck fractures in valgus position are treated initially with 3 weeks of bed rest with weekly x-rays during this time to confirm continued impaction.
    B. After this time, crutch walking without weight on the injured extremity is continued for at least 3 months.
    C. Weight bearing is not permitted until healing is evident on x-ray.
    D. If disimpaction occurs, or if impaction is not firm, internal fixation is performed.
    E. If impaction has occurred in varus position, internal fixation is performed because of the likelihood of disimpaction.
    F. Following internal fixation, usually with multiple pins, crutch ambulation without weight on the involved extremity is

permitted. Weight bearing is deferred until healing is evident on x-ray.

2. *Displaced Neck Fractures*

A. Displaced femoral neck fractures usually will not heal without accurate reduction and rigid fixation. Rigid fixation requires internal osseous fixation; hip spicas or traction are inadequate.

B. If accurate reduction cannot be achieved by closed means, open reduction should be done before insertion of an internal fixation device.

C. We use a sliding nail with a variable angle bar plate for internal fixation.

D. After operation, crutch walking is permitted without weight bearing on the involved extremity.

E. Healing must be visible on x-ray, usually after a minimum of 3 or 4 months, before weight bearing is resumed.

3. *Patients Over 65 Years of Age with Displaced Femoral Neck Fractures*

A. These fractures are treated by primary prosthetic replacement of the femoral head.

B. Occasionally, a patient who is chronologically 65 years of age but who appears physiologically younger warrants an attempt to save the femoral head by internal fixation.

C. Although immediate prosthetic replacement is still a controversial approach to this fracture, at our institution it has been the most satisfactory therapy.

D. The problem of ambulation in the elderly is simplified since full weight bearing is permitted one week after operation.

E. The problems of nonunion and avascular necrosis also are obviated in patients who might not be able to tolerate a second operative procedure for these complications.

F. Although prosthetic replacement provides a less satisfactory hip than the patient's own fully healed femoral head, it is a compromise born of necessity in this age-group.

4. *Intertrochanteric and Subtrochanteric Fractures*

A. The prognosis for healing in these fractures is good, provided that adequate stabilization can be achieved.

B. In the young patient, with adequate reduction, skeletal Russell's traction can be satisfactorily employed as definitive treatment.

C. Usually union is strong enough in 10 to 12 weeks to allow crutch walking without weight bearing on the involved side.

D. Since this method entails the risks attendant with prolonged bed rest, as well as the economic burden of extended hospitalization, operative fixation often is performed as an expedient alternative.

E. When adequate reduction is not possible by closed means, operative reduction and internal fixation are mandatory to achieve a satisfactory result.

F. In the elderly patient, operative fixation is undertaken in all cases except those previously nonambulatory patients mentioned below, in order to avoid the complications of prolonged immobilization in bed.

G. If possible, when internal fixation is performed in the elderly patient with an intertrochanteric fracture, a weight-bearing nail (Holt) is used to permit early weight-bearing ambulation postoperatively. As with the hip-replacement prosthesis, this is advantageous in aged patients who use crutches poorly, since healing on x-ray does not have to be achieved before full weight bearing can be begun.

H. The type of internal fixation with subtrochanteric fractures varies from a nail-long bar combination to an intramedullary nail or a Y nail, depending on the level and the comminution.

5. *Patients Who Are Extremely Elderly and Feeble:*

A. If these patients have not been ambulatory recently, fixation of the hip fracture or prosthetic replacement is unnecessary since there is little likelihood that these patients will ever walk again.

B. They are treated with small doses of analgesics, such as codeine, for the pain, and they are gotten out of bed into a chair daily. After a few days the pain becomes minimal and the patients are essentially back to their prefracture status.

## FRACTURES OF THE SHAFT OF THE FEMUR

### Basic Principles

Fracture of the shaft of the femur usually results from a direct blow to the femur but can occur from a sudden rotational force applied with the leg fixed. The latter results in a spiral, oblique fracture, while direct blows usually produce transverse or comminuted fractures. Femoral shaft fractures can occur at any age but are more common in the younger and middle-aged groups.

The large muscle groups surrounding the femur, with their abundant blood supply, are severely traumatized in femoral shaft fractures, resulting in significant blood loss into the soft tissues about the fracture site. The muscular attachments at the proximal and distal portions make displacement greater with fractures at these areas. Angulation and overriding are common at all levels. Lacerations of the femoral vessels by the sharp bony fragments may result in severe vascular injury.

### Criteria for Diagnosis

1. Pain and tenderness are routinely noted at the fracture site. In addition, obvious angulation is usually present.
2. The thigh at the fracture level may be ecchymotic and markedly swollen because of extensive bleeding into the soft tissues.
3. Accurate diagnosis of the fracture can only be made by x-rays taken in two planes. The entire length of the femur must be x-rayed since occasionally double shaft fractures can occur, as well as fractures or dislocations of the hip.
4. The distal portion of the extremity must be checked for color, warmth, arterial pulsations and sensation to rule out severe arterial or nerve injury.

### Management

#### Emergency Treatment

1. Immobilize the fractured extremity with a Thomas splint. If a Thomas splint is not available, strap long boards or rolled newspapers to either side of the extremity or a single board between the legs to fix the knee and bind both legs together.
2. Do not attempt to reduce deformity or retract protruding bone beneath the skin. Instead, splint in position if the vascular supply is good and cover open wounds, including bone, with sterile or at least clean dressings.
3. Check for impending or actual shock. Start intravenous fluid replacement immediately since femoral shaft fractures are often accompanied by considerable blood loss into the surrounding tissues.

#### Definitive Treatment

1. Once the level of fracture and degree of displacement are determined, definitive treatment may be begun.
2. Definitive treatment may be divided into three categories: (1) closed reduction and casting; (2) continuous skin or skeletal traction; and (3) open reduction.

   A. *Closed Reduction and Casting*

   *(1)* Primarily applicable to children and young adults

   *(2)* Requires general anesthesia, fracture table and x-ray control

   *(3)* Spica cast required

   *(a)* Single leg—snug fitting, above the nipple line and down to the toes with a 15- to 20-degree bend in the knee

   *(b)* One and one-half spica—to the nipple line above, to the toes on the ipsilateral side, and to the supracondylar region of the thigh on the contralateral side, with the hips abducted and the ipsilateral knee flexed. The cross bar between the thighs is placed posterior in males and anterior in females.

   *(c)* In both children and thin adults it is advisable to cut a large circular

hole over the abdomen to permit distention with meals.

(4) Check x-rays are taken at 24 hours, 72 hours and 10 days.

(5) If reduction is maintained, the patient may be discharged to be followed at monthly intervals until healing.

(6) Spica care includes turning of the patient frequently, maintenance of cast integrity and cleanliness, and relief of pressure points.

(7) Angular shifts may be corrected by wedging as in other extremity casts.

(8) Despite the weight, ambulation is possible for vigorous patients, especially with the one-legged spica.

(9) Change of the spica at three months is advisable both to check the fracture healing without the cast and to accommodate for patient obesity and muscle atrophy.

B. *Continuous Traction*

(1) Overhead bilateral leg traction through adhesive skin traction (Bryant's or gallows) is useful for children 2 years old and under.

(a) Sufficient weight need be applied to *just* lift the buttocks off the bed.

(b) Check rotary malalignment and correct early. If this is not accomplished, a closed reduction and casting should correct this deformity which *will not correct with age.*

(c) X-rays are taken at 24 hours, 48 hours, 96 hours and weekly until callus is present.

(d) When the fracture callus is nontender and/or the patient spins without discomfort in his traction, spica application with sedation but without anesthesia can be done. The fracture position should be rechecked by x-ray before the patient leaves the fracture room.

(e) The European variant, using an elevatable overbed frame on which the bent legs are strapped, offers the considerable advantage of greater extremity control, especially of rotatory deformity.

(2) Fixed traction is used in children over 2 years of age until cooperation for Russell traction is possible.

(a) Adhesive traction is applied to the skin of the lower thigh and leg. Avoid wrapping of the adhesive device below one inch above the malleoli.

(b) A standard tape spreader and rope are attached under the foot and tied to the notch of a full-ring Thomas splint.

(c) With the patient sedated, sufficient traction can be applied before tying the knot to effect the desired lengthening.

(d) The leg and thigh are then wrapped in the splint to increase immobility and maintain rotary alignment. The addition of anterior and posterior molded plaster splints over the thigh and leg may be required.

(e) The end of the Thomas splint is tied to the end of the bed, which is placed in steep Trendelenburg position.

(f) Check x-rays are done immediately, at 24 hours, 72 hours, and weekly thereafter.

(g) Good nontender callus or patient spinning is an indication for conversion to a full spica cast (*see* above).

(3) Russell's traction is applicable for children older than 5 years, in general, and for adults (Fig. 25-5).

(a) In children (before epiphyseal fusion), traction is done through an adhesive device applied to the skin of the leg (we still find moleskin adhesive plaster superior for this) to the level of the knee and wrapped with elastic bandage to a point 3 cm. above the malleoli.

(b) In an adult, especially with poor skin of the leg, traction is applied through a Kirschner wire placed through the calcaneus 2 cm. anterior to the back of the heel and 2 cm. proximal to the sole of the foot. Collodion pads placed over the site of entrance and exit of the wire will seal the skin openings. A proper-sized Kirschner wire spreader, gripping the wire close to the skin and adequately tensed, will prevent bending and breakage.

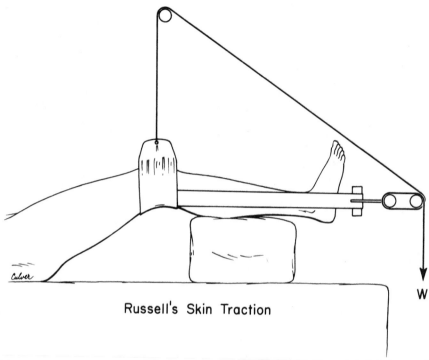

**Russell's Skin Traction**

Fig. 25-5. Russell's traction. Here traction is applied to the leg through moleskin adhesive applied to the skin. A Kirschner wire through the calcaneus may be substituted for long-term traction. Note the use of a double pulley at the bed end to permit parallel rope pull caudally.

(c) A padded sling is placed under the knee, and a traction rope (we prefer ordinary 1/4-inch cotton Mason Line) passes through a pulley directly over the knee with the patient properly positioned in bed, through one half of a double pulley at the foot of the bed extension, back to a pulley attached to the tape spreader or Kirschner wire spreader, then to the other half of the double pulley and to the traction weights.

(d) The use of the double pulley (Zimmer Catalog No. 99-6387) assures the continuous 2 x axial pull required in Russell's traction at all patient levels until the pulleys are locked.

(e) A tied pillow or folded sheet under the leg facilitates the maintenance of a comfortable position.

(f) Trendelenburg position of the bed enables the patient to maintain his proper location in bed so that the over-knee rope is vertical.

(g) Four to five pounds of weight are initially used in children and seven to eight pounds in adults, depending on muscle mass.

(h) Check x-rays are done at 24 hours and 72 hours (12 hours and 72 hours after each adjustment of weight) and weekly if position is stable.

(i) Well-leg Buck's traction may be required in children to compensate for valgus angulation due to pelvis tilt.

(j) Change to cast immobilization is dictated by fracture solidification on x-ray or the inability to correct axial alignment with traction.

(4) Balanced traction is direct axial skeletal traction with the leg maintained in

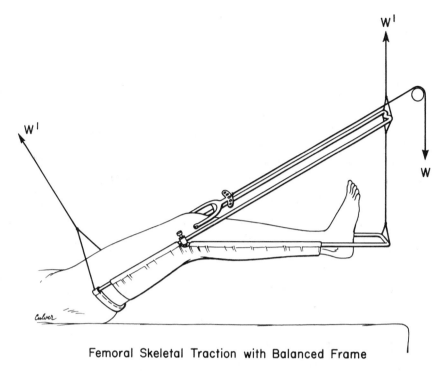

**Femoral Skeletal Traction with Balanced Frame**

Fig. 25-6. Axial skeletal traction for femoral shaft fracture (W). The Thomas splint with fixed Pearson extension is balanced (W$^1$) to provide both counter traction and upward mobility without loss of position.

position in a counterbalanced frame, usually a Thomas splint with a Pearson extension (Fig. 25-6).

(a) Traction is applied through a Kirschner wire drilled through the tibial tubercle area 1 cm. distal to the upper end of the tibial tubercle and 1 cm. deep to the palpable bone. Alternatively, direct femoral pull can be accomplished through a Kirschner wire drilled directly through the subcutaneously palpable femoral condyles 2 cm. above the medial joint line. A proper-size Kirschner wire spreader with adequate tension will minimize bend and breakage.

(b) The balanced frame should permit upward movement of the patient with maintenance of frame position. If the fracture is sufficiently proximal in the femur, the leg extension may be movable to permit knee exercise.

(c) Twenty pounds of traction usually are required initially for reduction. This may be reduced to 12 to 15 pounds to maintain reduction.

(d) Slings and antirotation traction may be necessary additions for reduction.

(e) Check x-rays are done in 24 hours and 72 hours (12 hours and 72 hours after weight change or fracture manipulation) and at weekly intervals once position has stabilized.

(f) Conversion to plaster immobilization is indicated only for uncorrectable deformity or for economic reasons to permit transfer out of the hospital.

C. *Open Reduction*

(1) Open reduction and internal fixation are indicated in femoral shaft fractures in the elderly as well as in those

patients in whom skeletal traction fails to achieve adequate reduction.

*(2)* Since operative fixation allows earlier ambulation and joint movement, its value in the elderly is obvious. It has become our treatment of choice for uncomplicated shaft fractures in other adults because of shortened hospitalization and earlier joint mobilization.

*(3)* Internal fixation may be accomplished by intramedullary nailing or compression plating, depending on the level and complexity of the fracture. We prefer intramedullary nailing with reaming by the modified Küntscher technique where possible.

*(4)* Infection is the obvious "běte noire" of open reduction. To minimize this complication, reduction should not be done in the presence of any open wound except as primary management where other modalities are not applicable.

## FRACTURES OF THE DISTAL END OF THE FEMUR

### Basic Principles

Fractures of the distal end of the femur usually result from severe direct trauma, except in the instance of pathologic bone. They may be supracondylar, intercondylar or confined to one condyle.

The fracture line in supracondylar fractures is transverse or oblique just above the condyles. If the obliquity of the fracture line runs posteriorly and superiorly, the distal fragment will be tilted posteriorly due to the pull of the gastrocnemius muscle with the posterior position maintained by the quadriceps pull. This angulation may cause injury to the popliteal vessels and nerves.

Intercondylar fractures (often referred to as T-fractures) are actually supracondylar fractures complicated by an additional fracture line extending downward between the condyles. In addition to the effects of the supracondylar element, this fracture produces bleeding into the knee joint, resulting in a marked hemarthrosis.

Isolated condylar fractures usually result from a direct blow and the fracture line is generally vertical, either in the sagittal or frontal plane. Hemarthrosis is common, and if the fragment of condyle retains no ligamentous or muscular attachment, it may be completely free within the joint.

### Criteria for Diagnosis

1. Pain, tenderness and swelling are evident at the fracture site.
2. Supracondylar fractures result in shortening of the femur and deformity at the supracondylar area.
2. Massive hemarthrosis may be evident in intercondylar fractures.
4. Check for vascular or neurologic deficit in the distal extremity.
5. Anteroposterior and lateral x-rays are essential for accurate diagnosis of the exact type of fracture present.

### Management

1. Emergency treatment involves Thomas splint immobilization and restoration of blood volume, especially if blood loss into local tissues is obvious.
2. For closed supracondylar fractures in a healthy adult, balanced skeletal traction with a pin through the tibial tubercle (*see above*) can result in a satisfactory reduction, but often is difficult. In those cases where reduction is unsatisfactory and in the elderly, who cannot tolerate prolonged bed rest with traction, open reduction and internal fixation are indicated. Blade-plate fixation provides the most satisfactory stabilization.
3. Intercondylar fractures require accurate reduction since joint spaces are involved. Unless displacement is insignificant, this can only be accomplished by open reduction and internal fixation, using a blade-plate and screw fixation.
4. Displaced, isolated condylar fractures also require anatomical reduction, and therefore open reduction and internal

fixation with screw fixation are indicated.

5. Immediate operative intervention is needed if signs of neurologic or vascular injury accompany the initial injury. A lacerated popliteal vessel or nerve will require repair, while compression or contusion will be relieved by reduction and fixation.

## DISLOCATION OF THE KNEE

### Basic Principles

Acute dislocation of the knee is a rare injury but can occur from direct or torsional trauma. Usually both cruciate ligaments and both collateral ligaments are torn in addition to tears in the semilunar cartilages. Displacement of the lower leg may be anterior, posterior, medial or lateral.

Commonly associated with knee dislocations is injury to the major vessels and nerves traversing the popliteal fossa. Popliteal artery injury results in a cold, pulseless lower leg and foot. Common peroneal and posterior tibial nerve injury produces anesthesia and motor deficits in the lower leg and foot.

### Criteria for Diagnosis

1. History of direct severe injury to the knee
2. Acute dislocation is obvious by the gross deformity produced. Dislocations which reduce spontaneously at the time of injury will present no deformity but will be evident by the complete instability of the ligamentous structures of the knee joint. Swelling and hemarthrosis may make the diagnosis difficult.
3. Two-plane radiography is essential for adequate diagnosis. X-rays of the femur and tibia are necessary to rule out associated fractures of these bones.
4. Always check for vascular and nerve injury.

### Management

1. Acute dislocations of the knee should be reduced as soon as possible after injury to relieve the stretching and compressive effects on the vessels and nerves in the popliteal area. Reduction should only be accomplished under general anesthesia and operative repair of the torn ligaments should be performed. Internal derangements of the knee are described more fully in Chapter 24.

2. Closed reduction followed by immobilization in a cylinder plaster cast for two months is an alternate method of therapy for those patients for whom operative repair is medically contraindicated. However, if signs of vascular injury persist after reduction, operative exploration of the popliteal vessels is indicated. While neurologic deficits often are due to nerve stretching or compression, they may be due to nerve disruption. Early operative exploration is indicated when signs of nerve damage are present.

## FRACTURES OF THE PATELLA

### Basic Principles

The patella is actually a large sesamoid bone within the tendinous portion of the quadriceps muscle. It protects the knee joint cavity and serves as a fulcrum to enhance extension of the leg. The patella may be removed completely or partially, with relatively little functional loss to the extremity.

Patella fractures usually occur from direct trauma to the flexed knee. This may result in two large fragments which may or may not be separated, while severe trauma may produce a totally comminuted fracture or comminution of one of the major fragments. Separated fractures are always accompanied by varying degrees of tear and separation of the extensor expansion on either side of the patella. Failure to repair this extensor apparatus will result in inadequate extension of the leg.

### Criteria for Diagnosis

1. Pain, tenderness and swelling are apparent.
2. Palpable defect over the patella

3. Joint effusion and hemarthrosis are marked.

4. Inability to extend the leg against resistance or inability to hold the leg extended when raised from the bed

5. Diagnosis is established by anteroposterior, lateral and axial radiographic views. Occasionally, a bipartite patella, with a superolateral fusion line resembling a fracture line, will cause confusion in diagnosis. Bipartite or tripartite patella is usually a bilateral finding and can be confirmed by x-ray of the uninjured knee.

## Management

1. Emergency splinting in extension in a Thomas splint

2. Unseparated fractures are treated in a cylinder plaster cast from upper thigh to ankle for a period of 6 weeks. Hemarthrosis should be aspirated before application of the cast. Weight bearing in the cylinder cast is permitted.

3. Separated fractures are treated by operative repair.

A. Where two large fragments are present, circumferential wire-loop fixation with an anterior tension wiring is performed.

B. Where one fragment is comminuted, it is removed and the tendon, either quadriceps or patella, is sutured to the remaining fragment.

C. Where the entire patella is severely comminuted, it is removed and the quadriceps tendon and patella tendon are sutured together.

D. In all operative cases, repair of the extensor expansion is essential. A postoperative cylinder cast is applied for 6 weeks.

## FRACTURES OF THE TIBIA AND FIBULA

*Fractures of the Proximal Tibia*

## Basic Principles

Fractures of the proximal tibia may in-volve either medial or lateral tibial plateaus, or both, and usually result from direct force or a fall.

1. Lateral plateau fractures are commonly called "bumper fractures" since they often result from the impact from an automobile bumper against the lateral aspect of the knee. This causes abduction of the knee, with crushing of the lateral plateau by the overlying lateral femoral condyle. The lateral plateau fragment may be single or comminuted, and often is depressed downward several millimeters. The medial collateral ligament is often torn and the lateral meniscus may be disrupted. In addition, the direct blow may damage the fibula head and adjacent peroneal nerve, causing foot drop and loss of sensation over the dorsum of the foot.

2. Medial plateau fractures are uncommon since they require the less frequently encountered forces which produce an adduction strain on the knee. Tears of the lateral collateral ligament and medial meniscus may accompany this fracture.

3. Both tibial plateaus may be fractured simultaneously by a fall, landing on the sole of the foot with the knee extended.

4. All tibial plateau fractures enter the knee joint and result in varying degrees of hemarthrosis.

## Criteria for Diagnosis

1. History of direct knee injury

2. Lateral tibial plateau fractures show valgus deformity of the knee, while medial plateau fractures will present a varus deformity.

3. Signs and symptoms of fracture of the knee are present.

4. Anteroposterior and lateral x-rays are the minimal views necessary for accurate diagnosis.

5. Check for peroneal nerve injury in lateral plateau fractures.

## Management

1. Emergency splinting with a Thomas splint should be performed at the accident site, before transport to the hospital.

2. Hemarthrosis should be treated early by aspiration.

3. Undisplaced tibial plateau fractures are treated by plaster immobilization in a long leg circular cast with the knee slightly flexed.

4. Lateral plateau fractures with mild displacement warrant an attempt at closed reduction. With the knee extended, lateral traction is exerted on the knee by the use of a sling, forcing the knee into adduction. Occasionally, a large fragment may be reduced by direct compression. Reduction is verified by x-ray and maintained by a long leg plaster cast.

5. When closed reduction of medial plateau fractures is attempted, the forces applied are opposite to those used for lateral plateau fractures.

6. When both plateaus are fractured with minimal displacement, manual traction in the long axis of the tibia, with bilateral compression at the knee, may achieve adequate reduction. If reduction is inadequate or difficult to maintain in plaster, skeletal traction through the calcaneus or lower tibia may be used.

7. Accurate congruity of the articular surfaces must be obtained in order to prevent subsequent arthritis and instability. If closed methods fail to achieve adequate reduction, open reduction and internal fixation are indicated. Single fragment plateau fractures can be secured with screw fixation, while comminuted fractures require more complicated procedures, including insertion of bone grafts to elevate severely depressed articular surfaces.

8. Regardless of the method of treatment, weight bearing must be avoided until soft callus has been supplanted by firm bony union. Premature weight bearing before at least three months may result in depression of the plateau.

9. Peroneal nerve injury, if present, usually will recover spontaneously, but during the healing period the foot should be fitted with a dorsiflexion splint.

## *Fractures of the Shaft of the Tibia and Fibula*

### Basic Principles

Fractures of the shaft of the tibia occur from direct trauma or torsional forces. Fractures resulting from direct trauma are transverse, comminuted or segmental, while those due to torsional injury are spiral or oblique. A large percentage of tibial fractures are open due to the subcutaneous position of the bone throughout most of its length. Usually both tibia and fibula are broken, but not necessarily at the same level. Less frequently, fracture of the tibia with an intact fibula may occur, as well as isolated fractures of the fibula.

### Criteria for Diagnosis

1. History of direct or indirect leg trauma

2. Clinical signs and symptoms of fracture are found on examination of the leg.

3. Anteroposterior and lateral x-rays are necessary for accurate diagnosis. The entire length of the tibia and fibula must be x-rayed because fibula fractures may occur at different levels than the tibial fractures.

4. Nerve and vessel injury is uncommon with tibial shaft fractures. Occasionally a fracture of the upper end of the fibula may result in peroneal nerve damage, with foot drop and loss of sensation over the dorsum of the foot.

### Management

1. Fractures of the tibia may be splinted with a Thomas splint, a pneumatic splint, in a pillow or with suitable lengths of folded newspaper or boards for transport to the hospital.

2. All manipulations and wound care should be performed under general or regional anesthesia.

3. Open fracture wounds are debrided thoroughly before reduction of the fracture is performed.

4. The preferred method of treatment, where possible, is closed reduction and immobilization in a long leg plaster cast.

A. Apposition of 50 per cent or more of the fracture surfaces is sought with good axial alignment and no rotation. Shortening of over 1 cm. is not acceptable.

B. The cast should hold the knee in moderate (20 to 35 degrees) flexion and the foot at a right angle.

C. Repeat x-rays during the first ten days are necessary to detect slipping of an unstable reduction.

5. Unstable oblique or spiral fractures and those fractures which redisplace after reduction and casting can be treated by external skeletal fixation. Pins placed through the proximal and distal tibia are incorporated into a long leg plaster after reduction.

6. Occasionally markedly comminuted fractures or fractures with extensive soft tissue loss can be treated by continuous skeletal traction with a pin in the calcaneus and the leg elevated on a Böhler-Braun frame.

7. When adequate reduction cannot be achieved by closed methods, open reduction and internal fixation are indicated. Compression plating is the most satisfactory method of fixation. Intramedullary nailing is used infrequently by us, reserving it for segmental fractures or where plating would not be feasible.

8. Closed methods of treatment, including external skeletal fixation, require maintenance of casting until evidence of union appears on x-ray. This length of time is extremely variable, depending on many factors such as age, type of fracture and associated soft tissue damage. It can vary from 4 and 8 months and in some cases even longer (delayed union). If union fails to occur after a prolonged period (nonunion), operative management usually is necessary.

9. Internal fixation often requires only a short period of casting, followed by early joint mobilization without weight bearing. Full weight bearing, however, must await x-ray evidence of healing, as in closed methods of treatment.

# FRACTURES OF THE ANKLE

## Basic Principles

The bony framework of the ankle joint consists of the tibia medially and superiorly, the fibula laterally and the talus distally. Strong ligaments connect these bones and provide stability for the joint. The large deltoid ligament fans downward from the medial malleolus of the tibia, while the lateral ligament joins the lateral (fibular) malleolus to the talus and calcaneus. The medial malleolus and lateral ligament prevent medial migration of the talus and keep it within the ankle mortise. Similarly, the lateral malleolus and deltoid ligament prevent lateral displacement of the talus. Posteriorly, a projection of the tibia, often designated the posterior malleolus, prevents posterior migration of the talus. The distal tibia and fibula are kept united above the ankle joint by the inferior tibiofibular ligament.

Injuries of the ankle are usually caused by indirect forces, rarely by direct trauma. Commonly, marked eversion (abduction) or inversion (adduction) forces are responsible for bony and/or ligamentous disruptions. In addition, rotational forces exerted with the foot fixed, as in a pivoting position during basketball, will produce injury. Least frequently, a vertical compression force resulting from a fall from a height produces a fracture of the distal tibial plafond (superior articular surface).

Since the ligaments are essential for the stability of the ankle, ligamentous injury must be evaluated in addition to bony injury in all trauma to the ankle. Severe eversion or inversion force will produce either a tear of the stressed ligament or the ligament will remain intact and the bone will break. If the ligament alone is torn, x-ray may fail to reveal the pathology, but clinical findings may suggest the defect. Stress films are needed for confirmation and usually will demonstrate the soft tissue injury.

*Unimalleolar Fractures*

## Basic Principles

1. Undisplaced fractures of the lateral or medial malleolus are held in place by surrounding periosteum and demonstrate no loss of ankle integrity since the major ligaments remain intact.

2. A displaced medial malleolar fracture can be produced by a strong eversion or inversion force.

A. Displaced medial malleolar fractures due to eversion are transverse avulsion-type fractures and often occur below the level of the upper border of the talus, leaving a "shoulder" of the medial malleolus attached to the tibia. The deltoid ligament remains intact. If the inferior tibiofibular ligament is torn, the talus will be displaced laterally. Occasionally, an eversion force will rupture the deltoid and inferior tibiofibular ligaments without any fracture occurring, but with resultant lateral displacement of the talus.

B. Displaced medial malleolar fractures due to inversion are produced by direct abutment of the talus against the inner surface of the medial malleolus. The medial malleolus is sheared off in an oblique manner, with the fracture line usually at or above the ankle mortise level. The lateral ligament is usually torn, allowing medial displacement of the talus.

3. A displaced fibular malleolus fracture is usually produced by an eversion force, combined with an external rotational stress.

A. Lateral displacement of the talus is associated with rupture of the deltoid ligament medially. The fracture line is oblique at the joint level, with the inferior tibiofibular ligament remaining intact.

B. Occasionally, the fibula will be fractured above the level of the joint, and in that instance the inferior tibiofibular ligament will rupture, producing a diastasis of the tibiofibular joint (classical Pott's fracture).

C. Isolated fibular fractures produced by inversion forces are not associated with displacement of the talus due to the buttress of the medial malleolus.

## Criteria for Diagnosis

1. History of inversion, eversion or twisting of the ankle

2. Clinical signs and symptoms of fracture. Gross deformity may be present but obscured by the swelling.

3. All ankle injuries, regardless of severity, should not be treated without adequate x-rays. This usually requires anteroposterior and lateral films, but oblique views may be needed for precise diagnosis.

A. Obvious displacement of the talus on x-ray will confirm loss of integrity of the medial or lateral ligaments.

B. If ligamentous injury is presumed but not obvious on plain x-ray, stress films should be taken. These are done by first anesthetizing the area of suspected ligament tear by local infiltration with Xylocaine. For medial ligament injuries the foot is everted, while for lateral ligament injuries the foot is inverted. Anteroposterior x-rays are taken while maintaining the forced position. If ligamentous injury has occurred, tilting of the talus in the ankle mortise will be noted.

## Management

1. All ankle injuries should be splinted in a pillow or between padded boards for transportation before x-rays are taken.

2. Undisplaced unimalleolar fractures are treated by immobilization in a short leg walking cast (toes to tibial tubercle) for 6 weeks. The ankle joint is kept at 90 degrees, in neutral version. If the swelling is significant, casting should be delayed, with elevation of the ankle for 3 to 4 days. This usually will result in sufficient subsidence of the swelling to allow casting without fear of vascular compromise or subsequent loosening of the cast.

3. All manipulative reduction of ankle fractures should be performed under general or regional anesthesia.

Displaced medial malleolar fracture due to an eversion stress, without displacement of the talus, may be reduced and casted in a short leg walking cast for 6 weeks. If after manipulation under general anesthesia perfect reduction cannot be obtained, minimal displacement may be accepted if the fracture line is below the level of the ankle mortise. If reduction is inadequate with the fracture at the joint level (usually because of interposed ligament and periosteum), immediate open reduction and internal screw fixation are indicated since fibrous union at this level will lead to instability of the ankle.

4. Displaced medial malleolar fractures due to eversion stress, with associated lateral displacement of the talus due to inferior tibiofibular ligament tear, are difficult to treat by closed methods. Closed reduction, if successful, is followed by application of a non-weight-bearing, long leg plaster cast for 6 weeks and then a short leg plaster cast for 2 weeks. If closed manipulation is inadequate or cannot be maintained, open reduction and internal fixation are indicated, to fix the medial malleolus and to restore the tibiofibular syndesmosis.

5. Displaced medial malleolar fractures due to inversion are reduced by closed means if possible. Since the fracture in these cases is usually at joint level, operative fixation is indicated whenever reduction is less than perfect, especially when medial displacement of the talus is also present.

6. Fractures of the lateral malleolus with displacement of the talus laterally can be treated by closed reduction if the torn deltoid ligament has not become interposed between the talus and medial malleolus. If, after an attempt at reduction, the gap between the talus and medial malleolus measures 4 mm. or more, open reduction is necessary to remove the ligament from the joint and to repair it. Internal fixation of the lateral malleolar fracture also is performed at that time.

## Bimalleolar Fractures

### Basic Principles

As with single malleolar fractures, bimalleolar fractures (fractures of medial and lateral malleoli) are produced by inversion, eversion or rotational stress. Inversion stress results in a shearing fracture of the medial malleolus and an avulsion fracture of the lateral malleolus. The ligaments remain intact and the talus is displaced medially. External rotational or occasionally eversion stress produces a spiral fracture of the lateral malleolus and an avulsion fracture of the medial malleolus. The ligaments remain intact and the talus is displaced laterally.

### Criteria for Diagnosis

Same as noted under Unimalleolar Fractures, above.

### Management

1. Closed manipulative reduction is attempted first under general or regional anesthesia.
2. The fragments are disimpacted by recreation of the injuring force and traction is applied to the foot.
3. The foot is dorsiflexed to 90 degrees (80 to 85 degrees in women with a tight tendo calcaneus) and reduction manipulation opposite to the injuring force is applied.
4. Manual pressure with the thumbs and heel of the hand may aid in pressing a displaced malleolus back into position.
5. Internal rotation of the foot (as differentiated from inversion) probably is the single most important maneuver since external rotation is the commonest injuring force.
6. If adequate position of the fragments is obtained, a long leg, non-weight-bearing plaster cast is applied and maintained for 8 weeks.
7. Repeat x-rays are imperative during the first two weeks to detect loss of reduction, since these often are unstable fractures.

8. If proper reduction cannot be obtained by closed means, or if reduction is lost while the ankle is in a cast, open reduction with internal fixation of both malleoli is indicated.

*Trimalleolar Fractures*

## Basic Principles

If the rotational stress producing a bimalleolar fracture is continued, the posterior lip (malleolus) of the distal tibia may be sheared off, resulting in the so-called trimalleolar fracture, and may be seen together with posterior subluxation of the talus. The fragment of "posterior malleolus" can vary in size from a small chip up to one the size of half of the articular surface of the tibia.

## Criteria for Diagnosis

1. In addition to the signs and symptoms of a bimalleolar fracture, varying degrees of posterior displacement of the foot may be present.
2. Adequate x-ray examination is essential for proper diagnosis. The posterior fragment and posterior talar subluxation will be seen best on lateral and oblique films.

## Management

1. If the posterior fragment is less than 10 per cent of the articular surface of the tibia, accurate reduction of the fragment is not essential. Usually posterior displacement of the foot will not be present with such a small fragment, and the treatment is identical to that for a bimalleolar fracture.
2. If the posterior fragment is 10 to 30 per cent of the articular surface, precise relocation of the fragment is advisable to obtain a congruous articular surface, preventing subsequent traumatic arthritis and posterior subluxation of the talus.
   A. In addition to the maneuvers described for bimalleolar fractures, downward and forward pressure is applied to the heel, both to reduce the subluxation and to tense the tendo calcaneus, which

will serve to reposition and maintain the posterior fragment.
   B. If closed manipulation is successful, a long leg, non-weight-bearing plaster cast is applied for 8 weeks.
   C. Repeat x-rays are imperative twice weekly for the first three weeks to assure maintenance of reduction.
   D. If displacement occurs in the cast, or if initial reduction was inadequate, open reduction and internal screw fixation of the posterior fragment, as well as the medial and lateral malleoli, are indicated.
3. If the posterior fragment constitutes one third or more of the articular surface, maintenance of reduction by closed means is usually inadequate, and immediate open reduction with internal fixation is recommended.

*Vertical Compression Fractures*

## Basic Principles

Falls from a height, with the patient landing on the heel, can produce severely comminuted fractures of the lower articulating surface of the tibia. The talus is driven upward as a wedge into the tibial plafond, resulting in marked disruption of the articular surface. Fractures of one or both malleoli may accompany this fracture.

## Criteria for Diagnosis

1. History of a fall, even from only a few feet
2. Signs and symptoms of a fracture about the ankle are present. The upward migration of the talus may produce an obvious shortening of the distance between malleoli and heel.
3. X-rays of the ankle are essential for proper diagnosis. Since the mode of injury may also result in other injuries, x-rays of the calcaneus, pelvis and lumbodorsal spine should be obtained.
4. Neurologic injury may be produced by a spinal fracture, making neurologic evaluation of the lower extremities essential in all vertical compression fractures of the tibia.

## Management

1. The degree of comminution will determine the therapy. If the articular surface is minimally disrupted, closed reduction may be sufficient to restore an adequate articular surface. A long leg plaster cast is maintained for 4 to 6 weeks, at which time it is removed for active ankle (tibial-calcaneal) exercises. Weight bearing is avoided for at least three months.

2. If reduction is unstable, a Kirschner wire may be inserted into the calcaneus for continuous traction on a balanced or Böhler-Braun frame, especially if severe swelling and local soft tissue injury are present. At a later date (or initially if swelling and local injury are minimal), another pin may be placed through the lower tibia, and, following traction reduction, casting is done incorporating the pins in the plaster for external skeletal fixation.

3. Moderately comminuted fractures of the distal articular surface, which cannot be reduced by closed means, should be treated by early open reduction and internal fixation. A functional articular surface often can be reconstituted by painstaking reapproximation of the fracture fragments.

4. Severely comminuted fractures usually represent an impossible task of restoration to any functional articular surface. In these cases, we revert to an extreme conservative approach, encouraging early active tibiocalcaneal motion and reserving arthrodesis for late symptomatology.

## FRACTURES AND DISLOCATIONS OF THE FOOT

*Fractures and Dislocations of the Talus*

### Basic Principles

The talus (astragalus) is the major link between the tibia and the foot, occupying the entire ankle mortise. The articular surface directly under the tibia forms the dome of the body of the talus. The narrower midportion is known as the neck. The blood supply of the bone is derived mainly from vessels entering distally in the neck and head. Severe dorsiflexion trauma is responsible for most of the common injuries of the talus. Fracture of the neck occurs as the neck of the talus impinges against the lower tibia. The fragments may be undisplaced or the distal fragment may displace dorsally. At the same time, the body may dislocate posteriorly. Isolated complete talar dislocation, without fracture, rarely may occur.

The pattern of blood supply to the talus makes fracture of the neck or total talar dislocation a more serious problem than just an anatomical derangement. Despite adequate reduction, loss of blood supply to the body can ultimately lead to avascular necrosis of the proximal portion of the talus, with crush of the body and subsequent disability and pain.

### Criteria for Diagnosis

1. History of sudden dorsiflexion of the foot (a vehicular crash with the foot on the brake, "aviator's fracture")

2. Signs and symptoms of fracture at the ankle area. Total dislocation of the talus usually occurs laterally, with a marked prominence evident anterior to the lateral malleolus. Frequently the overlying skin is torn, resulting in an open dislocation.

3. Talar fracture and fracture dislocation can only be diagnosed accurately by x-ray in at least two planes. Frequently two or more oblique views are needed to orient the surgeon to the pathology with total talar dislocation.

### Management

1. Undisplaced fracture of the neck of the talus is treated by a non-weight-bearing short leg plaster cast, with the foot in neutral position, for a period of 8 weeks. Weight bearing is not permitted until evidence of healing is present.

2. Displaced fracture of the neck of the talus is reduced under anesthesia by strong plantar flexion and eversion. A long leg, non-weight-bearing plaster cast is applied,

with the knee partially flexed and the foot plantar flexed and everted. After 8 weeks, a short leg cast in neutral position may be substituted for an additional 4 weeks. Weight bearing is avoided until evidence of healing is present, and periodic x-rays are taken to check for avascular necrosis of the body. If closed reduction is not possible, immediate open reduction and internal fixation are mandatory.

3. Total talar dislocation must be reduced without delay due to the danger of compromising the overlying skin. Closed reduction is extremely difficult but may be possible by plantar flexing and inverting the foot while applying strong pressure directly over the displaced talus. If closed reduction is not successful, immediate open reduction must be done.

*Fractures of the Calcaneus*

## Definition

*Tuberosity Joint Angle.* This is the angle formed by two lines, one from the anterior articulation to the subtalar joint, the other from the posterior tuberosity to the subtalar joint. The normal angle is 140 to 160 degrees. The complement angle (tuber or salient angle) is 20 to 40 degrees.

## Basic Principles

Fractures of the calcaneus (os calcis) usually result from a fall from a height with the patient landing on the heel. The importance of these injuries lies in the marked permanent disability they produce, consisting of decreased function and painful arthritis. Varying degrees of injury can result, from undisplaced fissure fractures to severely comminuted crush injuries involving complete disruption of the subtalar joint surface. Crush fractures demonstrate severe depression of the bone, with widening of the heel and loss of the normal tuber angle. Tongue-like avulsion fractures ("beak neck" fractures) of the posterior attachment of the Achilles tendon are also seen.

## Criteria for Diagnosis

1. History of direct trauma to the heel, as in a jump from a height
2. Signs and symptoms of fracture in the heel and ankle. Blisters may develop rapidly.
3. X-rays are essential for proper diagnosis. An axial and lateral view are the minimum needed to evaluate lateral spread.
4. X-rays of the lumbodorsal spine and pelvis should always be done because of the frequent association of fractures of these bones with this type of injury. Neurologic examination of the lower extremity likewise should be performed routinely and recorded.

## Management

1. All calcaneal fractures, regardless of type, are treated initially by elevation and compression dressing for 3 to 5 days to reduce the severe swelling which invariably occurs.
2. Undisplaced fractures are treated thereafter by crutch ambulation without weight bearing on the involved extremity for at least 6 weeks. If the fracture line extends into a joint, weight bearing may be delayed even longer. Joint exercises are begun early to minimize subsequent stiffness.
3. Depressed, comminuted fractures of the calcaneus with loss of tuber angle are difficult to reduce, either by closed or open methods.

A. If broadening of the heel is severe due to lateral and medial spreading of the fragments, closed manipulation by compressing the heel between both hands can correct this displacement; the subtalar disruption and depression usually are not amenable to reduction.

B. A compression dressing is applied after the lateral spread is narrowed, and the foot is elevated until pain and swelling subside.

C. Crutch ambulation without weight bearing on the involved foot is then begun, continuing the use of an elastic bandage on the foot and ankle.

D. Joint motion is encouraged but weight bearing is avoided for up to three months.

E. Despite the distressing appearance of the x-ray in these fractures, it is remarkable how often compression dressing, elevation and early mobilization will result in a reasonably functional foot.

F. If subsequent pain and disability are severe, a subtalar or triple arthrodesis may be necessary.

4. Dorsally displaced, tongue-like fractures of the posterior tuberosity are best treated by open reduction and internal fixation of the fragment to restore the insertion of the Achilles tendon.

### Fractures of the Metatarsals

## Basic Principles

Fractures of the metatarsal bones result from direct trauma or falls. One or multiple bones may be broken, with the fractures involving the shaft or neck of the bone. The closeness of the bones usually prevents displacement.

Insidious and often unrecognized fractures of the second, third or fourth metatarsal may occur without a history of injury due to prolonged stress such as occurred during initial recruit bivouac marches, hence the eponym "march" fractures. They are not displaced and usually show significant callus formation when first discovered.

Avulsion fractures of the base of the fifth metatarsal are due to severe inversion stress of the foot. The small fragment attached to the peroneus brevis tendon usually is not significantly displaced.

## Criteria for Diagnosis

1. History of acute direct or prolonged foot trauma
2. Signs and symptoms of fracture of the foot. In "march" fractures there is pain on standing and walking after prolonged exercise and frequently a palpable lump.
3. Anteroposterior and oblique views are necessary for proper diagnosis.

## Management

1. Undisplaced metatarsal fractures are treated by elevation until the swelling subsides. A short leg walking plaster cast is then applied for 6 weeks.
2. Displaced metatarsal fractures should be accurately reduced to maintain normal weight-bearing surfaces and to prevent subsequent painful disability. If closed reduction fails to achieve good position, open reduction and internal fixation with Kirschner wires are indicated. After reduction of displaced fractures, the short leg cast which is applied should not have a heel for weight bearing for the first two weeks.
3. March fractures are treated by a short leg walking cast for 3 to 6 weeks, depending on the extent of callus at the time the fracture is first discovered.
4. Fractures of the base of the fifth metatarsal may be treated by crutch ambulation and an elastic bandage until weight bearing without pain (usually after two weeks) is possible. A short leg walking cast may be applied instead for convenience in ambulation.

### Fractures and Dislocations of the Phalanges

## Basic Principles

Fractures of the phalanges occur from direct blows such as falling objects or striking the foot against a solid object. Fractures of the great toe and fifth toe are the most common. Displacement is unusual.

Dislocations of the phalanges are rare, occurring occasionally at the great toe metatarsophalangeal joint or at the interphalangeal joints of one of the toes.

## Criteria for Diagnosis

1. History of direct injury to the foot

2. Signs and symptoms of fracture in the toe or toes. In fractures of the distal phalanx, a subungual hematoma may be present. Dislocations display obvious deformity.

3. Anteroposterior and oblique views (or lateral view with a dental film and dental x-ray machine) are necessary for accurate diagnosis.

**Management**

1. Undisplaced fractures are treated by securing the fractured toe to the adjacent toe with adhesive tape, making sure to place gauze padding between the toes. The shoe is fitted with a one-half inch metatarsal bar behind the metatarsal heads to allow walking without pain. If a subungual hematoma is present and severely painful, a hole made in the nail under sterile conditions will permit drainage and relief of pain. An opened paper clip heated by a lighted alcohol sponge until red hot is the simplest method of draining subungual hematomas.

2. Displaced fractures of the toes can be reduced by closed means under digital block anesthesia. Occasionally, reduction of the hallux can only be maintained by application of continuous skeletal traction. This is accomplished by placing a pin through the distal phalanx, or by placing a steel suture through the nail, and applying traction to the pin or suture with a rubber band attached to a metal loop extending from a short leg cast. Reduction of displaced fractures of the smaller toes usually can be maintained by taping to adjacent toes and heel ambulation for 3 weeks.

3. Phalangeal dislocations should be reduced by closed methods and the position should be maintained by taping. Occasionally, open reduction may be necessary. Unreduced dislocations can result in permanent painful disability.

# 26. MAXILLOFACIAL FRACTURES

*In-Chul Song,* M.D.
*Bertram E. Bromberg,* M.D.

## Definition

Maxillofacial fractures generally are the result of severe trauma about the face and are frequently associated with varying degrees of soft tissue injury. Included in the facial skeletal complexes are the mandible, maxilla, zygoma, zygomatic arch and nose. The fracture may be single or multiple, depending on the direction and impact of the producing force.

## Basic Principles

The greater percentage of maxillofacial injuries are caused by speeding automobile and motorcycle accidents. The victims involved in a high-speed vehicular accident are most likely to have multiple body injuries in addition to the facial trauma. Obviously, these patients should receive immediate care for the urgent associated life-threatening injuries, such as those to the head, spinal cord, chest, abdomen and major skeletal system. The definitive repair of maxillofacial fractures can be delayed until the patient's general condition improves after administering essential immediate care.

Early reduction and dependable immobilization are the most important basic principles in the management of all fractures of the facial bones. Successful treatment of maxillofacial skeletal injuries must provide normal function and restoration of an acceptable external appearance. If strict and meticulous attention is not given to the initial adequate reduction and repair, permanent and tragic facial disfigurement and functional disability may result.

## Criteria for Diagnosis

1. *History.* Etiology is important in assessing the extent of the injury and in planning further management. The direc-

tion of the blow or fall and its speed, force and impact will often provide a fair pattern of the damage. An accurate history, including past traumatic history, will frequently eliminate unnecessary attempts at reducing a pre-existing deformity.

2. *Inspection*

A. A flattened or widened nasal dorsum or a markedly displaced nose is usually the result of a fracture.

B. A flattened malar prominence is generally the result of a displaced malar fracture.

C. Elongation of the midface is usually the result of a fractured maxilla.

D. Asymmetry, particularly in the malar and mandibular areas, represents underlying fractures. Local swelling may camouflage the deformity, but generally the irregularity can be diagnosed on palpation.

E. Malocclusion—occlusal relationship can be utilized effectively in diagnosing fractures of the maxilla and mandible.

3. *Malfunction*

A. Difficulty in opening the mouth can be caused by trismus, yet fractures of the mandible, especially of the condyloid process, or depressed fractures of the zygomatic arch impinging on the coronoid process of the mandible should be suspected.

B. Locking of the jaws in the open position may indicate a dislocation of the temporomandibular joint, a situation requiring prompt reduction.

C. Deviation of the chin point on opening the mouth frequently is indicative of a fracture of the mandible.

4. *Soft Tissue Injuries.* Ecchymosis of the skin, subconjunctival hemorrhage and edema in and around the orbit, nose, malar

complex, maxilla or mandible require further examination to rule out facial fractures.

5. *Ocular Signs*

A. Enophthalmos or eye level discrepancy may indicate a displaced fracture of the midface or a blowout type of fracture of the infraorbital plate.

B. Proptosis may indicate a possible retrobulbar hemorrhage.

C. A deep anterior chamber on globe examination may represent a dislocation of the lens or a rupture of the globe.

6. *Palpation.* Careful and systematic palpation of the facial skeletal structures, both externally and intra-orally, is one of the most important maneuvers in establishing the diagnosis of facial bone fractures. Gradual gentle pressure over the swollen soft tissue generally provides an outline of the bony framework. The examination by palpation should be accomplished with both hands when examining the patient's nose, orbit, malar prominence, zygomatic arch, temporomandibular joint and external mandible. The comparative evaluation of both sides of the face will provide a better appreciation of fracture displacement. The following findings are definite indications of fracture:

A. Displacement of a bony segment

B. Bony irregularity

C. Abnormal motion

D. Crepitus on palpation

E. Sensory deficiency within a particular nerve distribution

7. *X-ray Examination.* X-ray examination is absolutely essential in a patient with suspected facial bone fractures. When the patient has a concomitant major injury, x-ray evaluation should be delayed until the patient's general condition permits. Frequently, due to superimposition of the facial bone structures, fractures can be missed unless proper views and high-quality x-rays are obtained. Tomography is particularly valuable in the diagnosis of fractures of the orbital floor and condyle. Panoramic jaw x-rays are important in

eliminating superimposed bony structures, thus allowing easier identification of fracture sites.

*Suggested X-rays in Fractures of the Facial Bones:*

A. *Nasal Bone*

(1) Superior-inferior view

(2) Lateral view

(3) Occlusal view

B. *Mandible*

(1) Posteroanterior view

(2) Lateral oblique view

(3) Towne's view for ascending rami and condyles

(4) Occlusal view of the anterior mandible, particularly in symphysis fractures

(5) Tomography of the temporomandibular joint if further study is indicated

(6) Panorex view if needed

C. *Maxilla and Malar Complex*

(1) Water's view (30-degree and 60-degree occipitomental views of the face)

(2) Posteroanterior view

(3) Lateral view

D. *Zygomatic Arch*

Submental vertex view

## Management

### Early Emergency Care

1. *Establishment of an Adequate Airway*

A. Respiratory obstruction is common in severe maxillofacial injuries due to the following reasons:

*(1)* Massive edema and/or hematoma around the tongue, soft palate and pharynx

*(2)* Accumulating blood clots, vomitus or dentures in the oral cavity, especially in comatose or semi-comatose patients

*(3)* Retrodisplacement of the tongue in bilateral mandibular fractures

*(4)* Retrodisplacement of the palatal structures in maxillary fractures

B. Generally airway obstruction can be relieved by placing the patient in the prone or side position so that blood or secretions from the oral cavity can be evacuated and the tongue permitted to resume its forward position by the force of gravity.

C. Blood clots and secretions should be promptly suctioned and foreign bodies removed.

D. The tongue may have to be pulled forward manually to further clear the air passage. Frequently, a towel clip or heavy suture placed in the anterior third of the tongue will assist in this procedure.

E. In cases of airway obstruction due to severe retrodisplacement of maxillary or mandibular fragments, the fractured segment may have to be pulled forward to ensure a clear airway.

F. If the above maneuvers fail, tracheostomy should be performed immediately.

2. *Control of Bleeding*

A. Direct pressure or packing will usually control bleeding temporarily.

B. Severe hemorrhage from either the external maxillary or superficial temporal artery can be controlled by exposure and ligation.

C. Reduction of the displaced fractured segments may be necessary to control intra-oral bleeding.

D. Severe and uncontrollable bleeding arising from the internal maxillary artery may necessitate ligation of the external carotid artery.

3. *Treatment of Shock*

A. Shock is rare in the isolated facial skeletal fracture.

B. When a patient with non-hemorrhaging maxillofacial trauma is found in a state of shock, treatment must be undertaken immediately and the patient then evaluated for other concomitant injuries more apt to produce such a condition.

4. *Management of Pain*

A. Analgesic medication such as 50 mg. of Demerol every 4 hours or 65 mg. of Darvon every 4 hours should suffice for the control of pain.

B. Sedatives or analgesics should not be used in patients with respiratory distress or associated central nervous system injury.

## Management of Associated Trauma

Associated injuries which require the urgent attention of the surgeon prior to definite management of maxillofacial injuries are:

1. Cranial injuries
2. Spinal cord injuries
3. Thoracic and/or abdominal injuries
4. Skeletal injuries
5. Eye injuries
6. Massive soft tissue injuries

## FRACTURES OF THE NASAL BONE
### Classification

1. Simple fractures
2. Open fractures
3. Comminuted fractures
4. Fracture or displacement of the nasal septum

### Basic Principles

The nasal bones are the most commonly fractured bones of the face. If the patient is seen early, reduction and immobilization should be performed at once, but if marked edema is noted, it is better to wait until the edema subsides. Nasal bone displacements can be successfully reduced up to 2 weeks following the injury without undue difficulty.

### Criteria for Diagnosis

1. Local swelling
2. Tenderness
3. Ecchymosis
4. Deformity
5. Epistaxis
6. Crepitus
7. Movable nasal bones
8. Depressions and lateral displacements are the usual bony irregularities noted.

## Management

Undisplaced fractures or fractures with minimum displacement without apparent external deformity do not require treatment (Fig. 26-1).

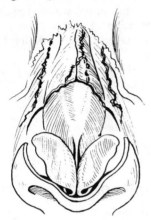

Fig. 26-1.

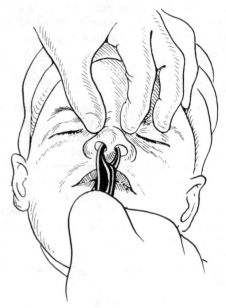

Fig. 26-2.

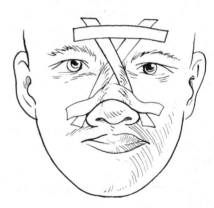

Fig. 26-3.

1. Provide local anesthesia with 1% lidocaine with 1:100,000 epinephrine, supplemented by topical anesthesia of the nasal mucosa with 10% cocaine and topical epinephrine in equal parts.

2. General anesthesia is preferable in children.

3. The majority of nasal fractures can be reduced by closed methods.

4. Generally, the fractures can be readily reduced by placing Asche forceps or the back of a long knife handle intranasally under the nasal bone along with external digital manipulation. In addition, if the septum is displaced as a result of the fracture, this structure should also be reduced by instrumentation (Fig. 26-2).

5. Open reduction is rarely required except in children if a fracture displacement of the nasal septum is associated with hematoma formation. In this instance, open reduction as well as evacuation of the hematoma should be carried out immediately.

6. Upon completion of the reduction, intranasal packing with Vaseline gauze strips is desirable.

7. An external splint device of some sort is generally indicated (Fig. 26-3).

8. The nasal packing is ordinarily removed in 2 to 3 days and the splinting device eliminated at 6 to 7 days.

9. In severely comminuted nasal fractures, the egg-shell-type fragments may have to be held together after reduction with metal plates or buttons placed on each side of the nose and fastened with wire transfixion sutures.

## FRACTURES OF THE MANDIBLE

### Classification

1. Closed fractures
2. Open fractures
3. Open comminuted fractures
4. *Anatomical Classification in Order of Frequency*
   A. Fracture of the condylar process
   B. Fracture of the body
   C. Fracture of the angle
   D. Fracture of the symphysis
   E. Fracture of the alveolus
   F. Fracture of the ascending ramus
   G. Fracture of the coronoid process

### Basic Principles

Fractures of the mandible are the second most common fracture seen in the facial bones despite the fact that the mandible is the strongest of the bones. The fracture sites are frequently bilateral and generally painful. Displacements of the fractured segments are more marked in this area due to the pull of the muscles of mastication in addition to the force of the offending trauma.

### Criteria for Diagnosis

1. Unlike other facial fractures, patients with mandibular fractures complain of pain on movement or manipulation of the lower jaw.
2. Mild to severe malocclusion is frequently noted as well as the displacement of the fractured segment. Patients usually are able to detect an abnormal bite.
3. Soft tissue edema, ecchymosis and hematoma are frequently observed at the fracture site.
4. Deformity with crepitation is readily noted or palpated, along with abnormal mobility.
5. Pain and/or crepitation in the temporomandibular joint region when the jaw is being opened and closed frequently indicate a condylar fracture. By placing the tip of the finger within the external auditory canal during opening and closing the jaw, lack of mobility of the condyle and

pain are frequently noted in fractures in this area.
6. Deviation of the jaw from the midline on opening the mouth is often indicative of a fracture displacement of the condylar neck. The jaw usually deviates to the fractured side.
7. All mandibular fractures should be confirmed by x-ray.

### Management

Prompt reduction and firm immobilization of these fractures should be achieved as soon as the patient's general condition permits. The ultimate goal is normal occlusion and satisfactory anatomical alignment.

1. *Barton's Bandage.* This measure can be utilized to limit jaw movement as an emergency procedure. Beware, however, of creating retrodisplacement and airway obstruction.
2. *Intermaxillary Fixation*
   A. This is the simplest and safest method of treatment of fractures of the body of the mandible.
   B. Closed reduction with intermaxillary fixation can be satisfactorily carried out with mild sedation with or without local anesthesia.
   C. Where teeth are present on either side of the fracture site, No. 25 stainless steel wires are twisted around the necks of the teeth of both jaws and then firmly fixed together.
   (1) Fixation can also be accomplished with orthodontic rubber bands and this method is an effective means of obtaining slow traction when further reduction is required. By properly directioned rubber-band traction, applied persistently and slowly, gradual satisfactory occlusal relationships can be obtained.
   (2) The rubber bands can be subsequently replaced with wire, because the wire provides better immobilization and ease in maintaining oral hygiene.
   (3) On the other hand, rubber bands can be more readily cut if the immobilization must be disrupted in an

emergency, such as a possibility of the patient aspirating after vomiting.

*(4)* The Water-Pik machine is helpful in maintaining oral hygiene, which is essential during all phases of care.

*(5)* Intermaxillary fixation may be used alone or in combination with open reduction and interosseous wiring.

D. When the patient is missing teeth or the dental condition is poor, arch bars are ligated to the necks of the teeth for support in fixation.

*(1)* The incisors should not be used for wire ligation because they possess unstable single conical roots and the danger of extraction is real.

*(2)* The arch bar is fashioned to conform to the root-crown junction of the teeth prior to ligation.

*(3)* Such arch bar fixation can be used in the great majority of mandibular fractures and even in some undisplaced unfavorable angle fractures and undisplaced symphysis fractures.

E. In partially edentulous patients, the arch bars can be incorporated into dental acrylic splints to prevent overriding of the edentulous segment.

*(1)* Frequently in edentulous patients, their own dentures or a manufactured acrylic splint can be used for space maintenance and fixation.

*(2)* Circum-mandibular wiring with a long Keith needle may be used for fixation of the lower dentures or splint.

*(3)* The upper denture or splint can be immobilized by circum-zygomatic wire suspension or direct wiring through the maxilla.

*(4)* Intermaxillary fixation should be maintained for 4 to 8 weeks, depending on the status of the bony union.

3. *Anterior Fixation*

A. This is a simple and effective technique which can be utilized for immobilization in mandibular fractures in the edentulous adult or the patient with extremely poor dental hygiene.

B. It is also applicable in young children with a deciduous dentition.

C. The fixation points are the buccal cortex of the anterior portion of the maxilla adjacent to the base of the nasal spine and the symphysis of the mandible.

*(1)* One No. 25 stainless steel wire is threaded through the buccal cortex of the anterior portion of the maxilla about ½ to 1 centimeter below the level of the nasal spine and the wire is snugged down in a clockwise direction.

*(2)* A circum-mandibular wire is then placed at the midsymphysis region and twisted at root level in between the lower central incisors.

D. When general anesthesia has been administered, intermaxillary fixation is delayed until the patient is fully recovered from anesthesia.

E. In local anesthesia cases, the wires from the upper and lower jaws can be immediately twisted together to obtain intermaxillary fixation in the proper alignment and occlusion.

F. If a denture or an acrylic dental splint is used for immobilization, it is placed in a position and locked between the maxilla and mandible.

G. The wire can be tightened or adjusted as required.

H. This method may also be used for supplemental intermaxillary fixation after open reduction.

4. *Open Reduction*

A. Open reduction with interosseous wiring is indicated in a displaced fracture which cannot be reduced and maintained by closed reduction. The open reduction should always be supported by intermaxillary fixation for 4 to 8 weeks in the most optimal occlusion and bony alignment.

B. Kirshner wire fixation is used in severe multiple fractures of the mandible. Insertion of a K-pin in shishkabob fashion in the early phase of trauma is useful. This method will suffice until the patient's general condition improves and more definitive reduction and immobilization can be obtained.

C. *External Skeletal Fixation.* In a

patient with a missing segment of bone, a Roger-Anderson-type of external fixation will maintain the space required for later reconstruction with a bone graft.

D. *Anesthesia.* In open reduction and for procedures carried out in children, it is advisable to administer general anesthesia. Intermaxillary fixation should be delayed until the patient is fully recovered from the anesthesia in order to avoid emesis aspiration.

E. *Postoperative Care*

(1) Antibiotics should be routinely administered for 2 weeks: ampicillin, 500 mg. b.i.d. for 2 weeks; streptomycin, 500 mg. b.i.d. for 1 week.

(2) Check on tetanus prophylaxis (*see* Chap. 10, Soft Tissue Injuries).

(3) Analgesics as necessary

(4) High-protein, high-caloric, liquid diet

F. *Oral Hygiene.* Cleansing of the mouth and teeth should be performed after each feeding and in between feedings. Commercial mouthwashes or ½-strength hydrogen peroxide can be used. The Water-Pik is extremely effective in maintaining excellent oral hygiene. Post-reduction x-rays must be obtained.

5. *Removal of the Intermaxillary Fixation*

A. After 4 to 8 weeks of jaw immobilization, radiographic examination is secured and a clinical evaluation made.

B. If sufficient evidence of bony union is present, the intermaxillary fixation between the upper and lower jaws may be removed, leaving the eyelets or arch bars in place.

C. Again, the patient is evaluated clinically for bony union. If the fracture is firm, the patient is placed on a soft diet and re-evaluated in 1 week. If the fracture remains firm over the next week, the patient's diet is gradually increased to normal within a 2-week period.

D. Any evidence of nonunion or delayed healing requires further intermaxillary fixation until bony union takes place.

## FRACTURE OF THE ANGLE OF THE MANDIBLE WITH DISPLACEMENT

### Basic Principles

When the line of the fracture runs in a direction parallel to the masseter muscle at the angle of the mandible, the proximal fragment is readily displaced upward due to traction of the masseter, external pterygoid and temporal muscles. This is called an unfavorable fracture of the angle and open reduction is indicated (Fig. 26-4).

### Management

1. Open reduction and interosseous wiring should be performed through a sub-mandibular incision located approximately a fingerbreadth below the border of the mandible.

2. The interosseous wiring is achieved by drilling 4 holes, 2 in each segment proximal and distal to the fracture site at the inferior one third of the mandible.

3. Wiring is performed in crisscross fashion to obtain firm maintenance of the reduction.

4. No. 25 stainless steel wire is used and always twisted in a clockwise direction.

5. The mandibular branch of the facial nerve should be preserved and the periosteum should be well reflected from the fracture site prior to wiring.

6. The evacuation of hematoma and foreign bodies is essential for an adequate reduction and ultimate successful bony union at the fracture site.

## FRACTURE OF THE SYMPHYSIS OF THE MANDIBLE

### Basic Principles

The pull of the digastric, geniohyoid and mylohyoid muscles tends to displace the fractures through the symphysis in a downward and backward direction (Fig. 26-5).

### Management

1. Fractures through the symphysis are best treated by open reduction with criss-

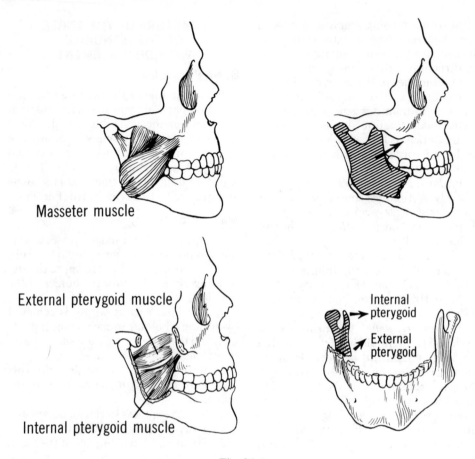

Masseter muscle

External pterygoid muscle

Internal pterygoid muscle

Internal pterygoid

External pterygoid

Fig. 26-4.

cross interosseous wiring along with inter-maxillary fixation for 4 to 8 weeks.

2. A curved incision about 1 finger-breadth below the border of the symphysis gives excellent exposure and a hidden scar postoperatively.

## DISLOCATION OF THE TEMPOROMANDIBULAR JOINTS

### Basic Principles

Acute dislocation or chronic habitual dislocation of the temporomandibular joint may occur without fracture. Yawning is a leading cause, locking the jaw bilaterally in a painful open position.

### Management

1. The reduction is performed under sedation by placing the gauze-wrapped thumbs of both hands intra-orally over the molar region and reducing by a downward and forward movement followed by a backward movement into normal position.

2. Occasionally a patient may require general anesthesia if the attempt at reduction under sedation fails.

3. Restricted jaw opening is obtained with an external elastic bandage for the next 2 weeks.

4. Chronic habitual dislocation may require eventual operative intervention.

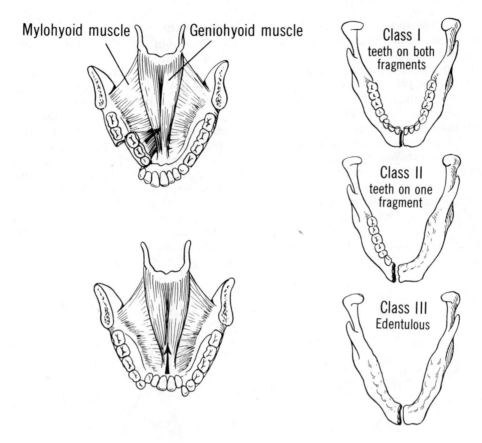

Fig. 26-5.

## FRACTURES OF THE ZYGOMA (MALAR BONE)

### Classification

1. *Simple Fractures.* The zygomatic complex fracture is usually tripod in type and is frequently associated with posterior, inferior and medial displacement.

2. *Comminuted Fractures.* Generally, these are similar to the simple fracture, but characteristically there is an egg-shell-type of fracture in the infraorbital plate as well as disruption of the infraorbital rim. In addition, the patient may disclose an obvious or palpable defect in the infraorbital region.

### Basic Principles

The zygoma is the third most commonly fractured bone in the facial skeleton. Fracture sites occur in the lateral orbit, the infraorbital margin and along the floor of the orbit. The anterior antral wall and the temporal process are frequently broken.

### Criteria for Diagnosis

1. Soft tissue swelling and ecchymosis are generally present, particularly in the periorbital region.

2. Flattening of the cheek prominence. Often by looking downward over the patient's forehead, a depression will be noted.

3. A depression or separation at the lateral or infraorbital rim is readily palpable.

4. Anesthesia of the upper lip and upper teeth may be present due to contusion or severance of the infraorbital nerve.

5. Diplopia may result if there is a depression of the orbital floor.

6. Difficulty in opening the mouth may be present from impingement on the coronoid process by a depressed fracture.

7. Intra-oral examination over the canine fossa may reveal a ridge or a depression at the zygomatic-maxillary suture line.

8. X-ray confirmation is necessary.

**Management**

1. *Reduction by the Temporal Approach* (Gillies' elevation, Fig. 26-6)

A. Simple depressed fractures of the zygoma and zygomatic arch can be reduced successfully by this method.

B. A ½-inch incision into the temporal fascia is made through a prepared shaved area in the temporal region.

C. Access is gained by sliding a Gillies' elevator under the heavy fascia and, with the fingertips of the other hand as a guide, the depressed fracture can be manually reduced.

D. For reduction of a simple W-shaped depressed fracture of the zygomatic

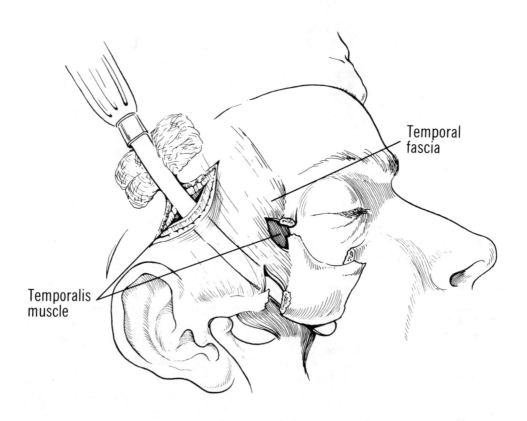

Temporal fascia

Temporalis muscle

Fig. 26-6.

arch, the elevator is similarly placed at the site of maximum depression and elevated.

2. *Reduction by the Antral Approach*

A. Through an incision in the upper buccal sulcus, an antral window is formed over the canine fossa after reflecting the mucoperiosteum.

B. A depressed fracture is reduced utilizing a Gillies' elevator (following evacuation of any hematoma or free bony fragments).

C. Irrigation of the antral cavity and inspection of the infraorbital plate for any bony disruption is an important next step.

D. The antral cavity is then packed with alcohol-washed, 1-inch iodoform gauze for support of the infraorbital floor and prevention of recurrent hematoma formation. The packing should be placed loosely and the end is brought out through the operative incision intra-orally or through a nasal antrostomy. Overpacking may cause overcorrection of the fracture and even proptosis.

E. The antral packing is usually removed in 7 to 14 days.

3. *Open Reduction*

A. An incision along a skin fold of the lower eyelid and a semicircular incision along the superior lateral orbital margin will provide excellent direct visualization of the fracture.

B. The periosteum is reflected at the site of bony irregularity and drill holes are made on both sides of the fracture.

C. The fractured segments are elevated and firmly brought together with stainless steel wire.

D. Elevation of an impacted fracture is achieved by placing an elevator behind the zygomatic complex through the lateral orbital incision.

E. In a blowout-type of infraorbital fracture with herniation of the orbital contents into the antral cavity, it is generally necessary to reduce the herniated orbital contents and place an infraorbital implant. The implants generally used are either autogenous iliac bone, cartilage or some

synthetic material such as Silastic or Teflon sheet.

F. When there is a badly comminuted fracture of the infraorbital plate along with a zygomatic complex fracture, open reduction with interosseous wiring can be supplemented by antral packing.

4. *Postoperative Care*

A. A protective device should be maintained over the operative site for 2 to 7 days.

B. Antibiotics are used when the fracture is associated with extensive soft tissue injury.

C. Tetanus prophylaxis is administered.

D. Analgesics are generally necessary.

E. Postreduction x-rays are necesary.

## FRACTURES OF THE MAXILLA

### Classification

Fractures of the maxilla are usually bilateral, although there are rare instances of unilateral fracture with separation of the midline of the hard palate. Maxillary fractures are generally classified according to the description of LeFort for convenience of diagnosis and treatment planning (Fig. 26-7).

1. *LeFort I Maxillary Fracture.* This is a transverse fracture of the maxilla and involves the entire segment of the palatal bone and alveolar process.

2. *LeFort II Maxillary Fracture.* This is a pyramidal fracture of the maxilla and involves the entire maxillary complex.

3. *LeFort III Maxillary Fracture.* This is a cranio-facial separation and involves the entire midface, including the nasal bones and both zygomatic and maxillary complexes.

### Basic Principles

Although maxillary fractures are the least common fractures of the facial skeleton, they bear significance since they are frequently associated with other facial

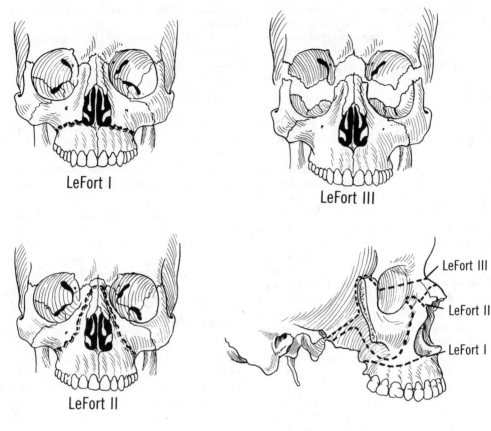

LeFort I

LeFort III

LeFort II

LeFort III
LeFort II
LeFort I

Fig. 26-7.

bone fractures and often with intracranial injuries. The leading causes of maxillary fractures are high-speed vehicular accidents, and the pattern of displacement is generally determined by the direction of the offending force and the anatomical strength and weakness of the bone itself.

## Criteria for Diagnosis

1. There is usually marked swelling and ecchymosis of the periorbital region and cheeks.

2. Malocclusion results from the displaced segments of the maxilla.

3. Epistaxis and/or cerebrospinal rhinorrhea are often present in cases of craniofacial dysfunction.

4. Elongation of the face or dish-face deformity is commonly noted in markedly displaced fractures.

5. Ordinarily there are mobility and crepitation at the fracture sites on examination. By grasping the anterior portion of the maxilla between the index finger and the thumb of one hand intra-orally while the other hand is stabilizing the head, the maxilla is gently rocked in and out or up and down. Motion is elicited in the majority of maxillary fractures if they are not seriously impacted.

6. Depression or separation at the orbital rims may be palpated in LeFort II and III fractures.

7. X-ray confirmation is necessary.

## Management

The objectives of therapy are re-establishment of the normal anatomical alignment of the maxilla, particularly facial length, and restoration of normal occlusion.

1. *LeFort I Maxillary Fractures*

A. Following reduction of the fracture with maxillary forceps, immobilization is obtained by the application of arch bars and intermaxillary fixation.

B. Further fixation can be obtained by circum-zygomatic arch or lateral orbital rim suspension to the arch bars.

(1) Percutaneous circum-zygomatic arch suspension is done with No. 25 stainless steel wire in the following manner.

(2) A long needle is fastened to each end of the wire and the needle is passed under the skin into the mouth.

(3) Both needles should enter the skin at the identical site, one needle passing over the arch and the other below the arch, entering the mouth through the buccal sulcus at the premolar level.

(4) The subcutaneous tissue caught between the wire and the zygomatic arch can be cut through by pulling both ends of wire back and forth prior to fixing to the arch bar.

(5) Lateral orbital suspension can be accomplished by making a small skin incision along the lateral orbital process of the frontal bone.

(6) After drilling a small hole through the lateral orbital rim above the anatomical frontozygomatic suture line, a No. 25 stainless steel wire is passed through the hole and passed behind the zygoma over the canine fossa into the buccal sulcus.

(7) Fixation is secured by anchoring the wires to the maxillary arch bar.

2. *LeFort II Maxillary Fractures*

A. Similar procedures as described for the LeFort I fractures can be utilized for the reduction and fixation of the pyramidal LeFort II fracture of the maxilla.

B. Fractures of the infraorbital rim can be treated by open reduction and direct interosseous wiring.

3. *LeFort III Maxillary Fracture*

A. Generally, it is advisable to disimpact and to reduce all of the fractured bones prior to fixation.

B. Direct bone wiring at the front-ozygomatic suture line or the lateral orbit should be performed as necessary.

C. Arch bar application and intermaxillary fixation should be established before suspending the maxillary segment to the nearest cephalad solid bony structure, which is generally the zygomatic process of the frontal bone.

D. Fractures of the nasal bones and the zygomatic complex should be reduced and immobilized as previously described during the same operation procedure.

E. Proper vertical dimension must be maintained so as not to shorten the midface as the maxillary segment is stabilized by tightening the suspension wires. Overtightening can also be dangerous if antral packing has been employed prior to the suspension of the maxilla.

F. If a mandibular fracture is associated with a LeFort III injury, the mandibular fracture should be reduced and immobilized and baseline occlusion established prior to reducing and immobilizing the maxillary fracture.

G. Fixation should be maintained for a period of 4 to 8 weeks, depending upon the healing process.

4. The technique of Kirshner wire fixation or external skeletal fixation with a head cap is rarely indicated in maxillary fractures.

5. *Postoperative Care*

A. Liquid diet is necessary during the intermaxillary fixation period.

B. Antibiotics are generally indicated if the fractures are compounded.

C. Tetanus prophylaxis should be administered.

D. Meticulous oral hygiene is necessary.

E. Analgesics are generally necessary.

F. Postreduction x-rays should be obtained.

# 27. DENTAL EMERGENCIES

*Martin Protell,* D.D.S.
*J. Gordon Rubin,* D.D.S.

## Definition

Dental emergencies involve either pain or discomfort, swelling, hemorrhage or esthetic problems of the teeth, gums, mouth or jaw.

## Classification

Dental emergencies may be classified as either traumatic, pathologic or miscellaneous.

## Basic Principles

Dental emergencies are usually caused by trauma, decay, neglect or postoperative sequelae. Treatment should be instituted as soon as possible in order to relieve the symptoms and prevent further aggravation of the acute problem.

A suggested armamentarium to treat dental emergencies in a general emergency department is as follows:

Instruments

1. Mouth mirrors
2. Explorers, No. 5DE and No. 7DE
3. College pliers, No. 317 regular and serrated
4. High-speed dental handpieces
   A. Straight
   B. Contra-angle (frictional grip)
5. Spoon excavators, No. 17 and No. 19
6. Plastic instruments, Ladmone No. 4 and Woodson No. 2 and No. 3
7. Root-canal probes and files, No. 10, No. 15, No. 20, No. 25 and No. 30
8. Scalpel blades, No. 10, No. 11 and No. 12
9. Tissue forceps
10. Hemostats
11. Needle holders
12. Disposable saliva ejectors
13. Forceps, No. 65, No. 286, No. 18R, No. 18L, No. 32, No. 32A, No. 62, No. 115, No. 116, No. 117 and No. 123

14. Periosteal elevators, No. 34, No. 34S, No. 46, No. OHL, No. MOLT9, No. 78, No. 79, No. 80, No. 301, No. 302 and No. 303
15. Rubber mouth props, small, medium and large
16. Aspirator—oral suction
17. Pulp tester—vitalometer
18. Mixing spatulas, No. 5 and No. 7
19. Mixing pads, glazed and glass
20. Bunsen burner
21. Scissors, No. 15, Kelly No. 264 and No. 268, Crown and Collar No. 110 and No. 111
22. Orthodontic pliers—Cone socket No. 102, Hau crown No. 110 and No. 111
23. Crown remover, Morrell No. 60 and No. 712
24. Bone spicule forceps
25. Rongeur forceps No. 5 and Mead No. 1A
26. Bone curette—Lucas No. 85 and No. 87
27. Bone files—Howard No. 10 and No. 12

Supplies

1. Tongue blades
2. Gauze, assorted sizes (2" x 2", etc.)
3. Dental floss and tape
4. Cotton pellets and dispenser
5. Cotton rolls, No. 2 and No. 3
6. Local anesthetics
   A. Xylocaine, 1:50,000, 1:100,000; Citanest forte
   B. Topical anesthetics—Xylocaine ointment, flavored
7. Syringes—carpule holders
8. Needles, short in 30 gauge, long in 25 and 27 gauges
9. Burs, No. 2, No. 4, No. 6, No. 8, No. 17, No. 19, No. 556, No. 557 and No. 171
10. Sutures—black silk 3-0 and green Ethiflex 5-0

11. Iodoform gauze, Johnson & Johnson, 5%, ½-inch and 1-inch sterile

12. Rubber dam drains

13. Articulating paper, thin and thick

14. Temporary crowns

    A. Aluminum, No. 10 through No. 20

    B. Polycarbon (assorted anteriors)

15. Gutta-percha—base plate and sticks

16. Assorted polishing strips, disks and wheels

17. Cements—oxyphosphate and EBA

18. Radiographic films—periapical DF58

### Medicaments

1. Isopropyl alcohol

2. Creosote, N.F.

3. Phenol, liquefied, U.S.P.

4. Eugenol, U.S.P.

5. Zinc oxide powder, U.S.P.

6. Cavit

7. I.R.M.

8. Temerex, temporary cement

9. Hemostatic agents—Oxycel, Hemodent and Gelfoam dental packs, No. 2 and No. 4

10. Triamcinolone acetonide—Kenalog in Orabase, 0.1%

11. Denture adhesives, either paste or powder

12. Tincture of myrrh and benzoin in equal parts

13. Metaphen

14. Silver nitrate, 3%

15. Ethyl chloride spray

16. Calcium hydroxide, Pulpdent

17. Hydrogen peroxide, 3%

18. Epinephrine, 1:100,000

19. Benzodent ointment

20. Solution of guiacol and glycerin

21. Protein precipitants (thymol and zinc chloride)

### Criteria for Diagnosis

1. A brief medical history should be taken to determine general health, cardiovascular history, drugs that are being taken, allergies and any other pertinent information. The history should include:

A. When did the difficulty start?

B. How did the difficulty start?

C. What, if anything, has been done up to the present?

D. Is the difficulty changing?

2. Clinical examination should include a thorough visual examination and palpation of the affected area. In cases of swelling or suspected infection, the temperature and vital signs are checked. X-rays should be taken if possible.

### Management

Treatment depends upon the nature of the emergency, its severity and the treatment facilities available. When antibiotics are recommended, either (1) penicillin I.M. 600,000 to 1.2 million units, (2) erythromycin, 250 mg. every 4 hours, or (3) tetracycline, 250 mg. every 4 hours, is chosen depending on patient sensitivity and suspected organism. Anti-inflammatory enzyme therapy usually is Ananase-50, 2 tablets stat and 1 tablet q.i.d. for 2 days.

## TRAUMATIC INJURIES

Injuries are treated by relieving pain, stopping hemorrhage, controlling swelling, and immobilization to prevent further damage.

### OSSEOUS AND DENTAL INJURIES

#### *Tooth Fractures*

### Criteria for Diagnosis

1. Pain will be present if the tooth is vital and the pulp is affected.

2. Pain will be present upon palpation or percussion of nonvital teeth.

3. Thermal sensitivity. If the pulp is vital, it will react to hot and cold.

4. There may be hemorrhage and/or swelling in the area.

5. Sharp edges will be present because of the crazing of the enamel.

6. Tooth mobility may be present.

7. The tooth, or teeth, may be discolored as compared to the adjacent dentition.

## Management

1. Smooth any sharp edges with rubber polishing wheels to prevent further soft tissue damage.

2. Treat the exposed dentin with a protein precipitant (thymol or zinc chloride) to seal the dentinal tubules.

3. Immobilize loose teeth with ligature.

4. Cover exposed or fractured teeth, which are extremely sensitive, with a temporary crown filled with zinc oxide and eugenol. Polycarbon crown forms can be used for anterior teeth, and aluminum shells can be used for posterior teeth.

5. If the pulp is exposed, use a local anesthetic and place calcium hydroxide over the exposure and adjacent dentin and treat as in paragraph 4 above.

6. If infection is suspected, start antibiotic therapy.

### *Avulsed Teeth*

## Criteria for Diagnosis

1. A bleeding socket and/or a tooth missing

2. Pain

## Management

1. If the patient has the tooth, anesthetize and clean and swab the area with sterile saline. Remove the clot in the socket and replace the tooth in the socket and immobilize. Refer the patient to a dentist.

2. Begin antibiotic therapy.

3. Tetanus prophylaxis should be considered if contamination is suspected.

### *Jaw Fractures*

*See also* Chapter 26, Maxillofacial Fractures.

## Criteria for Diagnosis

1. Pain; impairment of function and limitation of mobility

2. Swelling, crepitation, deformity

3. Change in intermaxillary occlusal relationships

4. Deviation of the jaw

5. At times, one will see sharp bony projections and/or displacements.

## Management

1. X-ray of the mandible

2. Debridement if necessary

3. If possible, attempt to reposition the fragments by occlusion.

4. Immobilization with a bandage or splints. Definitive closed or open reduction by an oral surgeon usually is needed later.

5. Place the patient on a liquid diet.

6. Antibiotic therapy.

### SOFT TISSUE INJURY

## Criteria for Diagnosis

1. Pain

2. Swelling

3. Hemorrhage

4. Obvious laceration of the gums, cheek palate or tongue may be seen.

5. Infection may be present.

## Management

1. Anesthesia, if possible, for debridement

2. Hemostasis with cautery or ligature

3. Ice packs

4. Antibiotic therapy

5. Tetanus-prone wounds should be left open when it is impossible to remove all foreign material.

6. Smooth hard tissue edges that may contribute to further irritation.

7. When hematoma only is present, institute enzyme therapy.

### SOFT TISSUE BURNS

### *Thermal Burns*

## Criteria for Diagnosis

1. History of thermal injury

2. Pain

3. Coagulation necrosis of the tissue of the mouth or slough or simple redness, depending on the degree of injury

## Management

1. Cold irrigation of the mouth to limit injury

2. Palliative treatment for pain
3. Cover with triamcinolone ointment (Kenalog).
4. Bland diet

### Chemical Burns

### Criteria for Diagnosis

1. History of chemical ingestion
2. Pain is present.
3. Whitish area of necrosis with a reddish base
4. Occasionally slough is seen.

### Management

1. Thorough irrigation of the mouth to remove the corrosive agent
2. All other procedures are the same as for thermal burns, above.

## SOFT TISSUE HEMORRHAGE

### Criteria for Diagnosis

1. Active and profuse bleeding
2. Postextraction oozing
3. Lowered blood pressure
4. Shock

### Management

1. Epinephrine, 1:100,000 concentration, applied locally under pressure
2. Apply pressure packs.
3. Apply ice packs for 5 minutes, then remove for 5 minutes. Repeat as needed.
4. Cauterize the area if necessary to seal off hemorrhaging capillaries.
5. Pack the area with coagulants, such as Gelfoam or Oxycel.
6. Suture as a last resort.

## INFECTIONS
### CARIES

### Criteria for Diagnosis

1. Pain
2. Sensitivity to thermal changes
3. Sensitivity (pain responsive) to sweets
4. Clinically visual decay

### Management

1. Carefully remove soft decay.
2. Place an obtundent into the cavity (creosote on a pellet of cotton).
3. Cover with zinc oxide and eugenol paste as a temporary filling until such time as the patient can see a dentist for more definitive procedure and treatment.

## PULPITIS

### Criteria for Diagnosis

1. Pain of a pulsating and severe nature
2. Thermal sensitivity. Heat increases the pain and cold relieves it.
3. Sensitivity to pressure
4. Reactive to percussion
5. Pain will increase at night when the head is lowered.
6. Temperature may be elevated.

### Management

1. Open the pulp chamber and establish drainage.
2. Relieve the pressures of occlusion.
3. Prescribe analgesics.
4. Antibiotic therapy
5. Hot saline rinses
6. Application of ice packs on the outside of the face

## PERIAPICAL ABSCESSES

### Criteria for Diagnosis

1. The x-rays will show a radiolucent area over the root of the affected tooth.
2. Swelling
3. The symptoms of a pulpitis

### Management

1. Incise and drain the abscess if the swelling is pointed.
2. Treat as for pulpitis.

## PERIODONTAL ABSCESSES

### Criteria for Diagnosis

1. Swelling
2. Not as severely painful as a periapical abscess

3. The surrounding tissues are hypertrophied.

4. The tooth may be elevated and/or mobile.

5. Sensitive to percussion

6. Pain when contacting the opposing tooth

## Management

1. Local anesthetic

2. Attempt to curette the periodontal pocket.

3. Incise and drain.

4. Relieve occlusion.

5. Hot saline rinses

6. Judicious use of analgesics

7. Antibiotic therapy

## PERIODONTAL PATHOLOGY

*Pericoronitis (Third Molar Flaps)*

### Criteria for Diagnosis

1. Acute pain

2. Fever—adenopathy

3. Swelling of tissue around the third molar

4. Pain on closure and/or trismus

5. There may be an exudate present.

### Management

1. Cauterization either with chemicals (phenol and iodine) or surgical removal of the flap

2. Analgesics

3. Antibiotic therapy

4. Hot saline rinses every 3 hours

5. Application of ice packs

*Aphthous Ulcer (Canker Sores)*

### Criteria for Diagnosis

1. There are small, white vesicles, usually found on the tongue, floor of the mouth, cheeks and alveolar gingiva. The base of these vesicles is usually depressed and surrounded by a reddish area.

2. Acute pain and soreness

3. Fever

4. Pain is further increased by the ingestion of spicy, acid foods.

## Management

1. Chemical cautery (3% ammoniacal silver nitrate or phenol and alcohol)

2. Alkaline mouth wash

*Acute Ulcerative Necrotizing Gingivitis (Vincent's Angina or Trench Mouth)*

### Criteria for Diagnosis

1. Pain and inflammation

2. Fever and general malaise

3. Greyish ulceration in the interdental spaces

4. Gingival margins bleed easily.

5. Increase in the viscosity of the saliva

6. A metallic taste and a fetid odor

7. In severe cases, there is adenopathy of the submaxillary glands, as well as a thick coating on the dorsum of the tongue.

### Management

1. Analgesics and sedatives

2. Oxygenating mouth wash (1 part 3% peroxide to 2 parts warm water)

3. Antibiotic therapy if severe

4. Tranquilizers.

5. A bland diet, no smoking and no alcoholic beverages, including ale or beer

*Glossodynia (Burning Tongue)*

### Criteria for Diagnosis

1. Severe burning sensation and pain in the tongue, together with a loss of taste

2. An absence of any visible lesions

3. Complaints are usually of long standing.

4. Usually of psychogenic origin

5. Usually found in patients who are depressed, in women who are going through menopause and in men who are having climacteric or sexual problems

### Management

1. The patient should be permitted to air complaints fully. A detailed and complete history is essential.

2. If possible, prescribe tranquilizers, particularly antidepressants. Constantly

check for mouth dryness as a result of the treatment, which complicates the clinical problem.

3. Therapeutic doses of vitamin B complex

4. The signs and symptoms should be treated symptomatically.

5. If the complaints persist, refer the patient to a psychiatrist.

### *Neuralgias*

#### Criteria for Diagnosis

1. Pain, severe and/or perverted, along the nerve paths

2. Pains are usually more severe at night.

3. The pain may be penetrating, intermittent, paroxysmal or of a burning nature.

4. Neuralgia does not have to present any obvious dental pathology.

5. Neuralgias are usually of long standing.

6. Neuralgias usually have trigger points or areas.

#### Management

1. Sedation

2. Analgesics

3. At times, hot, wet epsom salts compresses applied repeatedly to the external area for 5 minutes and off for 10 minutes afford symptomatic relief.

### *Neuritis*

#### Criteria for Diagnosis

1. Numbness, burning and tingling of short duration of the terminal nerve endings

2. It is often associated with some form of neuralgia.

3. Neuritis is usually of short duration and has no trigger points.

#### Management

1. Sedation

2. Hot, wet packs

3. Analgesics

## MISCELLANEOUS CONDITIONS

## TEMPOROMANDIBULAR JOINT SYNDROME

#### Criteria for Diagnosis

1. A limitation of motion of the jaw

2. Pain upon opening the mouth, possibly radiating into the ear and temporal muscle, as well as into the auricular area

3. There may be swelling over the temporomandibular joint.

4. There may be complaints of muscle spasm or trismus.

5. Tenderness upon palpating the temporomandibular joint area

#### Management

1. Sedation

2. Analgesics

3. Intermittent use and application of hot, wet packs

4. When acute symptoms have subsided, muscle exercise may be instituted.

## JAW DISLOCATION

#### Criteria for Diagnosis

1. The patient is incapable of closing his mouth.

2. Condyles are locked forward of the articular eminence.

#### Management

1. Place the thumb of each hand on the occlusal surfaces of the mandibular molars.

2. Support the inferior borders of the mandible with the fingers of the hand.

3. Pressure should be applied downward and backward to allow the head of the condyle to slip back into position.

4. *Note:* wrap thumbs with layers of gauze to prevent damage to the thumbs when the jaws snap closed.

# 28. EMERGENCIES INVOLVING THE EAR, NOSE AND THROAT

*Maurice Cohen,* M. D.
*S. S. Giovinda Swamy,* M.D.

## TRAUMA TO THE NOSE AND PARANASAL SINUSES

### INJURIES TO THE EXTERNAL SURFACES OF THE NOSE

**Classification**

1. Contusions
2. Lacerations
3. Avulsions

**Management**

The treatment for simple injuries to the external surfaces of the nose is the same as for other parts of the body (*see* Chap. 10, Soft Tissue Injuries).

### INJURIES TO THE INTERNAL SURFACES OF THE NOSE

*Hematoma of the Septum*

**Definition**

Hematoma of the septum is bleeding into the nasal system.

**Basic Principles**

This is usually associated with injury to the nasal pyramid. Immediate surgical evacuation is necessary to avoid septal necrosis and possible abscess formation.

**Criteria for Diagnosis**

1. Pain
2. Nasal obstruction
3. Intranasal examination reveals septal fluctuation, hematoma and tenderness.

**Management**

1. Application of topical anesthesia (4% cocaine or 2% Pontocaine topically; 1% Xylocaine by infiltration)
2. Incision and drainage
3. Insertion of a small Penrose drain

4. Nasal packing to splint the nasal septum
5. Appropriate antibiotics (erythromycin, 250 mg. q.i.d.)
6. Analgesics
7. Referral to ENT specialists, if available

### NASAL FRACTURES

**Definition**

A nasal fracture is a break or rupture of the nasal bone. It may be simple, compound or comminuted.

**Basic Principles**

The degree of nasal bony deformity and direction of dislocation depend upon the direction and force of the trauma received. Nasal fracture is usually associated with an injury to the nasal septum.

**Criteria for Diagnosis**

1. *Clinical Criteria*
   A. History of trauma
   B. Pain in the nasal region
   C. Bleeding from the nose. This is more severe in septal injuries and compound fractures.
   D. Swelling and ecchymosis
   E. Nasal deformity
   F. Possible nasal obstruction, usually unilateral, especially with associated septal fracture dislocations

2. *X-ray Studies*
   *Lateral View and Waters' View.* The lateral view may be negative. If one still clinically suspects a fracture, then a Waters' view is done, together with tunnel views of the nose.

**Management**

1. *Early.* If the patient is seen before

severe swelling and ecchymosis develop, closed reduction can be carried out.

2. *Late.* After swelling and ecchymosis develop, we must await subsidence of this swelling. Satisfactory closed reduction can be achieved as late as two weeks after trauma.

3. Patients in poor condition may have the closed reduction delayed while attempts are made to improve the patient's general condition before nasal fracture reduction.

4. In poor-risk patients, especially in the aged, if there is no obstruction to the airway, surgery may be deferred provided the patient is willing to accept a cosmetic deformity.

5. Old healed fractures with unacceptable deformity or airway obstruction will require open reduction.

### Techniques of Reduction

For Adults

1. *Closed Reduction*
   A. Topical anesthesia, 2% Pontocaine or 1% Xylocaine with epinephrine (if not hypertensive) by infiltration
   B. The septum is realigned with Walsham forceps; nasal fragments are brought into place by using a Goldman displacer and Walsham or Asch forceps.
   C. Intranasal packing is applied for support.
   D. External adhesive and plaster dressing are applied to prevent further injury.
2. *Open Reduction*
   A. This is necessary if closed reduction fails.
   B. Detailed technical knowledge requires specialist consultation.

For Children

1. General anesthesia is necessary.
2. The remainder of closed manipulation is the same as above for adults.

### FRACTURES OF SINUSES

### Basic Principles

Paranasal sinuses may be involved in nasofacial fractures. The ethmoid sinuses are most commonly involved. There may be escape of spinal fluid through the nose due to fracture of the cribriform plate of the ethmoid, which may lead to recurrent bouts of meningitis.

### Criteria for Diagnosis

1. It is difficult to demonstrate these fractures by x-ray.
2. Subcutaneous emphysema may be a clue to diagnosis.
3. With a cerebrospinal fluid leak, a unilateral, usually clear, colorless fluid is seen escaping through the nose, intermittently or constantly. A rise in intracranial pressure will increase its rate of flow.
4. This fluid can be distinguished from mucosal secretions by obtaining a positive glucose test, indicating that it is spinal fluid.
5. X-rays, including tomography and dye studies, may be necessary.

### Management

1. Proper nasal hygiene
2. Decongestants
3. Teach the patient to sneeze with the mouth open
4. Avoid forceful clearing of the nose
5. Appropriate antibiotics (ampicillin, 250 mg. q.i.d.)
6. Specialty consultations as appropriate
7. If drainage does not subside within two to three weeks, consider surgical intervention.

(Fractures of the facial sinuses are further discussed in Chap. 26, Maxillofacial Fractures.)

### CONGENITAL EMERGENCIES OF THE NASAL STRUCTURES

CHOANAL ATRESIA

*See also* Chapter 36, Pediatric Surgery.

### Definition

Choanal atresia is the persistent nasobuccal membrane that blocks the passage of air through the nose.

## Basic Principles

Blockage may be bony or membranous. It is usually found in the first-born and in females. Bilateral choanal atresia in the newborn is an emergency condition requiring the provision of a proper airway.

## Criteria for Diagnosis

1. Respiratory difficulty (The newborn has not learned to breathe through the mouth.)
2. Cyanosis may develop which improves with crying.
3. Difficulty in feeding
4. Increased mucus in the nose
5. Passage of catheters through the nasal orifices to establish patency or obstruction
6. Dye studies to establish and delineate the obstruction

## Management

1. Establish an oral airway. Use an oropharyngeal airway fastened with tape or a McGovern nipple.
2. Careful observation
3. If the infant is premature, he may require feedings through a gastric tube before definitive surgery is undertaken.
4. Membranous obstruction can be perforated with a stylet and a polyethylene tube inserted for several weeks.
5. Bony obstruction requires operative perforation, which is best approached by the transpalatine route.

## INFLAMMATORY CONDITIONS OF THE NOSE AND PARANASAL SINUSES

## Classification

1. Bacterial
2. Fungal
3. Viral
4. Iatrogenic (rhinitis medicamentosa)
5. Allergic (acute or allergic rhinitis)

(The latter two conditions are nonsurgical and beyond the scope of this discussion).

## BACTERIAL INFECTIONS
### *Furunculosis*

## Definition

Furunculosis is an inflammatory condition of the hair follicles and sebaceous glands of the vestibule of the nose, caused by *Staphylococcus pyogenes* organisms.

## Basic Principles

Prompt and vigorous therapy is necessary to avoid the more serious complications of thrombophlebitis leading to cavernous sinus thrombosis.

## Criteria for Diagnosis

1. Pain
2. Tenderness
3. Swelling of the nose
4. Rhinoscopic visualization of the furuncle

## Management

1. The patient is instructed not to pick or squeeze his nose.
2. Antibiotics: penicillin is the drug of choice, particularly those penicillins directed against staphylococci.
3. Continuous warm soaks
4. Analgesics and sedatives
5. The patient is advised that there is a strong tendency for recurrence and to use antibiotic ointment (e.g., bacitracin ointment) in the nasal vestibule.

### *Erysipelas*

## Definition

Erysipelas is an acute inflammation of the skin and subcutaneous tissues caused by streptococcal organisms.

## Criteria for Diagnosis

1. Pain, swelling and redness of the nose
2. Severe cases are associated with acute signs and symptoms of toxicity.

## Management

1. Analgesics and sedatives
2. Antibiotics: penicillin is the drug of choice.

## *Impetigo Contagiosa*

### Definition

Impetigo contagiosa is caused by staphylococcal organisms and consists of acute vesicular lesions involving the skin of the nose and other parts of the body.

### Management

1. Cleansing with pHisoHex
2. Local application of antibiotic ointment (bacitracin)
3. Systemic antibiotics as determined by culture sensitivity

## *Acute Sinusitis*

### Definition

Acute sinusitis is an acute inflammation of the mucosa of the nasal sinuses.

### Basic Principles

1. The common organisms are *Streptococcus pyogenes, Staphylococcus aureus,* pneumococcus and *Haemophilus influenzae.* The severity of infection depends on host resistance and the virulence of infecting organisms. Allergy and obstruction to drainage of the nasal sinuses play a prominent role in the development of infection. Carious teeth should not be overlooked. Nasal obstruction may be caused by:
   A. Deviated septum
   B. Nasal polyposis
   C. Hypertrophic turbinates
   D. Allergic rhinitis
2. Resistance of the host is lowered by:
   A. Viral infections of the nose
   B. General debility and avitaminosis
   C. Swimming during an upper respiratory infection

### Criteria for Diagnosis

1. Constitutional signs and symptoms associated with predisposing factors
2. Pain, usually aching in nature, exacerbated on "head-low" position (Region of pain depends upon the sinus involved.); fever and general lethargy
3. Nasal discharge, usually unilateral, thick, yellow, purulent
4. On examination, in the early phase, there is congestion and hyperemia of the nasal mucosa and turbinates. The characteristic nasal discharge should be sought.
5. Transillumination of frontal or maxillary sinuses reveals decreased or absent illumination.
6. Paranasal sinus x-rays: Caldwell, Waters', lateral and submentovertex views
7. Decongestion of the mucosa to search for pus from natural ostia
8. Smear of the discharge for culture and sensitivity

### Management

1. *Symptomatic*
   A. Bed rest
   B. Analgesics
2. *General*
   A. Push oral fluids
   B. Steam or nebulizer humidification inhalations
   C. Antibiotics (e.g., erythromycin, 250 mg. q.i.d.)
3. *Local*
   A. Topical decongestants
   B. Antihistaminics: Afrin nose drops; Neo-Synephrine, 1/2%, should be used with caution because of the danger of inspissating the discharge, with further blockage of natural ostia.

### Complications

1. *Intracranial*
   A. Cavernous sinus thrombosis
   B. Brain abscess
   C. Meningitis
2. *Orbital*
   A. Orbital cellulitis
   B. Orbital abscess
3. *Other*
   A. Oral-antral fistula
   B. Osteomyelitis

(The above complications of sinus disease may occur and will require the services of an ENT specialist. Orbital abscess also will require an ophthalmologic consultation since there is danger of loss of vision.)

## FUNGAL INFECTIONS

### Definition

Fungal infections are infections due to fungal organisms.

### Basic Principles

Mucumycosis of the paranasal sinuses is a fungal disease that occurs in intestinal, pulmonary or cranial form. The disease is usually associated with diabetic acidosis and carries a high mortality.

### Criteria for Diagnosis

This is established by a biopsy following a high index of suspicion.

### Management

1. Hospitalization
2. Simultaneous medical and ENT management
3. Amphotericin B is the drug of choice.
4. Surgical intervention for diagnosis and cure

## EPISTAXIS

### Definition

Epistaxis is bleeding from the nose.

### Classification

1. Traumatic (foreign bodies, nose picking, nasal fractures)
2. Inflammatory
   A. Acute inflammatory or allergic conditions. These cause local capillary and venous congestion.
   B. Chronic infections of the nose and paranasal sinuses
3. Septal perforations due to disease (e.g., tuberculosis, syphilis or recurrent aggressive cauterizations). This leaves raw areas which form crusts and bleed.
4. Hereditary telangiectasia (Rendu-Osler-Weber disease)
5. Deviated septum with spurs
6. Blood dyscrasias—leukemia, purpura, hemophilia

7. Chronic hepatic and renal disease, arteriosclerosis, hypertension, etc.
8. Neoplasia of the nose, paranasal sinuses or nasopharynx
9. Vicarious menstruation
10. Idiopathic

### Basic Principles

Although epistaxis is usually not serious, cases of near exsanguination have occurred due to improper management. It is most common in males and frequent between early childhood and puberty and in the elderly patient. The blood supply of the nose is derived from branches of the external carotid and to a lesser degree from the internal carotid artery (the ophthalmic artery gives the anterior and posterior ethmoidal branches which supply the roof of the nasal fossae).

### Criteria for Diagnosis

1. Bleeding from the nose
2. Diagnosis of the underlying condition

### Management

1. A good source of light is needed, along with nasal suction and instruments for nasal examination.
2. Prior to beginning the nasal examination the patient should have a general evaluation, with appropriate measures necessary to maintain vital signs.
3. Clear the nose of all blood clots. After clots are removed, a topical anesthetic on cotton gauze is applied. Pontocaine, 2%, with adrenaline is best if the patient is not hypertensive.
4. Establish the site of bleeding. In 75 per cent of the cases, bleeding from the anterior septum can be localized.
5. Control bleeding by chemical or electrocautery or by packing the anterior and posterior nasal chambers.
6. If bleeding persists, Vaseline gauze with tetracycline added is inserted. Sometimes bilateral deep anterior packing may be necessary.
7. Severe hemorrhage with posterior

bleeding will require posterior and anterior packing.

A. The conventional "posterior plug" with the string through the mouth and nose is usually used.

B. Alternatively, a Foley catheter with a 30-ml. bag inserted through the nose, with the balloon in the nasopharynx, is inserted; 8 to 10 ml. of water are injected and the catheter is pulled firmly against the posterior part of the nose by forward traction.

C. A pack is first wound around the Foley catheter to avoid trauma to the nasal vestibule and septum and to anchor the catheter, which is then fixed in place with adhesive. This can be removed in 4 to 5 days.

8. Rarely when proper packing fails, surgical intervention may be considered. This consists of ligation of the bleeding artery, which may be the sphenopalatine or ethmoid, depending on the bleeding site.

## TRAUMA TO THE EAR

### AURICULAR INJURIES

### Classification

1. *Mechanical*
   A. Contusions
   B. Lacerations
   C. Avulsions
2. *Thermal*
   A. Frostbite
   B. Burns
   C. Scalds

### Basic Principles

The exposed nature of the auricle predisposes it to sustain various injuries.

#### *Contusions*

### Criteria for Diagnosis

1. History of injury. Contusions of the auricle are commonly seen following accidents, fist fights, etc.

2. Pain and swelling of the ear. Usually the hematoma formation is due to the accumulation of blood between the cartilage and the perichondrium.

### Management

1. *Early Cases without Hematoma Formation*
   A. Analgesics
   B. Wet dressings
   C. Observation
2. *Cases with Hematoma Formation*
   A. Aspiration of the hematoma with a large bore needle
   B. Application of cotton packing and a tight mastoid pressure dressing
   C. If the blood cannot be properly evacuated, incision and drainage with the insertion of a Penrose drain should be done with the application of a pressure dressing.
   D. Analgesics
   E. Antibiotics: tetracycline, 250 mg. q.i.d. and zinc sulfate topical.

#### *Lacerations*

### Management

1. Simple lacerations without cartilage involvement should have primary repair of the wound.

2. With cartilage and skin involvement the perichondrium is sutured with 5-0 plain catgut before skin repair is attempted.

#### *Avulsions*

### Management

1. Complete avulsion of the auricle may be repaired primarily with good cosmetic result.

2. When there is extensive loss of tissue only primary debridement and cleansing are carried out, with cosmetic repair at a later date.

#### *Frostbite*

### Basic Principles

Frostbite is frequent because of the exposed nature of the auricle and the lack of adipose tissue to protect the blood vessels. The extent of damage depends upon the severity and time of exposure to cold. Initial vasoconstriction is followed by reactionary vasodilatation producing swelling and finally ischemia with necrosis of tissue.

## Management

1. Thaw gradually to room temperature.
2. Avoid pressure dressings.
3. Avoid rough cleansing or scrubbing.
4. Use protective ointment—bacitracin ointment.
5. Heparinization (*See* Chap. 18, Vascular Emergencies.)

### Burns and Scalds

*See* Chapter 34, Burns.

## FOREIGN BODIES AND INSECTS IN THE EXTERNAL AUDITORY CANAL

This is common in children. Vegetable foreign bodies should be removed under direct vision. Solid foreign bodies may be syringed. Before attempting forceps removal or syringing of insects from the external canal, the insect should be killed with mineral oil. The uncooperative child may require general anesthesia for removal of a foreign body.

## INJURIES TO THE TYMPANIC MEMBRANE (EAR DRUM)

### Perforations

## Classification

1. *Primary Perforations.* These are due to the accidental or deliberate introduction of sharp objects into the canal.
2. *Secondary Perforations.* These occur following head injury, temporal bone fractures or blast trauma.

## Criteria for Diagnosis

1. Pain, bleeding from the ear and hearing loss
2. Visualization by otoscopic examination

## Management

1. No cleaning or irrigations
2. Antibiotics, e.g., penicillin, 250,000 u. q.i.d. to avoid infections
3. Avoid ear drops or water entering the ear.

4. Careful follow-up; most of these perforations heal spontaneously within four weeks.
5. With the secondary type of perforation the management is the same as above plus ENT consultation.
6. Management of associated injuries which may be life-threatening

## INJURIES TO THE MIDDLE EAR

### Barotraumatic Otitis Media (Aero-otitis)

## Definition

Barotraumatic otitis media is a non-infective inflammatory condition due to the development of negative pressure within the middle ear cleft.

## Basic Principles

It is caused by failure or inability to open the eustachian tube. It is seen when flying (during descent) and diving. The common cold is a predisposing factor.

## Criteria for Diagnosis

Otalgia may be severe. There may be clogged ears, deafness and tinnitus; vertigo may occur occasionally.

## Management

1. Nasal decongestion by topical and oral routes, viz., e.g., Afrin nose drops, 4 drops in each nostril q.i.d.; Dimetapp, 1 tablet b.i.d.
2. Auto-inflation (Valsalva)
3. Politzerization; antibiotics if infection is present
4. Myringotomy if fluid is present.

## FRACTURES OF THE TEMPORAL BONE

## Basic Principles

Fractures of the temporal bone may be transverse or longitudinal. They are associated with head trauma.

1. Longitudinal fractures are more common and usually 80 per cent of these fractures are associated with rupture of the tympanic membrane, bleeding from the

canal, hearing loss and ossicular dislocation.

2. Transverse fractures usually involve the facial nerve and inner ear, leading to facial nerve palsy and sensory neural hearing loss.

### Management

1. Avoid ear drops or water in the ear canal.
2. Judicious sterile cleansing *or no* cleansing
3. Antibiotic coverage
4. Determine presence of cerebrospinal fluid in the external canal by the glucose dip-stick test.
5. ENT and neurosurgical consultations

## INFLAMMATORY CONDITIONS OF THE EAR

### Classification

1. Infections of the auricle
2. Infections of the external auditory canal (otitis externa)
3. Otitis media
4. Infections of the inner ear

### INFECTIONS OF THE AURICLE

*Impetigo*

### Basic Principles

Impetigo is often associated with inflammation of the external canal. It is usually due to staphylococcus and streptococcus. It is spread by auto-inoculation.

### Criteria for Diagnosis

Impetigo begins with a red spot which becomes papular, vesicular and then pustular.

### Management

1. Remove crusts with warm water.
2. Apply bacitracin ointment.

*Erysipelas*

### Criteria for Diagnosis

1. Spreading, superficial cellulitis extending to adjacent skin

2. Associated with constitutional signs and symptoms of sepsis

### Management

Penicillin, 500,000 u. q.i.d., is the drug of choice.

*Perichondritis*

### Definition

Perichondritis is infection of the perichondrium.

### Basic Principles

The infection may arise from trauma such as abrasion or laceration or following ear surgery. A furuncle may be a ready source of infection, especially in the postoperative ear. The causative organism may be staphylococcus, streptococcus or Bacillus pyocyaneus (in ears with chronic infections).

### Criteria for Diagnosis

1. Swelling
2. Tenderness
3. Redness of the auricle

### Management

1. Continuous soaks with Burrow's solution
2. Sensitivity and culture for organisms
3. Antibiotic coverage. The organisms are usually resistant to penicillin. Gentamicin may be used.
4. Topical polymyxin
5. Surgical intervention for evacuation of abscess and excision of necrotic cartilage
6. Zinc sulfate to promote better healing postoperatively. This condition may be stubborn and may lead to deformity of the auricle.

### INFECTIONS OF THE EXTERNAL AUDITORY CANAL (OTITIS EXTERNA)

*Furunculosis*

### Definition

Furunculosis is a staphylococcal infection of the hair follicles in the cartilaginous portion of the external canal.

### Criteria for Diagnosis

There is pain and tenderness, worse on motion of the auricle. The pain gets progressively worse, and the canal may become occluded. The postauricular lymph nodes may become enlarged.

### Management

1. Analgesics
2. Application of a wick with a topical anesthetic and use of Burrow's solution
3. Antibiotics (e.g., penicillin)
4. Abscess formation may require incision and drainage.

*Diffuse Otitis Externa*
*("Swimmer's Ear")*

### Basic Principles

This infection is common in hot, humid climates. It follows mild trauma causing abrasion of the external canal skin surface. The causative organisms are *B. pyocyaneus, B. picteus* or *Staphylococcus aureus.*

### Criteria for Diagnosis

1. Pain and swelling of the external canal
2. Slight discharge
3. Gradual obstruction of the entire lumen of the canal
4. Pain aggravated by jaw movements

### Management

1. Cleanse the external canal of debris.
2. Apply a wick with a topical anesthetic, followed by the application of Burrow's solution ear drops. Then start cortisone and neomycin ear drops.
3. Analgesics
4. Antibiotics may be considered for a staphylococcal infection after culture and sensitivity.

*Myringitis Bullosa*

### Criteria for Diagnosis

Myringitis bullosa has a viral etiology.

There is formation of purple blebs on the tympanic membrane and inner third of the external canal skin. The severe pain is not relieved by serosanguinous discharge (due to bursting of the blebs).

### Management

1. This is a self-limiting disease.
2. Analgesics
3. Antibiotics are of no value.

## INFLAMMATION OF THE MIDDLE EAR (OTITIS MEDIA)

### Definition

Otitis media is an inflammatory condition of the middle ear cleft and eustachian tube.

### Basic Principles

1. It is commonly a disease of childhood.
2. The causative organisms are hemolytic streptococcus, staphylococcus, pneumococcus and H. influenzae.
3. Predisposing factors are acute respiratory infections, allergy, eustachian tube malfunction, hypertrophic adenoids (in children) or nasopharyngeal tumor blocking the eustachian tube orifice.

### Criteria for Diagnosis

1. In the early stage, there are signs and symptoms of upper respiratory infection with a sensation of "blocked" ear(s) and otalgia. With low host resistance and high virulence the disease progresses with the development of severe otalgia, fever, nausea, vomiting and even cephalalgia. When the pressure of the purulent material rises in the middle ear cleft, it ruptures the eardrum, with a release of the exudate and relief of pain.
2. In the early stage, the tympanic membrane appears retracted due to eustachian tube occlusion. With fluid formation and accumulation of exudate, the eardrum appears red, congested and bulging.

### Management

1. Culture and sensitivity of pharynx with appropriate antibiotics

2. Decongestant nasal drops or oral decongestants

3. Myringotomy for bulging, painful eardrum

With rupture of the tympanic membrane, an exudate in the external canal and a perforation in the lower quadrant are seen on otoscopic examination.

1. Bed rest, symptomatic support, analgesics

2. Antibiotics—penicillin or ampicillin (drug of choice)

3. Topical decongestants, Neo-Synephrine, ½% nose drops, 3 drops in each nostril q.i.d. for adults (¼% strength for children)

4. Oral decongestants, e.g., Dimetapp, 1 tablet b.i.d.

5. ENT consultation

## INFLAMMATION OF THE INNER EAR

### Classification

1. Serous—hearing is reduced.
2. Suppurative—hearing is absent.
3. Circumscribed

### Criteria for Diagnosis

1. Symptoms may relate to hearing and equilibrium.
2. Dizziness and evidence of nystagmus
3. Various degrees of hearing loss
4. Vomiting may be present.

### Management

1. Hospitalization and ENT consultation
2. Large doses of antibiotics
3. Symptomatic supportive therapy
4. Work-up and consideration for possible surgical intervention by ENT staff

## COMPLICATIONS OF EAR DISEASE

### INTRACRANIAL COMPLICATIONS OF EAR DISEASE

#### Classification

1. Lateral sinus thrombosis
2. Epidural abscess
3. Brain abscess and meningitis
4. Petrositis or apicitis—reveals 6th nerve palsy

### Basic Principles

The history of ear disease is usually chronic. The patient may present with early intracranial symptoms or may be in a coma. Relatives or friends may provide a history of ear disease or history may not be available.

### Criteria for Diagnosis

The diagnosis is established by a high index of suspicion, ENT consultation and examination and neurologic consultations. A smear of the ear discharge will reveal the same organisms as cerebrospinal fluid.

### Management

1. The patient requires hospitalization.
2. ENT and neurologic consultations
3. Culture and sensitivity and smear of ear discharge
4. Cerebrospinal fluid studies
5. Appropriate massive antibiotics
6. Judicious decision as to the optimal time for operative intervention
7. These are dangerous conditions with a high mortality rate.

### FACIAL NERVE PARALYSIS

1. With facial nerve paralysis there is a history of ear disease, acute or chronic. Paralysis may follow an acute ear infection. The palsy usually clears spontaneously. In chronic otitis media, especially due to cholesteatoma, surgical mastoid intervention is necessary.

2. ENT consultation is important.

3. Bell's palsy and other causes of facial nerve palsy must be ruled out.

### VERTIGO

1. Vertigo is a sensation of spinning or motion. The sensation may be subjective (patient feels that he is spinning) or objective (the patient feels that objects are spinning).

2. It may be associated with severe vomiting and may be central or peripheral.

3. Common causes are:
   A. Acute labyrinthitis
   B. Meniere's disease
   C. Vestibular neuronitis
   D. Benign postural vertigo
   E. Vascular insufficiency
   F. Trauma
   G. Tumor

4. ENT consultation is required.

## SUDDEN HEARING LOSS

### Classification

1. External ear
   A. Impacted cerumen
   B. Impacted foreign body
   C. Hematoma
   D. Laceration
   E. Inflammation
2. Middle ear
   A. Perforated eardrum
   B. Dislocated ossicle
   C. Otosclerosis
   D. Infection
3. Inner ear
   A. Infection (i.e., mumps, measles, influenza)
   B. Noise—acoustic trauma
   C. Syphilis
   D. Ototoxic drugs and agents
   E. Vascular insufficiency
   F. Meniere's disease

### Basic Principles

Sudden hearing loss may be either conductive or sensory-neural in nature. In general, external and middle ear pathology gives rise to the conductive type and inner ear pathology gives rise to the sensory-neural type of hearing loss.

### Criteria for Diagnosis

It is important to ascertain the cause of the hearing loss by otoscopic examination and tuning fork test (lateralization to poor-hearing ear means probable conductive hearing loss).

### Management

ENT consultation for sudden sensory-neural loss is important in order to establish an immediate diagnosis and to start aggressive therapy.

## TRAUMA TO THE MOUTH, PHARYNX AND NECK

### STAB WOUNDS OF THE NECK

### Basic Principles

Even in the absence of progressive swelling and ecchymosis, neck exploration should be mandatory. Except in lower neck wounds which possibly go into the thorax, preliminary arch angiography is unnecessary. Neck emphysema indicates probable perforation into the oro-hypopharyngeal or possibly into the laryngo-esophageal spaces.

## INFLAMMATORY CONDITIONS OF THE MOUTH, PHARYNX AND NECK

### ACUTE TONSILLITIS

### Classification

1. Cryptic tonsillitis—nonmembranous
2. Follicular tonsillitis—usually membranous
3. Gangrenous tonsillitis—membranous

### Basic Principles

1. Most often caused by hemolytic streptococcus
2. In the membranous tonsillitis, the following must be ruled out:
   A. *Diphtheria.* The membrane causes bleeding on attempted removal (pneumococcal infection will also bleed).
   B. *Infectious Mononucleosis.* The membrane is usually thin, white and milky. The patient is usually on antibiotics without response, and the toxicity is less than anticipated from the degree of fever. Culture and sensitivity, smear and a general physical examination will help establish the diagnosis. ENT consultation may be required.

## Criteria for Diagnosis

There is malaise, fever, a sore throat and difficulty in swallowing; the patient may complain of otalgia. The tonsils are enlarged, hyperemic, and covered with a variable amount of exudate. In children, the cervical nodes may be enlarged.

## Management

Bed rest, analgesics, antipyretics, push fluids, antibiotics (Penicillin is the drug of choice.)

## PERITONSILLAR ABSCESS

### Basic Principles

1. A complication of tonsillitis
2. Some think it is a primary infection of the mucus-secreting glands of Weber in the supratonsillar space.
3. Usually unilateral and on the right side
4. Extremely rare in children

### Criteria for Diagnosis

1. Previous attacks of tonsillitis—same signs and symptoms as for tonsillitis
2. Severe dysphagia
3. Salivation
4. Fever and a variable degree of trismus (due to spasm of the internal pterygoid muscle)
5. By use of topical anesthesia the mouth can be opened and examination performed, revealing:
    A. Diffuse swelling of the palatine tonsil and adjacent soft palate
    B. The uvula is often edematous and pushed to the opposite side.

### Management

1. Aspiration of the region with an 18- or 15-gauge needle to avoid incision of an aberrant vessel
2. Incision and drainage
3. Culture and sensitivity and smear of the discharge
4. Antibiotic treatment is the same as for tonsillitis.

5. The patient will require tonsillectomy in 4 weeks to avoid recurrent bouts of peritonsillar abscesses.
6. ENT consultation

## PARAPHARYNGEAL ABSCESS

### Basic Principles

Parapharyngeal abscess is a rare complication of acute tonsillitis or it may spread from adjacent regional infections. The pus accumulates in the deep investing layer of the cervical fascia. There is a danger of the infection spreading to the carotid vessels, leading to fatal hemorrhage or spread to the mediastinum.

### Criteria for Diagnosis

Similar to peritonsillar abscess with severe toxemia

### Management

1. Hospitalization
2. Massive intravenous antibiotics prior to surgical drainage (usually external approach)
3. ENT consultation

## LUDWIG'S ANGINA

### Basic Principles

Ludwig's angina is an infection of the sublingual, submaxillary and submental spaces. This may follow dental infections, trauma to the floor of the mouth or tonsillar and peritonsillar infections. Male adults are affected more frequently. Streptococci are the common causative organisms.

### Criteria for Diagnosis

1. Fever, pain, difficulty in swallowing
2. Diffuse swelling in the submental and adjacent regions with associated redness and tenderness
3. The tongue is pushed forward, and there is a variable degree of restriction in tongue motion.
4. The floor of the mouth shows a variable degree of swelling.

## Management

1. There is a danger that the infection and swelling will cause respiratory difficulty; thus hospitalization is required.
2. Intravenous antibiotics
3. Local compresses
4. Careful observation of the airway. There should be a tracheostomy tray readily available.
5. Tracheostomy if there is airway obstruction
6. Incision and drainage
7. ENT consultation

### ACUTE RETROPHARYNGEAL ABSCESS

## Basic Principles

This is common in children. The abscess formation in the retropharyngeal space is due to suppurative breakdown of retropharyngeal lymph nodes. The source of the infection may be the tonsils and adenoids, trauma to the posterior pharyngeal wall or tuberculosis.

## Criteria for Diagnosis

1. Fever, sore throat, dysphagia or a feeding problem in the young child
2. The patient will exhibit variable degrees of general debility, dehydration and toxemia.
3. Neck movements may be restricted due to spasm of muscles.
4. Swelling in the posterior wall of the pharynx
5. The lateral x-ray view of the neck will reveal increased distance between the vertebral column and the laryngopharyngeal air space.

## Management

1. Hospitalization
2. Massive intravenous antibiotics (Penicillin is the drug of choice.)
3. ENT consultation
4. Incision and drainage are important.
5. *Danger:* spontaneous rupture in a sleeping child may lead to aspiration asphyxia!

## TRAUMA TO THE LARYNX

## Classification

1. *Closed Injuries.* These injuries (due to blunt trauma) may be undiagnosed in the early cases because there may be significant trauma to the larynx without evidence of soft tissue injury.
2. *Open Injuries.* These are caused by sharp or penetrating objects. They are dangerous because of hemorrhage, air embolism and aspiration.

## Basic Principles

Traumatic injuries to the larynx are less frequent than multiple injuries of the head and neck region. More than 50 per cent of the injuries are due to vehicular accidents and the remainder are due to sports or physical assault. The larynx receives some protection from the lower jaw. The common blunt trauma to the larynx is due to the impact of the neck against the dashboard during an automobile accident.

## Criteria for Diagnosis

1. There is a history of injury.
2. There may be various degrees of hoarseness, respiratory difficulty, dysphagia, hemoptysis and tenderness in the neck.
3. Examination may reveal:
   A. Swelling and tenderness in the anterior aspect of the neck
   B. Absence of the thyroid notch and cricoid cartilage (rare)
   C. Presence of air in the soft tissues
   D. Skin laceration and palpable cartilage fragments
4. Laryngoscopy may reveal:
   A. Variable laryngeal edema
   B. Ecchymosis
   C. Mucosal lacerations
   D. Fracture dislocations of normal structures

## Management

1. General life-supportive measures
2. Attention to possible head and chest injuries which may be life-threatening

3. Airway difficulty dictates an immediate "low" tracheostomy.

4. ENT consultation is needed for the decision whether conservative management or open reduction, which may be performed as late as one week after injury, should be undertaken.

## INFLAMMATORY CONDITIONS OF THE LARYNX

### ACUTE LARYNGITIS

#### Basic Principles

Hoarseness in a child is usually indicative of laryngitis and is usually associated with an upper respiratory infection. In the adult, laryngitis is usually caused by voice abuse, smoking and nonspecific infections. The adult must undergo indirect laryngoscopie examination to rule out neoplasm.

#### Criteria for Diagnosis

1. Noisy labored respirations
2. The child with hoarseness should undergo a complete physical examination, including the ear-nose-throat region.
3. Use of accessory muscles of respiration
4. Retrosternal, subcostal retractions or flaring of the nares

#### Management

1. The child should be admitted to the croup ward
2. Adequate hydration
3. Cool steam inhalation
4. Antibiotics (Ampicillin, 250 mg. every 4 hours, is the drug of choice.)
5. Steroids, e.g., Solu-Medrol, 1 mg./lb. of body weight, repeated q.i.d. for 2 days, depending on the degree of airway obstruction
6. Posteroanterior and lateral x-ray of the neck
7. Avoid sedatives because they may depress the respiratory center.
8. Consent is needed for direct laryngoscopy and tracheostomy.

9. A tracheostomy set should be available.

10. The clinical picture of laryngitis in children may be associated with tracheobronchitis as part of laryngo-tracheobronchitis. Maintenance and provision of an adequate airway are mandatory for life.

### ACUTE EPIGLOTTIDITIS

#### Basic Principles

This is less common and more serious than acute laryngitis. The causative organism is *H. influenzae.*

#### Criteria for Diagnosis

1. The symptoms are less dramatic; however, airway obstruction may occur rapidly without much warning.
2. Depressing the tongue with a blade will reveal a cherry-red epiglottis.

#### Management

1. Hospitalization
2. Consent and preparation for tracheostomy (especially in children)
3. Antibiotics. Ampicillin is the drug of choice, 250 mg. every 4 hours.
4. Solu-Medrol, 1 mg./lb. of body weight repeated q.i.d. for 2 days depending on the degree of airway obstruction.
5. Humidifier

### ACUTE LARYNGOTRACHEOBRONCHITIS

#### Basic Principles

Acute laryngotracheobronchitis is an acute inflammatory condition of the respiratory tract. It is common in children during the winter months. Causative organisms are streptococcus, staphylococcus and pneumococcus.

#### Criteria for Diagnosis

1. Sudden onset of a dry cough
2. Sore throat
3. Fever
4. Hoarseness and/or laryngeal stridor

## Management

1. *Mild Cases:*
   A. Humidifier
   B. Antibiotics (penicillin)
   C. Careful observation
2. *Moderate Cases:* same as for mild cases, plus cortisone
3. *Severe Cases:* same as for moderate cases, plus tracheostomy if indicated

## FOREIGN BODIES IN THE AIR AND FOOD PASSAGES

### Basic Principles

Accidental or intentional swallowing and inhalation of foreign bodies occur in adults and children. This causes approximately 2,000 deaths a year. Foreign bodies in the air passage are ten times more frequent in children than in adults. Types of objects include safety pins (most common up to 1 year of age) and nuts (most common from 2 to 4 years of age). Foreign bodies in the food passages occur twice as frequently in adults than in children. Children usually swallow coins, metallic objects, nuts, etc.; adults usually swallow bones and meat. The cricopharynx is the most frequent site for foreign bodies.

### Criteria for Diagnosis

1. Symptoms depend upon the age of the patient and the nature of the foreign body.
2. Initial symptoms usually are choking, gagging and coughing.
3. The final signs and symptoms depend upon the site of foreign body localization.
   A. *Laryngeal Foreign Body*
   (1) The patient may present with hoarseness or aphonia and respiratory difficulty.
   (2) Impacted foreign bodies may prove fatal immediately.
   B. *Tracheobronchial Tree Foreign Body*
   (1) Careful history of aspiration
   (2) The patient presents with choking, coughing, wheezing, dyspnea and cyanosis.
   (3) This acute phase is followed by a symptomless period with a nonobstructive foreign body.
   (4) The obstructive object gives rise to pulmonary signs of atelectasis, emphysema and lung abscess.
   (5) Organic foreign bodies (e.g., peanuts) cause severe reactional tracheobronchitis, especially in children.
   (6) X-rays of the chest, posteroanterior and lateral views
   C. *Esophageal Foreign Bodies*
   (1) Initial signs and symptoms of choking or gagging followed by difficulty in swallowing
   (2) In children, large foreign bodies lodged within the cervical esophagus may cause respiratory difficulty.
   (3) X-rays include lateral and posteroanterior views of the chest and neck; oblique views may also be needed. For nonmetallic objects, dye studies (e.g., a marshmallow soaked in barium) may be used.

## Management

1. *Airway Obstruction*
   A. Sharp objects and pins in areas threatening vital structures require immediate emergency removal.
   B. If asphyxia is threatened by a laryngeal foreign body, a stab cricothyroidotomy followed by a tracheostomy is in order.
   C. In other cases, keep the patient comfortable, do not slap him on the back in an attempt to dislodge the foreign body, and do not attempt to remove it by inserting the fingers into the throat because these maneuvers may obstruct the airway.
   D. Hospitalization and ENT consultation may be necessary to establish the type of foreign body, its location and proper removal.
2. *Pharyngeal and Esophageal Obstruction*
   A. Admit the patient to the hospital to follow the passage of the foreign body.
   B. If obstructed or if the object has not moved in 48 hours, instrument removal through an endoscope is necessary.

# 29. OCULAR EMERGENCIES

*Donald E. Willard*, M.D.

An ocular emergency exists whenever a patient's vision is in immediate danger. It is present in many eye conditions. Treatment must be instituted within minutes or hours of the onset of symptoms.

## GENERAL PRINCIPLES OF OCULAR EMERGENCIES

### Symptoms

1. Patients with ocular emergencies are either in acute pain or fear for their vision because of one or more of the following symptoms:

A. *Foreign Body Sensation.* "Something is in my eye."

B. *Redness.* "My eye is red."

C. *Vision Change.* "My vision is hazy," or "I see double," or "I see black spots in front of my eyes," or "I see haloes around lights."

2. Some conditions will produce additional symptoms related to the eyelids.

A. Eyelid spasm

B. Eyelid swelling

C. Eyelid discharge (including "runny eyes" and tears)

3. Systemic, nonspecific symptoms occasionally occur as prominent features of ocular emergencies.

A. Headache

B. Nausea or vomiting

C. Fever

### History

The treatment of all ocular emergencies may be delayed long enough for the development of a short history of the condition. It is important to place the symptoms in chronological perspective. The following information is usually necessary.

1. *Time of Onset.* When did the problem begin?

2. *Mode of Onset.* How did the symptoms begin?

3. *Prior Treatment.* What did the patient or other people do?

4. *Progression.* Is the condition becoming worse or better?

### Examination

An ocular examination is necessary to determine treatment of injury and can be carried out by using a small flashlight, ophthalmoscope and some reading material (e.g., newspaper). Whenever the patient is able to open his eyes voluntarily, his central visual acuity must be estimated for each eye. Do not forcibly open a patient's eyelids to test vision and do not allow him to do it himself. Carefully record all aspects of the examination, including, in sufficient detail, the type size and testing distance.

### Inspection

Systematically evaluate the integrity of the ocular anatomy, keeping in mind that an involuntarily closed eyelid may be protecting a lacerated eyeball. The following outline gives an examination routine that will disclose the important signs of ocular emergencies.

Eyelids

1. *Obvious Laceration, Hemorrhage or Edema*

A. Is an injury to the eyeball likely?

B. Can the patient open the eyelids voluntarily?

2. *Eyelid Symmetry* (eyes open)

A. Are the upper lid folds similar in both eyes?

B. Are the height and width of palpebral fissures the same in both eyes?

C. Do the midpoints of all four lids-touch the cornea?

## Pupil

1. In cases of obvious involuntary eyelid closure and a history of trauma or perforating eyeball disease:

A. Relax the orbicular muscle with Xylocaine.

(1) Find a point on the zygomatic arch midway between the orbital rim and the temporal artery pulsation.

(2) Subcutaneously inject 1 ml. of 2% Xylocaine above and below the point.

(3) Use a 23- or 25-gauge needle and direct it toward the eyebrow above and the tip of the nose below.

B. Gently separate the lids by placing one index finger on the patient's eyebrow and one index finger on his inferior orbital rim; press on the bone and slide the skin.

C. Allow an assistant to hold the flashlight.

2. When involuntary eyelid closure is due to obvious inflammation or the possibility of a perforated globe is remote:

A. Use self-retaining eyelid retractors or prepare eyelid retractors from ordinary paper clips as follows:

(1) Unfold the inner loop of wire 180 degrees.

(2) Bend one end of the loop back about 90 degrees.

(3) Wash the retractors in surgical prep solution or autoclave them.

B. Carefully insert the rounded ends of the retractors against the eyelid margins and gently open the lids.

C. Allow an assistant to hold the flashlight.

3. *Anatomy*

A. Is the pupil round, central and black?

B. Are the two pupils similar in size?

4. *Function*

A. Does each pupil constrict promptly upon direct stimulation with light?

B. If either pupil does not constrict to direct light, does it constrict when the other pupil is stimulated directly?

## Anterior Chamber

1. Is the iris surface bowed forward as the cornea is? Shallow chamber?

2. Is the iris flat and several millimeters behind the cornea? Deep chamber?

3. Is blood or pus present in front of the iris? Hyphema or hypopyon?

## Cornea

1. Is the cornea clear and transparent like a wrist-watch crystal?

2. Look for foreign bodies, abrasions and lacerations.

3. Do not mistake a nubbin of prolapsed iris for a foreign body.

4. Is there a large opaque area with an ulcerated center? Does the crater have a clear central bulge—a descemetocele?

## Conjunctiva

1. *Bulbar Conjunctiva*

A. Is white sclera visible through the normally transparent bulbar conjunctiva?

B. Are there areas of bright-red subconjunctival hemorrhage, boggy areas of edema or subconjunctival air?

C. Is superficial congestion present?

(1) Vessels are numerous and tortuous.

(2) The over-all color is bright red.

(3) The vessels move when the conjunctiva moves.

(4) Petechiae may be present.

D. Is deep congestion present?

(1) The vessels appear to radiate from the corneoscleral limbus and are straight.

(2) They produce a red-purple flush circumferentially around the cornea.

(3) The vessels do not move when the superficial conjunctiva moves.

2. *Palpebral Conjunctiva*

A. Press a finger against the inferior orbital rim and slide the eyelid skin toward the chin.

(1) Look for foreign bodies, exudates, pus or abnormal membranes.

(2) Is the color pale pink or bright red?

B. Eversion of the upper eyelid requires both hands.

*(1)* Have the patient look down with both eyes open.

*(2)* Grasp the eyelashes with thumb and finger and pull the lid down and away from the globe.

*(3)* Place an applicator stick or unfolded paper clip on the eyelid about halfway between the lid margin and the eyebrow; press gently toward the eyeball.

*(4)* Fold the eyelashes and the tarsal plate up and over the applicator stick; remove the stick and press the eyelashes against the eyebrow.

## Posterior Segment

1. Direct ophthalmoscopy is a clinical skill that must be acquired by examining many normal eyes prior to attempting it in an ocular emergency.

2. Set the ophthalmoscope lens at No. 1 black (plus 1 diopter).

3. If the patient's spectacles are available, have him put them on and look into the distance away from bright lights.

4. From a distance of about one foot, direct the light of the ophthalmoscope so that the pink-orange fundus glow fills the patient's pupil.

5. Hold the patient's eyelid open with the free thumb and lean forward until the examiner's forehead rests against the thumb.

6. Find the optic nerve head and then systematically inspect the fundus anatomy.

A. Are the disk margins distinct?

B. Are the vessels in focus on the disk with the same lens setting used to see them near the disk?

C. Do all the disk vessels appear to be filled with blood?

D. Follow each arteriole away from the nerve head and look for segmentation of the blood column.

E. Do the veins on the disk pulsate?

F. If there is a history of very recent total loss of vision, are the white fundus and bright-red fovea of central artery occlusion present?

G. Is the vitreous cloudy or opaque?

H. Small foreign bodies may be visible.

I. Is the crystaliline lens opaque or dislocated?

## Ocular Motility

1. Hold a penlight about an arm's length in front of the patient's nose.

A. Does the light reflex on the cornea seem to be in the same place on each cornea when the patient looks at the light?"

B. Ask, "Do you see one light?"

C. Slowly move the light horizontally, then vertically in the midline, then up and to the left and up and to the right.

D. Watch for asymmetry in the positions of the corneal light reflexes.

E. Say to the patient, "Tell me when you see two lights." Repeat the movements of the penlight.

F. Do not ask, "Do you see double?"

2. Move the light toward the patient's nose and ask him to look at it with both eyes; note any relative weakness of convergence.

## Peripheral Vision

1. Stand about one meter in front of the patient and ask him to look at the examiner's nose.

2. Ask the patient to cover one eye with his hand.

3. The examiner's arm is extended up and out about 45 degrees from the patient's line of sight.

4. Say, "Tell me when my fingers wiggle."

5. Systematically test the temporal and nasal fields both above and below the patient's line of sight.

## OCULAR TRAUMA
### CHEMICAL BURNS

**Definition**

A chemical burn of the eye is an ocular injury due to the chemical action of foreign liquids or solids which come in contact with the eyeball or eyelids.

## Classification

1. Alkali burns
2. Acid burns
3. Explosives
4. Irritants—liquids, gases, aerosols

## Basic Principles

1. Dilution of the chemical agent by copious irrigation is the main principle of first aid in chemical injuries to the eye.
2. Employ topical anesthesia and local infiltration as necessary to relieve the patient and permit atraumatic manipulations.
3. Alkali burns are usually more serious and more extensive than they appear to be at first.
4. Acid burn damage may turn out to be less severe than first appearances indicate.
5. Some organic chemicals such as anticholinesterase insecticides may cause minor eye injury when compared with the systemic effects of the agent when absorbed by the conjunctiva.

## Criteria for Diagnosis

1. History of injurious episode with acute ocular symptoms
2. Visible evidence of injury to the exposed ocular tissues

## Management

*All patients with a chemical burn of their eyes must have their eyeballs irrigated with copious amounts of the closest clean water. This is an imperative first-aid measure. All persons connected with patient care should be trained to minister to such patients without delay.* The very few exceptions to this rule are burns due to mustard gas and chemical refrigerants.

1. Assume that first-aid irrigation was inadequate.
2. Place the patient in a supine position with a pillow under the shoulders while directing an assistant to prepare a bottle of intravenous saline or water with a tubing set to be used for irrigating the eyes.
3. If the patient is unable to open his eyes or has pain, pull down the lower eyelid and instill several drops of a topical anesthetic (benoxinate as 0.4% Dorsacaine, proparacaine as 0.5% Ophthetic, or tetracaine as 0.5% Pontocaine).
4. Allow the water to run freely from the tubing set; direct the stream by holding the plastic adapter end.
5. Direct the water stream onto the eyeball and retract the upper eyelid as necessary. Insert the tip of the adapter under the lateral lid margins if holding the lids open proves difficult.
6. Continue irrigation in this fashion until 3 or 4 liters of water have been used.
7. A second setup and an assistant are necessary if both eyes are injured.
8. Topical anesthesia may be maintained by repeated applications of anesthetic.
9. Proceed to examine the patient according to the evaluation outline given on page 405.
   A. Evaluate the cornea by means of fluorescein.
      *(1)* Use only sterile paper strips or dropperettes.
      *(2)* Areas denuded of epithelium will turn green in white light and yellow in blue light.
   B. Diagram the areas of epithelial damage in the patient's record.
10. Consult with an ophthalmologist before beginning any definitive therapy.

## THERMAL BURNS

### Definition

A thermal burn of the eye is an ocular injury produced by heat.

### Classification

1. Burns of the eyelids only
2. Burns with injury to the eyeball
3. Burns associated with foreign bodies embedded in the cornea

### Basic Principles

1. Treat eyelid burns in the same way as any other burns of the face.

2. Evaluate the ocular status of the patient according to the general outline on page 405 as soon as the patient's general condition permits.

## Criteria for Diagnosis

1. History of injurious episode with acute ocular symptoms
2. Corneal staining with fluorescein
3. Presence of corneal foreign bodies

## Management

1. Press a sterile cotton-tipped applicator against the lower orbital rim and slide the skin toward the chin; instill several drops of a topical anesthetic into the conjunctival sac (0.4% benoxinate, 0.5% proparacaine or 0.5% tetracaine).
2. Lavage the cornea and conjunctiva with 1 liter of normal saline or Ringer's solution; direct the stream from the tubing set to wash out debris and any obvious foreign bodies.
3. Instill fluorescein (paper strip or sterile dropperette) and evaluate the integrity of the corneal epithelium.
4. If the cornea stains with fluorescein or contains an embedded foreign body, proceed according to management outlined under Chemical Burns, above.

## RADIATION BURNS

### Definition

A radiation burn of the eye is an ocular injury due to radiant energy.

### Classification

1. *Ultraviolet radiation injury* may be caused by exposure to a welding arc flash, ultraviolet sun lamps or sunlight reflected from snow.
2. *Infrared radiation injury* may be caused by exposure due to looking directly at sources such as the sun, atomic explosions and lasers.

### Basic Principles

1. The cornea absorbs ultraviolet radiation but transmits infrared radiation.

2. Infrared damage is usually permanent; ultraviolet damage is usually transitory.

### Criteria for Diagnosis

1. History of accidental or deliberate exposure to a radiation source
2. Ultraviolet radiation injury produces symptoms and signs of corneal injury: pain, blepharospasm, watery or sandy sensation, and photophobia associated with punctate, epithelial erosions, all beginning 3 to 6 hours after exposure.
3. Infrared radiation injury produces symptoms and signs of injury to the macular area of the retina: loss of central vision, producing central scotoma, with ophthalmoscopic evidence of hazy macula and bright-red fovea.

### Management

1. *Ultraviolet Radiation Injury.* Instill a topical anesthetic and proceed with ocular evaluation. Use sterile fluorescein to demonstrate the extent of epithelial damage. Patch one eye with a dry, sterile eye pad. Instruct the patient to go to bed for 8 to 12 hours after patching the second upon arrival home. Follow-up is not necessary if all symptoms are gone after 12 hours of patching.
2. *Infrared Radiation Injury.* No emergency treatment is necessary. Refer the patient to an ophthalmologist for evaluation.

## INJURY DUE TO FOREIGN BODIES

### Definition

A foreign body injury to the eye is an ocular injury due to solid substances from the external environment (foreign bodies) which adhere to or become embedded in the ocular tissues.

### Classification

1. External location
   A. Inert
   B. Chemically active

2. Intraocular location

## Basic Principles

1. Suspect a foreign body in all cases of ocular trauma.

2. Do not attempt to remove any foreign body which is wholly or partly intraocular.

3. Any foreign body can be a source of infection, and antibiotics are indicated in all cases.

## Criteria for Diagnosis

1. Direct visualization of the foreign body

2. Indirect visualization of the foreign body

    A. Roentgenographic localization

    B. Ultrasonographic localization

3. History of foreign body sensation. All people incur small externally located foreign bodies. The natural reaction is to attempt removal at once. Damaged epithelium, however, will continue to give a foreign body sensation even though the offending particle is gone.

## Management

1. Systematically inspect the ocular structures as outlined on page 405.

2. External foreign bodies may be treated as follows:

    A. Instill a local anesthetic such as 0.4% benoxinate or 0.5% proparacaine onto the conjunctiva.

    B. Ask an assistant to retract the upper eyelid.

    C. Irrigate the foreign body in an attempt to dislodge it.

    D. If necessary, dislodge the foreign body by pushing it with the bevelled edge of a sterile No. 20 hypodermic needle. Press the needle edge gently on the tissue adjacent to the particle and move it parallel to the surface.

    E. Irrigate again to flush out bacteria that may have been beneath the particle.

    F. Instill fluorescein by paper strip or dropperette; diagram the area of epithelial erosion in the patient's record.

    G. Instill an ophthalmic antibiotic containing polymyxin B and instruct the patient to continue using it 4 times a day.

    H. A dry, sterile eye patch may be used to increase the patient's comfort.

    I. The eye should be examined daily until there is no longer any staining with fluorescein.

    J. Always use a freshly opened container of antibiotic for each case; pathogenic bacteria such as *P. vulgaris* may be introduced with previously used containers.

3. Intraocular foreign bodies require specialized ophthalmologic management; emergency treatment may be instituted as follows:

    A. Absolute bed rest and NPO

    B. Antiemetic (Compazine, 10 mg. I.M.)

    C. Antitussive (codeine, 32 mg. I.M.)

    D. Bilateral eye patches, loosely applied, held in place with a strip of adhesive tape

    E. Consult with an ophthalmologist without delay.

## ACCELERATION (G-FORCE) INJURY

### Definition

An acceleration injury to the eye is an ocular injury produced by the force of a missile striking the patient or by the force with which the patient may strike a stationary object.

### Classification

1. *Blunt Concussion.* Any of the following manifestations of blunt concussion may occur in any combination.

    A. Ecchymosis of the eyelid

    B. Corneal epithelial abrasion

    C. Subconjunctival hemorrhage

    D. Folds or ruptures in Descemet's membrane

    E. Hemorrhage into the anterior chamber (hyphema)

    F. Iris damage

    G. Paralysis of the pupil (iridoplegia)

    H. Iritis

I. Disinsertion of the ciliary body
J. Dislocation of the crystalline lens
K. Vitreous hemorrhage
L. Cataract formation
M. Breaks in the choroid and retina
N. Retinal separation at the ora serrata (dialysis)
O. Macular edema
P. Optic nerve injury
2. *Laceration.* Any part of the ocular anatomy may be involved.
   A. Superficial (nonperforating) lacerations
   B. Deep (perforating) lacerations
3. *Perforation*
   A. Eyeball
   B. Orbital cavity
4. *Orbital Bone Fracture*
   A. Floor
   B. Roof
   C. Walls

## Basic Principles

1. Give first priority to any coexisting life-threatening injuries.
2. If perforating injury is found, stop all manipulations and seek ophthalmologic consultation.
3. Do not excise tissue of any type situated within the rim of the orbit.
4. Bullets and stab wounds may damage the posterior ocular structures even though the anterior anatomy is intact.

## Criteria for Diagnosis

1. History of injurious episode produced by the kinetic energy of objects in the environment
2. The presence of abnormal ocular anatomy and function

## Management

1. Systematically evaluate the ocular structures according to the outline on pages 405-407.
2. If evidence of eyeball perforation is found, emergency treatment may be confined to the following orders:
   A. Admit the patient to the hospital.
   B. Absolute bed rest and NPO
   C. Antiemetic (Compazine, 10 mg. I.M.)
   D. Antitussive (codeine, 32 mg. I.M.)
   E. Apply bilateral eye patches loosely with adhesive tape.
   F. Do not move the patient until he is seen by an ophthalmologist.
3. If no perforation exists, use copious irrigation, soap and cotton applicators to clean wounds of the eyelid.
4. Irrigate the cornea and conjunctiva with sterile saline solution.
5. Eyelid lacerations which parallel the lid margin may be repaired with fine, silk skin sutures.
6. All other manifestations of ocular injury require evaluation by an ophthalmologist; emergency treatment need consist only of ophthalmic antibiotic solution (with polymyxin B) onto the eyeball, followed by a dry, sterile eye patch held in place with adhesive tape.

# 30. UROLOGIC EMERGENCIES

*R. Keith Waterhouse,* M.D.
*Umeschandra B. Patil,* M.D.

## Classification of Urologic Emergencies

1. *Kidney*
   A. Acute pyelonephritis
   B. Carbuncle of the kidney
   C. Perinephric abscess
   D. Gross hematuria with clot colic
   E. Renal colic (calculus)
   F. Renal trauma
2. *Ureter*
   A. Ureteral colic (calculus)
   B. Rupture of the ureter
3. *Bladder*
   A. *Acute Urinary Retention in the Male*
      *(1)* Benign prostatic hypertrophy
      *(2)* Carcinoma of the prostate
      *(3)* Stricture of the urethra
      *(4)* Neurogenic bladder
   B. *Acute Urinary Retention in the Female*
      *(1)* Retroverted gravid uterus
      *(2)* Mass in the rectouterine pouch, ovary or fibroid
      *(3)* Hematocolpos or hydrocolpos
      *(4)* Hysteria
      *(5)* Neurogenic bladder
   C. *Rupture of the Bladder*
4. *Prostate Gland*
   A. Acute prostatitis
   B. Prostatic abscess (acute)
5. *Urethra*
   A. Periurethral abscess associated with urethral stricture
   B. Extravasation of urine associated with urethral stricture and periurethral abscess
   C. Rupture of the urethra
   D. Foreign body in the urethra
   E. Calculus in the urethra
6. *Penis*
   A. Balanoposthitis
   B. Paraphimosis
   C. Laceration or amputation of the penis
7. *Testis and Scrotum*
   A. Acute epididymoorchitis
   B. Torsion of the testis and appendages
   C. Rupture of the testis
   D. Laceration of the scrotum

## GENERAL PRINCIPLES OF UROLOGIC INVESTIGATION

### Physical Examination

1. *Kidneys.* The kidneys are deeply situated and are not normally easily palpable except in thin patients. They are best examined with the patient lying supine and breathing gently. Using two hands, one on the abdomen and one in the costovertebral angle, the kidney is examined during inspiration.

Tenderness over a kidney is best elicited with the patient sitting and the examiner percussing gently over the costovertebral angle. Differences in sensitivity to percussion will often indicate which kidney is involved in an inflammatory process.

The detection of perinephric abscesses by physical examination is also best accomplished with the patient sitting. Care must be taken that the patient is sitting straight and not slouching because of weakness, and having an assistant hold the patient's hands is often useful. A fullness in the flank will indicate the presence of an abscess.

2. *Ureters.* The ureters are not, for practical purposes, susceptible to physical examination. Occasionally a stone lodged in the lower third of the ureter can be palpated on vaginal examination in the parous patient.

3. *Bladder.* The normal bladder is not

413

palpable. If the bladder is palpable, the patient should be asked to void and then should be re-examined. If the bladder is still palpable, residual urine is present.

The amount of residual urine present may be determined by physical examination and without using a catheter. In this technique, the patient is placed supine with the knees flexed and abducted. The examiner's left index finger is well lubricated and placed in the rectum. The bladder is then percussed with a series of sharp taps in the abdominal wall, slowly descending from the umbilicus. The height of the tap above the pubis when a distinct fluid thrill is first felt by the finger in the rectum is noted.

Each centimeter above the pubis represents about 50 ml. of residual urine. Thus, if the thrill is first felt when the level of percussion is 3 cm. above the pubis, there are about 150 ml. of residual urine in the bladder.

4. *Prostate Gland.* The posterior lobe and the two lateral lobes of the prostate are accessible on rectal examination. It must be emphasized that the middle lobe is not palpable and that enlargement of the middle lobe causing acute urinary retention may be present in the face of a completely normal rectal examination.

Carcinoma of the prostate can be recognized with a high degree of accuracy on rectal examination, and the presence of a nodule in the prostate should always excite suspicion.

5. *Testes.* The testes and cord structures are easily palpable and can therefore readily be examined except in patients with acute inflammatory conditions of the testis and epididymis. In such cases, the cord structures may be infiltrated with 1% procaine prior to physical examination (*see* p. 429). Aspiration of a hydrocele may be required before the testis can be palpated, and this is sometimes indicated.

## Urinalysis

Urinalysis is an essential part of a urologic examination and should be carried out by the physician himself.

1. *Chemical Analysis.* Examination for sugar, acetone and protein by test tapes is entirely satisfactory. More elaborate chemical determinations such as urine urea, urine creatinine, urine sodium and osmolality are often needed in patients presenting with anuria.

2. *Microscopic Analysis.* A clean catch specimen should be centrifuged, the supernatant poured off and a drop examined under high power for formed elements. Red cells, white cells and casts should be noted and counted. The presence of crystals, except those of cystine, is rarely significant.

The urine should be stained with Gram's stain and examined for bacteria, and their presence in a carefully collected specimen is of great clinical significance.

3. *Culture.* Clean catch specimens of urine should be sent for culture and colony count. Sensitivity studies should be performed on organisms present.

Care should be taken in the interpretation of colony counts in patients who have been started on antibiotic therapy prior to the obtaining of urine for culture, because in these patients low colony counts may be significant. It is the practice in many laboratories to do sensitivity studies only if the colony count is greater than 100,000 colonies per ml. of urine. In patients who have been started on antibiotic therapy, sensitivities should be performed on all pathogenic organisms recovered regardless of the colony count.

## Blood Studies

1. *Chemical Analysis.* Determinations of serum electrolytes, blood-urea nitrogen and serum creatinine should be performed in patients with urologic emergencies.

2. *Microscopic Analysis.* A hematocrit and complete blood count are essential studies in patients being prepared for operation.

3. *Culture.* Blood cultures should be performed on patients with sepsis

suspected of having bacteremia. Multiple cultures are desirable since there are often relatively few circulating organisms.

## Radiologic Investigations

1. *Plain Abdominal Films (K.U.B.).* A plain film of the abdomen may be used alone or as part of the excretory urogram. The film should be examined with respect to:

    A. Outlines of the kidneys

    B. The psoas margins

    C. The presence of calcifications in the line of the kidneys, ureters or bladder

    D. Intestinal gas patterns and the presence of gas outside the bowel

    E. Bony abnormalities

2. *Excretory Urogram (IVP) and Tomogram.* Prior to the intravenous injection of contrast material, a plain abdominal film must always be obtained.

Contrast material should be injected in appropriate doses, 1 ml./kg. of body weight for adult patients. Exposures should be obtained at 5 minute and 15 minutes after injection. The need for oblique films and delayed films can be decided after study of the plain film and the 5- and 15-minute films. The incorporation of tomographic cuts at 5 minutes is invaluable.

3. *Retrograde Pyelography.* The retrograde passage of a ureteral catheter with the introduction of contrast material through the catheter is now used less than formerly. In the female it can be performed with local anesthesia, but in male patients and children general anesthesia is required.

The method is used in patients with a "silent" kidney on excretory urography. It has now been largely replaced by angiography.

4. *Angiography* (arteriography). Angiographic examination of the kidneys, the celiac axis and the hypogastric vessels may be accomplished by the percutaneous transfemoral introduction of a catheter through which contrast material can be injected (Seldinger technique).

This technique is invaluable in the examination of the severely injured patient, allowing the localization of injuries in the kidneys, liver and spleen and also the definition of bleeding points in the pelvis.

5. *Retrograde Cystography.* A No. 16 French Foley catheter is passed with full sterile precautions into the bladder. Any urine present is collected, sent for culture and the volume measured and recorded.

Contrast material, 150 ml. (we use 50 ml. of Hypaque-60 diluted with 100 ml. of normal saline), is then introduced into the bladder. Anteroposterior and oblique views are then made.

The bladder is then emptied and filled with 150 ml. of air, and a further anteroposterior view is made. The addition of this final study prevents small tears in the back of the bladder from being overlooked.

6. *Retrograde Urethrography.* A No. 12 French Foley catheter is inserted with full sterile precautions about 1 cm. into the anterior urethra. The balloon is inflated with about 2 ml. of water and the patient is placed in the oblique position with the lower leg flexed and the upper leg extended. About 10 to 15 ml. of contrast material are then gently injected and an x-ray exposure is made during injection.

## KIDNEY

### ACUTE PYELONEPHRITIS

#### Definition

Acute pyelonephritis is an acute bacterial infection of the pelvicaliceal system and parenchyma of the kidney.

#### Classification

1. Acute pyelonephritis
2. Chronic pyelonephritis

#### Basic Principles

Pathogenic organisms enter the kidney either from the bladder, for example, by the reflux of infected urine, or through the blood stream. Organisms commonly involved are *E. coli, Streptococcus faecalis, Pseudomonas aeruginosa* and *B. proteus.* In acute or chronic pyelonephritis, there is a history of previous attacks, of known urologic abnormalities and often of urologic surgery.

## Clinical Presentation

The patient has chills and fever often associated with involuntary shaking attacks known as rigors. There is pain in, and tenderness over, the affected kidney. There is dysuria, urinary frequency and urgency and often some hematuria, but this is rarely gross.

## Physical Findings

Tenderness over the affected kidney is the most constant finding. Tenderness over the bladder is not unusual, because many of these patients also have cystitis.

## Investigations

1. *Urinalysis.* Microscopic examination of the urine shows many white cells. There are also some red cells and bacteria. The urinary sediment should be examined after staining with Gram's stain or with methylene blue. It will show gram-negative rods in most instances. The urine should be sent for culture, colony count and determination of the sensitivity of organisms present.

2. *Blood Studies*
    A. Blood should be sent for culture.
    B. Blood-urea nitrogen, serum creatinine and serum electrolytes should be measured as soon as practicable.

## Management

1. Although acute pyelonephritis can be diagnosed on clinical grounds, and therapy may be initiated, an early part of the proper management is radiographic examination of the urinary tract by excretory urography. This will show either that the acute illness has occurred in an anatomically normal urinary tract, in which case operation is rarely, if ever, necessary, or it will show that the acute pyelonephritis is an illness superimposed on a more chronic disease, such as an obstructing stone, in which case operation will be required.

2. The management of acute, uncomplicated pyelonephritis is with bed rest, intravenous fluids and antibiotics. The latter may be given either by mouth, intramuscularly or intravenously. In the absence of information with respect to sensitivity, we currently start treatment with ampicillin, 2 gm. daily, in divided doses. In patients with severe, acute pyelonephritis and gram-negative septicemia, hypothermia, hydrocortisone, 1000 mg. daily, and support of the blood pressure with intravenous vasopressors may be required.

## CARBUNCLE OF THE KIDNEY

### Definition

A carbuncle of the kidney is an abscess in the kidney usually following suppuration elsewhere in the body.

### Basic Principles

Carbuncles usually occur 2 to 6 weeks after an acute suppurative lesion such as a furuncle, acute pharyngitis or a dental abscess. There is sometimes a history of trauma to the affected kidney. The causative organism is usually a staphylococcus.

### Clinical Presentation

Fever and pain in the affected loin are present. There are rarely any urinary symptoms.

### Physical Findings

There is tenderness over the affected kidney.

### Investigations

1. *Blood Studies.* There is a marked leukocytosis.
2. *Urinalysis.* Urinalysis is often normal, but there may be some white cells.

Culture may or may not show organisms.

3. *Radiologic Investigation. Excretory urography* shows a space-occupying lesion within the kidney.

## Management

A small abscess will resolve with vigorous antibiotic therapy. Larger abscesses require operative drainage. If the abscesses are multiple, nephrectomy is occasionally required.

## PERINEPHRIC ABSCESS

### Definition

A perinephric abscess is an abscess occurring in the perirenal fat.

### Classification

A perinephric abscess may be associated with the following:

1. An anatomically normal kidney
2. An anatomically abnormal kidney with spread of infection from the kidney to the perinephric space

### Basic Principles

While in some instances the origin of perinephric abscesses is clear, with spread either from some obvious lesion within the affected kidney or a lesion within the bowel such as acute appendicitis or acute diverticulitis, in many cases the origin of the disease is obscure. The causative organism is usually either *Escherichia coli* or *Streptococcus faecalis.* The disease is more common in diabetic patients.

### Clinical Presentation

Patients with perinephric abscesses present with fever and malaise. There is often little complaint of pain, and it is unusual for there to be symptoms drawing attention to the urinary tract.

### Physical Findings

If the patient is examined in a good light while sitting up, a swelling can be seen in the affected loin. This is often tender. Some pain of flexion and extension of the hip on the affected side due to spasm of the psoas muscle may be noted.

### Investigations

1. *Blood Studies.* There is leukocytosis, and the culture may be positive.

2. *Urinalysis.* Urinary findings are equivocal, sometimes being entirely normal in the presence of large perinephric abscesses.

3. *Radiologic Investigations*

A. *Plain Film.* Displacement of the large bowel toward the midline and gas outside the bowel and in the region of the kidney will often suggest the diagnosis. There is also lumbar scoliosis, due to spasm of the psoas muscle, toward the affected side. The psoas line is absent on the affected side.

B. *Excretory Urography* (intravenous pyelography). Excretory urography may show an obvious lesion within the kidney as a source of the perinephric abscess, but more often the kidney is anatomically normal. It has, however, lost its mobility due to the inflammatory reaction.

### Management

Incision and drainage of the abscess are required. If there are obvious causes for the abscess, these will need appropriate surgical attention.

## GROSS HEMATURIA WITH CLOT COLIC

### Definition

Clot colic associated with gross hematuria is colicky pain due to the passage of blood clots formed in the renal pelvis.

### Basic Principles

Bleeding from the kidney is usually painless, but on occasion clotting occurs in the renal pelvis, and the passage of these clots gives rise to acute colic.

## Clinical Presentation and Physical Findings

The patient presents with gross hematuria and colic.

## Management

The management of the immediate problem is with bed rest, forced fluids and sedation. Investigations to determine the origin of the hematuria should be begun as soon as practicable.

## RENAL COLIC

### Definition

Renal colic is acute colicky pain due to the presence of a stone in the upper urinary tract.

### Basic Principles

The passing of a stone from the kidney through the pelviureteral junction and down the ureter is associated with severe pain. It must be distinguished from acute cholecystitis, acute appendicitis, pneumonia and intestinal colic by a carefully taken history, physical examination and appropriate investigations.

### Clinical Presentation

1. The origin of the pain is usually acute. It begins in the loin and radiates forward and downward toward the groin. If the stone is moving down the ureter, the nature of the pain may gradually change, with the pain radiating to the testis or labium majus on the affected side. If the stone becomes fixed at some point, the colicky nature of the pain may change to a dull, constant aching in the loin.

2. There may be urinary symptoms of dysuria and frequency, and there is often some hematuria.

### Physical Findings

Patients seen at the time of renal colic are obviously in severe distress from pain and are usually restless. There is tenderness in the affected flank but none of the guarding and rigidity associated with peritoneal irritation. Some degree of ileus is not uncommon.

### Investigations

1. *Blood Studies.* Blood studies will usually be within normal limits except in patients with hyperparathyroidism and those with uremia. Patients passing uric acid stones may have an elevated serum uric acid level.

2. *Urinalysis.* It is dangerous to make the diagnosis of renal colic due to calculous diseases in the absence of hematuria, either gross or microscopic. Other findings in the urine are usually within normal limits. It should be noted that occasionally inflammation of the ureter due to retroperitoneal appendicitis can cause microscopic hematuria.

3. *Radiologic Investigations*

A. *Plain Film.* This may show an opacity in the line of the kidney or ureter. There is commonly some degree of ileus.

B. *Excretory Urography.* Urography shows not only the position of the stone in the collecting system but also the degree of obstruction in the affected kidney. It also is invaluable for studying the unaffected renal system. Care should be taken to obtain oblique films as well as the usual anteroposterior views to make certain that any radiopaque densities seen are within the urinary tract.

C. Nonopaque stones may be demonstrated by excretory urography, but additional studies such as retrograde pyelography are often required to make the diagnosis certain.

### Management

1. Stones less than 1.0 cm. in their longest axis will in many cases pass through the upper urinary tract and be voided spontaneously without operative interference. The attack of acute colic should be treated by generous analgesia with intramuscular meperidine. The patient is instructed to void into a clear

glass or plastic container to note if the stone is passed. This urine-catch should be done particularly at the time of moving the bowels, since this is a common time for the stone to be voided. When recovered, the stone should be submitted for chemical analysis.

2. Larger stones or stones which become impacted will require operation. Stones less than 1.0 cm. in their longest axis and lying in the lower third of the ureter may be considered for manipulation and possible extraction by cystoscopic methods. Larger stones and stones lying higher in the ureter need removal by open operation such as pyelolithotomy and ureterolithotomy.

## RENAL TRAUMA

### Definition

Renal trauma is damage to the kidney by external forces.

### Classification

1. Renal trauma may be due to:
   A. Closed injuries
   B. Penetrating injuries
2. The degree of trauma may be:
   A. *Contusion:* bruising only
   B. *Laceration*
      *(1)* Of the parenchyma
      *(2)* Of the parenchyma and collecting system
   C. *Avulsion:* when the kidney is torn from the renal pedicle

### Basic Principles

1. Injuries of a severity sufficient to cause renal trauma are commonly associated with injuries to other body systems. Injury to the spleen when the blow is on the left and lacerations of the liver when the blow is on the right are commonly seen. Care must be taken not to overlook associated injuries, the most important matter being to consider the possibility of their presence.

2. Some patients with modest injuries develop clinical signs suggesting a ruptured kidney. In these cases the kidney involved is often already the seat of a pathologic process, e.g., hydronephrosis, Wilms' tumor or hypernephroma.

### Clinical Presentation

1. In most instances, patients either give a history of injury to the flank or there are obvious penetrating wounds suggesting the possibility of injury to the kidney.

2. Hematuria is a constant finding, ranging from microscopic to gross with passage of clots.

3. Shock of varying degree, depending on the amount and rate of bleeding, is present.

### Physical Findings

A palpable mass may be felt in the flank, and there may be guarding and abdominal rigidity on the affected side. Lacerations, abrasions and wounds of entrance are often present.

### Investigations

1. *Urinalysis.* Examination of the urine will reveal the presence of blood.

2. *Blood Studies.* Measurement of the hematocrit as an estimate of the amount of bleeding is essential.

3. *Radiologic Investigations*
   A. An *excretory urogram* should be performed on an urgent basis. Only in the most life-threatening situations should a patient be taken to the operating room without this study, because it provides invaluable information with respect to the uninjured kidney.

   B. *Angiography.* The availability of angiography 24 hours a day has led to its increasing use in the study of the patient with an injured kidney. It is invaluable in studying patients in whom the injured kidney is "silent" on the excretory urogram.

   C. *Retrograde Pyelography.* Prior to the introduction of renal angiography, this was a common investigation. It is now much less commonly used, but it may be necessary in the study of the "silent kidney" if angiography is not available.

## Management

1. The management of the patient with an injured kidney is in the first instance conservative with bed rest and replacement of any blood loss with whole blood transfusion. Ninety per cent of cases of blunt renal injuries will respond to conservative management. In those patients who show subsiding signs, strict bed rest should be continued for 10 days. Insistence on carrying on with conservative therapy in the face of evidence of continued hemorrhage can be disastrous. Our standing rule is that patients who are still unstable after receiving 1500 ml. of whole blood must be explored.

2. Penetrating injuries much more commonly require exploration. In our experience, such exploratory operations are best performed through the transperitoneal route. This allows easy access to the renal vessels and thorough visualization of the other organs in the peritoneal cavity. The injured kidney should be carefully examined, because in many instances conservative debridement will suffice with partial renal salvage.

# URETER

## URETERAL COLIC

*See* Renal Colic, page 418.

## RUPTURE OF THE URETER

### Definition

Rupture of the ureter is damage to the ureter by external forces.

### Classification

Rupture of the ureter may be either partial or complete. The damage may be due to gunshot or knife wounds and occasionally to blunt trauma. Injuries to the ureter may occur during surgical procedures in the pelvis. Occasionally bilateral injuries occur.

### Basic Principles

Rupture of the ureter, either partial or complete, leads to extravasation of urine, and it is this extravasation which leads to the diagnosis—the urine either draining through recent surgical incisions or wounds or collecting to form a palpable mass ("uroma").

### Clinical Presentation

Patients usually give a history of a recent injury or an operation, suggesting that one or both ureters may have been damaged. It is important to consider ureteral injury both in the recently injured patient and also during operations in the abdomen and pelvis, because repair during the initial operation is easier and more satisfactory than delayed repair.

### Physical Findings

1. In the recently injured patient, there are no physical findings suggesting that the ureter has been damaged. Later in the course of the illness, extravasated urine may either drain from the surgical wounds or from the vagina in the case of patients with ureters damaged during hysterectomy, or it may collect in the abdomen. Encysted collections of urine are known as "uromas" and many produce palpable masses.

2. Patients with urinary extravasation, especially if infection has occurred, show signs of toxemia. Spiking fevers and rigors are common and should suggest the diagnosis.

### Investigations

1. *Urinalysis.* The urine may show red cells and white cells or may be completely normal. The urine should be cultured.

2. *Blood Studies.* Leukocytosis is present in later stages of the illness. The blood-urea nitrogen and the serum creatinine should be measured. If the blood-urea nitrogen is elevated and the serum creatinine is normal, it may be assumed

that the high levels are due to absorption of urea from the extravasated urine. If both the blood-urea nitrogen and the creatinine are raised, compromise of both kidneys should be suspected.

3. *Radiologic Investigations*

A. When damage to the ureter is suspected following bullet wounds or stab wounds, a *cystogram* should be performed. After the cystogram, the bladder should be drained of all contrast material and an *excretory urogram* done. If there is no extravasation on the cystogram, but there is extravasation on the excretory urogram, the ureter has been damaged.

B. In cases in which diagnosis has been delayed, excretory urography should also be performed. The side on which the injury has occurred will show hydronephrosis of a moderate degree. There is some element of obstruction with a fistula even if the ureter has been completely transected and urine is draining freely to the outside.

## Management

1. If the diagnosis of trauma to the ureter is made either before or at the time of exploration for injury, repair can be made at that time. The same principle applies to accidental transections during operation discovered at the time of injury. If the diagnosis is made later in the course of the disease, urinary diversion by nephrostomy, drainage of any collections and delayed repair 3 to 6 months later is the safest course.

2. Repair may be either by ureteroureterostomy, ureteroneocystostomy or by transureteroureterostomy.

3. It should be emphasized that all of the above remarks apply to complete transections. If it can be demonstrated by cystoscopy and the retrograde passage of a ureteral catheter that there is only a partial transection, then, provided that the extravasated urine is draining freely and the patient is not toxic, repair can be delayed

because in most instances spontaneous healing will occur.

# BLADDER
## ACUTE URINARY RETENTION
### Definition

Acute urinary retention is the inability to pass urine despite desire. It is usually associated with considerable discomfort.

### Classification

It is useful to consider acute urinary retention separately by sex.
1. Acute urinary retention in the male
2. Acute urinary retention in the female

*Acute Urinary Retention in the Male*
### Basic Principles

Urinary retention in the male has multiple causes.
1. Benign prostatic hypertrophy
2. Carcinoma of the prostate gland
3. Stricture of the urethra, with or without periurethral abscess
4. Neurogenic bladder
5. Calculus or foreign body in the urethra
6. Phimosis

### Clinical Presentation

The patient is acutely uncomfortable, with complaints directly referable to his inability to void. There is often a history of urinary difficulties with progressive slowing of the stream, hesitancy in the morning, nocturia and in some instances a history of a previous attack of retention. Small volumes may be passed, but they afford the patient no relief.

### Physical Findings

In all patients except the extremely obese, the distended bladder can be felt and often can be seen. Examination of the external genitalia may reveal an obvious cause such as a stone in the course of the urethra or impacted in the meatus, a periurethral abscess or severe phimosis. In a large number of patients, the diagnosis may be obvious on rectal examination, either an enlarged benign prostate being felt or there being an obvious prostatic malignancy. In patients in acute retention from urethral stricture, there are no physical findings.

## Investigations

The investigations required can be delayed until after the relief of the acute problem.

## Management

1. Management of acute urinary retention may be either by urethral catheterization or by suprapubic urinary diversion. The choice between these two methods is important, and an incorrect choice may be life-threatening.

2. Patients with obvious inflammatory involvement of the urethra should not be catheterized because gram-negative septicemia will commonly follow. Similarly, if gentle attempts at urethral catheterization are unsuccessful, they should be abandoned and suprapubic diversion performed, because again it is in this group of patients that iatrogenic injury to the urethra occurs.

3. Two techniques of relieving acute urinary retention must be considered.

A. *Technique of Urethral Catheterization*

(1) This must be a sterile procedure. The genitalia should be prepared with a suitable antiseptic and draped in a sterile fashion. The most suitable catheter is a No. 16 or 18 French Foley catheter. Smaller catheters are not rigid enough to pass the enlarged prostate, and larger catheters are unnecessarily traumatic. A 5-ml. balloon catheter should be chosen.

(2) In cases in which there is difficulty due to considerable prostatic enlargement, a Coudé catheter may pass more easily. In other instances a catheter guide (mandarin) may be used. This is a thin, flexible guide which is inserted into the lumen of the catheter. In experienced hands it is invaluable, but in those unskilled in its use it is a treacherous instrument, being a common cause of perforation of the urethra with the instrument passing into the rectum.

B. *Technique of Suprapubic Diversion*

(1) *Punch Cystostomy*

(a) Punch cystostomy should never be attempted in patients who have had previous bladder or prostatic operations by the suprapubic or retropubic route.

(b) The lower abdomen and genitalia should be shaved, prepared and draped. The bladder must be readily palpable. The area above the pubic symphysis is infiltrated with 1% procaine, additional 1% procaine being used to infiltrate the rectus sheath and the prevesical space. A short stab incision is made in the skin ½ inch above the pubic symphysis and a No. 24 French Campbell trocar is inserted. This is pushed through the rectus sheath into the bladder and the obturator is removed. A well-lubricated No. 16 French Foley catheter is then passed down the groove of the Campbell trocar and the balloon is blown up in the bladder. It is only after the balloon has been blown up that the trocar can be safely removed. The skin wound is closed with one or two stitches, and a sterile dressing is applied.

(c) This operation can safely be performed in the patient's bed or in the emergency department.

(2) *Formal Cystostomy*

(a) This operation should be performed in an operating room with good light. It is used in patients who have had previous bladder or prostatic surgery and require suprapubic diversion; in patients who have had these operations, the peritoneum is bound to the bladder and often even to the pubic symphysis.

(b) The patient is prepared as for

punch cystostomy, but a vertical 2-inch incision is made immediately above the pubis. This is deepened through the rectus sheath, and the recti muscles are separated bluntly. These muscles are retracted laterally, and the bladder is exposed by bluntly pushing the tissues above it in a cephalad direction. This should be continued until the characteristic crisscross muscle fibers of the bladder are seen. Good light and good retraction are essential.

*(c)* Once the bladder is recognized, the Campbell trocar can be used to introduce a No. 16 French Foley catheter as described under the technique of punch cystostomy. The recti muscles and the rectus fascia are closed with chromic 0 catgut interrupted sutures. The skin is closed with a number of silk sutures, and a dry dressing is applied.

*Acute Urinary Retention in the Female*

## Basic Principles

It is important to be aware that in almost all instances of acute urinary retention in the female the origin may be found in the gynecologic history and by pelvic examination.

## Causes

1. Retroverted gravid uterus
2. Mass in the rectouterine pouch, ovary or fibroid
3. Hematocolpos or hydrocolpos
4. Neurogenic bladder
5. Hysteria

## Management

Catheterization of the female urethra does not present technical problems, and there is no indication for suprapubic diversion of the urine.

## RUPTURE OF THE BLADDER

## Definition

Rupture of the bladder is damage to the bladder usually by external forces.

## Classification

Ruptures of the bladder are best considered as:
1. Extraperitoneal
2. Intraperitoneal
3. Spontaneous

## Basic Principles

In most cases there is a clear history of injury suggesting the possibility of rupture of the bladder, but it is important to be aware that intoxicated patients commonly rupture the distended bladder by falling and give little or no history. There is a small group of patients who develop a "spontaneous" rupture of the bladder. Many of these "spontaneous" ruptures may, of course, be traumatic, the trauma occurring during states of confusion, but there is a small segment of patients with bladder rupture in whom no such cause is suggested. While these "spontaneous," nontraumatic ruptures may occur in disease such as neoplasm, occasionally an apparently normal bladder will rupture spontaneously.

## Clinical Presentation

There is usually a clear history of trauma to the lower abdomen, suggesting the bladder may have been injured. Despite rupture of the bladder, many patients are able to void freely, the urine often showing signs of blood. Almost all extraperitoneal ruptures are associated with fracture of the pelvis.

## Physical Findings

There is tenderness in the lower abdomen, and, if the rupture is intraperitoneal, there may be evidence of peritonitis.

## Investigations

1. *Urinalysis.* The urine will always show blood either macroscopically or microscopically.
2. *Radiologic Investigation.* All patients suspected of having a ruptured

bladder should be investigated by retrograde cystography. It cannot be too strongly stressed that the instillation of a measured volume of sterile fluid into the bladder and the return of this measured volume does *not* rule out the diagnosis of ruptured bladder. (For the technique of cystography, *see* p. 415.)

## Management

The management of the patient with a ruptured bladder is operative. Urinary diversion by suprapubic cystostomy is essential. In intraperitoneal ruptures the tear in the bladder must be sutured with chromic 0 catgut. In extraperitoneal ruptures this is not essential, urinary diversion by cystostomy and drainage of the perivesical space being sufficient.

## PROSTATE GLAND
### ACUTE PROSTATITIS

### Definition

Prostatitis is an acute bacterial infection of the prostate gland.

### Basic Principles

In the past, acute gonococcal prostatitis was common. Although it still occurs, it is seen much less commonly, and the most usual causative organisms are *E. coli* and *Streptococcus faecalis.*

### Clinical Presentation

The patients are acutely ill with malaise and fever, often spiking to 104 to 105° F., and in some cases with rigors. There is urinary frequency and dysuria. There may be complaints of perineal pain and pain on defecation.

### Physical Findings

1. There are few physical findings except upon rectal examination. In patients suspected of having acute prostatitis, rectal examination should be performed with great gentleness, because a roughly performed examination will not only give the

patient great pain but also may cause gram-negative septicemia.

2. A complete urologic examination, including cystoscopy and urethral calibration, should be performed when the patient has recovered from the acute illness.

### Management

Treatment is the same as for acute pyelonephritis (*see* p. 415).

## PROSTATIC ABSCESS (ACUTE)
### Definition

A prostatic abscess is an abscess in the prostate, usually complicating acute prostatitis.

### Basic Principles

Since the advent of antibiotics, prostatic abscesses have become uncommon. The causative organism is almost always either *E. coli* or *Streptococcus faecalis.*

### Clinical Presentation

Physical findings and investigations are the same as in Acute Prostatitis, above.

### Management

Small abscesses will resolve with chemotherapy, but larger ones require drainage. This may be performed by exposure of the prostate perineally and drainage to the exterior or by rupture of the abscess into the urethra with the resectoscope. The choice of operation is dictated by surgical circumstances.

## URETHRA
### PERIURETHRAL ABSCESS ASSOCIATED WITH URETHRAL STRICTURE

### Definition

A periurethral abscess is a perineal abscess originating from the urethra.

### Basic Principles

Periurethral abscesses are associated

with strictures of the urethra. The strictures are gonococcal in origin, but the primary infection has occurred many years previously, often as long as twenty years ago, and the acute abscess is never gonococcal in origin. The causative organisms are usually *E. coli* and *Streptococcus faecalis*.

## Clinical Presentation

1. The patient presents with a midline swelling in the perineum, which usually is obviously inflammatory, and the swelling can vary from an acute inflammation with a history of only some hours to a more chronic process extending over several days. There is almost always some fever.

2. Urinary symptoms are variable, some patients being able to void freely whereas others are in almost complete retention. Many patients are aware that they have a urethral stricture because they have attended clinics for urethral dilatation.

## Physical Findings

There is a fluctuant swelling in the midline of the perineum, limited laterally by the attachment of the deep fascia to the inferior pubic rami and posteriorly by the attachment of the deep fascia to the pelvic diaphragm (triangular ligament). If diagnosis is delayed or frank rupture of the urethra occurs, the process may spread forward into the scrotum.

## Investigations

1. *Urinalysis.* Microscopic examination of the urine shows many white cells. There are some red cells and bacteria. The urinary sediment should be examined after staining with Gram's stain and in most instances will show gram-negative rods. The urine should be sent for culture, colony count and determination of the sensitivity of organisms present.

2. *Blood Studies*

A. Blood should be sent for culture.

B. Blood-urea nitrogen, serum creatinine and serum electrolytes should be measured as soon as practicable, because many of these patients have damaged urinary tracts.

C. The hematocrit and white blood cell count should be measured.

3. *Radiologic Investigations*

A. *Excretory urography* should be performed during the convalescence.

B. Under no circumstances should retrograde urethrography be attempted, because this will cause severe gram-negative septicemia and will not provide any information of value.

4. *Cystoscopy.* Cystoscopy is not indicated during the acute process.

## Management

Patients should be started on intravenous ampicillin and prepared for operation. The periurethral abscess is drained, and urinary diversion is obtained either by suprapubic cystostomy or perineal urethrostomy.

## EXTRAVASATION OF URINE ASSOCIATED WITH PERIURETHRAL ABSCESS AND URETHRAL STRICTURE

This is merely an extension of the process discussed under Periurethral Abscess Associated with Urethral Stricture, above.

The basic priniciples, clinical presentation, physical findings and management are similar except that in this case the process is more advanced. Extravasation of urine may have occurred, with dissection of the subcutaneous tissues not only of the scrotum but also of the abdominal wall. The fascial attachments between the superficial fascia and the deep fascia of the thighs prevent extension of the process into the legs.

## RUPTURE OF THE URETHRA

### Definition

Rupture of the urethra is damage to the urethra by external forces.

## Classification

Ruptures may occur either above or below the pelvic diaphragm (triangular ligament) and may be complete or incomplete.

## Basic Principles

It is important to distinguish between the two sites of rupture of the urethra (above or below the pelvic diaphragm), because they have different physical findings, are caused by different kinds of injury, require different treatment and have an entirely different prognosis.

## Clinical Presentation

1. Patients give a history of injury which will usually localize the site of the rupture. Blows between the legs from falling astride beams, scaffolding, loose manhole covers and the like are known as "straddle injuries" and cause rupture of the urethra distal to the pelvic diaphragm.

2. Injuries to the urethra above the pelvic diaphragm are almost always associated with automobile accidents, the injured person being a pedestrian, and the patient invariably has a fractured pelvis. "Seat-belt" injures also involve damage to the proximal urethra.

3. Patients with complete rupture of the urethra are unable to void.

## Physical Findings

1. In injuries below the pelvic diaphragm, there are physical findings in the perineum, with ecchymosis of the scrotum and perineal body. There may be blood at the meatus.

2. In injuries above the pelvic diaphragm, there are no physical findings in the perineum, all extravasated blood and urine being above the pelvic diaphragm in the pelvis. Rectal examination may show the prostate to be abnormally situated, having been displaced upward and backward by the injury and the unopposed pull of the levator muscles.

## Investigations

1. *Urinalysis.* Urine is unavailable for study, and patients should not be encouraged to void because voiding causes unnecessary extravasation of urine.

2. *Blood Studies.* Measurement of a hematocrit as an estimate of the amount of bleeding is essential.

3. *Radiologic Investigations.* Studies of the urethra by retrograde urethrography are invaluable for the accurate localization of the site of injury (for details of technique, *see* p. 415). Excretory urography is also useful in the general assessment of patients with a badly damaged urinary tract and should be performed if at all possible.

## Management

Treatment of the ruptured urethra is operative. Regardless of whether the rupture is above or below the pelvic diaphragm, suprapubic cystostomy should be performed. In ruptures below the pelvic diaphragm, the site of rupture is exposed and repaired; in those above the pelvic diaphragm, a Foley catheter is threaded through the urethra, across the tear and into the bladder. Light traction on this catheter will then bring the torn edges of the urethra into opposition. Traction should be maintained for 3 weeks so that healing can occur. Some surgeons prefer to repair ruptures above the pelvic diaphragm in 2 stages, performing a suprapubic cystostomy on the day of injury and repair of the urethra by urethroplasty about 6 months later.

## FOREIGN BODY IN THE URETHRA

### Definition

A foreign body in the urethra refers to the introduction of foreign objects into, and their subsequent incarceration within, the urethra.

### Basic Principles

1. Foreign bodies in the urethra are

limited to the male, since foreign bodies introduced into the urethra in the female do not lodge there but pass on into the bladder.

2. The range of sizes of foreign bodies introduced is enormous.

## Clinical Presentation

1. Patients may or may not give a history of insertion of a foreign object; many express surprise when told they have a foreign body in the urethra.

2. Patients may present with urinary retention, urethral discharge or the formation of an abscess in the line of the urethra.

## Physical Findings

The object may be palpable or there may be swelling and inflammation in the line of the urethra.

## Investigations

1. Radiologic examination of the urethra by plain film may show the location of a radiopaque foreign body. Retrograde urethrography should not be performed.

2. If there is a urethral discharge, it should be sent for culture.

## Management

1. Operative removal is usually easy and may be accomplished either through the lumen of the urethra, using endoscopic instruments, or by incision of the urethra overlying the foreign body. If the latter method is used, suprapubic cystostomy should be established to allow healing of the urethra.

2. Suitable broad-spectrum antibiotics should be administered if there is obvious superimposed infection.

## CALCULUS IN THE URETHRA

### Definition

This refers to the impaction of a calculus in the urethra.

## Basic Principles

This disease is limited to the male except in an occasional case in which a calculus occurs in a diverticulum of the female urethra. The stone usually lodges in the external meatus, but, in patients with urethral strictures, it may lodge in the pendulous urethra.

## Clinical Presentation

Patients may or may not have a history of stone disease. Most patients present with acute urinary retention, but in some cases there is acute pain during voiding and this causes the person to seek medical attention.

## Physical Findings

In almost all instances the stone can be seen at the external meatus. In those cases in which the stone is lodged in the urethra, it can be palpated.

## Investigations

Investigation of the local problem is usually unnecessary, but patients should be studied with respect to the general problem of stone disease in the urinary tract by excretory urography and blood studies.

## Management

1. Removal of stones impacted in the external meatus is usually very easy. In some patients external meatotomy may be needed.

2. Stones impacted behind strictures are more difficult to remove and usually require operation.

## PENIS

### BALANOPOSTHITIS

### Definition

Balanoposthitis is an inflammatory process between the foreskin and the glans penis.

### Basic Principles

This disease occurs in the uncircumcised

male when there is some degree of phimosis and the foreskin is not completely retractile. The infection is usually a mixed one, the causative organisms being *E. coli, Streptococcus faecalis* and organisms such as *Streptococcus viridans* which are normally present on the skin.

## Clinical Presentation

The patients complain of a purulent discharge and a painful nonretractile foreskin.

## Physical Findings

The foreskin is swollen, inflamed and nonretractile. Pus is seen to be present below the foreskin.

## Investigations

The purulent exudate should be cultured.

## Management

Free drainage is obtained by making a dorsal slit of the foreskin. General anesthesia is necessary and local anesthesia should be avoided. Complete circumcision should not be performed at this time since manipulation of infected tissue may lead to gram-negative septicemia. Sitz baths will lead to rapid improvement once free drainage has been obtained by the dorsal slit.

## PARAPHIMOSIS

### Definition

Paraphimosis refers to a swollen and edematous foreskin which has become fixed in the retracted position.

### Basic Principles

Paraphimosis only occurs in uncircumcised males with some degree of phimosis. After retracting the foreskin, the patient is unable to replace it, and the relative obstruction at the level of the glans penis causes edema in the connective tissue between the two layers of the foreskin. It is common in babies and young children, but it is also seen in adults.

## Clinical Presentation

The degree of swelling of the foreskin is often more than is expected, and the diagnosis is often overlooked because of the unusual visual aspect of the problem. The family, in the case of children, or the patient himself should be questioned as to whether or not the patient has been circumcised. The patient complains of gross swelling of the penis, but pain is not a marked feature of the disease. Progression to gangrene is very unusual.

## Physical Findings

There are no findings other than the previously described grossly edematous foreskin. The glans penis is uninvolved, but it may be partially hidden by the swelling.

## Investigations

No investigations are required.

## Management

1. Reduction of the paraphimosis can often be accomplished without operation. Firm pressure on the swollen foreskin will displace the edema fluid into the connective tissue below the shaft of the penis, and, following this, pressure on the glans will cause the foreskin to slip forward, reducing the paraphimosis.

2. In intractable cases, incision of the constricting band on the dorsal surface of the penis will allow both the escape of edema fluid and the easy reduction of the paraphimosis.

3. Episodes of paraphimosis are an indication for circumcision.

## LACERATION OR AMPUTATION OF THE PENIS

### Definition

Laceration or amputation of the penis is caused by damage to the penis by external forces.

### Basic Principles

Injuries to the penis may be due to

gunshot or knife wounds, to self-inflicted injuries or to industrial accidents. In the latter, workers usually have come too close to unprotected industrial or agricultural machinery and their clothes have become entangled. This results in stripping off the skin from the penis and testes. Blood loss is usually remarkably small.

### Clinical Presentation and Physical Findings

The nature and extent of the injury is obvious on inspection.

### Management

1. Treatment is operative and can best be carried out under general anesthesia. The skin of the glans is rarely affected and should be preserved. Minimal debridement of dead skin should be performed, and the skin should be replaced with interrupted nonabsorbable sutures. In cases of extensive loss of the scrotum, the testes may be placed in pockets of skin dissected in the thighs. In patients with extensive skin loss from the penis, the penis may be buried temporarily in the scrotum, being removed from the scrotum 3 to 6 months later. Skin grafting may be required at that time.

2. In patients in whom part or all of the body of the penis has been lost, toilet of the wound and urethrocutaneous anastomosis of the urethra should be performed.

3. In all patients, a small indwelling urethral catheter and a pressure dressing should be used for the first 72 hours after injury.

4. It should be unnecessary to stress the need for conservative surgery in the management of penile injury. In cases of self-amputation, if the distal stump is available, replantation should be considered.

## TESTIS AND SCROTUM
### ACUTE EPIDIDYMO-ORCHITIS

### Definition

Acute epididymo-orchitis is an acute inflammatory process in the testis and epididymis.

### Basic Principles

Acute inflammatory processes of the testis and epididymis are not always bacterial in origin, although in many instances the disease in the testis is secondary to urinary tract infection or acute prostatitis. The causative organism in such cases is usually *E. coli* or *Streptococcus faecalis*. Nonbacterial inflammation may be due to reflux of sterile urine down the vas deferens causing a chemical inflammation.

### Clinical Presentation

Patients with epididymo-orchitis complain of pain in the affected testis, swelling and fever. In bacterial infections, high fever is not uncommon and gram-negative septicemia may occur. Pain in the spermatic cord may indicate the presence of some degree of funiculitis. A recent history of urinary tract infection is often obtained.

### Physical Findings

1. The epididymis and testis become indistinguishable as a swollen, tender mass. Some thickening of the cord is often present.

2. Rectal examination may show the prostate to be tender.

### Investigations

A urine culture should be performed. In patients with a positive urine culture, complete investigation of the urinary tract should be undertaken after resolution of the acute process.

### Management

1. A great deal of symptomatic relief may be obtained by infiltration of the spermatic cord at the level of the external inguinal ring with 1% procaine. The skin should be infiltrated with a fine needle and then some 15 to 20 ml. of 1% procaine placed around the cord structures.

2. Pending the availability of the urine culture, treatment may be commenced with ampicillin, 500 mg. 4 times a day.

3. Local relief may be obtained by the wearing of a scrotal support.

## TORSION OF THE TESTIS AND APPENDAGES

### Definition

Torsion of the testis is the twisting of the testis on the spermatic cord, causing infarction. Similarly, the appendix testis may twist at its point of attachment to the testis.

### Basic Principles

This is usually a disease of children and young adults. There may be a history of previous muscular exertion, but torsion of the testis can occur at rest and even during sleep. There have been reported cases in the neonatal period. While usually unilateral, bilateral cases have been reported.

### Clinical Presentation

There is a sudden onset of pain in the affected testis without previous history of urinary tract complaints.

### Physical Findings

The testis and cord are involved in torsion of the testis. The testis is swollen and tender and the cord is thickened. The testis appears to be rather high in the scrotum. In cases of torsion of the appendix testis, the scrotum is swollen and edematous and there is tenderness localized to the small mass on the upper pole of the testis.

### Investigations

No investigations are required to diagnose these conditions, but routine preoperative studies of the blood and urine are required.

### Management

1. The treatment is operative. The twisted testis should be untwisted and fixed in position so that retorsion cannot occur.

In cases in which the diagnosis has been made late, orchiectomy may be required. At the time of operation, fixation of the normal testis should be performed.

2. Torsion of an appendix testis is treated by surgical removal of the structure. If the diagnosis is certain and the pain is easily controlled, torsion of an appendix testis may be treated conservatively.

## RUPTURE OF THE TESTIS

### Definition

Rupture of the testis is rupture of the tunica albuginea testis by external force.

### Basic Principles

Rupture of the testis is more common than is realized. Many patients thought to have a scrotal hematoma have in fact a ruptured testis.

### Clinical Presentation

There is a history of injury, followed by swelling of the scrotum.

### Physical Findings

The scrotum is swollen, tense and painful. The testis cannot be palpated.

### Investigations

No investigations are required to diagnose this condition, but routine preoperative studies of blood and urine are required.

### Management

Surgical exploration of the scrotum with evacuation of the hematoma and repair of the lacerated testis is required.

## LACERATION OF THE SCROTUM

### Definition

A laceration of the scrotum is an injury to the scrotum.

### Basic Principles

Laceration of the scrotum may be due to gunshot or knife wounds, to self-inflicted injuries or to industrial accidents. In the latter, workers have usually come too close to unprotected industrial or agricultural machinery and their clothes have become entangled. This results in the stripping off of the skin of the scrotum.

## Clinical Presentation and Physical Findings

The nature and extent of injury are obvious on inspection. There may be evidence of shock due to pain and blood loss.

## Management

Treatment is operative and can best be carried out under general anesthesia. Careful debridement should be performed and the lacerations repaired with nonabsorbable sutures. In cases with extensive skin loss, the testes can be implanted in pockets of skin dissected in the thighs. The scrotum should be drained for 48 hours with Penrose drains and a pressure dressing applied for 72 hours.

# 31. THE INJURED HAND

*Henry Burns,* M. D.

## INTRODUCTION

### Definition

Hand injury is a destruction of one or more of the structures that make up this complex unit (i.e., skin, bone, joint, nerve or tendon).

### Classification

1. Wounds of the integument alone
   A. Superficial
   B. Deep
   C. Perforating or nonperforating
   D. Crushed
   E. Avulsed
· 2. Compound wounds involving skin as well as one or more deeper structures, such as:
   A. Bone–joint
   B. Tendons
   C. Nerves
   D. Vessels
3. Closed or open fractures
4. Amputations
   A. Total
   B. Partial
5. Burns
   A. Thermal
   B. Electric
   C. Chemical
6. Frostbite
7. Vascular injuries
8. Volkmann's ischemic paralysis
9. Special wounds
   A. Wringer injuries
   B. Gunshot wounds
   C. Grease gun injuries
   D. Tear gas injuries

### Basic Principles

Hand injuries are a common form of injury and comprise up to one third of the injuries seen in the emergency departments of our hospitals. They are significant in that, while small in size, they incapacitate the individual and compromise his earning ability. Once severely injured, the hand which performs both simple and complex movements can never again do all its functions adequately. When reconstructing the hand, consider the hand's vital functions of *grasp* and *pinch* with *normal sensation* and *strength*. The most critical time in the treatment of hand injuries occurs when the assessment and initial definitive surgery are carried out.

Wound closure is probably the single most important factor in determining the final result. If the hand can be covered completely with viable skin, then edema and infection are reduced and healing by fibrosis is lessened. It is preferable for the skin to be flexible with adequate sensation. Next in importance is the skeletal reconstruction. Tendons and nerves can be repaired at a later date. The over-all consideration is toward the maintenance of the position of function and the prevention of edema and infection.

### Management

1. Initial management in the emergency department should consist of the following:
   A. Assess the damage. In the assessment of the type of reconstruction to be done consideration must be given to the patient's incentive, age and occupation, and the anticipated functional recovery of his hand, but in all injuries an effort is made to maintain length, movement and sensation to all digits.
   B. Apply a splint pressure dressing.
   *(1)* The pressure dressing serves a triple purpose:
   *(a)* It protects the hand from further trauma.

*(b)* It eliminates infection and further contamination.

*(c)* It produces adequate hemostasis.

*(2)* Applying a splint to the pressure dressing puts the hand in the functional resting position and alleviates much of the pain.

C. Elevation minimizes swelling.

D. Administer tetanus prophylaxis and antibiotics. The time since injury is less important since the advent of antibiotics.

E. Radiographic examination if osseous injury is suspected

F. Most injuries are usually worse than they appear. Exploration of severe wounds in the emergency department should be avoided.

G. Initial apparent injury is usually deceptive. Inapparent damage and ensuing edema are usually underestimated.

2. Definitive treatment of the severe acute injury is an operating room procedure.

A. General anesthetic or axillary block is necessary.

B. A bloodless field is advisable; a tourniquet should be applied.

C. The skin is scrubbed carefully.

D. The wound is copiously irrigated.

E. Meticulous debridement is essential since the hand is devoid of excess tissue.

F. All utilizable tissues should be preserved.

*(1)* Save all palmar skin since it is difficult to replace.

*(2)* When debriding tendons, nerves and bone, try, whenever possible, to leave them intact.

*(3)* Don't remove a fragment of bone which retains soft tissue attachment.

*(4)* Musculature should not be disturbed unless obviously necrotic or crushed. Obviously, judgment and experience are necessary to determine the viability of tissues.

3. Repair and closure follow standard principles.

A. Skin coverage is applied as the first consideration.

*(1)* It may be accomplished by primary suture, split graft or by flap.

*(2)* Split grafts are unsuitable for denuded tendons, nerves, bone or joint where flaps are necessary to cover these structures.

B. Fractures are reduced and immobilized, provided this will not compromise coverage.

C. Extensor tendons are repaired primarily, but contused flexor tendons and nerves may be saved for secondary suture. This is true if more than three of the five hand tissues are involved in injury. If only skin, nerves and tendons are involved, as in the wrist, primary repair of all these structures may be considered. Initial nerve repair appears to give the best results.

D. Despite the surgical skill, operation on the injured hand may result in post-traumatic edema with subsequent fibrosis, which will compromise the final result.

E. Amputation of a part of the hand is a difficult decision. The most important units to salvage in a hand are the wrist, thumb and index and middle fingers.

*(1)* Absolute indication for amputation is irreparable loss of blood supply.

*(2)* Relative indications are:

*(a)* Too many unfavorable aspects to the repair of a part

*(b)* The age of the patient and his profession

4. Delayed primary repair is indicated in the immediate care of severe injuries, especially on the battlefield, after three or four days when the wound begins to granulate. During this waiting period, the hand is elevated and maintained in the functional position with moist warm dressings and systemic antibiotics. When surgically clean, the skin may be closed. With this technique, debridement is more readily performed, complications are rare, postoperative rigidity is minimal and edema is reduced.

5. Postoperative care is directed toward preventing infection and minimizing edema, scarring and joint stiffness. Early motion is commendable, particularly of the noninjured parts. In the severely injured hand, further reconstructive surgery will usually be required.

6. In assessing the results, it is to be remembered that a painless hand, with grip and useful sensation, is generally superior to prosthesis. Remember Sterling Bunnell's aphorism: "When you have nothing, a little is a lot."

## WOUNDS OF THE INTEGUMENT OF THE HAND

### Definitions

1. *Incised Wound.* This is produced by a sharp cutting force.

2. *Superficial Wound.* This is a wound which is confined to the skin alone and does not go into the subcutaneous tissue.

3. *Clean Wound.* This is a wound without external contamination or devitalized necrotic tissue.

4. *Dirty Wound.* This refers to a wound with crushed or avulsed tissue or obvious external contamination.

5. *Abrasion.* This wound of the skin is superficial to the dermis.

6. *Perforating Wound.* This is usually a deep wound with a small skin incision.

7. *Avulsed Wound.* This refers to full- or partial-thickness elevation of the skin from its base with or without attachment to surrounding skin.

8. *Fresh Wound.* This is a wound less than 8 hours old or 12 hours old with the use of antibiotics administered soon after injury.

9. *Old Wound.* This refers to any wound older than 8 to 12 hours if antibiotics have been used.

### Basic Principles

All wounds must be treated for prevention of infection and edema and for restoration of adequate function. Copious irrigation, tetanus prophylaxis and antibiotics are routine.

Wound debridement should be performed cautiously, particularly on the palmar surfaces due to the sparsity of skin. All injuries in the hand should be evaluated for nerve and tendon function, no matter how minor the injury appears. Whenever there is doubt in the emergency department as to the extent of the wound, minimal exploration is done in the operating room with a tourniquet without enlarging the wound.

Fresh wounds are closed primarily. Older wounds, if clean, may be debrided and closed primarily, but without tension. If not clean, these wounds may be closed by primary delayed repair or allowed to heal in secondarily.

Splinting is indicated after treatment wherever extensive wounds exist or when a wound crosses a crease line where motion will delay wound healing.

### Criteria for Diagnosis

1. Visual inspection of the wound usually will suffice to classify it.

2. Viability of hand skin is surprisingly good and even complete avulsions may survive if infection is avoided.

### Management

#### Superficial Wounds

1. Cleanse with antiseptic solution (Zephiran).

2. Closure is done with Steristrips or 5-0 monofilament suture.

3. Dress with a single layer of non-adherent gauze (Adaptic, Telfa, Furacin, Vaseline) and a pressure dressing.

4. Antibiotics are given only if the wound is very dirty.

#### Deep Wounds

1. Soak and cleanse the wound with antiseptic solution (Zephiran or Betadine).

2. Test for sensation by pin-prick test.

3. Test motor function by asking the patient to flex and extend the digit or hand.

4. Test joint function by forcibly abducting, adducting, hyperextending and hyperflexing the joint involved.

5. X-rays if indicated.

6. *Local Anesthesia for Repair of Wounds*

A. *For Finger Lacerations*

(1) *Ring Block*. Injection of 1 or 2% Xylocaine without epinephrine along either side of the base of the proximal phalanx and in the dorsum of the base of the proximal phalanx.

(2) *Web Space Block*. Injection of 1 or 2% Xylocaine without epinephrine into the web space on either side of the injured finger and in the dorsum of the base of the proximal phalanx.

(3) *Intermetacarpal Block*. Injection of 1 or 2% Xylocaine without epinephrine on either side of the metacarpal with which the finger is continuous and one injection in the dorsum of the base of the proximal phalanx.

B. *For Lacerations Over the Dorsum of the First or Second Metacarpals*

(1) Superficial radial nerve block by injecting 1% Xylocaine without epinephrine into the subcutaneous tissue dorsal, lateral and volar to the distal radius at the wrist.

(2) Field block by infiltrating the skin and subcutaneous tissue surrounding the wound with 1% Xylocaine without epinephrine

C. *For All Other Lacerations*

(1) Field block (*See* above.)

(2) Infiltration of skin edges with 1% Xylocaine

7. *Repair of Wounds*

A. Fine sutures (5-0 or 6-0 nylon) are used to reapproximate skin edges.

(1) For palmar skin and lateral borders of the fingers, simple interrupted sutures will suffice.

(2) For dorsal skin it is best to use vertical mattress sutures.

B. If the wound is relatively old but clean:

(1) Debride the skin edges minimally.

(2) Close without tension.

C. If the wound is dirty, debride without closure.

D. If the laceration crosses the volar crease line of the proximal or distal interphalangeal joint, it should be repaired with a Z-plasty (Fig. 31-1).

*Z-Plasty*. The Z-plasty relaxes the tension in a wound closure by transposing flaps made by two cuts at 60-degree angles on either side of the wound. In this manner:

(1) The scar line is broken.

(2) Wound tension is redistributed.

(3) Wound length is equalized.

E. Once the wound is closed:

(1) Apply a pressure dressing.

(2) Splint if:

(a) The laceration is extensive.

(b) The laceration crosses a crease line or joint

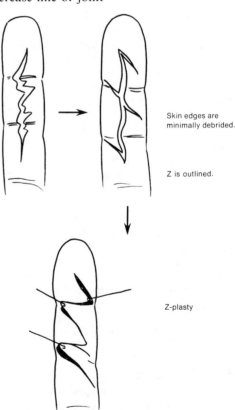

Skin edges are minimally debrided.

Z is outlined.

Z-plasty

Fig. 31-1. Z-plasty.

*(c)* The patient is not reliable or is a child.

*(3)* Antibiotics are given routinely:

*(a)* Tetracycline, 250 mg. b.i.d. for relatively clean wounds

*(b)* Ampicillin, cephalosporins or lincomycin for more extensive or dirtier wounds

## Crushed Wounds

1. Clean thoroughly.
2. X-rays, as indicated
3. Pressure dressing
4. Splint if a large surface is involved or if joints or crease lines are involved.

## Avulsed Wounds

1. If some skin attachment is present, *and*:

A. If the pedicle length is more than one and one-half times the width of the base:

*(1)* Detach the base, defat the skin and suture as a free full-thickness graft with 5-0 nylon.

*(2)* Apply a small localized pressure dressing with a stent (Fig. 31-2).

*(3)* Immobilize the stent with 4-0 black silk sutures.

B. If the length of the pedicle is less

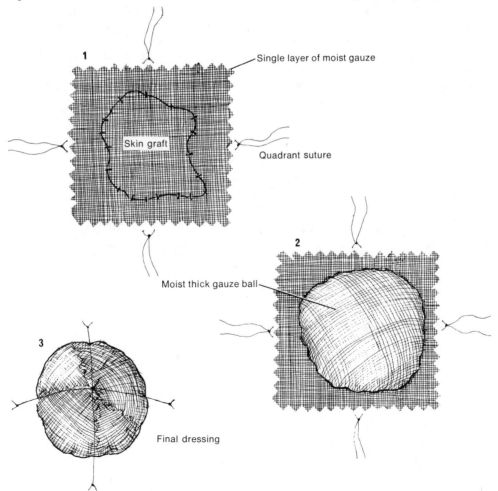

1

Single layer of moist gauze

Skin graft

Quadrant suture

Moist thick gauze ball

2

3

Final dressing

Fig. 31-2. Pressurized dressing with a stent.

than one and one-half times that of the base:

*(1)* Resuture skin which is minimally debrided to surrounding skin with 5-0 nylon sutures.

*(2)* Apply a pressure dressing.

*(3)* Give antibiotics as above.

2. If the skin is completely detached, *and*:

A. If the thickness of the avulsed skin is partial and thin:

*(1)* Apply a pressure dressing with a single layer of nonadherent gauze.

*(2)* Give antibiotics as above.

B. If there is full-thickness loss:

*(1)* Without exposure of bone, tendons, nerves or joints, and with an adequate bed of fat or paratenon (i.e., if the extensor tendon is involved), a split-thickness graft should be used to close the defect with a stent dressing. If avulsed skin is available and if it is clean and uncrushed, it can be used, after defatting, as a free graft.

*(2)* Skin grafts can be used to cover minimally exposed bone, as on the dorsal aspect of the terminal phalanx.

*(3)* Nail bed avulsions should not be covered with skin grafts. If the defect is small, allow it to granulate in and heal secondarily.

*(4)* If bone, tendon, joint or nerves are exposed, the area must be covered with a flap (*see* Chap. 10, Soft Tissue Injuries).

*(a)* Full-thickness avulsions from the dorsum of the hand may be repaired by local sliding flaps, especially if the defect is small.

*(b)* In infants and children, circumferential defects of the fingertips may be treated as superficial avulsions even if bone is exposed.

*(c)* Defects crossing volar or lateral crease lines must be darted (Fig. 31-3) before grafting to avoid future scar contractures.

*(5) Postoperative Care of Grafts*

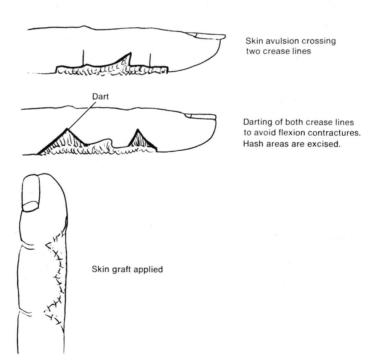

Skin avulsion crossing two crease lines

Dart

Darting of both crease lines to avoid flexion contractures. Hash areas are excised.

Skin graft applied

Fig. 31-3. Darting.

*(a)* Change the dressing by the third or fourth day.

*(b)* Evacuate any accumulation of fluid under the graft (i.e., serum or blood).

*(c)* Remove sutures after 10 days.

## CRUSH INJURIES OF THE HAND

### Definition

Crush injuries are multiple tissue injuries caused by a crushing or tearing force.

### Basic Principles

Crush injuries of the hand are a demanding therapeutic problem. Skin, bone, joints, tendons, nerves and vessels are usually all involved in various degrees of severity. Amputations, partial or complete, are often present. The restoration of skeletal architecture, skin coverage and sensation is a primary consideration. Too much done too soon can be as detrimental as too little done too late. Again, remember that the only absolute indication for amputation is *irreparable* loss of blood supply.

### Criteria for Diagnosis

1. History of crushing trauma. Explore if heat as well as crush was involved.
2. Physical assessment including motor and sensory deficits
3. X-ray to evaluate the extent of osseous damage

### Management

#### Emergency Treatment

1. Wounds are thoroughly cleansed with Zephiran or Betadine.
2. Tetanus prophylaxis is given.
3. Antibiotics of broad-spectrum-type are begun immediately.
4. There is minimal exploration to determine the extent of injury.
5. Pressure dressing with a splint is applied.

#### Operative Treatment

1. The patient or extremity is anesthetized.
2. The wound is thoroughly cleansed again with antiseptic solution, elevated and a tourniquet applied.
3. Following copious irrigation with cool saline, meticulous debridement is performed.
4. Since skin availability is limited in the hand, only obviously necrotic skin is excised.
5. Repair and closure follow the standard principles outlined previously.
6. The entire hand, wrist and forearm are placed in a pressure dressing with a splint.
7. *Postoperative Care*
   A. Antibiotics
   B. Analgesics
   C. Elevation (essential)
   D. With severely crushed tissues, particularly muscles, watch for gas gangrene.
   E. Change dressings at 48 to 72 hours or as soon as clostridial infection is suspected.
8. Plan the timing and sequence of secondary reparative procedures.

## TENDON INJURIES

### FLEXOR TENDON INJURIES

### Definition

Flexor tendons can be lacerated or ruptured. Acute rupture occurs only at the insertion of the flexor profundus tendon.

### Basic Principles

Flexor tendon lacerations are treated according to the level of injury to the tendon. Although strict rules do apply to most tendon repairs, a margin of flexibility in the treatment of these injuries is based on the surgeon's experience and judgment.

With the possible exception of injuries in "no man's land," which is Zone 2 in the thumb and in the fingers and Zone 4 in the

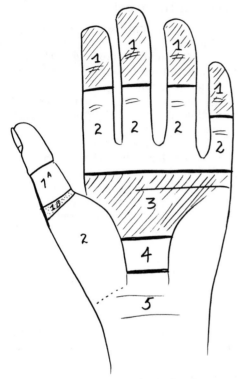

Fig. 31-4. Zones in the hand.

hand (Fig. 31-4), all tendon injuries should undergo primary or delayed primary repair (up to 72 hours from time of injury). The sooner the repair is done the better.

While clean wounds give better results than crushed and dirty wounds, nevertheless repair in the latter cases can be done primarily.

## Criteria for Diagnosis

1. History of injury
2. *Physical Examination*
   A. *Lacerations at the Level of the Finger*
   *(1)* Isolated sublimus laceration (uncommon)—the patient cannot flex the proximal interphalangeal joint when the other fingers are held back.
   *(2)* Isolated profundus laceration—the patient cannot flex the distal interphalangeal joint.

*(3)* Laceration of both tendons—there is absence of all flexion.

*(4)* Occasionally, in an isolated laceration of the profundus tendon, flexion may be present due to a small remnant of intact tendon or due to pulling through intact vinculum.

B. *Lacerations at the Level of the Palm*

There are the same findings as in the fingers except that isolated sublimus laceration is common.

C. *Laceration at the Level of the Wrist*

*(1)* Same findings as in laceration of the tendons in the palm

*(2)* Laceration of both wrist flexors will prevent strong wrist flexion.

*(3)* If there is a laceration of only the flexor carpi ulnaris or flexor carpi radialis, the involved tendon is not palpable when the wrist is flexed.

## Management

Zone 1

*Profundus Lacerations Only*

1. Primary tenorrhaphy with end-to-end anastomosis, using 5-0 Tevdek suture
2. If the laceration is close to the insertion into the bone, a pull-out wire with a button is used.
3. If the laceration is at the upper limit of Zone 2, one can perform a tendon advancement of up to 1½ cm. with excision of the distal pulley.
4. No extensive dissection of synovia or other soft tissue is done at this time.

Zone 2

1. *Profundus Laceration Alone (Uncommon)*
   A. Unless tendon advancement is indicated, the skin wound is closed and the patient is scheduled for tendon graft in 10 to 12 days if the wound is clean, or 3 weeks later if the wound is less than satisfactory.
   B. With experience we have been successfully doing primary profundus tendon repairs in this area.

*(1)* Tendon ends are simply identified.

*(2)* No resection of synovia or pulleys is performed at this time.

*(3)* All tissues are minimally handled or dissected.

*(4)* For a peritenon repair, 6-0 Tevdek is used.

2. *Sublimus Laceration Alone*

A. The laceration can be partial, involving only one slip, and may be treated by excision of the involved slip or resuturing with a single 5-0 Tevdek suture.

B. Other partial lacerations are usually repaired.

C. For complete transection, the sublimus ends are excised.

3. *Profundus and Sublimus Combined Lacerations*

A. If the wound is sharp, the patient is seen and operated on early, and the laceration is at the level of the distal half of the proximal phalanx or proximal half of the middle phalanx, the recommended procedure is:

*(1)* Excise the sublimus, distal pulley and portion of the proximal pulley.

*(2)* Utilize a box suture (Fig. 31-5) with 5-0 Tevdek to approximate the profundus end-to-end.

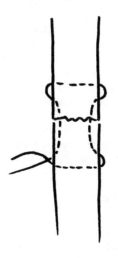

Fig. 31-5. Box suture.

*(3)* Several 6-0 Tevdek epitendinous sutures are then used to approximate the edges accurately.

*(4)* An alternative method for lacerations involving the distal portion of "no man's land" is Z-lengthening of the profundus at the level of the wrist and advancement of the profundus tendon out of "no man's land." This is actually a form of primary free graft and the lumbricales will be out of balance. There also will be two areas of scarring at the wrist and at the finger.

*(5)* Primary tendon repair with excision of sublimus, although it may require secondary tendolysis later, gives better results than later tendon grafting.

B. If the wound is crushed or grossly contaminated, the skin is closed and the patient is scheduled for a tendon graft in 3 weeks.

### Zone 1B

*Thumb*

1. This is a relative "no man's land." Usually advancement of the flexor pollicis longus is possible.

2. The entire flexor sheath is excised at the level of the metacarpophalangeal joint.

### Zone 3

*Lacerations of the Sublimus or Profundus or Both, Involving Single Digit or Multiple Digits*

1. The treatment consists of repair of all tendons end-to-end.

2. Unsatisfied ends of sublimus allowed to retract into the wrist may cause more adhesions than the scar from multiple tendon repairs.

3. If the injury is close to the carpal tunnel, the latter should be incised to prevent scar adhesions.

### Zone 4

This is a relative "no man's land" of the hand.

1. For sublimus lacerations only, all structures are repaired.

2. If both sublimus and profundus are lacerated, only the profundus is repaired.

3. In this zone, all procedures are accompanied by resection of the carpal ligament.

## Zone 5

Injuries in this level are usually complex, involving nerves as well as tendons and arteries.

1. Usually all structures, except the palmaris longus (if present), are repaired primarily. This includes the sublimus tendon lacerations as well as the profundus tendon lacerations.

2. The transverse carpal ligament is transected if the tendon lacerations are close to the carpal tunnel.

## Additional Considerations

1. In children, all lacerations of tendons are repaired primarily with the exception of the sublimus in "no man's land" when both sublimus and profundus are lacerated.

2. Ruptures of the profundus at its insertion are treated as Zone 1 lacerations with pull-out button and wire.

3. *Complex Injuries to Flexor Tendons*

A. Whenever flexor injuries are accompanied by comminuted fracture or loss of skin, the primary considerations are skin coverage and restoration of skeletal architecture.

B. Tendon repairs can be done secondarily.

4. *Postoperative Care*

A. Pressure dressing

B. Dorsal plaster splint maintaining the wrist in mild palmar flexion

C. Elevation

D. Antibiotics

E. Immobilization for flexor tendon injuries is 3 weeks. Thereafter the patient is allowed active movement. Passive movements are allowed after 6 weeks.

F. Pull-out buttons are removed on the sixth week.

## EXTENSOR TENDON INJURIES

### Definitions

1. *Mallet Finger.* This refers to a drop of the distal phalanx of the finger following sudden forced flexion of the distal phalanx, resulting in:

A. A laceration of the common terminal tendon over the tendon joint

B. A fracture avulsion of the tendon insertion or a tear in the tendon insertion

C. A laceration of both lateral bands of the extensor tendon over the middle phalanx

2. *Boutonniere Injury.* This is a deformity characterized by proximal interphalangeal (PIP) joint flexion and distal interphalangeal (DIP) joint hyperextension due to a laceration or rupture of the central tendon insertion on the base of the middle phalanx. The DIP joint hyperflexion is not seen early and is due to the volar slippage of the lateral bands which also increase the PIP joint flexion.

### Basic Principles

Extensor tendons may be lacerated or torn from the insertion at the distal interphalangeal joint or the proximal interphalangeal joint. Lacerated extensor tendons can all be repaired primarily even with severe crushing injuries with fractures present. The one exception to primary repair would be loss of skin or a portion of tendon which would require bridge grafting or tendon transfers.

A laceration of the central tendon at the level of the metacarpophalangeal joint (Fig. 31-6, 3) has minimal retraction, and primary repair is simple and may be done in a well-equipped emergency department. All other lacerations should be repaired in the operating room.

### Criteria for Diagnosis

1. History of injury

2. On examination of the hand:

A. An isolated drop of the distal interphalangeal (DIP) joint indicates tendon

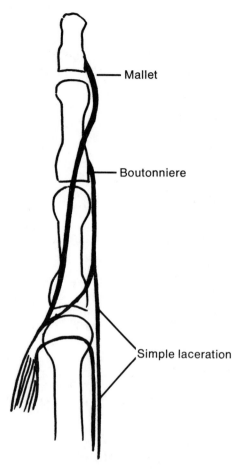

Fig. 31-6. Lacerations of the extensor tendon.

injury distal to the insertion of the middle extensor slip on the base of the middle phalanx.

    B. A drop of the proximal interphalangeal (PIP) joint alone indicates an injury to the middle slip of the extensor tendon.

    C. Loss of extension of the metacarpophalangeal (MP) joint indicates injury in the tendon proximal to the joint. With this joint supported in extension, extension of the DIP and PIP joints is possible through lumbrical and interossei insertion.

    D. In the thumb, loss of extension of

the interphalangeal joint indicates a laceration of the extensor pollicis longus.

    E. Loss of independent extension of the MP joint of the thumb suggests a laceration of the extensor pollicis brevis.

    F. Inability of abduction of the thumb indicates laceration of the abductor pollicis longus.

## Management

    1. *Mallet Finger*
        A. *Lacerations*
        *(1)* Primary tenorrhaphy with Kirschner wire fixation of the DIP joint in mild hyperextension
        *(2)* Kirschner wire is removed after 6 weeks.
        *(3)* Mallet thumb, due to laceration of the extensor pollicis longus over the proximal phalanx, is treated in the same manner.
        B. *Fracture Avulsion*
        *(1)* Reinsertion of the fragment with pull-out wire and Kirschner wire fixation of the DIP joint in mild hyperextension
        *(2)* Kirschner wire and pull-out wire are removed after 6 weeks.
        C. *Tear*
        *(1)* Percutaneous intramedullary wire fixation through the DIP joint in mild hyperextension for 6 weeks
        *(2)* Frequently closed splinting of the DIP joint in hyperextension for 6 weeks also will produce a satisfactory result (Fig. 31-7).

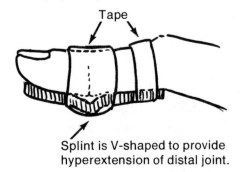

Splint is V-shaped to provide hyperextension of distal joint.

Fig. 31-7. Splinting for mallet finger.

2. *Boutonniere Injury*

A. *Lacerations*

(1) Primary tenorrhaphy

(2) For 3 weeks the entire finger and wrist are immobilized in hyperextension.

(3) For the last 2 to 3 weeks, only the PIP joint and wrist are immobilized.

B. *Fracture Avulsion*

(1) Reinsertion of the fragment with a pull-out suture

(2) Kirschner wire fixation of the PIP joint for 5 to 6 weeks with light external splinting

C. *Tear*

(1) If picked up early, the finger is splinted in extension from tip to forearm for 3 weeks, followed by another 3 weeks of splinting of the finger from the MP joint to the DIP joint.

(2) Late tears require tenorrhaphy.

3. *Laceration of the Central Tendon at the Metacarpophalangeal Joint*

A. Primary tenorrhaphy

B. Splint, in extension, from the PIP joint to the wrist for 3 weeks.

4. *Laceration of the Communis Tendon, Extensor Indicis Proprius or Extensor Digiti Quinti at the Level of the Metacarpals*

A. Primary tenorrhaphy with splinting in hyperextension for 3 weeks

B. The splint extends from the proximal phalanx to the forearm. The proximal interphalangeal joint and the distal interphalangeal joint need not be immobilized.

5. *Laceration of the Extensor Pollicis Longus*

A. Primary tenorrhaphy

B. If the laceration is close to the wrist, the proximal end may have retracted. Do not explore but do a primary extensor indicis proprius transfer.

6. *Laceration of the Extensor Pollicis Brevis at the Level of the Metacarpophalangeal Joint*

A. Primary tenorrhaphy

B. The thumb is splinted in extension from the distal joint to the wrist for 3 weeks.

7. *Laceration of the Abductor Pollicis Longus and Extensor Pollicis Brevis at the Level of the Wrist*

A. Primary tenorrhaphy with excision of the first dorsal aponeurotic canal

B. If the injury is old and the tendon ends have retracted, tendon transfer is indicated.

8. *Complex Injuries*

A. Repair all extensor tendon injuries even in the presence of crushing injuries or fractures.

B. With loss of substance and the inability to approximate ends, a primary bridge graft is done with the palmaris longus tendon or the ulnar half of the extensor digiti quinti minimi tendon.

C. End-to-side anastomosis also may be done with the intact communis tendon. These tendons usually act as a unit and therefore a communis tendon can activate several fingers at the same time without any loss in function.

D. Complex injuries with loss of substance over the DIP joint or the PIP joint must be deferred for secondary repair if graft is necessary.

## NERVE INJURIES

### Definition

An injured nerve is a nerve which does not fulfill its sensory or motor function properly. The injury can be a contusion with temporary loss or partial or total laceration or tear with permanent deficit.

### Basic Principles

Whenever possible, nerves should be repaired primarily because this gives the best results measured by return of function. Contraindications to primary repair are poor skin coverage and multiple tissue injuries requiring the placement of the hand or fingers in a position detrimental to the repair of nerves.

In multiple injuries of tendons, nerves,

vessels, bone and skin, only skin coverage, vessel restoration and possibly reconstitution of the skeletal architecture take priority over digital nerve repairs. In laceration of major nerves (median, ulnar and radial), if a primary repair is not possible, tagging the cut ends of the nerve together at the time of injury is worthwhile to prevent retraction of the nerve, simplifying secondary neurorrhaphy.

## Criteria for Diagnosis

*See also* Chapter 33, Peripheral Nerve Injuries.

1. *Digital Nerve*

A. Anesthesia distal to the laceration. The pin-prick test is a good test.

B. In children, where it is difficult to evaluate loss of sensation, diagnosis is by exploration or repeated clinical reevaluation.

2. *Median Nerve*

A. *Sensory:* pin-prick test for sensory deficits. The areas involved may be the palmar surface of the thumb, index, and middle fingers and the radial half of the ring finger and the radial half of the palm. The dorsum of the distal phalanges and portion of the middle phalanges of those fingers are also involved.

B. *Motor Deficits*
(1) *Low Median*
*Loss:* Thumb opposition
(2) *High Median*
*Loss:* Pronation
Radial deviation of wrist
All flexor sublimus function
Flexor profundus of index and middle fingers
Thenar muscles (opposition)
Lumbrical to the index and middle fingers
*Clinical Appearance:* flattened "ape" hand
C. *Anterior Interosseous Nerve*
*Loss:* Flexor pollicis longus
Flexor digitorum profundus of the index and sometimes middle fingers

3. *Ulnar Nerve*

A. *Sensory:* the areas involved may be the palmar and dorsal surfaces of the little finger and the ulnar half of the ring finger.

B. *Motor Deficits*
(1) *Low Ulnar*
*Loss:* Abduction, adduction of the fingers
Adduction of the thumb
Primary flexion of metacarpophalangeal joints of the ring and little fingers
*Clinical Appearance:* the patient has claw hand and cannot pinch properly between the thumb and index fingers.
(2) *High Ulnar*
*Loss:* Same as for Low Ulnar with the addition of loss of the flexor digitorum profundus of the ring and little fingers and flexor carpi ulnaris

4. *Radial Nerve*

A. *Sensory:* there may be loss of sensation over the dorsum of the hand from the thumb to a portion of the ring fingers excluding the distal one and one-half phalanges.

B. *Motor Deficits*
(1) *Low Radial*
*Loss:* Extensor digitorum communis of the index, middle, ring and little fingers
Extensor indicis proprius
Extensor digiti minimi
Extensor pollicis longus
Abductor pollicis longus
Extensor pollicis brevis
Extensor carpi radialis brevis
*Clinical Appearance:* inability to extend all the fingers and abduct the thumb
(2) *High Radial*
*Loss:* Same as for Low Radial with the addition of extensor carpi radialis brevis and brachioradialis
*Clinical Appearance:* wrist drop and loss of extension of all digits

5. *Combined Median/Ulnar Nerve Injuries*

A. *Sensory:* total anesthesia of the palmar surface of the hand

B. *Motor Deficits*

(1) *Low Motor*

*Loss:* Opposition

Abduction and adduction of all fingers

Pinch

*Clinical Appearance:* flattened clawed hand

(2) *High Motor*

*Loss:* Opposition

Abduction and adduction of all fingers

Pinch

Flexion of all digits

Flexion of wrist

Pronation

*Clinical Appearance:* flattened clawed hand

## Management

For specific technique of nerve repair, *see* Chapter 33.

1. *Digital Nerves*

A. These nerves contain only sensory fibers and are found slightly below the midlateral line of the fingers, which is just below the level of the ends of the crease lines of the finger.

B. The laceration in the distal third of the middle phalanx is usually difficult to repair due to numerous branchings. An attempt at repair should be made despite variations in anatomy.

C. In case of avulsion of the nerve with loss of substance, some distance can be gained by hyperflexing the digit.

D. If this is not possible, secondary repair with nerve graft should be considered later.

E. *Postoperative Care.* Immobilization for the digital nerve is from 3 to 4 weeks in neutral position.

2. *Major Mixed Laceration at the Level of the Wrist*

A. Repaired by standard perineural or epineural technique

B. Immobilized for 4 weeks in moderate flexion position to relax tension and then 2 weeks in neutral position

3. *Laceration of the Radial Nerve or Injuries to the Radial Nerve at the Level of the Upper Arm*

A. In a penetrating wound of the arm, transection of the nerve is probable; therefore it is explored and repaired if necessary.

B. In fracture of the humerus not requiring open reduction, the nerve may be observed for 8 weeks before exploration. If the injury is just a neurapraxia, it should show moderate recovery during this period of time.

4. *Other Factors in Management*

A. The prognosis in mixed nerve lacerations is fair to poor in adults, particularly with high lesions.

B. The best results are with repair of the radial nerve because of the short distance between the lacerated nerve and the muscle to be innervated.

C. In spite of the poor prognosis with injury of the median and ulnar nerves, it is essential to repair them to gain as much sensory return as possible.

D. Tendon transfers are done if there is no sign of motor return after 6 months.

E. In high nerve lesions, the muscle will often be atrophic or fibrosed by the time its nerve regenerates. It is therefore advisable to do tendon transfers sooner in these cases.

## FRACTURES

### Basic Principles

In severe crush injuries, skin closure takes priority and fractures may have to be reduced secondarily. Often, however, good skin coverage requires maintenance of a stable reduction. In partially amputated fingers requiring reduction and pinning, manipulation should be minimal and the simplest reduction possible should be performed to avoid losing the finger. Intra-articular fractures should always be reduced open, particularly if more than 30 per cent of the joint surface is involved.

The first, fourth and fifth metacarpals are mobile or semimobile units. The second and third metacarpals are fixed units. Additionally, the second, third, fourth and fifth metacarpals are well-padded units. Deformities which create functional difficulties with the metacarpals are malrotation and shortening. Fracture of the neck of the fifth metacarpal is one of the most common hand fractures (boxer's or battler's fracture).

## Criteria for Diagnosis

1. Clinical signs and symptoms of fractures (*see* p. 323).

2. *X-ray:* anteroposterior, lateral and oblique views for all suspected fractures. Fine detail of the DIP joint and distal phalanges is often better visualized using dental film and dental x-ray units.

## Management

1. *Terminal Phalanx*
   A. Fracture of the tuft heals without special treatment. A pressure dressing and a splint are applied for support and protection. Subungual hematomas must be drained for relief of pain (*see* p. 367).

   B. These fractures are usually open and often involve the nail bed. In this case, remove the nail to expose the nail bed and repair it if necessary to avoid uneven wound. (*Editor's Note:* we prefer to retain the nail by resuturing it to the eponychium as a splint for the fracture.)

   C. Open fractures through the shaft or base of the distal phalanx often may be reduced by good skin closure. A splint and dressing are applied as usual.

   D. If the fracture is unstable, transfix the fracture percutaneously with a Zimmer pin (Fig. 31-8).

   E. Rarely a patient may require open reduction in the operating room.

   F. Fractures of the dorsal lip with avulsion of extensor tendon insertion have been discussed under tendon lacerations.

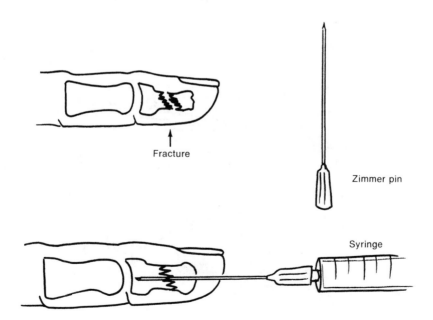

Fracture

Zimmer pin

Syringe

Zimmer pin introduced percutaneously

Fig. 31-8. Zimmer pin fixation of fracture of the terminal phalanx.

G. Intra-articular fractures with displacement or involvement of more than one third of the joint surface require open reduction. Kirschner wire fixation is used for large intra-articular fractures which are displaced or if the fragment that is avulsed contains a collateral ligament or tendon attachment. Smaller fragments may be sutured with fine monofilament steel or may be satisfactorily managed in a splint in functional position for 3 weeks.

2. *Middle Phalanx*

A. The angulation of fractures depends on location and tendon attachment (Fig. 31-9, B and C). Stability is variable so that closed reduction over a volar splint should be tried initially.

*(1)* Apply a short arm cast or splint from the proximal forearm to mid palm and incorporate an aluminum and foam rubber splint into the plaster. Bend the splint into the functional position.

*(2)* Anesthetize the finger with a metacarpal block.

*(3)* Two strips of ½-inch tape are applied along the lateral border of the finger after painting the skin with tincture of benzoin.

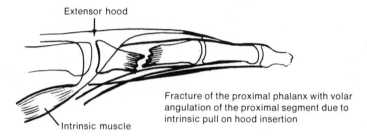

Extensor hood

Intrinsic muscle

Fracture of the proximal phalanx with volar angulation of the proximal segment due to intrinsic pull on hood insertion

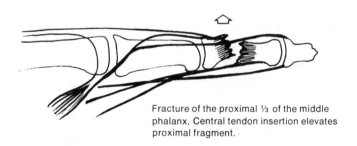

Fracture of the proximal ⅓ of the middle phalanx. Central tendon insertion elevates proximal fragment.

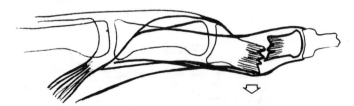

Fracture of the distal ⅓ of the middle phalanx. Sublimus insertion angulates the proximal segment volarly.

Fig. 31-9. Fractures of the proximal and middle phalanges.

(4) The fracture is manipulated and reduced.

(5) Tension is maintained on the tape, which is then anchored by further tape to the cast.

(6) The finger is then taped gently to the splint (Fig. 31-10).

(7) If properly applied, this traction should not create any ischemia or pressure necrosis of the skin.

(8) Nondisplaced fractures do not require traction for maintenance of reduction.

B. Open reduction with axial or crossed Kirschner wire fixation or the use of ASIF small fragment plates is necessary if satisfactory alignment is not obtained.

C. Open fractures are treated by debridement and closed reduction if possible.

3. *Proximal Phalanx*

A. The fracture tends to angulate volarly due to intrinsic pull (Fig. 31-9, A). Lateral angulation also may occur.

B. Treatment is the same as with the middle phalanx.

C. Fractures of the base of the proximal phalanx are often difficult to manipulate and we can accept small angular deformities in our reduction.

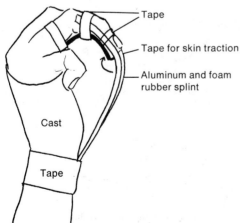

Fig. 31-10. Traction splinting for unstable fractures of the middle and proximal phalanges.

4. *Thumb*

A. Fractures of the thumb, if simple, are best handled with closed reduction and a molded cast rather than a splint.

B. Severe open fractures require open reduction.

5. If multiple digits are involved, splinting becomes cumbersome and open fixation is the best treatment.

6. *Metacarpal Fractures*

A. *Neck of the Metacarpal*

(1) Closed reduction is accomplished under anesthesia by flexing the MP joint to a right angle and pushing up on the flexed PIP joint. This should elevate the depressed knuckle.

(2) Splinting in this position can be done with plaster molded over heavy felt and incorporated into a forearm splint or cast.

(3) Correct rotation is maintained by including the adjacent finger in the cast and making certain that the fingertip points to the tuberosity of the navicular.

(4) Immobilization in this extreme position may be discontinued after 8 to 10 days and the MP joint splinted at a 45-degree angle for an additional 2 weeks.

(5) The result of healing with angulation but without tendon adhesions is primarily cosmetic and rarely functional.

(6) A severe comminuted fracture which is unreduced, however, will cause permanent joint stiffness and pain, primarily due to tendon adhesions involving the extensor tendon and occasionally the flexor tendons.

(7) When severely displaced or comminuted, fractures cannot be maintained following closed reduction. Internal fixation with an axial intramedullary Kirschner wire drilled through the articular surface is necessary. The finger and hand are then splinted in functional position.

B. *Shaft of the Metacarpal*

(1) Fractures of the shaft of the metacarpal may be oblique, transverse or comminuted.

*(2)* They may or may not be stable.

*(3)* Closed fractures or those with minor open wounds are manipulated under local anesthesia and a cast applied from the distal forearm to the mid palm. A splint is incorporated into the cast, and the involved finger and an adjacent finger are splinted together in functional position with immobilization of the MP and PIP joints.

*(4)* The cast remains on usually for 3 to 4 weeks until healing is seen radiographically.

*(5)* Open reduction and internal fixation with single or multiple Kirschner wires (Fig. 31-11) or ASIF small fragment plates and screws are necessary if there is shortening, uncorrected angulation or rotation.

C. *Fracture of the Shaft of the First Metacarpal*

Management is identical to other metacarpal shaft fractures.

D. *Fracture of the Base of the First Metacarpal*

*(1)* Without dislocation of the carpal metacarpal articulation, it is treated as a fracture of the shaft.

*(2)* With articular involvement and proximal displacement of the distal frag-

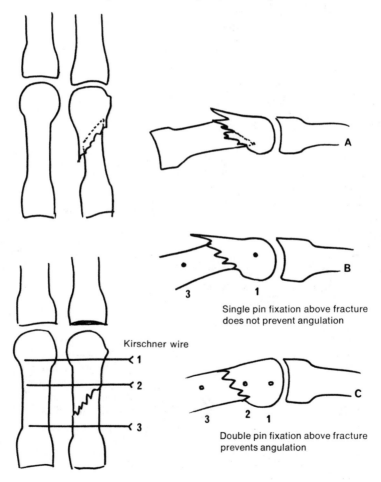

Kirschner wire

Single pin fixation above fracture does not prevent angulation

Double pin fixation above fracture prevents angulation

Fig. 31-11. Transverse fixation of unstable metacarpal fractures.

ment (Bennett's fracture dislocation), this may be treated by:

*Closed Reduction*

*(a)* The thumb is anesthetized with a median nerve block.

*(b)* Reduction of the dislocation is done by pulling on the thumb and pressing medially over the base of the first metacarpal.

*(c)* Application of a molded cast with the first metacarpal abducted and the IP joint flexed

*(d)* If the reduction does not hold, traction, in an axial direction applied through a Kirschner wire drilled through the distal first metacarpal or the distal proximal phalanx and attached to a wire outrigger incorporated in the cast, may maintain an anatomical position.

*Open Reduction*

*(a)* Through an incision over the dorsolateral aspect of the base of the metacarpal, the fracture is exposed and reduced.

*(b)* The articular surface reduction should be perfect.

*(c)* A fine Kirschner wire is drilled from the distal fragment through the small proximal fragment into the greater multangular bone.

*(d)* Cut the Kirschner wire so that the end protrudes under the skin and immobilize the thumb in a short arm plaster mold for 4 to 6 weeks, at which time the wire may be removed.

*(e) Caution:* carefully avoid injuring the sensory branch of the radial nerve.

E. *Epiphyseal Fractures*

*(1)* For all fractures of the epiphysis, closed reduction is done with splinting in functional position, incorporating an adjacent normal digit to prevent rotation.

*(2)* Healing usually occurs within 3 weeks.

*(3)* In fractures involving the base of the proximal phalanx of the finger, lateral angulation often occurs and is reduced by placing a pencil in the web

space and applying pressure against the fracture site.

## JOINT INJURIES

### Classification

1. Intra-articular fractures
2. Dislocations with or without fracture
3. Capsular tears
4. Crushing injuries with or without fracture or tendon injury
5. Infections

### Basic Principles

A joint can be injured either directly or indirectly. Indirect involvement is due to the proximity of a joint to the area of trauma such as fractures, lacerations of tendons or crushing injuries. With injury there will be swelling, stiffness and pain in the joint, which will aggravate the original trauma.

### Criteria for Diagnosis

1. *Intra-articular Fractures*

A. Signs and symptoms of fracture

B. Confirmation by excellent x-ray visualization

2. *Dislocations*

A. *Without Fracture*

*(1)* Visible deformity of joint

*(2)* Pain

*(3)* Inability to flex or extend joint

*(4)* Discoloration of skin

*(5)* Palpation of deformity

*(6)* X-ray with the beam centered on the joint, showing a dislocation

B. *With Fracture*

*(1)* Same as above

*(2)* X-rays reveal fracture in addition to articular incongruity.

3. *Capsular Tears*

A. Swelling and pain on palpation

B. Stiffness with limited range of active motion

C. Lateral or extension instability

4. *Crushing Injuries*

A. Discoloration of skin

B. Break in skin with or without skin avulsions

C. Pain and swelling

D. X-rays will reveal fracture, if present.

E. Tendon function is difficult to evaluate in the early period.

5. *Infections*

A. Recent history of trauma—laceration, puncture wound or crush injury

B. Pain and swelling

C. Redness and stiffness

## Management

1. *Intra-articular Fractures*

A. *Closed Intra-articular Fractures.* If the fracture involves less than 30 per cent of the joint and is not accompanied by collateral ligament injury, treat conservatively with splinting in the position of function.

B. *Open Intra-articular Fractures.* Large fragments or those with collateral ligament involvement require open reduction.

2. *Dislocations without Fracture*

A. *Metacarpophalangeal Joint*

(1) Closed reduction under regional block

(2) Apply a volar plaster splint in position of function for 3 weeks.

(3) Occasionally, the head of the metacarpal locks within the fibrous and tendinous complex of the volar surface of the metacarpophalangeal joint and closed reduction is impossible. Open reduction through a palmar incision is necessary. This is especially true of index metacarpophalangeal dislocations.

B. *Proximal Interphalangeal Joint*

(1) The dislocation is usually posterior and reduction is easily done closed under regional block.

(2) Posterior molded plaster extending into the palm in functional position is needed for 3 weeks.

(3) The rarer anterior dislocation is usually accompanied by an extensor tendon tear, so that after reduction it is splinted for 6 weeks in extension.

C. *Distal Interphalangeal Joint*

(1) *Closed Dislocation without Fracture.* Same as posterior PIP joint dislocations.

(2) *Closed Dislocation with Fracture.* Open reduction with Kirschner wire fixation if the fragment is displaced.

(3) *Open Dislocation with or without Fracture.*

(a) Debridement, open reduction and internal fixation if indicated

(b) Posterior molded plaster for 3 weeks in functional position

(c) Broad-spectrum antibiotics or combination (Keflin and Kantrex)

3. *Capsular Tears.* Treatment is always conservative when the tear is acute, with splinting in the functional position.

4. *Crushing Injuries*

A. Immobilize with a volar padded splint for 2 to 3 weeks and start on active exercises thereafter.

B. If the joint remains painful, continue night splinting for as long as 8 to 12 weeks.

C. Associated tendon injuries may require prolonged initial immobilization.

D. Intra-articular corticosteroid injection is reserved for chronic capsulitis.

5. *Infections*

A. Drain the joint through a lateral incision.

B. Culture and smear exudate for organisms and sensitivity.

C. Insert a Penrose drain down to the joint.

D. Splint in functional position and elevate the hand.

E. After 12 hours apply continuous warm saline soaks.

F. Broad-spectrum antibiotics are given until organism-specific antibiotics can be started based on the culture report.

## ACUTE INJURIES OF THE WRIST

### Definitions

1. *Midcarpal Dislocation.* This is dislocation of the hand and distal row of carpal bones on the proximal row.

2. *Perilunar Dislocation.* This is dorsal dislocation of all the carpal bones except the lunate and usually the triquetrum, which retain their normal radial articulation.

3. *Radiocarpal Dislocation.* This is dislocation of the entire carpus dorsal to the radio-ulnar articulation.

## Basic Principles

1. The wrist is composed of a proximal and distal row of carpal bones, the proximal row consisting of the navicular, lunate, triquetrum and pisiform bones and the distal row composed of the greater and lesser multangular bones, the capitate and the hamate. The navicular acts as a bridge between the two rows.

Kaplan has shown that motions of the wrist occur in three places—the radiocarpal, intercarpal and midcarpal joints. In the normal wrist:

A. Volar flexion occurs primarily at the radiocarpal articulation and secondarily at the midcarpal articulation.

B. Dorsiflexion occurs primarily at the midcarpal articulation and secondarily at the radiocarpal articulation. The lunate slides under the dorsal lip of the radius, pointing its distal articulation surface dorsally. The head of the capitate remaining in contact with the distal articular surface of the lunate permits the long axis of the capitate to attain a position perpendicular to the long axis of the radius.

C. Radial deviation occurs primarily at the midcarpal articulation and ulnar deviation at the radiocarpal articulation.

2. Most dislocations and fractures, except severe crushing injuries, can be treated by closed means; however, occasionally open reduction and internal fixation are necessary.

3. The possible combinations of fractures and dislocations are almost innumerable. Common associated injuries are:

A. Midcarpal dislocation with navicular fracture

B. Radiocarpal dislocation with dorsal lip of the radius fracture (Barton's fracture)

C. Perilunate dislocation with navicular fracture and occasionally also a capitate fracture

4. Most carpal fractures and dislocations are due to falls on the dorsiflexed wrist with the hand in different positions of lateral deviation. The navicular fracture, the most common carpal fracture, is a special problem since the entire blood supply enters distally, and the more proximal the fracture line, the better is the possibility of aseptic necrosis of the proximal fragment despite excellent reduction.

## Criteria for Diagnosis

1. All injuries have a history of direct or indirect trauma. A specific mechanism of injury may greatly assist in diagnostic evaluation.

2. *Physical Findings*

A. *Dislocations*

(1) *Midcarpal*

(a) Wrist deformity

(b) Pain, swelling, limitation of motion

(c) X-rays — three views — anteroposterior, lateral and oblique, plus comparison with similar views of the other wrist

(d) On x-ray look for possible fracture of the navicular, radial or ulnar styloid.

(2) *Radiocarpal*

(a) Same signs, symptoms and x-rays as above

(b) On x-ray look for possible fracture of the rim of radius, radial or ulnar styloid.

(3) *Perilunate*

(a) Same signs, symptoms and x-rays as above

(b) On x-ray the triquetrum and lunate remain attached to the forearm bones while the navicular dislocates with the remaining carpus. The capitate and carpus are displaced dorsally over the lunate and occasionally may pinch the lunate and thrust it volarward. This may be accompanied by fracture of the navicular.

(4) *Navicular*

(a) Pain and swelling in the wrist and snuffbox

(b) Limitation of motion; pain with movements of the thumb

(c) X-rays—four views—anteroposterior, lateral, oblique and navicular, and comparison with comparable views of the other wrist

(d) On x-ray look for a transverse lie of the navicular and a widening of the navicular-lunate articulation.

(5) *Greater Multangular*

(a) Pain, swelling, limitation of motion and localized tenderness at the base of the thenar eminence; pain with movements of the thumb

(b) X-rays—three views—anteroposterior, lateral and oblique, plus comparison with the other wrist

(c) On x-ray look for posterior dislocation.

(6) *Pisiform, Hamate*

(a) Pain, swelling, limitation of motion and localized tenderness in the base of the hypothenar area

(b) X-ray—four views—anteroposterior, lateral, oblique and carpal tunnel view, and comparison views of the other wrist

(c) On x-ray look for posterior dislocation over the triquetrum. Often the fourth and fifth metacarpals are fractured.

(7) *Lesser Multangular*

(a) Pain, swelling, limitation of motion and localized tenderness at the base of the thenar eminence; pain with movements of the thumb

(b) X-rays—three views—anteroposterior, lateral and oblique

(c) On x-ray look for the commonly accompanying Bennett's fracture.

(8) *Lunate*

(a) Pain, swelling, limitation of motion with localized tenderness in the volar wrist

(b) Median nerve compression symptoms are (1) hypoesthesia in the thumb, index and middle fingers and half of the ring fingers, (2) pain in the volar wrist, and (3) positive Tinel's sign.

(c) X-rays—four views—anteroposterior, lateral, oblique and carpal tunnel view, if possible, and comparison views of the other wrist

(d) On the lateral view the lunate is displaced volar and faces backward.

B. *Fractures*

(1) *Navicular*

(a) Pain, swelling, limitation of motion and localized tenderness in the snuffbox

(b) Pain with movements of the thumb

(c) X-rays—four views—anteroposterior, lateral, oblique and navicular views, and comparison views of the other wrist

(d) Fracture is not always obvious at the time of injury. Repeat x-rays are essential if the initial x-ray was negative but symptoms persist.

(e) Acute clinical symptoms, if severe, dictate treatment as a fracture even though x-rays are negative.

(2) *All Other Bones of the Wrist*

(a) Signs and symptoms of fracture

(b) X-rays—anteroposterior, lateral, oblique, and comparison views of the other wrist

(c) Persistent symptoms require repeated rotational views with comparable comparison views of the uninjured wrist.

C. *Sprains or Ligamentous Tears*

(1) Pain, swelling, limitation of motion

(2) Localized tenderness

(3) No x-ray evidence of fracture or dislocation

(4) Special stress views might reveal abnormal separation of bones.

## Management

### Dislocations

1. All dislocations must be reduced under general anesthesia or regional block.

2. With complete muscle relaxation, traction is exerted on the hand and direct pressure is exerted on the dislocated bone or bones until a sudden reduction with restoration of normal appearance is achieved.

3. With the forearm suspended by the fingers, x-rays are taken to ascertain reduction before plaster is applied.

4. A snug-fitting unpadded forearm cast, extending from the distal palmar crease to just below the elbow, with the wrist in neutral position, is applied. Repeat x-rays are taken after application of the cast.

5. In navicular dislocations, the forearm cast is extended to include the thumb up to the interphalangeal joint.

6. High elevation of the hand postoperatively should prevent swelling necessitating splitting of the cast because of vascular compromise.

7. Lunate dislocations require prolonged traction and hyperflexion of the wrist before the volarly displaced lunate can be pressed back into position.

8. The failure of closed reduction is an indication for immediate open reduction and transfixion in anatomical position with Kirschner wires. In general, dislocations of the pisiform, hamate and navicular will require open reduction. Additionally, associated fractures, if not perfectly reduced with the reposition of the dislocation, should have open reduction immediately.

### Fractures

1. *Navicular*

A. Undisplaced fractures of the navicular may be treated with a snug-fitting forearm cast, incorporating the thumb with the metacarpal abducted and the proximal phalanx flexed at the MP joint (drinking-glass position).

B. Displaced fractures may be reduced by traction and manipulation under general anesthesia, and immobilized in a long arm cast down to the interphalangeal joint of the thumb, as above, with the wrist in mild radial deviation and slight volar flexion.

C. The initial cast change for both fractures is at 6 weeks, at which time healing is judged by clinical signs of pain on axillary compression (*see* Chap. 25) and x-ray evidence of osseous continuity.

D. If additional immobilization is required, a forearm cast, including the thumb, is reapplied. This is removed every 6 weeks for repeated clinical and radiographic examination.

E. Open reduction with Kirschner wire or compression screw fixation is necessary when good anatomical reduction cannot be obtained or maintained.

2. *Other Carpal Bone Fractures*

A. Most other fractures of the carpal bones are minimally displaced and only require protection in a forearm cast for 3 to 6 weeks until there is x-ray evidence of healing.

B. Open reduction with internal fixation is mandatory for displaced fractures not amenable to closed reduction.

3. *Crushing Injuries of the Carpus*

A. Since the primary consideration is the restoration of the transverse carpal arch, open reduction with Kirschner wire fixation is usually needed in all these injuries.

B. Following open reduction, a padded long arm cast is applied to the metacarpal heads, including the thumb.

C. Immobilization is continued for 3 weeks, at which time the cast is removed for x-ray check of healing.

D. If healing is sufficient at this time, the percutaneously placed Kirschner wires may be removed through small incisions under local anesthesia.

E. Active physical therapy is then commenced, with night splinting to maintain the osseous architecture.

## Sprains and Ligamentous Tears

1. If no fractures or dislocations are noted, a volar splint in neutral position, secured with a pressure dressing, will suffice for immobilization. If symptoms are severe, a complete forearm cast may be preferable.

2. Elevation of the arm to minimize swelling

3. Butazolidin Alka, 100 mg. q.i.d. for 5 days

4. Discontinue immobilization after 3 weeks and begin active patient physical therapy unless symptoms remain severe.

5. Local corticosteroid injections are only used if chronic symptoms persist.

## TRAUMATIC AMPUTATIONS

### Definitions

1. *Traumatic Amputation.* This is total or partial loss of tissue substantial enough to reduce the size of a digit or the hand in its diameter or its length.

2. *Total Amputation.* This is interruption of all vascular supply.

3. *Partial Amputation.* This is retention of some vascular supply together with some soft tissue attachment.

### Basic Principles

Loss of length in the thumb, index and middle fingers primarily affects pinch and fine movements. Loss of length in the ring and little fingers primarily affects grip. Loss of width of the palm primarily affects grasp of large objects.

Loss of length distal to the distal interphalangeal joint is detrimental to pinch in the thumb, index and middle fingers, and affects grip in the ring and little fingers. Therefore, all attempts at maintaining length should be made in these amputations. On the other hand, maintenance of length is less useful when the amputation is proximal to the DIP joint, since amputation below the midportion of the middle phalanx is equivalent to total loss of function for pinch and fine movements. Amputation of a single digit close to the metacarpophalangeal joint not only loses the function of that digit but often constitutes a hindrance to normal function of the remaining fingers.

The exception to the above principles is in the management of multiple proximal phalangeal amputations. Here, all available length should be maintained to give the hand maximum return of function and permit later transfer as appropriate.

All return of function of an amputated digit depends on the quality of skin, the hypo- or hypersensitivity of that skin and the stiffness of that finger. Therefore, in all amputations between the proximal and distal joints, both nerves are identified and resected below the level of amputation. As in all hand trauma, the age of the patient and his occupation and economic status are always considerations. Amputations through the hand, wrist, forearm or arm are problems of replantation.

### Criteria for Diagnosis

1. History of cutting, avulsing or crushing injury

2. Visual inspection of the injured hand
    A. *Total Amputation*
        *(1)* Total separation of tissue or structure from its origin
        *(2)* Total loss of blood supply but retaining some attachment (tendon or very narrow bridge of skin)
    B. *Partial Amputation*
        *(1)* Partial separation of tissue or structure from its origin
        *(2)* Partial loss of blood supply with partial or total separation from its origin. Thus, a finger may be totally severed except for a single neurovascular bundle.

### Management

#### Digits

1. *Total Amputation.* All fingertip amputations with full-thickness loss of skin and exposure of bone, tendon or joint require local or distant flaps.

A. For amputations involving 30 per cent or less of the fingertip:

*(1) Moberg Slide.* The volar skin is totally released and advanced over the amputated tip with or without bone resection. This procedure is best for oblique amputations involving mostly the dorsal half of the fingertip and is ideal for the thumb.

*(2) Kutler Flap.* This is an excellent procedure for guillotine-type amputations. Two triangular flaps are outlined on the lateral borders of the finger and, remaining attached to their blood supply, are slid distally over the fingertip where they are sutured to each other and the surrounding skin in V-Y-plasty fashion.

It is best *not* to undermine the flaps to give them added mobility. Some resection of bone is usually necessary.

*(3) Kleinert Flap.* A single triangular flap, remaining attached to its blood supply and taken volar and proximal to the amputated tip, is advanced over the defect. This is not as satisfactory a procedure as the Kutler flap.

B. For amputations involving more than 30 per cent of the fingertip, or where the loss of tissue is very extensive or involves the lateral borders of the fingertip:

*(1)* Cross-finger flap

*(2)* Palmar flap

C. For multiple amputations:

*(1)* Multiple cross-finger flaps

*(2)* A combination of palmar and cross-finger flaps

*(3)* Abdominothoracic flaps

*(4)* Occasionally, the above procedures may be indicated for amputations involving less than 30 per cent of the fingertip.

D. Amputations below the distal interphalangeal joint are usually treated with primary closure, without flaps, unless multiple digits are involved.

E. For multiple amputations, consideration toward maintenance of length is more important.

*(1)* Tailored abdominal flaps are indicated for multiple midphalangeal amputations.

*(2)* Multiple cross-finger flaps or a combination of cross-finger and palmar flaps are indicated for fingertip amputations.

*(3)* Occasionally, if the amputation is distal to the midportion of the middle phalanx, one can do primary closure with minimal bone resection.

F. In infants and the very young, circumferential or guillotine-type amputations can be treated by simple pressure dressing or resuturing of the amputated pulp or tip.

G. *Special Procedures*

*(1) Neurovascular Island Pedicle Transfer.* This is usually a secondary reconstructive procedure.

*(2) Cross-finger Sensory Flap.* This is indicated for thumb amputations where the ulnar half of the pulp or tip is involved. A dorsal flap on the radial side of the proximal phalanx of the index finger is transferred as a pedicle with an intact sensory branch of the radial nerve which terminates in the flap. Thus a sensory cross-finger flap is transferred on the thumb. The flap is detached 15 to 21 days later.

2. *Total Amputation of Specific Digits*

A. *Thumb*

*(1)* Always try to maintain length.

*(2)* For tip amputations, the Moberg slide is excellent.

*(3)* For larger amputations:

*(a)* Sensory cross-finger flap

*(b)* Nonsensory cross-finger flap. This flap is taken from the dorsum of the middle phalanx of the middle finger.

*(c)* Thoracico-abdominal flap. If substantial bone resection is necessary and local flaps are not possible, a tailored abdominal flap is performed.

B. *The Index Finger*

*(1)* For amputation through the distal interphalangeal joint:

*(a)* Resect a portion of the head of the middle phalanx and its articular surface.

*(b)* Resect condyles to eliminate flare and thus obtain a more fusiform, cosmetic appearance.

*(c)* Resect neurovascular bundles as far proximally as possible from the area of amputation.

*(d)* The lacerated profundus tendon is withdrawn, transected and allowed to retract into the palm. Leaving the lacerated profundus tendon in the finger may produce a checkrein phenomenon—that is, the scarred profundus will hold back proper flexion of the intact profundus tendons in other digits. Since, except for the index finger, they have a common muscle origin, problems of one will affect the others.

*(e)* Extensor tendons are not resected if lacerated.

*(2)* For amputations below the distal interphalangeal joint, resection of bone with primary closure is done, unless we are dealing with multiple amputations.

*(3)* For amputations close to the metacarpophalangeal joint, the index finger, when repaired and healed, usually becomes a hindrance to the patient, who will transfer all function of pinch to the middle finger.

*(a)* Primary ray resection is done in these cases, if the wound is clean.

*(b)* The first dorsal interosseous also is transferred to the middle finger at the same time.

*(c)* Ray resection is deferred for a secondary procedure if the wound is not clean.

C. *The Middle Finger and Ring Finger*

*(1)* Same treatment as for the index finger

*(2)* For amputations close to or through the metacarpophalangeal joint, ray resection with transfer of index or little finger ray is recommended as a secondary procedure.

D. *The Little Finger*

*(1)* Same treatment as for the index finger.

*(2)* If amputation is near or through the metacarpophalangeal joint, primary ray resection with transfer of

hypothenar muscles to the ring finger should be considered in clean wounds.

3. *Partial Amputation*

A. Repair all lacerated structures.

B. If properly trained, the digital artery may be repaired under the microscope.

C. Flexor tendons are usually not repaired in "no man's land."

D. In a severely crushed finger with a viable distal segment, the primary consideration is viability.

*(1)* Manipulation is contraindicated because it will further traumatize the tissue.

*(2)* Reduction of a fracture (one or two attempts at most) should be simple and done only as a means of stabilizing the finger.

*(3)* Skin closure is often the only procedure done to avoid unnecessary trauma and insure viability of the finger.

## Hand, Wrist, Forearm and Arm

1. *Total Amputation. See* pages 464-465 on replantation.

2. *Partial Amputation*

A. Repair all major arteries.

B. Repair all other lacerated structures.

## BURNS

*See also* Chapter 34, Burns.

### Basic Principles

In the care of all burned hands, the primary objective is restoration of function. Since the hands represent only a small percentage of body surface, the general principles of fluid replacement and intensive care play no role in isolated burns of the hand.

### Criteria for Diagnosis

*See* Chapter 34.

### Management

1. Basic emergency treatment is:

A. *For First-Degree Burns:* application of soothing ointment and moderate pressure dressing with splinting

B. *For Superficial Second-Degree Burns*

*(1)* Wash hand in saline solution or immerse in ice water.

*(2)* Blisters are left intact unless they are already broken. These can be minimally debrided at that time.

*(3)* Apply Furacin ointment with pressure dressing and splint.

*(4)* Antibiotics, tetanus prophylaxis and analgesics

*(5)* The patient is sent home with a sling.

C. *For Deep Second-Degree Burns*

*(1)* Saline wash or immersion in ice water

*(2)* Minimal debridement of broken blisters only

*(3)* Admit the patient and treat with topical antibacterial regimen (Chap. 34).

D. *For Third-Degree Burns*

*(1)* Immersion in saline or ice water

*(2)* Antibiotics, tetanus prophylaxis and analgesics

*(3)* Admit the patient to the hospital and institute antibacterial treatment.

*(4)* Debridement of eschar is done early in the operating room and autologous grafts applied as soon as possible.

2. *Problems Peculiar to Second- and Third-Degree Hand Burns*

A. Burned tendon, bone and joints are left exposed until they slough or sequester. As soon as an adequate bed is available, these areas are grafted.

B. If the digit is severely burned, it is often best to totally amputate the denuded or charred portions.

C. A destroyed joint and tendon mechanism, such as the extensor mechanism, requires secondary flaps and tendon/joint reconstruction. A stiff finger is the usual sequel.

D. Scar contractures in burns of the dorsum of the hand are fairly common and difficult to prevent. Splinting with the MP joints at 90 degrees or the use of the "hay rake" Kirschner wire immobilization may minimize contracture until grafting is completed.

## FROSTBITE

*See* Chapter 18, Vascular Emergencies.

## ACUTE VASCULAR INJURIES

*See also* Chapter 18, Vascular Emergencies.

### Criteria for Diagnosis

1. History of injury, usually penetrating, but occasionally thrombosis can follow blunt trauma

2. Signs and symptoms of vascular insufficiency

A. Absent or diminished pulse

B. Massive blood loss, occasionally with obvious arterial spurting

C. Cyanosis or blanching, with lack of capillary refill

3. Brachial arteriogram followed through the venous phase, usually done by a percutaneous injection

4. Further evaluation of the type and extent of injury must be done by direct inspection at operation.

5. Differentiation between vascular injury and reactive vasospasm can also frequently only be made at exploration.

### Management

1. *Emergency Treatment*

A. Whenever a patient enters with a laceration of the forearm or hand and arterial bleeding is noted, never attempt "blind" clamping. This frequently damages additional vessel length and other vessels and nerve.

B. Apply a pressure dressing to the area of bleeding and a tourniquet to the arm if necessary to control the bleeding.

C. With the bleeding controlled, minimal exploration of the wound can be done and the open ends of lacerated major vessels can be finely clamped.

D. The patient then can be taken to the operating room where the vessels may be repaired, if possible.

2. *Definitive Management*

A. All hand and forearm vascular repairs are done in the operating room.

B. With the possible exception of the digital arteries, all other injured arteries should have repair attempted.

C. Both the radial and ulnar arteries in the forearm should be repaired when injured. Although a single artery laceration in the forearm is often considered adequately treated by simple ligation, since the remaining major artery with the abundant collateral circulation will suffice to obviate gangrene, we prefer repair of the artery, because intermittent claudication may occur when only one major vessel is functioning. When both forearm arteries are lacerated, both should be repaired, since the chances of thrombosis of either one is more than 50 per cent.

D. In clean, sharply divided injuries of palmar or digital arteries, anastomosis repair should be attempted. Success depends on the duration since injury, the condition of the vessels and the skill of the surgeon. Microsurgical technique is essential.

E. Similarly, venous lacerations when no other venous drainage exists should be repaired with fine suture technique under magnification.

F. All other lacerated vessels in a traumatized arm or hand should be identified and ligated to avoid future aneurysms or arteriovenous fistulae.

3. *Postoperative Care*

A. Loose pressure dressing exposing the nail beds for inspection

B. Splint with molded plaster away from the repair and use joint flexion to avoid anastomotic kinking or tension.

C. Moderate elevation of the entire arm for good venous drainage

D. Antibiotics as above

E. Anticoagulants are of questionable value, although in small vessel repair we use systemic intermittent intravenous heparinization and 100 ml./day of low-molecular-weight dextran (Rheomacrodex 40) in saline for 2 days.

F. Stellate ganglion blocks may be done in the presence of vasospasm but probably are worthless.

## VOLKMANN'S ISCHEMIA

### Definition

Volkmann's ischemia is a consequence of vascular insufficiency of a main extremity artery (in the instance of the hand, the brachial), in which there is muscle and nerve necrosis.

### Basic Principles

1. Volkmann's ischemia can be due to primary arterial injury or secondary arterial spasm. The spasm is the single most important factor responsible for muscle necrosis. Seddon has noted that the lesion is a true infarct, in some cases involving skin and bone in addition to the muscle and nerves.

2. Four clinical pictures are recognized:

A. *Impending ischemia* which occurs within 6 to 12 hours following the injury. Here, arterial spasm may not yet be present and the process is still reversible. Hypoesthesia without paralysis is the hallmark of this stage.

B. *Early ischemia* usually is seen 24 to 36 hours following the injury. Arterial spasm is already present with the onset of muscle and nerve ischemia, although the extent of involvement may be mild to moderate and is reversible by prompt treatment.

C. *Late ischemia.* Muscle and nerve death is extensive but not necessarily complete in that return of some function is possible with revascularization.

D. *Established Ischemia.* Contractures are present, fibrosis is extensive, and nerve death is partial or total.

3. Prevention of Volkmann's ischemia is much easier than the treatment (*see* Supracondylar Fractures of the Humerus, Chap. 25).

4. Remember that Volkmann's ischemia can begin even 3 days after the manipulation and application of cast in a supracondylar fracture.

5. Three major compartments in the upper extremity involved in Volkmann's ischemia are the extensor and flexor compartments in the forearm and the intrinsic muscle compartment in the hand; the flexor compartment in the forearm is the most commonly involved.

6. In all compartments, the deeper muscles are affected first, followed by the ischemia of the involved nerves, the median, ulnar and radial. The median nerve is the most susceptible to this ischemia.

7. Besides loss of major arterial flow, the increased pressure due to muscle swelling in the fascial compartments causes venous congestion with more edematous swelling that eventually totally obliterates the collateral circulation.

## Criteria for Diagnosis

1. The classical picture is represented by the 4 P's.
   A. Pain
   B. Paralysis
   C. Pallor
   D. Pulselessness

It is important to remember that when these signs are present, it is already fairly late.

2. All of the signs need not be present to make the diagnosis. Volkmann's ischemia can occur without any loss of distal pulse.

3. Retrograde catheter arteriography from the femoral or other brachial artery may be helpful in locating the area of arterial occlusion.

4. The most ominous sign is pain on extension of the fingers, since this indicates severe muscle ischemia.

## Management

1. *Impending Ischemia*

A. Immediate total decompression of the involved fascial compartments with decompression of the nerves at the various points of muscular constriction

*(1) For the Median Nerve*

*(a)* An aberrant head of the pronator teres or the supracondylar process can cause pressure.

*(b)* In the forearm, constriction may occur where the nerve passes between the heads of the pronator teres or in the fascia of the sublimus muscle in which the median nerve lies.

*(c)* At the wrist, it can be in the carpal tunnel.

*(2) For the Ulnar Nerve*

*(a)* At the elbow, the pressure point can be in the ulnar groove at the medial epicondyle.

*(b)* In the forearm, constriction may be found where the nerve passes between the two heads of the flexor carpi ulnaris.

*(c)* At the wrist, the pressure may be in the ulnar tunnel of Guillon.

*(3) For the Radial Nerve*

*(a)* In the arm, the pressure point for the radial nerve is in the spiral groove of the humerus.

*(b)* In the forearm, constriction may occur at the entrance of the radial nerve into the supinator muscle or distally at the exit of the superficial nerve through the brachioradialis muscle in the distal forearm.

B. If after decompression of the fascial compartments the pulse and muscle color does not return, the brachial artery must be isolated in the antecubital space and investigated for occlusion both by inspection and Fogarty catheter thrombectomy.

*(1)* Areas of injury must be resected and end-to-end anastomosis performed.

*(2)* Arterial spasm not responding to local warmth, intra-arterial procaine and local papaverine should be dilated either with a Fogarty balloon or by the hydraulic dilatation described by Mustard.

C. Following decompression, it may not be possible to close the wound primarily:

*(1)* Allow the wound to granulate until conditions are stable.

*(2)* Secondary skin closure or grafting is then done.

D. *Postoperative Care*

*(1)* Mild elevation

*(2)* Splinting in functional position

*(3)* Antibiotics intravenously, of broad-spectrum-type or combination

*(4)* Daily change of bandages to assess viability of the extremity

E. In cases of supracondylar fracture:

*(1)* Initial treatment should consist of removing the cast, extending the elbow and stellate ganglion block.

*(2)* If the condition of the extremity does not improve immediately, exploration of the brachial artery in the antecubital space is emergently necessary.

2. *Early Ischemia*

A. Immmediate decompression and arterial exploration as above

B. Do not debride any questionably viable muscle.

C. Same postoperative care as above

D. The patient may require secondary debridement of muscles.

3. *Late Ischemia*

A. Decompression and arterial exploration as above

B. Debride only obviously necrotic sloughing muscle.

C. Same postoperative care as above

D. Will require secondary muscle debridement

E. May require secondary coverage with abdominal flaps or split-thickness skin grafts if nerves and tendons are exposed and the wound is clean

F. May require secondary nerve reconstruction and tendon transfers

4. *Established Contractures.* This is not an emergency condition. Secondary neurolysis, tendolysis and epimysial fasciotomy are done. Secondary nerve and tendon reconstructions are done according to the extent of damage.

5. *To summarize:*

A. *Early recognition is essential.* Unfortunately this is still not commonly done.

B. Arterial spasm most often is the offending mechanism.

C. Immediate and complete decompression of all involved muscle and nerve region compression must be done, as well as assurance of main channel arterial flow as soon as impending ischemia is recognized.

D. In supracondylar fractures of the humerus, close observation of the patient following reduction and cast application is most important since Volkmann's ischemia can occur as late as three days after reduction.

E. Numerous operations are available for the established case, but the philosophy should be not to get into the situation where this is necessary.

## SPECIAL WOUNDS
### WRINGER INJURY

#### Definition

A wringer injury is a crush injury due to the hand or arm being caught between the rollers of a machine such as a wringer of a home washing machine.

#### Classification

1. *Simple.* Crushing, avulsing injury involving mostly skin and subcutaneous tissue.

2. *Compound.* Involvement of muscles, tendons, nerves and bone.

#### Basic Principles

Wringer injuries are more common in children, although in industry rollers of all kinds can create similar injuries. The basic trauma in home accidents can involve the hand, forearm and/or arm, while industrial injuries usually are limited to the hand and forearm. Typically, the childhood injury is in the upper arm where the ingress of the upper extremity is stopped by the axilla. The avulsed skin, if present, usually is based distally due to the effort of the patient to withdraw the extremity from the wringer or the rollers. Hot rollers in industry add to the problem by causing second- and third-degree burns.

## Criteria for Diagnosis

1. Typical history of injury
2. Ecchymosis, edema and abrasive injury to the skin, usually in the upper arm
3. There may be an avulsing injury to the skin with the flap based distally.
4. Despite marked swelling and apparent cyanosis, pulses are present.
5. X-rays of the entire extremity from the shoulder to the hand must be done to rule out osseous injury.

## Management

1. Nonadherent antibiotic dressing (Furacin stretch gauze) over the abraded skin
2. Marked elevation to the entire extremity except the fingertips, with the arm resting in a padded Thomas arm splint
3. Tetanus prophylaxis
4. Broad-spectrum antibiotics as above
5. Analgesics for pain
6. Avulsing injuries should have the following:
   A. Questionably viable skin should be sutured lightly into place, and the viability reevaluated later.
   B. Split-thickness skin grafts are applied to replace obvious skin necrosis or loss.
7. Increased intrafascial pressure (impending Volkmann's ischemia) requires total fasciotomies of the involved compartments, as noted above.
8. If fractures are present, they can be reduced closed if the viability of the extremity is not compromised. Avoid encircling casts.
9. *Tendons and Nerves*
   A. If covered by a suitable bed, these may be repaired secondarily once the patient's condition has stabilized.
   B. If no suitable cover is present, immediate flaps or skin grafts must be used to close the wound.

10. *Arterial Injuries*
   A. If the extremity's viability is in question, a stellate block may be of value. Hypothermia and vasodilators have not been proven to be beneficial.
   B. If sympathetic blockade does not improve apparent viability, manage the arterial injury as noted above.

## GREASE GUN INJURIES

### Definition

A grease gun injury is an injury due to the ejection of grease under high pressure through a small orifice.

### Basic Principles

Grease enters the digit, the palm or the web space and will travel into the subcutaneous tissue along tissue planes and through tendon sheaths and bursae. It causes a difficult, severe injury with extensive residual crippling.

### Management

1. In the operating room, under anesthesia and tourniquet control, immediate incision and drainage are done of all spaces and sheaths involved, with culture of the material.
2. Copious irrigation of all the exposed structures with peroxide and saline. *Do not use a grease solvent.*
3. Mechanical debridement of all affected areas
4. Place numerous drains in the incision, and close the wounds lightly if at all.
5. Apply a light pressure dressing; splint and elevate the hand.
6. Tetanus prophylaxis and broad-spectrum antibiotics are given.
7. Analgesics as necessary
8. Continuous saline soaks are started 24 hours postoperatively.

## PAINT GUN, TEAR GAS GUN AND CEMENT GUN INJURIES

Treat as Grease Gun Injuries, above.

## REPLANTATION

### Definition

Replantation is the anatomical restoration of an amputated extremity so that it remains viable.

### Basic Principles

The first cardinal principle considered in replantation is whether the amputated extremity will be better from a functional viewpoint than a prosthesis. The technical considerations of vascular, nerve and tendon reconstruction present no additional difficulties over those sustained from simple lacerations. The period of ischemia of the extremity, equivalent to tourniquet injury, and the severity of the crush of the amputated part determine in large measure whether replantation is worthwhile. Occasionally, replantation may be done to salvage a joint even though the remaining distal extremity is not expected to be functional. Replantations are probably only of value in the upper extremity, especially the hand, and microsurgical techniques have provided excellent results even with amputated digits. The replantation of digits where amputation is distal to the wrist requires special technique, and such patients after emergency care should probably be referred to centers skilled in these techniques.

### Criteria for Diagnosis

Evident total amputation of the digit, hand, forearm or arm, with this as an isolated injury and the amputated part in reasonably untraumatized condition

### Management

1. *Emergency Treatment*
   A. Place the amputated extremity in a plastic bag together with a dilute solution of antibiotic if available. This is then put into a container filled with water and ice. Such hypothermia can prolong the ischemic interval before replantation will become unsuccessful.

   B. The patient together with the amputated extremity, after resuscitation, is taken immediately to the operating room.
2. *Operative Management.* General principles of management are:
   A. Perfuse the amputated extremity with cooled heparinized saline and/or low-molecular-weight dextran (Rheomacrodex 40).
   B. Debridement of both wounds is meticulously done and the bone is shortened, if necessary, to allow vascular anastomosis without tension.
   C. The skeleton is stabilized with plates and screws or with intramedullary wires, as appropriate, to the level of amputation.
   D. Two veins are repaired for each artery to be repaired.
   E. The arterial repairs are accomplished with fine suture technique, using magnification as necessary.
   F. Blood flow through the amputated extremity is then permitted by removing the proximal arterial-occluding clamps. Additionally, divided vessels are ligated and meticulous hemostasis must be obtained.
   G. If the general condition of the extremity appears satisfactory and the wound is comparatively clean, nerve repair should be done, followed by tendon repair if the patient's condition permits.
   H. If definitive repair is not possible, the ends of the nerves and tendons should be tagged together for repair at a later date.
   I. Skin coverage, preferably by closure of intact skin, must be accomplished. The use of flaps or split-thickness skin grafts may be necessary in some instances.
3. *Postoperative Care*
   A. A loose pressure dressing is applied to the entire extremity, with an antibiotic nonadherent dressing (Furacin mesh gauze) over the wound. The fingertips and the region for palpation of the radial pulse must be left out for inspection and determination of main channel vascular flow.

B. The extremity is splinted with a molded plaster in the functional position and elevated moderately above heart level to permit good venous drainage.

C. An intravenous broad-spectrum antibiotic combination is used for the first five days or until sepsis provides a culture for type-specific antibiotics.

D. Low-molecular-weight dextran (Rheomacrodex 40 in saline), 1,000 ml./day, is given starting 24 hours after replantation; anticoagulation with heparin is used only in digital replantation.

E. The patient's blood volume must be restored to an optimal value and maintained with whole blood transfusion if necessary. An hourly check of the nail bed color, capillary filling and distal pulse must be done, with immediate re-exploration and repair if there has been a loss of arterial inflow or venous outflow.

F. The wound should be inspected daily until healing has occurred.

G. If primary nerve or tendon reconstruction was not accomplished, this should be done as soon as local wound conditions permit.

# 32. ACUTE HAND PROBLEMS

*Julian Zweig,* M.D.

Surgery of the hand has established itself as a specialty because improper management of even minor hand problems may result in serious sequelae. This is true of all forms of hand trauma as well as of infections of the hand.

## INFECTIONS OF THE HAND

### Definitions

1. *Cellulitis.* This is a diffuse inflammatory swelling of infectious origin, producing the usual signs of redness, heat, swelling and pain.
2. *Abscess.* This is a localized collection of pus within an anatomical compartment or closed space.

### Classification

1. Superficial infections and infections of subcutaneous tissues
   A. Furuncles and carbuncles
   B. Subungual abscess
   C. Subcutaneous abscess of a finger or hand
   D. Paronychia
   E. Felon
2. Tenosynovitis
3. Subfascial space infections
   A. Web space
   B. Midpalmar space
   C. Thenar space
   D. Hypothenar space
   E. Lumbrical space
   F. Dorsal subaponeurotic space
   G. Quadrilateral or Parona's space
4. Osteomyelitis
5. Acute suppurative arthritis

### Basic Principles

1. Untreated cellulitis will usually progress to abscess formation.
2. An abscess whose internal pressure is not relieved by surgical drainage will eventually erode through its confines to other anatomical spaces.
3. Tendons bathed in pus will lose their sliding mechanism. Deposition of fibrin on tendon surfaces stimulates scar formation and results in dense adhesions.
4. Stiffness of the hand results from the formation of dense scar, tendinous adhesions and fibrous ankylosis.
5. Nerves may be damaged from pressure within closed spaces, and muscle and soft tissue may be destroyed by pressure necrosis.

### Criteria for Diagnosis

#### Cellulitis

1. Diffuse, poorly limited erythema
2. Increased warmth of the affected area
3. Moderate pain and tenderness
4. Moderate swelling without fluctuation
5. Either no loss or minimal loss of motion

#### Abscess or Closed-Space Infection

1. Well-limited erythema, and swelling which is fluctuant and under tension
2. Marked pain of a throbbing nature, with severe tenderness on palpation
3. Voluntary splinting because of severe pain

### Management

#### Cellulitis

Treatment is conservative but must be vigorous to prevent abscess formation.
1. Antibiotics such as:
   A. Penicillin V, 250 mg. every 6 hours
   B. Ampicillin, 250 to 500 mg. every 6 hours
   C. Lincomycin, 500 mg. 3 times a

day, for patients who are allergic to penicillin

2. Warm compresses to the area of cellulitis

3. Elevation of the arm

4. Immobilization

## Abscess or Closed-Space Infection

1. Antibiotics are continued as before until results of culture and sensitivity tests are obtained.

2. The mainstay of treatment is adequate surgical drainage.

3. Packing of dead spaces within the hand should be avoided. Gauze packing retards drainage and acts as a dam, and in addition the internal pressure created causes further tissue destruction. We prefer the insertion of soft rubber drains into the wound and the application of a well-padded compression dressing to control any further bleeding.

4. Incisions should be planned to avoid injury to important underlying structures and to avoid the formation of subsequent scar contractures.

5. Intermittent warm saline soaks through the dressing plus antibiotics are continued until all drainage has stopped.

6. Penrose drains are usually removed after 48 hours.

7. Specimens for culture and sensitivity tests are taken at the time of surgical drainage. Specific antibiotics are then given according to the results of sensitivity tests.

## SUPERFICIAL INFECTIONS AND INFECTIONS OF SUBCUTANEOUS TISSUES

### *Furuncles, Carbuncles and Subcutaneous Abscesses of Finger or Hand*

### Definition

These are abscesses of the skin or superficial subcutaneous tissues, usually occurring around a hair follicle or as a result of penetrating trauma.

### Classification

1. *Folliculitis.* This is an infection within a hair follicle. It usually responds to antibiotics alone; surgical drainage is not required.

2. *Furuncle.* This is an abscess involving the base of the hair follicle and the sebaceous gland.

3. *Carbuncle.* This is a confluence of several furuncles.

4. *Subcutaneous Abscess.* This abscess is deeper than the other forms of superficial infections, arising either by direct extension from another focus of infection or as a result of penetrating injury.

### Criteria for Diagnosis

1. Localized pain, swelling and erythema, often capped by a "head" or crust, under which necrotic or purulent material may be found

2. There is no evidence of tendon or deep space involvement.

### Management

1. Conservative management is begun as previously described under Cellulitus.

2. If the abscess becomes tense and fluctuant, surgical incision and drainage are indicated.

3. Penrose drains are left in place for 48 hours.

4. Soaks and antibiotics are continued until all signs of infection have subsided.

### *Subungual Abscess*

### Definition

A subungual abscess is a collection of pus under the fingernail, often due to a splinter or other foreign matter penetrating between the fingernail and the nail bed.

### Classification

1. *Acute.* This is due to penetrating injury underneath the fingernail.

2. *Chronic Recurring.* This is due to the presence of heaped-up keratin, a foreign body or a plug of necrotic material beneath the fingernail.

## Basic Principles

All foreign matter must be evacuated along with the drainage of purulent material. The nail bed should be left smooth and clean. Recurrences occur if foreign material is present at the time that the newly forming fingernail advances.

## Criteria for Diagnosis

1. The fingernail is often raised and loosened from the nail bed and there is visible purulent material underneath the nail.

2. Exquisite tenderness upon compression of the fingernail

## Management

1. The fingernail in its entirety, or a portion thereof, should be removed under digital block anesthesia.

2. The pus, foreign material and debris are evacuated, the nail bed is curetted until smooth, and an ointment-impregnated gauze is applied to the nail bed and covered by a compression dressing.

3. The patient should wet the dressings with warm water four times a day. This is continued for one week, at which time the dressings are changed and soaks are stopped.

4. After the second week, the nail bed is allowed to dry by exposure to air and with the aid of painting the nail bed with Mercurochrome.

5. Once the nail bed is dry, dressings are no longer required.

6. The fingernail grows back completely in approximately four months.

### *Paronychia*

## Definition

Paronychia is inflammation of the periungual tissues.

## Classification

1. Acute purulent
2. Chronic
   A. Bacterial
   B. Retained foreign material
   C. Mycotic (onychomycosis)

## Basic Principles

1. Infection will not subside if pus, debris or other foreign matter is not evacuated.

2. Inadequate treatment results in complications such as sloughing of skin or extension into the pulp space.

## Criteria for Diagnosis

Swelling, erythema, and throbbing pain of the periungual tissues

## Management

### Acute Purulent Paronychia

1. Early cases may be treated with antibiotics and soaks, as mentioned previously under Cellulitis.

2. In addition, the patient should repeatedly retract the paronychial tissues while soaking the finger. This encourages spontaneous drainage of purulent material and prevents further necrosis due to pressure of the edge of the fingernail upon the soft tissue.

3. Advanced cases should be treated by removal of a portion of the fingernail, allowing drainage of pus from the paronychial and eponychial tissues. Incisions into skin and soft tissue are unnecessary. After removal of the portion of the fingernail, the cavity is opened through the periungual border by the spreading action of a hemostat. A sliver of Penrose drain is then inserted into the cavity for 48 hours. A nonadherent gauze dressing followed by a compression dressing is then applied. Soaks and antibiotics are continued for one week, after which the nail bed should be allowed to dry.

4. If a felon is also present, this may be drained through the paronychial border by following the sinus tract which is almost invariably present.

### Chronic Paronychia

1. If debris and foreign material are present, these should be removed by excising the overlying portion of fingernail.

2. Heaped-up keratin is curetted from the surface of the nail bed.

3. Onychomycotic infections can be treated by oral griseofulvin, 0.5 gm. twice a day, and topical applications of 1% Tinactin cream until the fingernail grows back.

### *Felon (Whitlow)*

### Definition

A felon is an infection of the pulp space of the terminal phalanx of a digit.

### Classification

1. From penetrating injuries to the pulp space
2. From direct extension of a severe paronychia
3. From necrosis and superinfection of pulp tissues
4. As a result of a crushing injury

### Basic Principles

1. The tissues of the pulp space cannot swell due to the presence of fibrous septa. Internal pressure is therefore not tolerated, and as a result the pulp tissue quickly becomes necrotic.
2. Unrelieved internal pressure may also cause the infectious process to spread either to the bone of the terminal phalanx, resulting in osteomyelitis, or to the nearby flexor tendon sheath, resulting in a suppurative tenosynovitis.
3. Relief of pressure by incision and drainage must be done whenever the pulp of the finger is felt to be under tension.

### Criteria for Diagnosis

1. Throbbing intense pain in the pulp space of a digit
2. Acute tenderness to light palpation of the pulp space
3. Unyielding tension of the pulp tissues
4. Discoloration of the skin, progressing to sloughing of the skin with spontaneous drainage

### Management

1. A very early felon, which has not yet produced tension of the pulp tissues, may be treated by antibiotics and warm soaks.

2. As soon as unyielding tension of the pulp space has developed, incision and drainage are mandatory.
  A. An incision is made along the midlateral line of the terminal phalanx. This is deepened with the scalpel blade along the volar aspect of the bone. Remaining fibrous septa are ruptured, and the entire pulp space is opened with the spreading action of a hemostat.
  B. All pus and necrotic material should be evacuated.
  C. The wound is irrigated with saline, and a sliver of Penrose drain is inserted.
3. Antibiotics and soaks are continued until subsidence of drainage and until all signs of infection have gone.
4. If postinfection wounds are healing by secondary intention, epithelialization can be hastened by drying of the surface of the wound—by exposure to air and with the aid of painting of the wound with Mercurochrome or Betadine.
5. The following forms of treatment unnecessarily complicate the postoperative course:
  A. Internal packing of gauze in the pulp space. The gauze acts as a dam, preventing further drainage, and in addition the internal pressure causes further necrosis of skin and soft tissue.
  B. The fishmouth incision is unnecessary and, upon healing, leads to deformity and tenderness of the fingertip.
  C. If two midlateral incisions are made on either side of the phalanx, the insertion of a through-and-through Penrose drain should be avoided. This also acts as a dam, preventing further drainage. It is better to place two slivers of Penrose drain, one in each wound.

## TENOSYNOVITIS

### Definition

Tenosynovitis is a close-space infection of a tendon sheath or of a synovial bursa of a tendon.

### Classification

1. Acute bacterial suppurative

2. Chronic

   A. Mycobacterial (e.g., tuberculous synovitis)

   B. Fungal

## Basic Principles

1. Infection of a tendon sheath can be caused by:

   A. Puncture wounds inoculating the synovia with pathogenic bacteria

   B. Extension from a contiguous infection

   C. Hematogenous spread

2. As in any closed-space infection, internal pressure must be relieved by incision and drainage in order to prevent further destruction and to allow the healing process to commence.

3. Exudate upon the surface of a tendon incites the production of rigid scar tissue adhesions.

## Criteria for Diagnosis

### Acute Suppurative Tenosynovitis

The cardinal signs of Kanavel are diagnostic.

1. Swelling of the palmar aspect of the entire finger, from the distal interphalangeal joint to the midpalmar crease

2. The finger is held in a position of semiflexion.

3. Tenderness over the entire tendon sheath

4. Severe pain on attempted extension of the finger, or attempted isometric flexion

### Chronic Tenosynovitis

1. Swelling of the entire palmar aspect of the digit but without the tenderness present in the acute form

2. Loss of motion of the digit

## Management of Acute Tenosynovitis

1. Antibiotics are begun, and the patient is prepared for incision and drainage of the tendon sheath under anesthesia and with proper tourniquet control.

2. The classical procedure for acute suppurative tenosynovitis has been to incise the flexor tendon sheath over its entire length through a midlateral incision. The wound is either left open, packed with gauze or closed loosely with the insertion of multiple Penrose drains. The patient is placed on soaks and antibiotics. The packing is removed gradually over several days, and the wound is allowed to heal by secondary intention.

3. Since results from the above form of treatment have been less than ideal, a less radical form of surgical drainage has evolved. This consists of:

   A. Opening the tendon sheath at both extremities

      *(1)* At the level of the middle phalanx

      *(2)* In the palm at the level of the metacarpal head

   B. The tendon sheath is then flushed with copious amounts of saline or tetracycline solution (100 mg. in 1000 ml. of saline).

   C. Penrose drains are inserted in both wounds, which are closed loosely.

   D. The Penrose drains are removed after purulent drainage has ceased. Active exercises are encouraged as soon as tolerance to pain allows.

## SUBFASCIAL SPACE INFECTIONS

### *Web Space Infection*

## Definition

The web space is a fat-filled space existing between the proximal portions of the proximal phalanges of adjacent fingers. The spaces are bounded by vertical septa which extend from the palmar fascia.

## Criteria for Diagnosis

1. The web spaces are wedge-shaped and oblique dorsally.

2. When infected, the web space becomes rounded, swollen and tense, and the fingers cannot be approximated.

3. Other signs of abscess formation are

present, such as redness, pain and tenderness.

## Management

1. Longitudinal incisions are made on the dorsum of the involved web space.
2. The incision is deepened by blunt dissection with a spreading hemostat until the abscessed cavity is reached and drained.
3. Palmar incisions are usually unnecessary.
4. Penrose drains are inserted, and compression dressings are applied.
5. The patient is placed on soaks and antibiotics, as previously described.
6. Drains are removed in 48 hours, and soaks are stopped when all evidence of drainage has ceased.

### Midpalmar Space Infection

## Basic Principles

The midpalmar space extends from a septum overlying the third metacarpal to the radial border of the hypothenar muscles. This space is often infected whether by a penetrating injury or by contiguous extension from a purulent tenosynovitis or a web space infection.

## Criteria for Diagnosis

1. The midpalmar space abscess bulges into the palm.
2. It is exquisitely tender, red and hot, and finger motion, especially of the middle, ring and little fingers, is extremely painful.

## Management

1. The incision should be placed in the distal palmar crease.
2. This is deepened through the subcutaneous tissue.
3. The palmar fascia must be carefully incised in order to avoid injury to the underlying nerves and vessels.
4. After evacuation of purulent material, the midpalmar space is irrigated with saline or antibiotic solution, and Penrose drains are inserted.

5. The skin incision is loosely closed and a compression dressing is applied.
6. Soaks and antibiotics are instituted and early finger motion is begun.
7. The drains are removed usually in 48 hours, and saline soaks are continued until all drainage has ceased.

### Thenar Space Infection

## Basic Principles

The thenar space lies radial to the septum, overlying the third metacarpal bone. The floor of this space is occupied by the abductor pollicis muscle. Infection of this space is frequently caused by extension from a purulent tenosynovitis of the index finger or thumb, by a direct penetrating injury, or by extension from a midpalmar space infection.

## Criteria for Diagnosis

1. There is marked swelling and tenderness in the spaces between the first and second metacarpals.
2. The thumb is held in a position of abduction.

## Management

1. The incision should be made parallel to the thenar crease.
2. Dissection should be blunt with a spreading hemostat until the abscess cavity is reached.
3. Care must be taken not to injure the motor branch of the median nerve or the two sensory digital nerves to the thumb and index finger.
4. For a thenar space infection and first web space infection, which is bulging dorsally, a longitudinal dorsal incision may be made along the radial border of the first dorsal interosseous muscle. Dissection into the abscess cavity is performed with a spreading hemostat until the purulent collection is encountered.
5. Postsurgical treatment is the same as for other closed-space infections.

## *Hypothenar Space Infection*

### Basic Principles

The hypothenar space is that space occupied by the hypothenar muscles and contained by an aponeurotic covering.

### Criteria for Diagnosis

1. There is swelling, tenderness and erythema of the ulnar portion of the hand.
2. The abscess may point into the palm or toward the dorsum of the hand near its ulnar border.

### Management

1. Drainage may be performed through a midlateral incision on the ulnar border of the hand or through a curved longitudinal palmar incision along the radial border of the hypothenar musculature, depending upon the site of greatest fluctuance.
2. The ulnar digital nerve to the little finger is very superficial and easily injured if not identified and protected.
3. Drainage is followed by soaks and antibiotics as previously described.

## *Lumbrical Space Infection*

### Basic Principles

The lumbrical spaces follow the passage of the lumbrical muscles, extending from the midpalmar and thenar fascial spaces obliquely toward the dorsum of the proximal phalanges of the fingers.

### Criteria for Diagnosis

1. Infection of the lumbrical spaces is by direct extension from midpalmar, thenar or web space infections along the course of the lumbrical muscles.
2. If infection of any of these spaces exists, along with signs of infection of the dorsum of the proximal phalanges, it must be assumed that pus has tracked along the lumbrical muscles.

### Management

1. Drainage is through a dorsal longitudinal incision placed over the proximal phalanx.

2. The midpalmar, thenar or web space infection must also be drained. The tracts along the lumbrical muscles must be opened, irrigated and drained. This is followed by soaks and antibiotics as previously described.

## *Dorsal Subaponeurotic Space Infection*

### Basic Principles

The dorsal subaponeurotic space is the space between the extensor tendons on the dorsum of the hand and the fascia covering the metacarpals and interosseous muscles. Infection of this space is caused either by penetrating injuries, superinfection of a hematoma, or by extension from a midpalmar space infection through the interosseous spaces, a web space infection or a dorsal subcutaneous abscess.

### Management

1. Drainage is through a dorsal longitudinal incision extending between the extensor tendons.
2. If caused by extension from a midpalmar space infection, this space also must be opened through a palmar incision, and the tract through the interosseous space must be widely opened and drained.
3. Soaks and antibiotics are continued as previously described.

## *Quadrilateral or Parona's Space Infection*

### Basic Principles

The quadrilateral space (Parona's space) lies above the pronator quadratus muscle and under the flexor digitorum profundus and flexor pollicis longus group of muscles, extending from the carpal tunnel proximally to the origin of these muscles. Infection of this space is often caused by extension from a purulent tenosynovitis of the thumb or little finger, with involvement of the radial or ulnar bursae, or from extension from a midpalmar space infection which has spread proximally through the carpal tunnel. It may also be caused by direct trauma to the forearm with superinfection.

### Criteria for Diagnosis

1. There is severe swelling and tenderness of the volar aspect of the distal forearm.
2. The wrist and fingers are held in flexion, and attempted extension is painful.

### Management

1. Drainage is obtained through a longitudinal incision on the volar aspect of the distal forearm, paralleling either the flexor carpi ulnaris tendon or the flexor carpi radialis tendon.
2. The antebrachial fascia is incised, and dissection is carried around the flexor tendons until the quadrilateral space is reached.
3. Pus is evacuated, the space is irrigated with saline, and Penrose drains are inserted.
4. The incision is then closed loosely with nylon sutures.
5. Soaks and antibiotics are continued until drainage stops, at which time the drains are removed.
6. Other infected spaces must be concomitantly drained.

## OSTEOMYELITIS

### Definition

Osteomyelitis is an infection of bone.

### Classification According to the Cause of Bone Involvement

1. Hematogenous spread from a distant focus of infection (rare in the hand)
2. Direct inoculation from a compound fracture
3. Extension from an adjacent closed-space infection

### Basic Principles

Infection of bone causes necrosis of the involved portion of bone. Antibiotics cannot enter the devascularized necrotic bone;

therefore sequestrectomy and saucerization are essential for cure.

### Criteria for Diagnosis

1. An infection that persistently drains despite adequate soft tissue incision and drainage
2. X-ray evidence of bone necrosis, that is, increased density or cavitation with sclerotic borders

### Management

1. Incision and drainage, plus sequestrectomy of all necrotic bone with saucerization of the remaining viable bone
2. A Penrose drain is left in the wound, which is closed loosely.
3. Soaks and antibiotics, active against gram-positive organisms (e.g., Prostaphlin, ampicillin, lincomycin), which are changed according to the results of sensitivity tests
4. The drain is removed when purulent drainage has ceased.
5. Soaks are continued until all drainage has ceased, and antibiotics are stopped when there is no longer any evidence of infection.

## ACTIVE SUPPURATIVE ARTHRITIS

### Definition

Active suppurative arthritis is infection of a joint space.

### Classification

Same as for osteomyelitis

### Basic Principles

Pressure and bacterial activity will rapidly destroy the joint cartilage and cause fibrosis of the periarticular structures unless the purulent material is quickly and adequately evacuated.

### Criteria for Diagnosis

The articulation is swollen, tender, and held immobilized because attempted motion is extremely painful.

## Management

1. The articulation must be opened, drained, and irrigated with copious amounts of saline or antibiotic solution.

2. An opening should be left in the joint capsule to allow continued egress of fluids, and the surrounding soft tissues should be drained with a sliver of Penrose drain.

3. Early motion should be instituted in an attempt to prevent fibrous ankylosis.

4. Soaks, antibiotics and removal of drains are the same as for osteomyelitis.

## STENOSING TENOSYNOVITIS

### Definition

Stenosing tenosynovitis is a painful inflammatory condition of a tendon due to a discrepancy in the size of the tendon and the size of its fibrous sheath.

### Classification

1. Trigger or snapping finger (including trigger or snapping thumb)
   A. Idiopathic
   B. Post-traumatic
      *(1)* Acute injury
      *(2)* Repeated microtraumata
   C. Rheumatoid
   D. Congenital
2. De Quervain's Tenovaginitis
   A. Idiopathic
   B. Post-traumatic
      *(1)* Acute injury
      *(2)* Repeated strain

### Basic Principles

Both trigger finger and De Quervain's tenovaginitis occur at a point where a tendon angulates upon the edge of a nonyielding retinaculum. In the case of trigger finger, the flexor tendons angulate over the bulbous head of the metacarpal bone. At the level of the neck of the metacarpal bone the flexor tendon sheath begins, with the proximal pulley forming the entrance to the tunnel. It is at this point that the tendon becomes irritated. In De Quervain's tenovaginitis, the extensor pollicis brevis and abductor pollicis longus tendons pass over the radial styloid on their way to the points of insertion on the thumb. At the level of the radial styloid the tendons are held to the bone by a portion of the dorsal retinaculum, forming the first dorsal compartment. The tendons angulate over the edge of this retinaculum when the thumb is in motion. Ulnar deviation of the wrist places an even greater strain upon these tendons. In both conditions the angulation and irritation to the tendon initiate an inflammatory response within the tendon, producing a local swelling of both the synovial lining and the tendon substance. This swelling makes the available space even tighter, producing more irritation, and thus a vicious cycle is produced.

### Criteria for Diagnosis

#### Trigger Finger

1. Pain on motion of the involved finger, localized over the metacarpal head in the palm or sometimes referred to the proximal interphalangeal joint

2. A history of snapping of the finger on motion, or of actual locking in either flexion or extension. This is due to the catching of the intratendinous nodule on the proximal pulley of the flexor tendon sheath.

3. A palpable nodule on the flexor tendons overlying the metacarpal heads. The nodule moves as the patient flexes and extends the finger. It is frequently tender to palpation.

#### De Quervain's Disease

1. Severe pain in the region of the radial styloid, with radiation up the forearm, especially on motion of the thumb and wrist

2. Finkelstein's sign—severe pain when the patient grasps the thumb in the fingers and then ulnar deviates the wrist

3. A tender, hard swelling in the region of the radial styloid is sometimes present. X-rays are frequently taken to rule out a bony prominence, but these are usually negative.

## Management

In both trigger finger and De Quervain's tenovaginitis, an early and late stage can be distinguished. The significance of this is that in the early stage conservative forms of therapy may be tried with about a 50 per cent success rate. In the late stage only surgery will help. Surgical decompression is curative.

The two stages are distinguished in trigger finger by the presence or absence of locking and by the size of the tendon nodule.

In De Quervain's tenovaginitis, the early stage is differentiated from the late stage by the fact that pain is brought about only after the patient has been using his thumb for some time. In the late stage, any motion of the thumb will elicit severe pain, and there is usually a large tender swelling in the region of the radial styloid.

The following is an outline of our form of treatment for these conditions.

### Trigger Finger

1. *Conservative Nonoperative Treatment*

A. Rest by splinting the finger with all joints by 30-degree flexion

B. Steroid injections into the tendon sheath

(1) We have been using a 1:1 mixture of 1% Xylocaine with Decadron, 4 mg. per ml., although other steroid preparations may be used with equally good results.

(2) Through a 25-gauge needle, 0.5 to 1.0 ml. of this solution is injected through the proximal pulley of the flexor tendon sheath in the palm.

(3) If the needle moves on finger motion, the point of the needle is in the tendon substance and should be withdrawn until it no longer moves.

(4) At this point the solution is injected slowly, after which the finger is extended and flexed in order to distribute the liquid along the tendon sheath.

(5) The patient should be warned that pain may be aggravated for approximately 24 hours following the injection but will subside spontaneously.

(6) The injection is repeated at intervals of two weeks for a maximum of three injections. If there is no improvement, operation is recommended.

(7) If improvement has occurred but is not yet complete, conservative treatment may be continued until cure or until there are no further signs of improvement.

2. *Operative Treatment.* All operations are done under tourniquet control at 300 mm. of mercury, with either general, regional, intravenous or local anesthesia.

A. A transverse incision is made in the palm about 1 inch in length, centered over the tendinous nodule. If an adjacent finger also is to be treated, the incision can be extended to expose both flexor tendon sheaths.

B. Care is taken to expose and retract the digital nerves lying on either side of the tendon sheath.

C. The proximal portion of the tendon sheath is excised up to the base of the finger. One must observe free clearance of the nodular portion of the tendon on full flexion and extension of the finger.

D. Compression dressings are applied and the hand is elevated.

E. Early active motion is encouraged.

F. A Penrose drain is often placed in the wound and removed 24 to 48 hours after surgery.

### De Quervain's Disease

1. *Conservative Nonoperative Treatment*

A. Splinting should first be tried for a period of two weeks. The thumb is splinted in a position of extension in line with the radius, and the wrist is splinted in 30-degree dorsiflexion.

B. Phenylbutazone may be tried in a dosage of 100 mg. 4 times a day for a period of 5 to 7 days.

C. Steroid and local anesthetic agents may be injected in a manner similar to that described for trigger finger. In this condition the first dorsal compartment is injected.

D. *Caution:* one must be certain that the injection is within the tendon sheath, because a steroid injection in the vicinity of the branches of the radial nerve can produce a severe and stubborn neuritis. In our experience, injections have not been very successful in the treatment of De Quervain's tenovaginitis. The reason for this is often observed clearly at operation. The extensor pollicis brevis tendon frequently lies within its own separate compartment, and on numerous occasions we have found this compartment to be so tight that a needle could not be inserted under direct vision. This would explain the frequency of poor results following steroid injections for De Quervain's tenovaginitis.

2. *Operative Treatment*

A. A transverse incision is made about 1 inch in length and 1 inch proximal to the radial styloid.

B. The subcutaneous tissue is divided by blunt dissection in order to expose and avoid injuring the branches of the radial nerve.

*(1)* These branches lie immediately above the first dorsal compartment.

*(2)* If these branches are cut, very painful and neuromas result, which are disabling and difficult to treat.

C. The retinaculum of the first dorsal compartment is completely excised, freeing the abductor pollicis longus and extensor pollicis brevis tendons.

D. Two anatomical peculiarities of this region frequently mislead the surgeon into an incomplete surgical decompression.

*(1)* The first anatomical peculiarity is that the extensor pollicis brevis is often in a separate compartment. The tendon is thin and it is frequently overlooked.

*(2)* The second peculiarity is that the abductor pollicis longus does not usually exist as a single tendon but is composed of 2 to 6 separate tendon units. See-

ing multiple tendons, the unsuspecting surgeon does not search out the extensor pollicis brevis, thinking that he has already freed it.

*(3)* If one of the two tendons remains compressed within its compartment, the condition will persist.

E. Following operation, the thumb and wrist are splinted for 1 to 2 weeks, after which active motion is begun.

## ACUTE CALCIFIC TENDINITIS

### Definition

Calcific tendinitis is an inflammatory condition of a tendon, manifested by severe pain, swelling and erythema with marked restriction of motion. Roentgen examination frequently reveals a deposit of calcium within the substance of the tendon. The cause is unknown, although repeated minor traumata are suspected.

### Classification

In the hand and wrist, acute calcific tendinitis has been known to occur in the following locations:

1. The flexor carpi ulnaris tendon near its insertion into the pisiform bone
2. The digital flexor tendons within the carpal tunnel
3. The extensor carpi radialis brevis tendon near its insertion
4. The lumbrical tendons in the web spaces
5. The abductor pollicis longus tendon near its insertion
6. The collateral ligaments of proximal interphalangeal joints

### Basic Principles

Acute calcific tendinitis is easily mistaken for an acute infectious process because of its sudden onset, swelling, localized pain, redness, warmth and loss of mobility. X-ray evidence of calcification in a tendon or ligament helps to differentiate this from an infectious condition.

Treatment in general is nonsurgical. The

disease is self-limiting, although sometimes prolonged, and the calcium deposits eventually disappear. Only rarely is surgical excision necessary.

## Criteria for Diagnosis

1. Sudden onset of well-localized pain directly over the involved tendon or ligament, accompanied by marked swelling, redness and warmth, suggesting an acute infectious process
2. Immobility due to the production of intense pain by the slightest motion
3. Calcium deposits visible on x-ray confirm the diagnosis.

## Management

1. Splinting of the involved part for at least two weeks or longer if necessary
2. Needling of the calcium deposit, aspiration if the deposit is large, and injection of a mixture of a local anesthetic and a steroid preparation (such as 1% Xylocaine with Decadron, 4 mg. in 1 ml.). Approximately 1 ml. of a 1:1 mixture is used.
3. Physical therapy, including ultrasound, diathermy and whirlpool and paraffin baths
4. Radiotherapy, 200 rads on 3 alternate days
5. If in spite of adequate conservative therapy the symptoms continue and the calcium deposit is still present, surgical excision is indicated. The timing for surgery may vary according to the severity of the symptoms, but usually six months is an adquate trial of conservative therapy.

## ACUTE GOUTY ARTHRITIS

### Definition

Gout is a disease of uric acid metabolism, the mechanism of which is still poorly understood. The manifestations of the disease are due to the deposition of monosodium urate crystals in the synovial tissues, cartilage, bursa, tendon and ligament, as well as in bone.

## Classification

1. Acute gout
2. Chronic gout

## Basic Principles

As stated above, the mechanism of the disease is poorly understood, but what is known is that the sum of the ingestion and endogenous production of uric acid exceeds the sum of the excretion and utilization of uric acid. Acute attacks of gout are managed by the administration of a drug which prevents the deposition of urates in the tissues, e.g., colchicine, as well as an anti-inflammatory drug which helps terminate the acute attack. Chronic gout is managed by controlling the dietary intake of uric acid, by favoring its urinary excretion, e.g., with uricosuric drugs, and by inhibiting the synthesis of uric acid, e.g., with allopurinol. Operation is indicated when gouty deposits threaten to destroy functional structures, become infected, ulcerate or interfere with function by their mere presence, or when they are the cause of severe pain. Operation, however, should be deferred until a normal serum urate concentration is achieved.

## Criteria for Diagnosis

1. *Acute Gout*
   A. Sudden onset of severe pain, usually after some sort of provocation such as emotional or physical stress, excesses of food or alcohol, and certain drugs
   B. Swelling and a purple-red color resembling cellulitis
   C. Sudden disappearance after about 6 or 7 days, with desquamation over the area of inflammation
2. *Chronic Gout*
   A. Similar to osteoarthritis, but affecting mainly the small peripheral joints
   B. Punched-out lesions on x-ray in epiphyseal areas of bone
   C. Clinical finding of tophi, consisting of monosodium urate, in periarticular regions, the ear, olecranon bursa and Achilles tendon

D. History of previous articular attacks, renal stones, hematuria or albuminuria

3. Elevation of serum uric acid above 6 mg.%, leukocytosis and elevated erythrocyte sedimentation rate are found in both acute and chronic forms and are strongly suggestive.

## Management

The objectives of management are:

1. To terminate an acute attack with anti-inflammatory drugs or colchicine

2. To prevent a recurrence of acute attacks by the daily use of colchicine until other therapy is established

3. Prevention of further deposition of monosodium urate as well as the resolution of existing tophi by increasing the urinary excretion of uric acid and by inhibiting the synthesis of uric acid

## The Acute Attack

1. Colchicine, 0.5 mg. by mouth every hour until complete relief has been established or until diarrhea and vomiting have developed. Not more than 7.0 mg. should be given in a 48-hour period. A maintenance dose of 1 to 2 mg. per day should then be started.

2. ACTH gel (a long-acting repository gel), 40 to 80 units intramuscularly. It is used as an alternative to hourly colchicine, but it is recommended to give colchicine concomitantly in the dosage of 0.5 mg. twice a day or three times a day.

3. Phenylbutazone (Butazolidin), for patients who are intolerant to, or unresponsive to, colchicine. The dosage is 400 mg. to start, and then 200 mg. 4 times a day after meals for 2 to 3 days.

4. Indomethacin (Indocin), 50 mg. by mouth 3 times a day after meals until symptoms have disappeared

5. Corticosteroids are not recommended in the treatment of gout since the response is inconsistent and rebound attacks are common.

## Chronic Gout

1. Colchicine, maintenance doses of 0.5 mg. by mouth twice a day to 4 times a day

2. *Uricosuric Therapy*

A. Probenecid (Benemid), 0.5 mg. once a day to 4 times a day

B. Sulfinpyrazone (Anturane), 100 mg. once a day to 4 times a day. Adjust the dose to maintain a normal serum uric acid level. Avoid salicylates since they antagonize the uricosuric effects of these agents.

C. Salicylates in doses of more than 3 gm. a day are uricosuric and may be used.

3. *Inhibition of Uric Acid Synthesis.* Allopurinol (Zyloprim), 200 to 600 mg. a day. The dose varies according to the serum uric acid concentration.

4. The medical management of chronic gout should be accompanied by the following:

A. A diet poor in high-purine foods such as liver, kidney, sweetbreads, anchovies and gravies. Excesses of fats and alcohol should be avoided.

B. An abundant fluid intake is recommended in order to prevent precipitation of urates in the kidneys.

C. Operation is indicated when tophi begin to present the threat of complications.

(1) These complications may consist of ulceration, drainage, superinfection, erosion and destruction of tendons, ligaments and bone, compression of nerves, production of pain, and the mechanical interference of function.

(2) Tophi are surgically excised along with any existing drainage tracts.

(3) It is not necessary to remove all tophaceous material if by doing this functional structures will be destroyed. It is only necessary to remove the bulk of the material and to gently curette any material which happens to be infiltrating skin, tendon or bone.

(4) Digital nerves frequently pass through, and are completely surrounded

by, tophaceous material. The nerves must be carefully dissected out of these large tophaceous deposits.

(5) Wounds should be closed loosely and drained.

(6) To avoid the precipitation of an acute gouty attack by the stress of surgery, colchicine should be given prophylactically 2 to 3 days preoperatively and postoperatively. In addition, ACTH should be given since some patients will develop flare-ups in spite of colchicine administration.

## ARTERIAL EMBOLIZATION

### Definition

Emboli are fragments of blood clot which obstruct vessels at a distance from their point of origin. Most emboli occurring in the brachial artery result from clots arising from the left atrium due to atrial fibrillation and mitral stenosis or as a result of a previous myocardial infarction or ventricular aneurysm.

### Basic Principles

Most emboli lodge at sites of arterial bifurcation. In the arm the most common site is at the origin of the deep brachial artery. Next in frequency is the site of origin of the radial and ulnar arteries. Although the collateral circulation in the arm is good, distal propagation of thrombus can obliterate collateral vessels. Embolectomy therefore should be performed without hesitation. Following embolectomy, consultation with the cardiac surgery team should be obtained, since it might be advisable to follow the embolectomy with a mitral commissurotomy, excision of a ventricular aneurysm or other cardiac surgical procedures.

### Criteria for Diagnosis

1. Sudden onset of pain in the hand and upper extremity
2. Change of color, either blue or pale, of the involved hand, as well as a drop in temperature

3. Absence of peripheral pulses
4. Loss of sensation due to ischemia
5. Arteriography is helpful but is not always necessary, since the site of embolization can be deduced from the level of color and temperature changes.

### Management

1. Embolectomy may be easily performed under local anesthesia, with an approach to the distal portion of the brachial artery through a longitudinal incision just proximal to the antecubital fossa. This same incision should be used regardless of the site of arterial obstruction.
2. The distal soft clot is milked proximally through the arteriotomy site. Fogarty catheters are then used to evacuate both distal and proximal blood clots.
3. Following embolectomy, the patient is heparinized.
4. The wound is protected from hematoma formation by a mild compression dressing.

## MEDIAN CARPAL TUNNEL SYNDROME

### Definitions

1. *The Carpal Tunnel.* This is an anatomical space in the hand, bounded on three sides by bone (navicular, lunate and hamate), forming a trough, the fourth side being formed by the transverse carpal ligament composing its roof. Through this tunnel pass nine flexor tendons plus the median nerve, which is its most superficial structure.
2. *Median Carpal Tunnel Syndrome.* This is a compression syndrome of the median nerve as it passes through the carpal tunnel.

### Classification

1. *Chronic Median Carpal Tunnel Syndrome.* This is the usual form of carpal tunnel syndrome and has a variety of causes. The most common cause is idiopathic. It is known to predominate in postmenopausal women, and it is caused

by a nonspecific synovial thickening within the carpal tunnel. It may be related to hormonal changes, since it also has been observed to occur during pregnancy. Other causes of carpal tunnel syndrome are:

A. Post-traumatic

*(1)* Colles' fracture

*(2)* Lunate or perilunate dislocation

*(3)* Fracture of navicular bone

B. Space-occupying lesions

*(1)* Dislocated lunate

*(2)* Ganglion

*(3)* Tumor within carpal tunnel

*(4)* Gouty deposit along flexor tendons

C. Synovitis

*(1)* Rheumatoid flexor tenosynovitis

*(2)* Mycobacterial tenosynovitis

*(3)* Mycotic tenosynovitis

2. *Acute Carpal Tunnel Syndrome.* This form is less frequent. It is due to:

A. Sudden swelling of the contents of the carpal tunnel, such as:

*(1)* Sudden massive edema following a crushing injury to the arm or as a result of certain medical conditions producing generalized edema (e.g., acute nephrosis, acute glomerulonephritis or the late stages of cirrhosis)

*(2)* Infection

*(3)* Hemorrhage, traumatic or due to bleeding tendencies

*(4)* Acute tenosynovitis

B. Sudden bony deformities

*(1)* Dislocated lunate bone

*(2)* Smith's fracture

## Basic Principles

1. In acute compression of the carpal tunnel, relief of pressure upon the median nerve is urgent in order to prevent permanent damage to nerve fibers.

2. In the chronic carpal tunnel syndrome, reduction in local swelling by the injection of steroid preparations into the carpal tunnel may be performed in early cases (those presenting with paresthesias and only minimal hypoesthesia).

3. In later cases of chronic carpal tunnel syndrome, where hypoesthesia is marked or has progressed to anesthesia, or where there is atrophy of the thenar muscles, surgical decompression of the median nerve should not be delayed. The longer the period of compression, the greater the intraneural scarring, with a lesser likelihood for a good postoperative result.

## Criteria for Diagnosis
### Acute Compression

1. The diagnosis is suspected when there is a sudden onset of paresthesia, hypoesthesia or anesthesia in the sensory distribution of the median nerve (e.g., the palmar aspect of the thumb and index and middle fingers, the radial half of the ring finger, and the radial half of the distal palm).

2. Tenderness may be elicited by tapping the median nerve as it enters the carpal tunnel (Tinel's sign).

3. There is frequently a swelling in the distal forearm.

### Chronic Compression

1. Paresthesias and wrist pains which characteristically are aggravated at night and awaken the patient. Relief is obtained by shaking and massaging the hand.

2. The same symptoms are produced by holding the wrist in an acutely flexed position for at least one minute (Phalen's sign).

3. Hypoesthesia leading gradually to anesthesia in the median nerve distribution

4. Positive Tinel's sign at the entrance to the carpal tunnel

5. Atrophy of the thenar muscles (abductor pollicis brevis and opponens pollicis) and loss of opposition of the thumb. This is a late sign and indicates severe constriction of the median nerve.

6. Electromyography (EMG) is helpful when the clinical picture is confusing. Increased latency across the wrist localizes the lesion.

## Management
### Acute Compression

1. Preliminary measures should im-

mediately be instituted, such as elevation of the arm and, depending upon the etiology, diuretics, salt and water restriction and correction of any clotting abnormalities.

2. If the cause of the acute compression is traumatic, or if there is no response within 1 to 2 hours after onset from medical causes, then surgical decompression should be performed.

3. Drains are left within the carpal tunnel, and a compression dressing is applied as well as a plaster splint. The hand is kept elevated postoperatively.

4. Penrose drains are removed 48 hours after operation.

5. Early active motion of the fingers is begun as soon as possible.

## Chronic Compression

1. *Early Cases*

A. Injection of 1 ml. of a steroid preparation such as Decadron (4 mg. per ml.) into the carpal tunnel is frequently helpful. Addition of a local anesthetic is not necessary.

B. Injection may be repeated at 2-week intervals until cure, or for a maximum of 3 injections. If there is no response, operation would be indicated.

2. *Later Cases*. Surgical decompression of the median nerve within the carpal tunnel is indicated.

A. The incision is a curved or S-shaped incision placed directly over the carpal tunnel and paralleling the thenar crease.

(1) The incision need not extend more proximally than the proximal wrist crease.

(2) It should not be extended too far radially, because there is a danger of cutting the palmar cutaneous branch of the median nerve, which runs superficially within the subcutaneous tissue near the flexor carpi radialis tendon. Injury to this nerve will result in a painful surgical scar.

B. The median nerve is found by incising the volar carpal ligament, a thickening of the antebrachial fascia, on the ulnar side of the palmaris longus tendon. The nerve will be found underneath and is easily recognized by the presence of the artery of the median nerve.

C. The transverse carpal ligament, which forms the roof of the carpal tunnel, is then incised under full visual control, and a segment of it is excised to prevent recurrence.

D. If there has been atrophy of the thenar muscles, the motor branch of the median nerve should be isolated.

(1) It is the first branch on the radial side of the nerve before it exits from the carpal tunnel.

(2) This branch frequently perforates the transverse carpal ligament through a separate aperture. This must be individually decompressed if muscle function is to return.

E. The floor of the carpal tunnel must be inspected for the presence of a space-occupying lesion. If found, this must be appropriately handled by excision.

F. The presence of a rheumatoid or other synovitis mandates a longer incision, which is extended proximally so that a complete flexor tendon synovectomy can be performed.

G. *Postoperative Management*

(1) Penrose drains are removed from the incision after 48 hours.

(2) Compression dressings and a volar splint are continued for 2 weeks.

(3) After 2 weeks, sutures are removed and active exercises are begun. Paresthesias and night pains are the first symptoms to disappear. The patient is advised, however, that improvement in sensation is slower, depending upon the degree and duration of nerve compression. The return of motor function is slowest and, depending upon the duration of symptoms, may never be complete.

# 33. PERIPHERAL NERVE INJURIES

*Michael J. McAlvanah*, M.D.

## Definitions

1. *Nerve.* This is a collection of axons and their surrounding fascia following an anatomical pathway.

2. *Nerve Funiculus.* This is the smallest macroscopically visible component part of a nerve, composed of one or more nerve fascicles with their supporting connective tissue.

3. *Nerve Fascicle.* This is the smallest collection of axons visible as a distinct entity with surgical magnification.

4. *Epineurium.* This is the layer of fascia surrounding each individual nerve.

5. *Perineurium.* This is the fascia surrounding the nerve funiculi and their contained fascicles.

6. *Neurapraxia.* This refers to loss or decrease of axonal conduction without loss of anatomical nerve continuity.

7. *Nerve Laceration (Neurotmesis).*

This refers to disruption of part or all of the nerve continuity by injury.

## Basic Principles

### Peripheral Nerve Anatomy

Figure 33-1 shows the cross-sectional area of a peripheral nerve. The loose surrounding epineurium is a thickened layer of fascia investment surrounding a peripheral nerve, carrying minute blood vessels which enter it perpendicularly from the mesoneurium. The epineurium is quite strong yet loosely attached to the underlying nerve fibers and easily dissected from them.

Within the epineurium and bundled into more or less distinct areas are the nerve funiculi. These are separated from each other by surrounding layers of fascia called perineurium, which are extremely thin but very strong. Each funiculus is subdivided

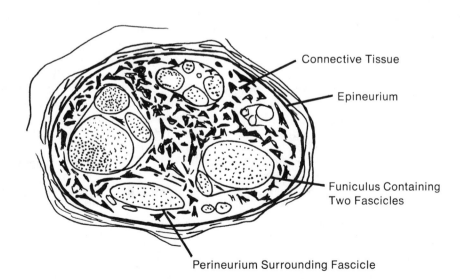

Fig. 33-1. A cross section of a peripheral nerve.

Connective Tissue

Epineurium

Funiculus Containing Two Fascicles

Perineurium Surrounding Fascicle

into distinct nerve fascicles also surrounded by perineurium. The fascicles are easily separated from each other and each contains up to 10,000 axons for neural transmission. In smaller and more distal nerves, funiculi may contain only one fascicle.

The connective tissue within the fascicles is the endoneurium. It is primarily collagen which is loose and extremely vascular, for contained within it are the fine arterioles and capillary system responsible for axonal nutrition.

There is a double blood supply of a peripheral nerve. Besides the longitudinal vessels which run the entire length of the nerve, there are multiple segmental small blood vessels going into it from the connective tissue attachment of the surrounding areas, forming a pseudomesentery, the mesoneurium. The perpendicular vessels eventually anastomose with the longitudinal vessels within the epineurium.

## Types of Injuries

1. Neurapraxia is a lesion of peripheral nerve in which there is a decrease or loss of axonal conduction while complete anatomical continuity of all structures remains. The neuron and end-organ are axonally connected and, therefore, Wallerian degeneration does not occur. This is a temporary situation following trauma, and recovery can be anticipated in a variable amount of time, from a few days to several months, unless the source of trauma persists. Examples of this injury are: (1) acute closed nerve contusions; (2) chronic nerve pressure (one's leg falling asleep, "crutch" palsy, "Saturday night" paralyses); and (3) operative tourniquet injuries. Etiologically the lesion is felt to be secondary to direct nerve compression or transient nerve ischemia. Compression neurapraxias show swelling, notching and vacuolation of nerve axons leading to edema and further secondary compression and dysfunction. Ischemic neurapraxias seem to show earlier reversibility and less

tendency to advance on to permanent defects.

2. Axonotmesis is axonal disruption or injury of such extent that the axon fails to survive distal to the lesion and for a small but variable distance proximal to it. The endoneurium and neurolemmal sheaths do remain intact. Disintegration of the axon is accompanied by myelin breakdown and degeneration, producing classical distal Wallerian degeneration. This myelin degeneration is usually completed by the end of two weeks, and a variable amount of time ranging from one to three months is necessary for phagocytic removal of the degenerated myelin. Although the peripheral end-organ has been isolated from axonal innervation, there is still neurolemmal continuity. With effective regeneration of the intact proximal axon, after a few days' delay, growth then proceeds in a distal direction with assurance of proper axonal alignment in the distal segment. Axonotmesis follows similar but more severe injury than that which leads to neurapraxia. The clinical picture is that of complete loss of motor, sensory and sympathetic innervation along the distribution of the injured nerve.

The interval between injury and recovery is influenced by the level of the injury and the rate of advancement of the regenerating axon, which is usually from 1 to 1.5 mm. daily. Individual muscular function restoration occurs on a strictly anatomical basis, with the more proximal muscles along the path of the nerve returning first. This differs from functional restoration in neurapraxias, which is variable and not subject to any anatomical distribution.

3. The third type of peripheral neurologic injury, termed neurotmesis, refers to injuries producing axonal injury or disruption as well as separation of the connective tissue elements of the nerve structure. This loss of physical integrity of the nerve occurs from sharp injury, gunshot wounds or severe thermal or

chemical burns. After disruption of the nerve, there is proximal and distal retraction of the divided ends, producing an over-all gap of up to 2 to 3 cm. in some cases. For effective reinnervation to occur, this gap must be eliminated and the proximal and distal axonal sheaths realigned in close proximity to allow the regenerating axons to pass undisturbed into the distal recipient tubes. This is the purpose of operative repair: to hold the nerve ends in close proper rotational alignment until axons have crossed the junction and connective tissue strength across the gap is sufficient to maintain contact.

## Timing of Repair

1. If conditions are acceptable, primary suture of peripheral nerve lacerations is preferable to secondary repair.

A. Besides strong laboratory evidence favoring it, the technical aspects of primary repairs are simpler than those of late repairs. Once surrounding blood and hematoma are removed, dissection is anatomical and usually simple.

B. On the other hand, secondary repairs require dissection through scar tissue to find and free the nerve structures which may be firmly adherent to surrounding tissue.

C. Secondary nerve repair also requires resection of the proximal and distal neuromas which have formed on the cut ends of the lacerated nerve before repair can be attempted. Resection of neuroma ends perpendicularly with a razor blade must be done until a normal-appearing funicular pattern devoid of scar tissue is visible at both ends. Unless the segment of resection is extremely short, the funicular patterns proximally and distally will no longer be matching mirror images.

D. Since secondary resections usually require removal of at least 1 cm. proximally and distally, a 2-cm. gap is produced. Repair, therefore, will be under tension, which is relieved either by placing nearby joints in position of acute flexion or by freeing-up long segments of the nerve proximal and distal to the anastomosis, removing the mesoneurium and lessening the blood supply in the region of the repair.

2. Certain types of peripheral nerve injuries are best treated by secondary nerve repair and must therefore be individually judged. If an excessive period of delay has elapsed from the time of an open injury until the patient first seeks medical treatment, secondary repair may be best suited. In these cases, the contamination to the wound may have already become proliferative and may have provided the milieu for a local infection despite irrigation and antibiotic administration. The same would be true for wounds initially greatly contaminated: wounds received with ground-in dirt, feces, solvent or chemicals. Here again, the high risk of a postoperative infection spreading down the new tissue planes opened up by the operation outweighs the advantages of a primary repair.

The most common indication for secondary repair which we employ is for gunshot-wound lacerations of peripheral nerves. The tissue injury produced by the shock waves preceding and following a high-speed projectile is impossible to evaluate completely at the time of initial injury and may extend far beyond the boundaries of visible damage. In these cases primary repair would be inappropriate because of the risk of either excising unidentifiable viable nerve or leaving irreparably damaged fascicle.

3. In certain injuries, mitigating circumstances may prevent immediate repair when the patient is first seen. Examples of situations may include: delay in obtaining operative consent for children and adolescents; other surgical or medical conditions which may require priority treatment; or alcoholic or drug intoxication producing an uncooperative patient.

## Criteria for Diagnosis

1. All lacerations are evaluated for

nerve injury as well as being examined for the wound proper.

2. Diagnosis of peripheral nerve injuries is suggested by either acute motor or sensory defects of the involved nerve.

A. Sensory defects may be seen as paresthesias, anesthesia or burning pain over the sensory area of the nerve involved.

(1) Median nerve distribution is localized to the radial half of the palm of the hand, plus the volar surface of the thumb, index, middle and radial side of the ring finger.

(2) Ulnar nerve loss above the wrist gives loss of sensation of the ulnar half of the palm and dorsum of the hand, as well as the entire little finger and ulnar half of the ring finger.

(3) Radial nerve sensation is limited to a variable area overlying the thumb and index metacarpal, occasionally only reliably localized to the region of the anatomical snuffbox.

(4) Complete transection of sensory nerves usually allows for discernment of fingertip pinprick as deep pressure, but ability to elicit pain is commonly absent.

B. Motor loss is reflected in loss of function of the muscle innervated distal to the nerve injury.

(1) *Median Nerve.* High injury produces loss of thumb flexion and opposition, loss of index and middle finger flexion at the PIP joint and DIP joint, and loss of independent flexion of the PIP joint of the ring and little fingers.

*Low* injury is manifested only by loss of thenar opposition. This must be carefully tested because some people can attain minimal opposition with the ulnar-innervated thenar muscle (deep head of the flexor pollicis brevis). Attempts to oppose the thumb should be palpated along the radial border of the thumb metacarpal. When median nerve function is intact, the firm muscular contraction of the abductor pollicis brevis muscle may be easily felt. Its absence should raise a high index of suspicion for median nerve injury.

(2) *Ulnar* nerve injury produces loss of hypothenar musculature innervation with inability to abduct the little finger in the plane of the palm, loss of intrinsic interosseous musculature and ability to abduct all fingers in the plane of the palm, especially evident in loss of index abduction from loss of the first dorsal interosseous and loss of thumb abduction. A high ulnar lesion (above the elbow) would also give inability to flex the distal IP joint of the little and ring fingers.

(3) *Radial Nerve.* High injury produces loss of all wrist and finger extensors.

*Low* injury only has loss of finger extensors and ulnar wrist extension.

C. It must be emphasized that all of the functions of a nerve should be tested in a questionable lesion. The presence of one normal function or sensation does not rule out a possible major deficiency from a partial laceration, which will only be noted with a complete examination. Conversely, be careful not to diagnose extensive nerve injuries preoperatively when the inability to flex a distal joint is due to multiple tendinous injuries.

3. Examination of the wound may reveal evidence of partial or complete tendon injury, where there is a high incidence of concomitant nerve laceration. We consider evidence of partial laceration of any tendon in the forearm, wrist or palm, with the occasional exception of the isolated palmaris longus tendon, as indication for exploration at operation. In keeping with this, evidence of laceration through the brachial fascia of the forearm requires exploration.

4. Once examination is done and operative treatment appears necessary, a sterile dressing is applied which is not removed until the patient is in the operating room. Multiple examinations of the wound only serve to further contaminate the area and are, in general, no more beneficial than one competent examination.

## Management

1. Neurapraxia and axonotmesis are best managed by conservative observation, with eventual recovery expected. Distal tendon transfers may be necessary in cases of high ulnar or median nerve axonotmesis, where muscular fibrosis will have occurred before reinnervation occurs. This fibrosis may be delayed to some extent by external electrostimulation, but it is essentially irreversible beyond 24 months.

2. Where immediate repair cannot be done when the patient is first seen or the delay from injury until the operative procedure will exceed 4 or 5 hours, patients with "tidy" lacerations should be treated as follows while awaiting the opportunity for primary nerve repair.

A. After the decision of the necessity for operation is reached, the wounds are inspected and copiously irrigated with physiological saline to remove blood, debris, and collected hematoma.

B. Subcutaneous bleeders may be tied off with fine 5-0 chromic ties or merely twisted with a small hemostat until controlled. Injuries beneath the fascia are not tied off, and hemostasis is obtained by means of a proximal pneumatic tourniquet.

C. The skin is closed with interrupted simple sutures of 5-0 nylon; 6-0 nylon is used for lacerations distal to the wrist crease.

D. The patient is placed in a firm pressure dressing with gauze, gauze roll, and a plaster splint for counter pressure. This also serves to immobilize the extremity and prevent motion of injured structures.

E. The patient is placed on immediate high doses of any broad-spectrum antibiotic, unless there are specific indications or known allergies.

F. This treatment is preferable to merely covering the wound with a sterile dressing while awaiting operation, because it removes the contaminated hematoma, which may act as a nidus for infection.

3. Acute repair of nerve lacerations should always be performed in a well-managed, brightly lit operating room.

A. Under appropriate anesthesia, either general or regional block, after sterile prep and draping, the arm is exsanguinated by means of an Esmarch bandage in a distal to proximal direction and maintained bloodless by a well-padded, proximal pneumatic tourniquet.

B. The skin laceration is extended by appropriate incisions for adequate exposure into the wound.

C. In general, all other structures (muscle, tendons, arteries and veins) should be repaired first, saving the neural repairs for last. In this way, no inadvertent traction will be placed upon the delicate, structurally weak nerve anastomosis, and motion will be kept minimal at the nerve anastomosis so as not to malalign the accurate funicular placement.

4. Instrumentation can be minimal. Several fine jeweler's pickups (which are quite inexpensive), spring-worked needle holders and fine scissors are all that is essential. Sutures may range from 6-0 to 10-0, all on extremely fine-tapered needles. Monofilament nylon pulls smoothly and is least reactive.

5. The type of nerve repair done is dependent upon the ability and experience of the surgeon. Epineurium can be sutured together, as can funicular bundles or even individual fascicles. Suggested suture material would be 6-0 or 7-0 for epineurium, 8-0 or 9-0 for funicular sutures, and 9-0 or 10-0 for fascicular stitches. *Caution:* one should be extremely hesitant to attempt suture techniques which are beyond one's abilities. These most delicate structures can be irreparably harmed by inadequate (or indiscreet) handling. Any advantages of fine suture use and techniques will be lost because of this.

6. Regardless of the technique employed, all methods will benefit from— in fact, proper funicular and fascicular

sutures require—the use of magnification. Most desirable is a dual eyepieced operating microscope (Diploscope), which enables an assistant to follow the procedure well. Small portable individual microscopes are also available which have the advantage of light weight, ease in maneuvering and ability to clamp onto the edge of the operating hand table. Although not as effective as an operating microscope, portable magnifying loupes, worn like regular eyeglasses or over prescription eyeglasses, give manifications of 2.5x to 4x, are helpful and very popular.

Nerve repairs should attempt to leave as little foreign material as possible within the nerve structure itself.

A. Large fascicles or funiculi can be aligned with one or two tiny sutures, which are instrument tied under magnification with two throws and cut off at the knots.

B. The repair should be performed without tension so that the nerve ends lie in proximity to each other before anastomosis.

C. The epineurium should always be closed with slight eversion to prevent the ingrowth of scar tissue from this structure.

D. The nerve may be rotated in the normal manner for suture of the posterior wall.

8. The pneumatic tourniquet should be released prior to skin closure to obtain hemostasis and prevent any blood clot from accumulating between the anastomosed ends of the nerve which would prevent axonal passage.

9. The skin is then closed with the extremity so flexed as to remove all tension from the site and fixed in sterile dressings with plaster splint immobilization.

10. The arm is elevated postoperatively for 1 to 4 days, depending upon the extent of injury.

11. The extremity is kept immobilized for a minimum of three weeks, more if other structures require it. Skin sutures are not removed until the first cast removal, at three weeks at the earliest.

## Postoperative Evaluation

Evaluation of nerve regeneration following injury and/or repair is done by either of two methods:

1. *Hoffman-Tinel Sign*

A. This classical sign of progressing nerve axons was first described by P. Hoffman in 1915 and later that same year, independently, by J. Tinel. It is elicited as paresthesias over the distal sensory innervation pattern of the tested nerve when light taps are made over the advancing distal axon buds.

B. Lightly tap with your finger on the skin over the anatomical course of a repaired nerve, moving from a distal point toward the area of repair.

C. It is advantageous to place a flat object, as the edge of a tongue blade, between the area tapped and the region of the nerve anastomosis to decrease pressure transmissions to the nerve anastomosis (where some axonal endings are inevitably trapped), preventing a falsely positive response.

D. When a good nerve repair permits axonal growth, the axons progress distally at the classical rate of one millimeter daily, one inch per month. The area of Hoffman-Tinel paresthesia response likewise should continue distally at this rate, until the final sensory and motor end-organs of that nerve are ready.

E. Failure of advancement of the Hoffman-Tinel sign is indicative of poor axonal progression and a poor prognosis for recovery.

2. *Electrodiagnostic Studies.* Electromyography is the measurement of the electrical muscular response to a proximally applied electrical stimulus to the nerve normally innervating that muscle. If axonal regeneration has reached the muscle tested, there will be a sharply, peaked-action potential recorded. Lack of response with just minor background electrical activity or muscular fibrillations is indicative of lack of reinnervation. Sensory

conduction studies are performed either orthodromically (along the normal path of conduction of a nerve) or antidromically (opposite to normal conduction path, i.e., stimulate the ulnar nerve at the wrist while recording over the little finger). While this test is valuable for sensory evaluations, it must always be performed (as a standard) comparing the normal nerve to the opposite uninjured extremity.

# 34. BURNS

*In-Chul Song*, M.D.
*Bertram E. Bromberg*, M.D.

## Definition

Burns are caused by thermal, chemical, electrical and radioactive agents.

Thermal burns produce the most common form of tissue injury resulting from local hyperthermia. The most common heat sources are flame, hot water and steam. The intensity of the heat, the duration of contact or exposure, and the speed or dissipation of the heat energy by the burned surface determine the extent and depth of tissue destruction.

## Classification

Burn injuries are classified by depth and extent. The estimation of both the depth and extent of tissue damage is important in the appraisal and subsequent management.

### Classification by Depth

1. *First-Degree Burn.* First-degree burn is a superficial mild form of thermal injury such as sunburn and generally results in the formation of skin erythema and edema. The erythema is caused by dilatation of capillaries and small blood vessels, and the edema is a result of translocation of intravascular fluid into the interstitial space due to increased permeability of the capillary walls.

2. *Second-Degree Burn.* In second-degree burn, the destructive process penetrates beyond the epidermis into the dermis. Blisters may form from accumulation of fluid beneath the epidermis. Scalds and flash burns are good examples of second-degree thermal burns.

If further progressive cell destruction from infection is prevented, second-degree burns will heal spontaneously in 2 to 3 weeks by re-epithelialization from residual viable skin appendages.

3. *Third-Degree Burn.* In third-degree burn, the destruction involves the full thickness of skin and frequently even deeper structures. Flame and contact burns are usually full-thickness in nature and give the appearance of a leathery, white dry surface, often with visible thrombosed vessels. Large third-degree burns require skin grafting to obtain surface closure.

### Classification by Extent

1. *Minor Burns.* Minor burns include all first-degree burns and second-degree burns of less than 15 per cent of the body surface. Also included in this group are small third-degree burns of less than 1 per cent of the body surface.

These burns can generally be treated on an outpatient or office basis except in infants and elderly patients. Small areas of full-thickness burn may be treated on an outpatient basis while the eschar is separating. Thus, only a short hospitalization is required for the actual skin grafting.

2. *Moderate Burns.* Moderate burns represent second-degree burns of 15 to 30 per cent of the body surface and third-degree burns of 1 to 10 per cent of the body surface.

These patients should be hospitalized for systemic supportive therapy and local burn wound care. Burn wound infection may convert a moderate burn into a major catastrophe.

Consideration should be given to immediate surgical intervention by tangential excision of the eschar in a deep partial-thickness burn or escharectomy in limited full-thickness burns, with either delayed or immediate split-thickness skin grafting. Where delayed grafting is employed, temporary biological dressings are used.

3. *Major Burns.* Major burns encompass second-degree burns of over 30 per cent of the body surface and third-degree burns of over 10 per cent of the body surface. Full-thickness burns of the face, hands, feet, genitalia and perineum should be included in this category. Burns associated with inhalation injury or other associated major skeletal or soft tissue injury are managed as serious burns. Included in this group are high-tension electrical and total body irradiation burns.

Major burns are best treated in a burn care center where the planning management is handled by experts.

## Basic Principles

1. A major burn represents the ultimate traumatic insult. Despite major advances, burn mortality has been but slightly improved in recent years. Increased knowledge of early resuscitative care, chemotherapy, both local and systemic, bacteriology and temporary biological dressings, etc. have added immeasurably to improving prognosis. A tremendous body of knowledge has been accrued but much remains to be done.

2. Thermal injury in infants and older individuals carries an increased risk, morbidity and mortality. A 30-per cent full-thickness burn in infants and older people will produce a relatively high mortality, whereas in a young adult full recovery is expected. It is prudent to hospitalize the extremes of age even with a lesser burn.

3. Functional disturbances and cosmetic disfigurements may result from late burn scar contractures and hypertrophic scars. Consequently, these defects may lead to permanent disability and emotional instability.

4. The areas of special concern in full-thickness burns are the face, neck, hands, feet, joint surfaces and genitalia. These anatomical locations merit special care once the lifesaving initial critical phase has passed. Past and present illness and associated injuries—obesity, alcoholism, drug addiction, epilepsy, diabetes, cardiac and renal diseases and associated major skeletal or soft tissue injuries—may alter the course of the burn. Serious consideration should be placed on these systemic diseases and any associated bodily trauma in the determination of the course of therapy.

## Criteria for Diagnosis

1. *Etiology.* Information as to the etiological agents is valuable in determining the depths of tissue damage. Hot liquid scalds, hot steam and flash fire burns usually result in partial-thickness skin injury. Burns caused by boiling oil or liquid fat tend to cause deeper second-degree burns.

Flame burns, particularly when clothing is ignited, contact burns produced by heated metals or liquids at extreme temperatures, such as molten metal or hot tar, burns from prolonged immersion in hot water, chemical burns without adequate hydrotherapy and electrical burns generally result in the full-thickness destruction of the skin. The thickness of skin also affects the depth of the burn. Infants and older age-groups are inflicted with deeper burns compared to young adults injured by the same agent.

2. *Depth of Burns.* Estimation of the depth and extent of the burn is essential in appraising the magnitude of the injury and planning of the therapeutic regimen.

Second-degree or partial-thickness burns are red, weeping and hypersensitive and generally covered with blisters or bullae.

Third-degree or full-thickness burns are flat, pale, dry, brown or charred, leathery, waxy and anesthetic. As a result, the body's first line of defense against microorganisms is lost as well as the heat-regulating function and the water-vapor barrier.

3. *Extent of Burns.* This is generally expressed as percentage of the total body sur-

face burned. A reasonably accurate and easily remembered guide is the "rule of 9's." The body surfaces are divided into anatomical regions, each representing 9 per cent, or a multiple of 9 per cent, of the body surface.

#### Rule of 9's

| | |
|---|---|
| Head and neck | 9% |
| Upper extremities (9 × 2) | 18% |
| Lower extremities (18 × 2) | 36% |
| Anterior trunk | 18% |
| Posterior trunk | 18% |
| Perineum | 1% |
| | 100% |

It is necessary to alter the rule of 9's, particularly in infants and children, because the head in children occupies considerably more of the body surface and the lower extremities occupy less. Body surface determination as related to age is a much more accurate estimation in thermal injury.

## Management

### First Aid

Emergency care should be established immediately in all major burns.

1. Secure an adequate airway.

   A. Hypoxia due to airway obstruction from secretions or carbon particles should be cleared by immediate suctioning.

   B. Airway obstruction caused by bronchospasm or mucosal edema from thermal or chemical irritants to the respiratory tracts should be treated with intravenous steroids and humidified oxygen.

   C. Tracheostomy should be a last resort and endotracheal intubation may be utilized for maintenance of the airway, especially where assisted ventilation is required.

2. Establish a lifeline.

   A. An intravenous infusion of Ringer's lactate solution should be instituted immediately to combat hypovolemia and acidosis from the thermal injury.

   B. An 18- or 19-gauge needle should be inserted into the most available vein. Do not attempt to do a cutdown at this time in adults because valuable time may be lost. In children, however, where veins are difficult to enter, a cutdown may be the more rapid approach.

   C. Blood samples must be obtained for baseline hematology and blood chemistry prior to the infusion of Ringer's lactate.

3. Protect the burn wound from contaminations. Prevent cross-contamination by covering the burn wound with a sterile, dry sheet.

### Initial Care of Minor Burns

Aseptic precautions are essential. All personnel in contact with burn patients should use cap, mask, gown and sterile gloves.

1. First- and second-degree burns involving less than 15 per cent of the body surface may be treated with occlusive dressings or open-exposure therapy.

   A. A culture of the burn wound is taken and the wound is cleaned gently with luke-warm or cold water and mild surgical soap and irrigated with saline.

   B. In occlusive therapy, sterile, nonadherent, water-permeable fine mesh gauze (which may or may not be impregnated with antibacterial agents) is applied over the burn surface, followed by a bulky absorbent gauze fluff, a moderate pressure dressing.

   C. In exposure therapy, the cleaned areas of burn are left open to the air, permitting a coagulum to form.

2. Elevation of involved extremities will minimize postburn edema.

3. Tetanus prophylaxis is routine.

4. Narcotics or sedatives are given if needed for the alleviation of pain or discomfort.

## Table 34-1. Relative Proportions of the Body Surface According to Age

|  | Infant | Ages 1–4 | Ages 5–9 | Ages 10–14 | Adult |
|---|---|---|---|---|---|
| Head | 19% | 17% | 13% | 11% | 7% |
| Neck (1 × 2) | 2% | 2% | 2% | 2% | 2% |
| Upper Extremities (10 × 2) | 20% | 20% | 20% | 20% | 20% |
| Lower Extremities | 27% (13.5 × 2) | 29% (14.5 × 2) | 33% (16.5 × 2) | 35% (17.5 × 2) | 39% (18.5 × 2) |
| Anterior trunk | 13% | 13% | 13% | 13% | 13% |
| Posterior trunk and buttocks | 18% | 18% | 18% | 18% | 18% |
| Perineum | 1% | 1% | 1% | 1% | 1% |
|  | 100% | 100% | 100% | 100% | 100% |

## Initial Care of Severe Burns

1. The care of moderate and major burns is included in this plan of therapy, which is as follows:

A. Obtain an adequate airway.

B. Perform venipuncture.

C. Evaluation of the patient (Include a history and past illnesses.)

D. Insert an indwelling Foley catheter

E. Estimate the weight of the patient and the extent and depth of the thermal injury.

F. Fluid replacement

G. Tetanus immunization

H. Prophylactic antibiotics if indicated

I. Nutrition

J. Psychological uplift

K. Initial local wound care (escharotomy when indicated)

2. Obtain an adequate airway.

A. The establishment and maintenance of a patent airway is of prime importance in a comatose burn patient and in burn victims with concomitant servere inhalation injury.

B. The possibility for inhalation injuries exists in patients with:

(1) Burns of the face, neck and oral mucosa

(2) Burns or hyperemia of the postpharygeal wall

(3) Singeing of the hair in the nostrils

(4) Carbon particles in the oral cavity or in the respiratory tract

(5) History of a burn sustained in an enclosed space

C. Noxious gases and the carbon particles in smoke, as well as heated air, play a major role in the production of inhalation injury.

D. Thorough suctioning or even saline lavage of the tracheobronchial tree may be needed in some severe inhalation injuries to clear out carbon particles.

E. A large dose of steroid is administered for bronchospasm when indicated.

F. Determination of the carbon monoxide level may be valuable in evaluating the oxygen-carrying capacity of hemoglobin in a patient with suspected inhalation injury.

G. Tracheostomy may be necessary in a patient requiring assisted tracheal toilet and ventilation. Administration of humidified oxygen and endotracheal inhalation, however, may eliminate the need for a hazardous tracheostomy.

3. Perform venipuncture.

A. An initial venipuncture is performed with a large bore needle (17- or 18-gauge). Blood is obtained for typing and crossmatching, baseline hematology and blood chemistry.

B. An arterial blood sample is obtained for serum pH, $pO_2$ and $pCO_2$, particularly if inhalation injury is suspected. Ringer's lactate solution is initiated immediately and continued until the plan of replacement therapy is established.

C. Initial sedative is best administered intravenously when needed.

D. A venous cutdown should be performed in all major burns, especially in children, as soon as the urgent initial care is given. Convenient sites for a cutdown are at the medial malleolus for the long saphenous vein and at the shoulder or wrist level for the cephalic vein.

4. *Evaluation of the Patient*

A. Information regarding the cause, the circumstances and the time of burn and any initial therapeutic measures given prior to reaching the hospital should be obtained.

B. The age of the patient, pre-existing diseases, the medications which the patient has received or is receiving and the status of immunization are all important factors in establishing the therapeutic regimen.

5. Insert an indwelling Foley catheter.

A. A Foley catheter is inserted in all major burn patients upon admission to the hospital, and a urine specimen is obtained for examination.

B. The urinary output should be recorded hourly since it is the most reliable indicator available at present for the adequacy of fluid replacement. An hourly urinary output of 30 to 50 ml. is minimally adequate for the adult, and an hourly output of 15 to 30 ml. should be just sufficient for infants and small children.

As a rule of thumb, remember that 1 ml. of urinary output per minute is adequate for an adult (60 ml. per hour), and an output of 0.5 ml. per minute is sufficient for children (30 ml. per hour).

C. A fall in urinary output is most frequently associated with inadequate fluid therapy during the first 48 hours after thermal injury. If the output drops, the rate of fluid infusion should be increased accordingly.

D. Dehydration may manifest as:

  *(1)* Thirst

  *(2)* Increased irritability

  *(3)* Vomiting

  *(4)* Increased pulse rate and a fall in blood pressure

  *(5)* Decrease in urinary output

E. In questionable cases, a water-load test is performed to establish a differential diagnosis between dehydration and organic renal failure.

  *(1)* A water-load test is done by rapid infusion of 1,000 ml. of 5% glucose in water within 30 minutes.

  *(2)* If the urinary output is increased, the fall in urinary output is generally a result of dehydration or insufficient fluid replacement.

F. Accurate measurements of body weight and central venous pressure monitoring can be used as additional guides for fluid replacement.

G. The indwelling catheter should be removed as soon as the intake and output are stabilized. Prolonged use of a catheter may predispose to urinary infection.

6. Estimate the weight of the patient and the extent of thermal injury.

A. The weight of the patient, the depth of the burn and the per cent of body surface burned are essential factors in calculating the fluid requirements.

B. A clinical impression of the depth and extent of the burn must be charted on admission to the hospital.

7. *Fluid Replacement*

A. The objectives of fluid replacement in the acutely burned patient are to maintain adequate tissue perfusions and to prevent hypovolemic shock.

B. The required amount of fluid is determined by the size of the patient and the extent of the thermal injury.

C. The type and quantity of fluid to be given are adjusted to the age and medical status of the victim and are altered by the various parameters such as urinary output, body weight and central venous pressure.

D. Translocation of fluid from the vascular tree and intracellular space into the interstitial space is maximum during the initial several hours and then gradually spreads over the next 2 days; accordingly, the fluid replacement should follow the pattern of fluid loss.

*(1)* Half of the estimated fluid should be given during the first 8 hours and then half of the remaining fluid is administered during the next 16 hours.

*(2)* The most widely accepted and used guide in fluid replacement is the Brooke formula, which is the Brooke Army Hospital modification of the Evans' formula and was established in 1953.

*Brooke Formula:*
*(a) First 24 Hours:*

Electrolyte (Ringer's lactate)    1.5 ml. × kg. of body weight × per cent burned
Colloid (blood, plasma or dextran)    0.5 ml. × kg. of body weight × per cent burned
Water (5% G/W)    Maintenance:
    Adult:    2000 ml.
    Children: 1 year, 80 ml. × kg. of body weight
        5 years, 60 ml. × kg. of body weight
        8 years, 40 ml. × kg. of body weight

Half of the total volume is administered over the first 8 hours and the second half of the fluid is infused during the ensuing 16-hour period.

*(B) Second 24 Hours:* electrolyte and colloid are reduced to one half of the volume administered in the first 24 hours. Maintenance water is the same as in the first 24 hours. If more than 50 per cent of the body surface is burned, calculations should be based on 50 per cent. It is rarely necessary to administer more than 10,000 ml. of total volume during the first 24 hours. Colloids are not essential in the treatment of a second-degree burn.

*Example:* 60 kg. man with 30% burn

*First 24 hours*

Electrolyte         1.5 × 60 × 30 = 2700 ml.
Colloid             0.5 × 60 × 30 =  900 ml.
Maintenance water   (5% G/W)       = 2000 ml.

                    Total = 5600 ml.

Rate of fluid administration:

First 8 hours = 2800 ml.
Remaining 16 hours = 2800 ml.

*Second 24 Hours*

Electrolyte         1/2 of 2700 ml. = 1350 ml.
Colloid             1/2 of  900 ml. =  450 ml.
Maintenance of water   (5% G/W)     = 2000 ml.

                    Total = 3800 ml.

In the selection of an electrolyte solution, Ringer's lactate is favored over normal saline. Ringer's lactate reduces the acid load and at the same time eliminates overloading of chloride as in saline. Colloids and whole blood are not widely utilized in the initial resuscitating phase except in extensive full-thickness burns.

*(3)* It must be remembered that all formulas are used as guidelines in estimating the volume to be replaced and the volume must be adjusted to the individual patient and to the systemic response.

8. *Tetanus Immunization*

A. Patients actively immunized within a 5-year period should receive 0.5 ml. of tetanus toxoid booster.

B. Patients without active immunization should be passively immunized with 250 units of human immune globulin (Hyper-Tet).

9. *Prophylactic Antibiotic Therapy*

A. Prophylactic antibiotics should not be used in minor burns.

B. In major burns, 600,000 units of procaine penicillin are administered twice a day for 4 to 5 days to prevent bacterial colonization, particularly of beta-hemolytic streptococci. A broad-spectrum antibiotic is given for the patient with hypersensitivity to penicillin.

C. Cultures of the burn wound and sensitivity testing should be done at the time of admission, and the antibiotic regimen should be altered according to the results of the culture and sensitivity testing.

10. *Nutrition*

A. All patients with severe burns should not be fed orally for 24 hours to avoid acute gastric dilatation, water intoxication and resulting hyponatremia. Paralytic ileus may develop secondary to thermal injury, and abdominal distention, hyperperistalsis and nausea and vomiting may ensue.

B. Usually by the second day, the patient may be placed on a limited liquid diet.

C. The food intake is gradually increased beginning with a soft diet, and eventually at the end of the first week the patient should be on a high-calorie and high-protein diet.

D. High doses of vitamin B and C are advised.

11. *Psychological Assistance.* This is one of the neglected aspects of burn care. The initial shocking experience of a severe burn, underscored by the constant fear of death and by the uncertain prospect of a functional disability and physical disfigurement, may drive the patient into a state of emotional instability and demoralization. The physician who is treating a burn patient should attempt to meet this psychological need and reassure the patient during the entire course of therapy.

12. *Initial Local Wound Care*

A. The skin is the first line of defense against bacterial invasion into the human body. When this protective barrier is destroyed by thermal injury, a prime objective should be the prevention of invasive burn wound sepsis.

B. Strict aseptic precautions are essential in burn wound care to prevent not only invasive infection but also the conversion of partial-thickness burns into full-thickness burns.

## Escharotomy

1. Circumferential inelastic constricting eschar resulting from full-thickness flame burns often requires immediate decompression incisions to relieve hypoxia distal to the constricted area.

2. The decompression incisions are generally made into the subcutaneous tissue and carried down to a bleeding level or on occasion to the fascia.

3. Anesthesia is not needed in the majority of cases.

4. Escharotomy of the extremities is performed along the entire axis of the constricting band, generally at the medial or lateral aspect or both. The straight incision should be broken at the knee or elbow level to minimize any eventual scar contracture.

5. Incisions of the chest wall are done

transversely along the ribs and in a vertical direction at the mid and anterior axillary line.

## Burn Wound Cleansing

1. All personnel who come in contact with the patient must wear masks, caps, gowns and sterile gloves.

2. The majority of flash burns, charred flame burns and full-thickness contact burns do not require cleansing of the wound.

3. In high-risk patients with extensive third-degree burns, cleansing the wound should be deferred until the patient's condition improves.

4. The burn wound should be gently but thoroughly cleaned with a bland soap and luke-warm water or saline. Further irrigation of the burn wound is carried out with saline in a warm draftless room.

5. All large blisters and broken blisters are debrided.

6. Chemical burns, particularly acid or alkali, should be copiously irrigated immediately with water for a minimum of 4 to 8 hours.

7. Mild sedation or intravenous analgesics may be given to relieve any pain or discomfort during the cleansing process.

## Occlusive Dressing

1. The occlusive compression dressing is one of the oldest methods and is extremely effective in certain situations. This technique is widely utilized for the local therapy of circumferential burns of the trunk or extremities. It is useful in children and in minor burns and for ambulatory care.

2. Burns of the hands and feet are best treated with occlusive dressings. The hands are immobilized in a position of function, the digits must be separated by gauze, and the entire hand must be splinted.

3. The occlusive dressing is applied to protect the wound from further cross-contamination, to aid in proper positioning and to put the injured part at rest.

4. Standard occlusive dressings are applied in layers. Nonadherent, water-permeable, fine mesh gauze is placed on the burn wound. This inner layer is covered with an even, resilient layer of fluffed gauze which is held in place by stretch gauze bandages. The dressing should be absorptive and bulky.

## Exposure Therapy

1. An open technique is preferred in burns involving the face, neck, axillae and perineum, and in single surfaces.

2. The hard coagulum from the exudate of partial-thickness burns and the dry eschar in full-thickness burns serve as a natural protective barrier to microorganisms.

3. The open method also permits constant daily inspection of the wound. Cracks developing in the eschar should be covered with pieces of fine mesh gauze to eliminate potential avenues of infection.

4. In partial-thickness burns, regeneration of epithelium is completed under the dry coagulum in 14 to 21 days.

5. In full-thickness burns, exposure therapy is no longer effective when the eschar begins to slough from autolysis at the interface of devitalized and viable tissue. Therapy should then be changed to aggressive debridement and saline soaks should be changed at least every 6 to 8 hours.

6. Occlusive compression dressings and exposure therapy are complementary techniques and combined methods can be applied in the same patient.

## Topical Chemotherapy

The recent use of topical chemotherapeutic agents in the management of the local wound has proven effective in controlling bacterial colonization, especially by *Pseudomonas aeruginosa*.

1. *Sulfamylon Acetate (10%)*

   A. *Advantages*

    *(1)* Sulfamylon acetate diffuses rapidly into the burn wound and underlying tissues, and it is rapidly excreted and lacks toxicity.

*(2)* It reduces bacterial proliferation, especially Pseudomonas.

*(3)* It prevents conversion of deep dermal burns to full-thickness losses.

*(4)* It decreases the incidence of Pseudomonas septicemias.

*(5)* It promotes a sense of well-being and permits early ambulation and physiotherapy.

*(6)* It does not cause any electrolyte derangements.

*(7)* It is easy to apply and markedly reduces the burden of patient care.

B. *Disadvantages*

*(1)* Causes some mild discomfort upon application

*(2)* There appears to be an increased colonization of Klebsiella and Aerobacter organisms.

*(3)* Hypersensitivity reactions occur in a small percentage of cases.

2. *Silver Nitrate Solution (0.5%)*

A. *Advantages*

*(1)* Judicious use of silver nitrate soaks in the burn wound has proven to be effective in controlling Pseudomonas and overcoming the vapor loss through burn wounds.

*(2)* It also prevents conversion of deep dermal burns to full-thickness burns.

B. *Disadvantages*

*(1)* Requires frequent wetting of dressings (every 3 to 4 hours)

*(2)* Black discoloration of the patient and the equipment

*(3)* Rapid loss of soluble minerals from the patient, causing deficiencies in sodium, potassium, chloride, calcium and magnesium. Supplementary electrolytes are therefore essential.

3. Other topical agents being commonly used are gentamicin and silver sulfadiazine.

## Immediate Excision of Full-Thickness Burns and Split-Thickness Grafting

1. Full-thickness burns of less tha 10 per cent of the body surface may be effectively' treated by immediate excision of the eschar and split-thickness skin grafting.

2. The grafting procedures can be delayed 24 to 48 hours if excessive bleeding is encountered.

3. This procedure is particularly valuable in the restoration of function in deep dermal burns of the hand.

## Temporary Biological Dressings

1. In recent years, the immediate application of temporary biological dressings to partial thickness burns, particularly burns of the hand and scald burns in children, has added a significant dimension to burn wound care.

2. Commercially available porcine xenografts are immensely useful in these instances.

# 35. BITES OF ANIMALS, REPTILES AND INSECTS

*David H. Harshaw*, M.D.

## RABIES

### Definition

Rabies is an encephalitis caused by a large virus and is transmitted by the bite of mammals. Unless treatment is initiated prior to the onset of symptoms, death is inevitable.

### Classification

The disease as seen in different mammalian species tends to vary in some symptoms, but the manifestations of the disease can be roughly classified into two phases:

. 1. The first phase is the excited or furious phase.

2. If the animal survives, the first phase is followed by the paralytic or stuporous phase.

### Basic Principles

1. Animal bites, aside from the wound itself and the introduction into the wound of pathologic organisms such as tetanus, always present the problem of whether the biting animal is rabid or not.

2. In animals (e.g., dogs), the disease follows a similar course as in man except that dogs rarely get hydrophobia. It is in the excited stage that the animal bites, it is highly nervous, anxious and, with little provocation, will bite. As the excited state progresses, the animal becomes insane, biting and attacking any other animal, including his master. It is in this phase of extreme excitement that wild animals normally fearful of humans will attack a man.

3. After being bitten by a rabid animal, the time of onset of clinical rabies is related to the amount of virus inoculated into the wound and the distance of the local nerves from the central nervous system. Thus, severe or multiple bites about the head and neck should receive treatment immediately even though the animal is apparently healthy.

4. The onset of clinical rabies may precede the development of immunity. Those patients with bites which would be prone to have an early onset of the disease should receive hyperimmune serum in addition to the vaccine. These include massive or multiple bites and bites in the region of the head and neck. Despite the objection that the hyperimmune serum may interfere with the antibody response to the vaccine, it is still recommended since it no doubt decreases the amount of the infecting virus. It should be given only once and preferably as soon after the bite as possible. If the patient is seen later, the dose of hyperimmune serum should be increased over the usual dose of 40 international units/kg. of body weight.

5. The quarantine of the animal is based on the fact that an apparently healthy animal (with rabies) that bites a person will in practically all cases show symptoms of clinical rabies within 10 days. It is entirely possible that at the time of biting the animal's saliva harbored the rabies virus.

6. The incubation period for rabies in most domestic animals (especially dogs) is about 30 days but may be longer with a very small virus inoculation. About 20 per cent of animals will have shorter incubation periods. The bite of a wild animal (wolf, fox, bat, skunk, etc.) tends to inoculate a more virulent virus than the bites of domestic animals and should be treated by immediate vaccination and hyperimmune serum. This more virulent virus tends to have a shorter incubation period.

7. A thorough washing of the wound with soap and irrigation with Zephiran has been shown experimentally to reduce the development of rabies by about 90 per cent.

## Criteria for Diagnosis

1. One of the earlier symptoms of rabies is an abnormal sensation at the site of the bite, either numbness or intermittent sharp pains. This appears in a prodromic phase prior to excitement.

2. The outstanding clinical symptom of rabies is related to swallowing, in which liquid, food or saliva irritates the oropharynx sufficiently so that extremely violent, painful contractions of the swallowing mechanism are produced, resulting in the expulsion of the material. The victim tends to avoid swallowing; thus there is a drooling of saliva from the mouth. It was this symptom that gave rabies the alternate name of hydrophobia.

3. The inability to swallow occurs in the excited stage and is preceded by an increasing nervousness and anxiety.

4. Eventually tremors and fibrillar muscular contractions begin and these progress to convulsive episodes.

5. The act of swallowing will bring on bouts of apnea.

6. Between seizures, a patient will show a maniacal behavior.

7. Most patients and animals die in this phase, but they can go on to the next, or paralytic, phase, when many of their symptoms will disappear, including the inability to swallow.

8. This apparent remission is followed by a progressive paralysis of the flaccid type. The paralysis is caused by degeneration of the motor nuclei and is often first manifested by ocular palsies, facial weakness and weakness of phonation, or hoarseness of voice. Vertigo and nystagmus develop, the pulse rises and Cheyne-Stokes breathing begins.

9. The blood has a leukocytosis of 20,000 to 30,000/mm.[3], which is largely polymorphs and large monocytes.

10. The urine may contain protein, sugar and acetone.

11. The analysis of animals thought to have rabies is classically done by looking for Negri bodies in brain tissue, using slides stained with a mixture of basic fuchsin and methylene blue. The Negri bodies stand out as cherry red with a deep blue inner structure. The problem with this technique is that it is only accurate in about 80 per cent of cases. Negri bodies tend to be more abundant in the area of Ammon's horn in the brain. (Dogs with distemper can also demonstrate an inclusion body which may be confused with the true Negri body.) At the same time, some of the brain tissue of the animal should be ground and suspended in 1% saline, then mixed with penicillin and streptomycin and inoculated intracerebrally into mice. False negative tests for Negri bodies can develop either early in the course of the disease or if the animal lives with a long paralytic phase (2 to 3 weeks). Thus, the practice of quarantining the animal and examining the brain when the furious symptoms develop will tend to give the best chance of finding the Negri bodies. Recently an immunofluorescent antibody test has been developed which is said to be more accurate than looking for Negri bodies.

## Management

1. The bite wound should be thoroughly washed with a soap solution (20%) and then irrigated with a 1% Zephiran solution. After thoroughly cleansing the wound, it should be treated as any other wound, including the use of tetanus toxoid or hyperimmune human tetanus antiserum.

2. The animal involved should be apprehended and examined by a veterinarian as to its state of health. If it appears ill and there is the slightest suspicion of its being rabid, the treatment of the patient should be initiated immediately. The animal should be quarantined for 10 days out of contact with any other animal. During this period, if it gets better, the treatment of the patient can be discontinued. On the other hand, if the animal progresses in its illness, treatment of the patient should be continued as if the animal were rabid, the animal should be sacrificed and its brain

examined for Negri bodies. Some of its brain should be injected intracerebrally into mice and an immunofluorescent antibody test done on the brain tissue. Animals may show an atypical clinical course and the laboratory analysis may give false negative results. The longer the animal progresses in its disease, the greater the chance of getting a true positive laboratory test. The clinical course of the animal is most valuable since rabies is 100 per cent fatal if untreated.

If the biting animal is healthy and remains so for 10 days, no treatment need be given the patient except for bites of the head and neck region and massive bites. If the animal, although initially healthy, develops symptoms suggestive of rabies, treatment of the patient should begin.

3. The dose rate of hyperimmune serum is 40 international u./kg. of body weight in a single intramuscular dose, with one fourth of the total dose given into the tissue about the site of the bite. If the bite is massive or in the head and neck, 50 to 100 international u./kg. of body weight should be given. If the bite is seen 3 or more days after infliction, larger doses should be used. The hyperimmune serum is horse serum and the patient should be checked for allergy to the serum by a 1:1000 dilution injected subcutaneously. A sensitive patient should receive the hyperimmune serum by a desensitizing procedure, giving diluted serum injected at 20-minute intervals and slowly increasing the amount of serum until the entire dose has been given.

4. The vaccine used today is duck embryo vaccine, which has an extremely low incidence of postvaccination encephalomyelitis. It is given as 2 ml. of a 5% tissue emulsion subcutaneously for 14 days and for severe bites should be extended to 21 days. Booster doses should be given 10 days and 20 days after the last of the daily doses, especially if hyperimmune serum has been given, in order to overcome the interference effect. The site of injection is usually the abdominal wall.

## REPTILE BITES

### Definition

Venenation is the injection of a toxic venom into a victim by a poisonous reptile, usually a snake.

### Classification

1. *Type of Snake.* There are five groups of poisonous snakes in the world:
   A. True vipers
   B. Pit vipers
   C. Cobras and kraits
   D. Sea snakes
   E. Rear-fanged snakes

In North and South America, all the poisonous snakes are of the pit viper group except for the coral snake, which is in the cobra group. The venom of the vipers and pit vipers is primarily hematotoxic and affects the blood vessels and blood coagulation system. The venom of the other groups is primarily neurotoxic, affecting neuromuscular control and respiration.

2. *Degree of Venenation.* Every strike by a poisonous snake does not necessarily mean that venom was injected, and, when venom is injected, it can be injected in varying amounts. In order to give antivenin, the bites by the pit vipers have been classified:

*Grade 0:* No venenation, fang or tooth marks; minimal pain, with less than 1 inch of surrounding edema and erythema

*Grade I:* minimal venenation, fang or tooth marks; severe pain, 1 to 5 inches of surrounding edema and erythema in the first 12 hours, no systemic symptoms

*Grade II:* moderate venenation, fang or tooth marks; severe pain, 6 to 12 inches of surrounding edema and erythema in the first 12 hours. Systemic symptoms are present, such as nausea, vomiting, dizziness, shock and neuromuscular symptoms.

*Grade III:* severe venenation in first 12 hours; greater than 12 inches of surrounding edema and erythema, with similar systemic symptoms as in grade II

## Basic Principles

1. Not all snakes are poisonous and not all poisonous snakebites have venom injected. The reaction the victim has to the venenation is a balance between size of snake, site of the bite, size of the victim, age of the snake and the victim, and the particular toxicity of the venom. All reptile bites that are poisonous come from snakes except the bite of the gila monster lizard of the American Southwest and Mexico. This lizard injects a neurotoxin-type venom by chewing it into the victim. No antivenin is as yet available against it.

2. Upon injection of pit-viper venom into a soft tissue mass, local destruction of tissue and blood vessels occurs from the powerful enzymes composing the venom. These proteins attack red blood cells, lysing them. They attack blood vessel walls, allowing leakage of blood and fluids into surrounding tissues. Intravascular thrombosis occurs and fibrinogen is used up, causing further systemic effects. Local muscles and nerves are lysed by cytolysins. The local swelling becomes of such an intensity that blood supply to the local area is impaired, resulting in tissue and skin necrosis. Treatment is aimed at:

   A. Preventing spread of venom
   B. Preventing local necrosis
   C. Combating systemic effects

3. The spread of venom, which primarily proceeds through lymphatics, is done by incising the area of the bite, suction removal of the venom, application of a tourniquet below arterial pressure and cooling the local area with ice. The local necrosis is prevented by use of local and systemic antivenin, fasciotomy and debridement, and cortisone. The systemic effects are combated by use of antivenin intravenously, cortisone, fluid support and antibiotics.

4. The most important treatment is the use of antivenin. This is horse serum for the pit vipers and can cause anaphylaxis. Thus the patient must be skin-tested with a 1:50 dilution of the antivenin. The development of serum sickness is directly proportional to the amount of antivenin injected. About 90 per cent of those patients receiving more than 200 ml. of antivenin will get serum sickness. A severe bite may require 1 to 5 vials of antivenin every 6 hours.

5. The spread of venom is accelerated by exercise and alcohol whereas cooling with ice will retard it by 10 times and a tourniquet will cut the absorption in half. The tourniquet should be below arterial pressure, proximal to the erythema, and used only until the cooling can be put into effect. The cooling is done with ice in plastic bags and can be continued up to 48 hours, beyond which it has little effect. The cooling should be done dry so as not to macerate or necrose tissues.

## Criteria for Diagnosis

1. *Poisonous or Nonpoisonous Snake.*

   A. Most of the poisonous snakes in the United States are pit vipers and they have the following characteristics:

   *(1)* Large prominent retractile fangs in the upper jaw
   *(2)* A small pit between the nostril and eye
   *(3)* An elliptical pupil to the eye
   *(4)* A diamond-shaped head
   *(5)* Rattles at the tip of the tail in the rattlesnakes, and in all pit vipers there is only a single row of caudal plates beyond the anal plate on the ventral surface.

   B. The nonpoisonous American snakes have:

   *(1)* Round pupils
   *(2)* Oblong-shaped heads
   *(3)* Multiple teeth
   *(4)* Double row of plates just beyond the anal plate

   C. The brightly colored coral snake resembles in appearance several brightly colored and banded nonpoisonous snakes. However, only the coral snakes have a red ring next to a yellow ring. The coral snake chews its venom into its victim rather than injecting it.

2. *Envenomization.* The injection of venom by a pit viper produces severe to ex-

cruciating pain at the site of the bite, which is quickly followed by erythema and edema at the site. This erythema and edema then spreads in a radial fashion. The lethal toxicity of the venom of most of the pit vipers is about 1 mg. of dried venom per kilogram of body weight. Many of the pit vipers have considerably less toxicity. However, if a large rattlesnake injects its entire venom into an adult human, it is lethal. In general, snakes seldom inject this amount. An adult eastern diamondback rattler has about 450 mg. of venom, well above the lethal amount.

3. *The Symptoms.* A strike onto a bony prominence may have little venom injected, whereas one into a large muscle mass usually gives maximum venenation. Recently fed snakes may have little venom left over to inject again. An intravenous injection is usually rapidly fatal.

The symptoms of bites from snakes with a neurotoxin consist of blurring of vision, ptosis, drowsiness, increased salivation and sweating. The victim may notice paresthesia about the mouth and throat, slurring of speech, nausea and vomiting and respiratory difficulty. If a patient has none of these symptoms 30 minutes after a bite by a supposedly neurotoxic snake, venenation did not take place.

## Management of Pit Viper Bites

1. Make a cruciate incision between the fang marks. The depth of the bite is about three fourths of the distance between the puncture sites. By suction, up to 50 per cent of the venom can be removed if done within 15 minutes of the bite, and suction should be instituted as long as 2 hours after venenation. The incision should extend as deep as the fangs have penetrated. If oral suction is used, there should be no open wounds or sores in the mouth.

2. Apply a tourniquet which is kept below systolic pressure and placed above the developing edema and erythema. The tourniquet should be released every 15 to 20 minutes for 1 minute and moved higher as the edema progresses.

3. As soon as ice is available, the site of the bite and/or the extremity is placed in it. The skin should be kept dry by placing the ice in plastic bags. Once cooling has been instituted, the tourniquet is no longer needed. The purpose of the ice is to cool the extremity, not to freeze or macerate it. The cooling should be continued for 24 to 48 hours, which is usually the time it takes for the edema to reach its maximum.

4. If a large muscle bundle has been bitten and the bite is of grade II or III, the skin over the muscle bundle should be incised its entire length and, if the bundle is swollen, a fasciotomy of that bundle is done. The muscle is then irrigated with saline and any necrotic tissue is debrided. During the next 48 hours, the incision and fasciotomy are inspected for further swelling and more debridement is carried out. Early use of the fasciotomy will prevent extensive muscle loss from a severe bite. The wound is covered with an antibiotic dressing and kept moist and cool.

5. Hydrocortisone is injected intravenously for grades II and III bites at a rate of 100 mg. every 4 hours for the next 48 hours.

6. Antivenin is given by injecting half of a vial (5 ml.) into the edema around the bite. If the bite is on the fingers or toes, do not inject antivenin into these sites. Another half vial is injected deep into the proximal muscles. A vial is then given by intravenous drip in saline over a 30-minute period. A grade I bite usually requires no more than 1 to 2 vials of intravenous antivenin. A grade II bite requires 3 to 4 vials and a grade III bite requires 5 or more vials. The antivenin is given at 30-minute to 2-hour intervals to keep systemic symptoms from progressing. The use of antivenin is no longer necessary after 48 hours. The patient should be skin-tested for allergy to the antivenin prior to its use, using a 1:50 dilution subcutaneously.

7. The patient may lose considerable amounts of fluids into the tissues surrounding the bite and therefore his state of hydration should be maintained using

Ringer's lactate and plasma. His blood pressure, pulse, respiration and urine output should be carefully monitored each hour. Laboratory tests should include hemoglobin, hematocrit, white blood cell count, red blood cell count, platelets, differential blood count, serum hemoglobin, $Na^+$, $K^+$, $Cl^-$, $CO_2$, bilirubin, blood-urea nitrogen, fibrinogen, clotting time, prothrombin time, partial thromboplastin time, and other clotting factors if indicated. These should be checked twice a day for the first 48 hours and then daily for the next week. Serum sickness, wound complications and clotting defects can occur many days after the initial bite.

8. Antibiotics should be given systemically to cover any wound infection. Tetanus prophylaxis is also given. The wound is treated finally by delayed closure or skin grafting only after it is thoroughly clean and all necrotic areas have been removed.

## INSECT BITES

In addition to acting as vectors of disease, insects can also inflict injury to man by their bites and stings. This injury is usually in the form of a toxic or an allergic reaction. Insects within the same general order tend to have similar reactions upon man with their bites and stings. It is therefore important in treating an insect bite to identify the type of insect involved. The bites have been grouped into 6 groups.

### BEES AND WASPS

#### Basic Principles

Both these insects are divided into solitary and social groups. The solitary bees and wasps live alone, with each female preparing her own nest composed of several adjoining cells. The solitary bees live only one season, and they are commonly named for their way of life. Thus there are the miner bees, carpenter bees, mason bees, etc. The social bees include the bumblebee and the honeybee. In a similar fashion, the solitary wasps include the cicada killer, mud dauber, etc., and the social wasps include yellow jackets and hornets. The stinging apparatus of the bee is a hollow needle 2.5 mm. in length. It is located at the tip of the abdomen and has a barb at the end. Venom glands secrete both an acid and alkaline material, which is forced into a poison sac and then by muscle contraction through the stinger. Two lancets alongside the stinger, by moving forward and backward, work the stinger even deeper into the tissue, the barb making withdrawal impossible. In trying to free itself after a sting, the bee avulses the entire apparatus and soon dies. However, even after avulsion, reflex action of the muscles attached to the lancets continues to drive the stinger deeper into the tissue. The stinger when left attached should therefore be scraped away, since pulling it may only squeeze more venom from the poison sac into the flesh. The stinger, once embedded, cannot be absorbed and may serve as a constant source of irritation. The stinging apparatus of the wasp is similar to that of the honeybee except for the absence of barbs; therefore it is unusual to find an embedded wasp stinger.

The venom contains histamine, hyaluronidase, acetylcholine and high-molecular-weight proteins. The local reaction is due to the various chemical components; the allergic reaction is due to the protein. Some of these proteins are species-specific while others share reactivity with other species. Thus reactivity has been shown from wasp stings in bee-sensitive individuals. The bumblebee only shows reactivity with the honeybee.

#### Criteria for Diagnosis

1. *Normal Reaction.* After the initial sting, a small area of erythema begins which eventually develops into a wheal. The wheal usually subsides in a few hours. Stings about the eyes can be hazardous if they provoke extensive local reaction resulting in atrophy of the iris, lens

abscess, globe perforation or glaucoma or corneal ulcer. Injury to the eye can occur months later from a stinger working its way through the eyelid, causing irritation to the eye underneath.

2. *Toxic Reaction.* Multiple stings even without sensitivity can lead to death. The symptoms are those of systemic poisoning, with vomiting, faintness, diarrhea, generalized edema, drowsiness and convulsions. In an adult human, the lethal dose is about 500 to 1000 stings.

3. *Infection.* Hornets are scavengers and along with venom they may inject bacteria, including tetanus, gas gangrene, etc.

4. *Immediate Hypersensitive Reaction.* The symptoms of anaphylaxis come within 2 to 3 minutes of the sting. They begin as a cough and tightness in the chest and throat due to bronchospasm. The massive urticarial reaction follows along with tachycardia and hypotension. The reaction can be mild or may progress to fatal shock.

5. *Delayed Hypersensitive Reaction.* This reaction occurs 10 to 14 days after the sting and consists of fever, lymphadenopathy, urticaria, polyarthritis and malaise.

## Management

1. *Local Reaction.* In order to prevent further squeezing of the venom into the tissue, an avulsed stinger should be scraped away with a sharp knife. The site of the sting is then washed with soap and water. Ice packs can reduce the intensity of the swelling. Rest and elevation of the part prevent spreading of the wheal. Oral antihistamines are useful to a limited degree for pruritus that may follow. Topical steroid may combat the inflammatory reaction. An embedded stinger should be removed.

2. *Toxic Reaction.* Supportive care such as intravenous fluids, intravenous antihistamines and sedation are the usual measures for multiple bites. Calcium gluconate intravenously is the most effective agent against massive stings. In shock, large doses of hydrocortisone, 0.5 to 1.0

gm. every 4 hours, are useful. The airway must be observed and, if compromised, a tracheotomy is done.

3. *Infection.* Soaks and antibiotics are used if an infection is thought to have developed after a sting. Tetanus toxoid booster, etc., is often indicated after a hornet sting.

4. *Generalized Hypersensitive Reaction.* A mild reaction such as bronchospasm can be relieved by an Isuprel inhaler combined with systemic oral antihistamines. A severe reaction demands:

A. A dose of 0.3 to 0.6 ml. of 1:1000 epinephrine subcutaneously, with the site of injection massaged. This may have to be repeated every 15 to 20 minutes.

B. Aminophylline, 500 mg. in 100 ml. of 5% glucose in water by intravenous drip in 10 to 15 minutes for severe bronchospasm

C. Benadryl, 50 mg. intravenously over a 15- to 30-minute period, repeated every 4 to 6 hours

D. If the subcutaneous epinephrine does not seem to be controlling the hypotension, then Levophed, 1 or 2 ampules in 500 ml. of 5% glucose in water by intravenous drip, is used to titrate the blood pressure.

E. If the patient requires intravenous pressors and he has massive urticaria, dextran and plasma should be administered.

F. Hydrocortisone, 0.5 to 1.0 gm. every 4 hours, should be given initially and then tapered when the reaction subsides.

G. The central venous pressure, blood pressure, respiration and urine output should be monitored.

H. If the bronchospasm does not respond to the aminophylline, steroids and intravenous pressors, then tracheostomy and a volume ventilator should be used to ventilate the lungs. The effectiveness of the ventilation is monitored by blood gas studies. The volume ventilator will also tend to keep the fluid out of the lungs.

I. After subsidence of the initial shock, steroids and antihistamines should be continued for a week or so. Upon recovery, the patient should be desensitized.

5. *Desensitization.* A solution of mixed antigens to bee and wasp venom is usually used. A scratch test is used at a dilution of 1:1,000,000 and, if negative, *intradermal* skin tests are done in ever-increasing concentrations until a reaction is obtained. Beginning at the dilution which gives a wheal and a flare, a series of *subcutaneous* injections are done at weekly intervals, using ever-higher concentrations until a full dose can be tolerated, that is, a dose which gives a 4-cm. wheal with no systemic reaction. This should be at about 0.3 ml. of a 1:10 dilution. If any subcutaneous injection gives a greater reaction, the dosage must be dropped back and worked up at weekly intervals to that level again before proceeding further. The injection should be given in the arm where a tourniquet can prevent systemic spread. The patient should be observed for 30 minutes after the injection for any reaction. A patient who has had a severe hypersensitive reaction after being able to tolerate a 1:10 dilution should get biweekly injections during the summer and monthly injections during the winter, and the injections should be continued indefinitely.

## FLIES

### Basic Principles

Although the common housefly can neither bite nor sting, he has relatives which are capable of inflicting a painful and reactive bite upon humans. Such flies are the stable fly, horsefly, deer fly, black fly and sand fly. Each of these varieties of flies has many subvariations. The pain from the bite of a fly is actually due to enzymes and salivary secretions, injected along with its stylet-like proboscis, in order to break down tissues and make them easier to aspirate and digest. The injection of the proboscis itself is painless. The flies that give painful bites are all bloodsuckers and can also transmit anthrax, tularemia, trypanosomiasis, etc.

### Criteria for Diagnosis

The reactions can be merely a wheal but they may progress in some individuals to a local area of sensitivity. The black fly bite is notorious for developing a site of extreme pain and intense pruritus in about one hour. This is followed either by a vesicular reaction or hard pruritic nodules. Anaphylactic reactions can develop.

### Management

Since flies can transmit infection, the site of the bite should be washed and inspected for the subsequent development of infection. Topical steroids will reduce the local reaction. A localized area of reaction with wheals and pruritus can be treated with oral antihistamines in addition to topical steroid. An anaphylactic reaction to a fly bite is treated like that to a bee sting. Attempts at desensitizing individuals to fly bites have been unsuccessful.

## ANTS

### Basic Principles

The bites and stings of most ants rarely present more than a nuisance, except for the fire ant, which has invaded the southern United States from tropical climates. This ant is about 0.5 cm. long and builds nests in the ground, the entrance to which consists of shallow mounds of dirt up to 3 feet in diameter. The fire ant is a voracious eater, destroying germinating seeds, young crops, eggs and young of ground-nesting birds. They have a very rapid reproduction rate, and an infested area may contain hundreds of nests. When a nest is disturbed, the ants literally bubble forth, inflicting a very painful sting due to a unique toxin.

### Criteria for Diagnosis

A single ant may inflict multiple stings, each insertion of the stinger giving instant pain as with a bee sting. Several minutes later, a 0.5-cm. wheal will develop and expand over the next several hours. In the area of the wheal, a vesicle eventually develops which further develops into a small umbilicated pustule surrounded by a halo of erythema. The pustules may last up to one week, and on subsiding they are replaced by a pigmented macula or in some more sensitive person by hard fibrotic nodules or an eczematoid dermatitis.

## Management

At the present time there is no known local treatment which can prevent the development of the pustules. Severe systemic toxicity or anaphylaxis is treated like that due to bee stings. Desensitization has been unsuccessful.

## SPIDER BITES

Of the several thousand species of spiders, including tarantulas, only two are dangerous to man: the brown recluse spider and the black widow spider. Both are found within the United States.

### *Brown Recluse Spider*

## Criteria for Diagnosis

This spider is about 1 to 1.5 cm. long and about 0.5 cm. wide. It is brown to light tan and has a darker violin-shaped band extending back from the eyes. Brown recluse spiders can be found in or out of doors and spin irregular webs in remote, poorly frequented places. There is no initial pain from the bite, the pain occurring later. A transient erythema develops at the site of the bite and this becomes a blister surrounded by a blanched ischemic zone. Three to four days later, the blistered area begins to show evidence of necrosis and, in one to two weeks, a well-demarcated area of dry gangrene exists. This eventually sloughs, leaving an ulcer extending into the corium. A systemic reaction may occur, especially in children. This consists of fever, chills, vomiting and joint pains, along with a generalized petechial rash. Hematologic disturbances may ensue such as hemolytic anemia and thrombocytopenia. Jaundice, migratory phlebitis and convulsions have been reported.

## Management

1. Intravenous steroid, 100 to 200 mg. of hydrocortisone every 4 hours for about 3 days
2. Systemic antihistamines and antibiotics
3. Subcutaneous Regitine at the site of the bite to reduce the local ischemia
4. Despite the above measures, the ischemic changes may progress. An early incision of the blistered ischemic area may prevent further extension of the necrosis. A bite over a joint such as on a finger can lead to exposure and eventual destruction of the ligaments, tendons or joint capsule. An early excision of the impending necrosis and then covering with a skin graft can preserve the mobility of the joint.

### *Black Widow Spider*

## Criteria for Diagnosis

This spider is found throughout the United States except for Alaska. It is identified by a black shoe-button body, 1.5 cm. long, with a red hour-glass figure on the undersurface. Its web is an irregular arrangement of thick fibers which is quite distinctive and unlike any other spider's web. The bite of the spider is immediately painful, very much like a pin prick. Shortly after the bite, a local pain or discomfort occurs in the region of the bite and is followed by pain and rigidity of the abdominal and extremity muscles. The rigidity of the abdominal muscles resembles that of an acute abdomen. This abdominal rigidity may also have some degree of tenderness. The muscle spasms will eventually involve all the muscles of the body. These pains and spasms are poorly responsive to sedatives and narcotics, and they may last 2 to 4 days, although with decreasing intensity. The mortality is about 3 per cent.

## Management

Despite its being self-limited, the intensity of the pain demands some relief for the patients. The use of tourniquets, incision and suction have little effect on limiting the toxin. Ice packs may reduce the local pain.

1. Intravenous 10% calcium gluconate tends to relieve muscle spasms, although it usually needs to be repeated every 4 hours.

2. Ten ml. of methylcarbinol intravenously, followed by a slow intravenous drip of methylcarbinol in saline, may give some pain relief.

3. Antivenin, which is hyperimmune horse serum, is the best treatment. Two to three ml. of the reconstituted serum are given intramuscularly and may need to be repeated once more. It is most effective when given as soon after the bite as possible.

4. Muscle relaxants have been used but, in order to stop the contractions, respiration may be depressed and ventilatory support should be available before using this treatment.

## TICK BITES

### Basic Principles

Ticks are bloodsuckers which, on attaching themselves to a victim, may take 2 to 3 weeks to completely fill themselves. The tick can attach itself to its victim with a cement-like substance, and although it can detach itself, any forcible attempt in removing it leaves the mouth parts embedded in the tissue. The tick has the ability to regenerate its lost parts. Forcible removal also squeezes more toxin into the victim. The damage from ticks comes not only from its being a vector, but certain ticks are also able to elaborate a neurotoxin which can cause its victim to develop an ascending paralysis. Other ticks of the same sex and species may not be able to induce this paralysis.

### Criteria for Diagnosis

Tick paralysis is an acute, ascending flaccid paralysis, which is preceded by malaise, anorexia, paresthesias, lower extremity pain and an apathetic attitude by the patient. Several hours later a rapid ascending paralysis begins. This progresses to a bulbar-type paralysis, with dysphagia and respiratory failure. Once the tick is removed, the paralysis rapidly clears. In contrast to an encephalitis of viral origin, tick paralysis produces an apathetic, painless, afebrile patient with a normal peripheral blood and spinal fluid.

### Management

Any patient with a rapidly progressing ascending paralysis should be carefully searched for a tick which has become engorged with blood. The search should particularly include the scalp, axilla and pubic regions where a tick can easily hide. The tick is detached by applying ether to it or warming it with a lighted cigarette. This will cause the tick to detach itself.

## SCORPION STINGS

### Basic Principles

The venom of the scorpion is either of two types. One has effects which are purely local and nonlethal. It causes a sharp, burning pain, swelling and a spreading erythema. Anaphylaxis is rare. The other type of venom is a potent neurotoxin which can give a fatal reaction. The particular neurotoxin causes no local swelling or discoloration.

### Criteria for Diagnosis

The pain of the sting is followed by paresthesia in that area, which rapidly spreads. The area becomes hyperesthetic and then hypoesthetic. The patient becomes drowsy, his speech becomes sluggish, and twitchings begin and progress to convulsive episodes. In these seizures, the patient has laryngospasms, opisthotonos and respiratory and circulatory depression. The convulsive episodes come in waves of increasing severity. The entire process may last as long as 2 days but usually reaches its maximum in 3 to 4 hours. If the patient survives beyond the peak of the reaction, he usually will recover. Children, the elderly and weakened victims are usually exhausted by the wave-like seizures and usually are the fatal victims.

## Management

Of the over 30 species found in the United States, only two are of the type possessing a neurotoxin. If the patient is bitten by a scorpion and there is little local swelling and erythema, this is a danger signal of the impending neurotoxic reaction. Prompt treatment should be given to lessen the degree of reaction.

1. Apply a tourniquet near the site of the sting.

2. If a limb is the site of the sting, immerse the limb completely in ice water; then intermittently release the tourniquet every 15 minutes for 1 to 2 hours. If the bite is on the body proper, the area should be covered with crushed ice.

3. Narcotics increase the toxic effects.

4. Specific antivenin is available for the two dangerous species of scorpions and should be used if available.

5. Calcium gluconate should be given intravenously.

6. Barbiturates intravenously will tend to lessen the intensity of the seizures.

# 36. PEDIATRIC SURGICAL EMERGENCIES

*Peter K. Kottmeier*, M.D.

## Surgical Emergencies in the Neonate

Most surgical emergencies in the neonate, in view of their complexity, ranging from congenital anomalies to various types of neoplasm, require the cooperation of an experienced team of neonatologists, radiologists and pediatric surgeons, together with chemotherapists in the instance of certain malignant tumors. Additionally, specialized ancillary facilities for the care of the newborn, as well as anesthesiologists well-prepared and well-equipped for operations on infants during the early weeks of life, make it better to manage most neonatal emergencies by lifesaving emergency care and the transfer to appropriate institutions with the facilities and experience to care for these children.

This chapter will therefore deal only with the diagnosis and immediate treatment of those problems commonly encountered or when transfer of the patient may be inappropriate. These are marked with an asterisk in the schema below.

### Classification of Neonatal Surgical Emergencies

Neonatal Respiratory Emergencies

1. Cerebral
2. Abdominal
3. Metabolic
4. Respiratory
    A. *Nonsurgical*
       (1) Prematurity
       (2) Atelectasis
       (3) Aspiration
       (4) Respiratory distress syndrome
    B. *Surgical*

(1) Head and Neck
    (a) Choanal atresia
    (b) Enlargement of the tongue (macroglossia or tumor)
    (c) Lingual thyroid or cysts
    (d) Laryngeal obstruction
(2) Tracheobronchial obstruction
    (a) Intrinsic
       Stenosis
       Malacia
       H-fistula
    (b) Extrinsic
       Neoplastic (thyroid)
       Congenital
       Duplications
       Stenosis
       Vascular ring
(3) Pulmonary
    (a) Atelectasis
    (b) Lobar emphysema*
    (c) Congenital pulmonary cyst
    (d) Hypoplasia or agenesis
(4) Intrathoracic
    (a) Simple pneumothorax*
    (b) Tension pneumothorax*
    (c) Interstitial emphysema and pneumomediastinum
    (d) Chylothorax
    (e) Diaphragmatic hernia*
    (f) Eventration
    (g) Phrenic nerve paralysis
(5) Mediastinal masses

Neonatal Intestinal Obstruction

1. Nonbiliary Vomiting
    A. *Intrinsic Causes*
       (1) Esophageal atresia*
       (2) Chalasia
       (3) Achalasia

*(4)* Hiatal hernia
*(5)* Esophageal stenosis
*(6)* Congenital pyloric stenosis*
B. *Extrinsic Causes*
   *(1)* Vascular ring
   *(2)* Duplication
2. Biliary Vomiting
  A. *Duodenal obstruction*\**
    *(1)* Diaphragmatic web
    *(2)* Atresia or stenosis
    *(3)* Annular pancreas
  B. *Malrotation*\**
  C. *Small bowel atresia*\**
  D. *Meconium ileus*\**
  E. *Meconium plug*\**
  F. *Duplication*
  G. *Hirschsprung's disease*\**
  H. *Imperforate anus*
  I. *Intussusception*

## Neonatal Peritonitis

1. Gastric perforation*
2. Enteric perforation*
3. Enterocolitis with Hirschsprung's disease*
4. Volvulus
5. Appendicitis*
6. Perforated Meckel's diverticulum*
7. Duplication
8. Bile peritonitis
9. Intraperitoneal hemorrhage*

## Neonatal Gastrointestinal Bleeding

1. Secondary bleeding*
2. Systemic bleeding disorders*
3. Esophageal bleeding*
4. Gastroduodenal bleeding*
5. Intestinal*
  A. *Volvulus*\**
  B. *Meckel's diverticulum*\**
  C. *Small intestinal polyps*\**
  D. *Intussusception*\**
  E. *Enteritis*\**
  F. *Colonic polyps*\**
6. Anal fissures*

## Neonatal Abdominal Masses

1. Mesenteric cyst
2. Duplication

3. Hydronephrosis
4. Cystic kidneys
5. Hydrocolpos
6. Abdominal Tumors
  A. *Neuroblastoma*
  B. *Wilms' tumor*
  C. *Rhabdomyosarcoma*
  D. *Liver*
    *(1)* Hepatoma
    *(2)* Hemangioma
    *(3)* Hamartoma
    *(4)* Cyst
    *(5)* Hematoma

## Neonatal Jaundice

1. Physiologic
2. RH incompatibility
3. Hemolytic disease
4. Biliary atresia
5. Extrahepatic obstruction
6. Intrahepatic obstruction
7. Choledochal cyst

## Neonatal Abdominal and Chest Wall Defects

1. Omphalocele*
2. Gastroschisis*
3. Exstrophy of the cloaca
4. Chest wall fusion defects
5. Upper sternal cleft
6. Distal sternal cleft
7. Prune belly
8. Urachal anomalies
9. Omphalo-enteric duct
10. Umbilical infection*
11. Umbilical hernia*

## Neonatal Genitourinary Problems

1. Female
  A. *Hydrocolpos*
  B. *Labial fusion*
  C. *Adrenogenital syndrome*
  D. *Urethral prolapse*
2. Male
  A. *Meatal stenosis*\**
  B. *Torsion of the testis or (appendages)*\**
  C. *Epididymitis and orchitis*\**
  D. *Undescended testis*

## NEONATAL RESPIRATORY EMERGENCIES

### Basic Principles

Respiratory difficulties in the neonate present the most serious threat to an infant's life, yet the clinical signs and symptoms may be minimal until cardiorespiratory collapse has occurred. Prompt diagnostic work-up and continuous observation are therefore essential in all neonates displaying signs of even "minor" respiratory difficulties.

### Management

The general management in neonates with respiratory difficulties without proven diagnosis should include the following:

1. *Improved Oxygenation.* Oxygenation can be improved by providing an atmosphere of increased oxygen concentration by either tent, mask, endotracheal tube or tracheostomy.

*Caution:* regardless of the type of oxygen administration, concentration should usually be kept at an atmosphere of 40 to 60 per cent to avoid a prolonged elevation of the arterial $pO_2$ over 80 mm./Hg, since this may lead to retrolental fibroplasia. The short-term administration of 100 per cent oxygen may be indicated in infants with dire respiratory emergencies if immediate diagnostic work-up followed by definitive therapy is contemplated.

2. *Aspiration of the Tracheobronchial Tree.* In patients in whom either aspiration, mucous plugs or retained secretions are suspected, tracheal aspiration with a soft plastic catheter should be performed.

*Caution:* during the period of aspiration, the infant is unable to inspire and aspirations have to be limited to short intervals. The instruction of personnel responsible for tracheobronchial aspiration to hold their *own* breath while introducing the catheter will prevent undue prolonged aspiration.

3. *Humidity.* Increased humidity may help in the liquefaction of retained secretions although no definite proof exists. Humidity is indicated when oxygen is provided to compensate for the desiccating effect of $O_2$.

*Caution:* the use of nebulizers may assist in the application of humidity, but extended use of ultrasonic nebulizers may lead to water intoxication if used indiscriminately.

4. *Assisted Ventilation*

A. Mouth-to-mouth or mask ventilation is preferable to intubation in the absence of experienced personnel.

*Caution:* the positive pressure applied to a bag should be under 25 to 30 cm. of water. If higher pressures are required, the positive-pressure phase should be short to avoid alveolar distention and rupture. A short high-peak pressure is more easily tolerated by the infant than a prolonged positive-pressure phase. Whenever mask or mouth-to-mouth ventilation is used, gastric decompression is indicated to avoid diaphragmatic elevation and the danger of gastric regurgitation and aspiration.

B. Mechanical Ventilators, either pressure or volume respirators, can be used if they are properly designed for infants.

*Caution:* adaption of adult ventilators is only possible if the disproportionately large dead space can be avoided. Although positive pressures up to 35 cm. of water may be required in some infants, a pressure of 25 cm. is usually adequate and preferable to avoid overaeration which may lead to alveolar rupture and pneumomediastinum or pneumothorax.

*Caution:* in patients with suspected pneumothorax, pneumomediastinum or tension pneumothorax, the use of a ventilator may aggravate the patient's condition unless the involved area is promptly decompressed through an appropriate thoracostomy tube.

C. *Continuous Positive-Pressure Breathing.* A continuous positive-pressure respiration (approximately 5 cm. of water) can be used through either an endotracheal tube or a mask. Although the indications vary, it appears to be most valuable in infants with respiratory distress syndrome.

5. *Thoracostomy*. Needle aspiration to relieve·the pressure created by tension pneumothorax may have to be performed in patients with suspected tension pneumothorax before the diagnosis can be corroborated by x-ray. The technique and indications for thoracostomy are discussed under Common Emergency Pediatric Surgical Procedures, page 616.

6. All infants displaying signs and symptoms of respiratory difficulties should be worked-up promptly, even though their symptoms may improve after they have been placed in an enriched-oxygen environment. Once the infant's condition deteriorates while in a high-oxygen environment, the opportunity for a proper diagnostic work-up and effective treatment may be lost.

# PULMONARY PROBLEMS

## *Lobar Emphysema*

### Definition

Congenital lobar emphysema is caused by overaeration due to trapping of the inspired air.

### Basic Principles

The formation of congenital lobar emphysema is based on a ball-valve mechanism, probably secondary to a deficiency of bronchial cartilagenous rings which allow air to enter the involved lobe without escape during expiration. *This is a dire surgical emergency.*

### Criteria for Diagnosis

#### Clinical

The development of respiratory distress with hyperresonance on one side and mediastinal shift to the contralateral side is indicative of either tension pneumothorax or congenital lobar emphysema. Due to the rapid mediastinal shift, the contralateral, normal, lung, will be compressed leading to further deterioration.

#### X-ray

Overaeration on the involved side, with mediastinal shift towards the contralateral side is the radiographic picture. In contrast to tension pneumothorax, pulmonary markings are still present in the overaerated side.

### Differential Diagnosis

Tension pneumothorax, diaphragmatic hernia, lobar overaeration due to mucus plugs (ball-valve mechanism).

### Management

1. In patients with rapidly expanding congenital lobar emphysema, immediate operative intervention is indicated. Although the patients will require intubation to maintain aeration of the compressed contralateral lobe, forceful ventilation is contraindicated, since it will further expand the emphysematous lobe and increase the compression of the contralateral lobe.

2. Needle aspiration of the emphysematous lobe has been reported to temporarily improve the respiratory embarrassment.

3. In patients who are close to or in respiratory arrest, an emergency thoracostomy through the fourth or fifth intercostal space, permitting the emphysematous lobe to prolapse through the chest incision may be life saving.

4. In most infants, intubation administration of 100% oxygen and rapid transportation to the operating room will suffice to allow thoracotomy with lobectomy of the involved lobe.

5. In patients who are not *in extremis,* with moderate lobar emphysema, preoperative bronchoscopy is indicated to rule out the presence of a mucus plug producing the ball-valve mechanism.

## INTRATHORACIC NONPULMONARY PROBLEMS

### *Simple Pneumothorax*

### Definition

Simple pneumothorax is the presence of air in the intrapleural space, with partial or complete pulmonary collapse.

### Basic Principles

The most likely cause of neonatal pneumothorax is the spontaneous rupture of small emphysematous blebs. In patients with atelectasis or aspiration, resuscitative maneuvers with overinflation can lead to an iatrogenic rupture.

### Criteria for Diagnosis

#### Clinical

Neonatal pneumothorax is common in the newborn infant. The clinical signs and symptoms do not necessarily relate to the size of the pneumothorax, but may be related more to the underlying cause, such as pre-existing respiratory distress due to atelectasis, amniotic aspiration, etc. The clinical findings include:

1. Auscultation: decreased or absent breath sounds on the involved side, with normal breath sounds on the contralateral side unless the pneumothorax is bilateral or contralateral disease exists.
2. Cardiac impulse: either no mediastinal shift or a shift toward the contralateral side
3. Tachycardia
4. Tachypnea
5. Cyanosis
6. Alar flare and retractions, usually mild to moderate unless coexisting disease is present

#### X-ray

X-ray shows accumulation of air in the pleural space with partial or complete collapse of the ipsilateral lung.

### Management

1. Mild to moderate degrees of spontaneous pneumothorax in infancy, without clinical signs of respiratory embarrassment or deteriorating blood gases, can usually be treated nonoperatively under close observation.
2. If a complete pulmonary collapse exists, if the pneumothorax increases under observation or if clinical signs or symptoms of respiratory distress exist, tube thoracostomy should be employed.
3. Although an anterior chest tube is adequate in older children and adults, in view of the close proximity of major vascular structures, a tube thoracostomy is better inserted through the fifth or sixth interspace in the midaxillary line in infants. The tube usually can be removed within 24 hours after complete pulmonary expansion if no active leak is present.
4. In patients who are treated conservatively, close attention should be paid to the contralateral side, since an additional pneumothorax may develop if pre-existing diseases, such as aspiration, pneumonia or atelectasis, exist.

### *Tension Pneumothorax*

### Definition

Tension pneumothorax is an accumulation of air under pressure in the pleural cavity, with compression of the ipsilateral lung followed by mediastinal shift and compression of the contralateral lung.

### Basic Principles

Air escaping into the pleural cavity through a ball-valve mechanism without an exit accumulates under pressure, first compressing the lung on the involved side, then shifting the mediastinum and compressing the contralateral side. The result is a combined respiratory and cardiac insufficiency with decreased cardiac return.

### Criteria for Diagnosis

#### Clinical

1. In contrast to the simple tension pneumothorax, mediastinal shift to the

contralateral side is marked, leading to a compression of the contralateral lung.

2. On auscultation, breath sounds are absent on the involved side and with expanding pneumothorax become decreased on the contralateral side.

3. The cardiac impulse is shifted to the contralateral side.

4. Clinical signs of acute respiratory distress, with cyanosis, tachypnea, tachycardia and eventually shock, develop.

5. If a tension pneumothorax is suspected clinically, without radiologic proof, an 18- or 19-gauge needle attached to a 20-cc. syringe should be introduced into the fifth or sixth intercostal space in the midaxillary line. In the presence of a tension pneumothorax, the piston in a syringe will usually be pushed backward. The needle is then turned in a position where it lies parallel to the chest wall to avoid laceration or puncture of the lung.

## Laboratory

Blood gases reflect a rapidly increasing degree of pulmonary insufficiency.

## X-ray

X-ray shows radiolucency of the involved side without pulmonary markings, mediastinal shift and finally compression and atelectasis of the contralateral side.

## Differential Diagnosis

1. *Ipsilateral Side:* congenital lobar emphysema, expanding congenital lung cyst, ipsilateral diaphragmatic hernia

2. *Contralateral Side:* Simple pneumothorax, atelectasis

## Management

1. Before respiratory and cardiac deterioration has occurred, insert a thoracostomy tube immediately.

2. When signs of acute deterioration occur, needle aspiration of the involved pleural cavity should be performed immediately.

3. After the pneumothorax has been decompressed, a thoracostomy tube is inserted and connected to 10 to 15 cm. negative water pressure (suction). In most cases the expansion of the lung will seal off the pulmonary leak. The chest tube can be removed within 24 to 36 hours after complete lung expansion and cessation of the pulmonary leak.

### Diaphragmatic Hernia

## Basic Principles

The cause of the diaphragmatic hernia is probably related to a fusion failure of pleural-peritoneal folds. The development of the intestine within the thoracic cavity in patients with posterolateral hernia not only leads to the development of a pulmonary hypoplasia on the involved side, but also to an inadequate development of the abdominal cavity.

The swallowing of air after delivery leads to a gaseous distention of the intestine. This explains the absence of findings immediately after birth, with increasing cyanosis and respiratory distress developing proportionately to the accumulation of gas within the intestine. Since the ipsilateral side is usually atelectatic, an arteriovenous shunt is present. With increased intestinal expansion within the chest, secondary interference with the ventilation of the contralateral lung can lead to a rapidly developing respiratory insufficiency. In patients with anterior mediastinal hernia, neither lung is compressed; symptoms are therefore minimal if present at all.

## Criteria for Diagnosis

### Posterolateral Diaphragmatic Hernia

1. Symptoms occur within the first few hours or days of life.

2. The extent of the herniation and the prognosis are related to the acuteness of the onset of symptoms.

3. Infants with apparent respiratory distress within several hours after delivery usually have the entire intestine within the hemithorax.

4. Depending on the side, either the liver or spleen may also reside within the thoracic cavity.

5. The newborn infant is asymptomatic until enough gas has entered the intestinal tract to lead to distention with symptoms and signs indistinguishable from a tension pneumothorax.

6. Not only is the involved, usually hypoplastic, lung compressed, the expansion of the gas-filled intestine leads to a mediastinal shift and compression of the contralateral lung.

7. This sequence leads to symptoms of rapid deterioration of respiratory efficiency.

8. In contrast to patients with tension pneumothorax or lobar emphysema, the abdomen of patients with posterolateral diaphragmatic hernia is scaphoid or flat.

9. Although bowel sounds may be present within the thoracic cavity on auscultation, their absence does not rule out the presence of a diaphragmatic hernia.

10. Blood gases will reveal a respiratory insufficiency with increased $pCO_2$ and decreased pH and arterial $pO_2$ in large hernias.

11. The accumulation of gas within the intestine, leading to mediastinal shift and contralateral pulmonary compression, is readily apparent on anteroposterior and lateral films.

## Differential Diagnosis

1. Diaphragmatic eventration
2. Phrenic nerve paralysis

## Management

1. The infant's intestinal tract should be decompressed through a nasogastric tube.

2. The treatment of the respiratory acidosis consists of endotracheal intubation and increased oxygenation, with rapid preparation for the operative procedure.

3. Type and crossmatch blood.

4. Venous cutdown

5. Emergency operation is rarely indicated for anterior diaphragmatic hernia but is indicated for all posterior hernias with respiratory distress.

6. Operation consists of reduction of the herniated viscera through an abdominal approach and closure of the diaphragmatic defect primarily or with a synthetic graft. Malrotation necessitating a Ladd procedure may be an associated finding.

7. *Postoperatively:*

A. Rapid expansion of the hypoplastic lung is contraindicated since pneumothorax may result.

B. A chest tube is placed on the involved side and connected to straight water-seal drainage without negative pressure.

C. The intestinal tract is decompressed to avoid distention and compression of the uninvolved lung.

D. Slow expansion of the lung over several days is preferred.

E. Prolonged endotracheal or nasotracheal intubation with ventilatory assistance and close attention to serial blood gases is indicated in all infants.

F. Nasogastric feedings should not be attempted until the respiratory condition has been stabilized.

G. Hyperalimentation may be necessary in the immediate postoperative phase.

## Postoperative Complications

1. Pneumothorax
2. Persistent pulmonary atelectasis with arteriovenous shunting
3. Intra-abdominal distention with secondary diaphragmatic elevation and respiratory embarrassment
4. Uncorrected malrotation with intestinal obstruction

# NEONATAL INTESTINAL OBSTRUCTION

## Basic Principles

The signs and symptoms of neonatal intestinal obstruction vary markedly depending on the site and cause of the obstruction, associated anomalies or secondary involvement of other systems. Numerous nonsurgical entities can lead to signs and symptoms suggestive of either intestinal obstruction or peritonitis which the pediatric surgeon must be familiar with. Although regurgitation is common in neonates, persistent vomiting, even if nonbiliary, is abnormal and should be investigated. Regurgitation, probably related to the incompetent gastroesophageal sphincter mechanism in neonates, results only in regurgitation of a small part of the ingested formula; it does not interfere with the baby's nutrition, development or state of hydration.

## Criteria for Diagnosis

1. The inability to feed
2. Biliary or persistent nonbiliary vomiting
3. Diffuse or partial abdominal distention
4. Abdominal tenderness
5. The presence of an abdominal mass
6. Inability to pass meconium or the presence of abnormal meconium
7. External gastrointestinal anomalies (imperforate anus, cloaca, gastroschisis)
8. Chest x-ray in supine and upright position and lateral decubitus abdominal films and contrast studies may be indicated.
9. Nonsurgical causes simulating intestinal obstruction should be ruled out.
   A. Neurogenic causes (subdural or cerebral hemorrhage)
   B. Sepsis
   C. Respiratory distress
   D. Cardiac anomalies
   E. Systemic causes (RH incompatibility, endocrine anomalies such as adrenogenital syndrome)
   F. Enteritis
   G. Enteropathies: disaccharide or protein
   H. Adynamic ileus

## Management

1. Nasogastric decompression
2. Measure serum electrolytes, blood gases, and serum and urine osmolarity.
3. Measure hematocrit, and white blood cell count.
4. Hydration
5. Measure urinary output.
6. Weight every 8 hours
7. *Rehydration.* The dehydration resulting from intestinal obstruction or peritonitis is usually an isotonic dehydration requiring isotonic rehydration. In patients with nonbiliary vomiting, chloride and hydrogen ions are lost in excess of sodium, leading to a metabolic alkalosis with a hypochloremia and hypokalemia. In patients with biliary vomiting, the acid–base state is usually normal or slightly acidotic. With marked abdominal distention, a superimposed respiratory acidosis may occur.
8. If Gastrografin is used, the osmotic pressure of Gastrografin has to be considered and adequate intravenous isotonic fluid administered to counteract this osmotic loss.
9. Type and crossmatch blood (including the mother's blood).
10. Give 1 mg. of vitamin K intramuscularly.
11. Temperature control
12. Respiratory assistance if diaphragmatic elevation exists
13. Broad-spectrum antibiotic coverage

## ESOPHAGEAL ATRESIA

### Definition

Atresia of the esophagus with or without associated tracheoesophageal fistula.

### Basic Principles

The most common type (80%) consists of an atresia of the upper esophagus with a tracheoesophageal fistula of the lower esophagus originating at the level of the carina. Other forms include esophageal atresia of both the upper and lower end, and tracheoesophageal fistula of the upper esophagus with atresia of the lower esophagus. Interference with fetal absorption of amniotic fluid leads to maternal polyhydramnios in over 40% of cases.

Associated anomalies are frequently found in the gastrointestinal, skeletal, and cardiac systems.

## Criteria for Diagnosis

### Clinical

1. History of maternal polyhydramnios
2. Excessive salivation
3. Inability to swallow
4. Inability to pass a nasogastric catheter
5. Aspiration or cyanosis during feeding
6. A scaphoid, gasless abdomen indicates that there is no lower tracheoesophageal fistula.
7. Gas in the abdomen indicates the presence of a fistula.

### X-ray

1. Anteroposterior and lateral chest films and abdominal flat film
2. Instillation of 1 ml. of contrast material (Lipiodal or Gastrografin) into the upper esophagus to determine the level of the atresia.

## Management

1. Nasoesophageal tube on intermittent suction
2. Type and crossmatch (including mother's blood)
3. Vitamin K, 1 mg. intramuscularly
4. Broad spectrum antibiotics
5. Venous cut-down with intravenous fluids 65 ml./kg./24 hours of a one-third isotonic solution (either all bicarbonate or half bicarbonate and half saline)
6. Operation in the full term infant with upper esophageal atresia and tracheoesophageal fistula includes:
   A. Ligation or transsection of the fistula
   B. End-to-end or end-to-side esophageal anastomosis
   C. Gastrostomy in difficult cases
   D. Drainage of the anastomotic site if it is extrapleural

E. Feedings may be started on the 4th postoperative day and progress to full feedings by the 6th day
F. Postoperative complications include:
   (1) Anastomotic leak
      (a) If an extrapleural dissection has been made these leaks will clear spontaneously with drainage.
      (b) After transpleural repair, a secondary repair is often necessary. If not possible, cervical esophagostomy, ligation of lower esophagus, and gastrostomy should be performed.
   (2) Recurrent tracheoesophageal fistula requiring secondary repair
   (3) Esophageal stenosis requiring retrograde dilation
7. In a premature infant primary repair may not be tolerated. Management is directed at preventing chemical pneumonitis by:
   A. Gastrostomy alone with esophageal suction
   B. Ligation of the tracheoesophageal fistula, gastrostomy and nasoesophageal suction
   C. Double ligation of the stomach with placement of proximal and distal gastrostomy tubes
8. In the full term infant without a fistula, operation consists of:
   A. Gastrostomy
   B. Measurement of length of gap by catheters in upper and lower esophagus
   C. In the presence of a large gap, the upper esophagus is dilated daily with a mercury-filled dilator
   D. Primary repair may be made if the gap is small or has been reduced significantly by stretching.
   E. If the gap is too large, a secondary colonic interposition may be necessary.

## CONGENITAL PYLORIC STENOSIS

## Definition

Congenital pyloric stenosis is hypertrophy of the muscles surrounding the pyloric canal, leading to mechanical gastric outlet obstruction.

## Basic Principles

The etiology is unknown but the previously accepted theory of aganglionosis has been discarded. Since pyloric stenosis is known to have an increased incidence within families, a genetic tendency can therefore be assumed. It is most often seen in first-born males and usually apparent at 2 to 3 weeks of age. The hypertrophy of the pyloric muscles leads to a gastric outlet obstruction with resulting projectile nonbiliary vomiting, usually within 20 to 30 minutes after feeding. Gastric fluid loss leads to a hypochloremic, hypokalemic alkalosis and dehydration.

## Criteria for Diagnosis

### Clinical

1. Nonbiliary projectile vomiting, usually at 2 to 3 weeks of age
2. Failure to thrive
3. Loss of weight
4. Visible gastric peristalsis
5. A palpable olive-shaped mass in the epigastrium
6. Occasional coffee-ground or slightly blood-stained vomiting
7. Occasionally mild jaundice
8. Dehydration

### Laboratory

Serum electrolyte values are compatible with a hypochloremic, hypokalemic alkalosis.

### X-ray

1. Gastric distention
2. Contrast material swallow shows a "string sign" or "railroad track," gastric retention and gastric hyperperistalsis.

## Management

1. *Correction of Dehydration and Alkalosis.* Dehydration and alkalosis can be corrected by initial administration of isotonic saline, followed by two-thirds isotonic saline and finally half isotonic saline with potassium after urinary output has been established. The total amount of fluid given ranges between 2,500 to 3,000 ml./square meter of body surface/24 hours and correction can usually be accomplished within a 24 hour period.

2. Nasogastric decompression to reduce gastric distention

3. Type and crossmatch blood (although blood is rarely given, bleeding may occur following the pyloromyotomy).

4. Intake and output measurement

5. Weight every 8 hours

6. *Operative Procedure*

A. The Fredet-Ramstedt pyloromyotomy is the accepted procedure of choice through either a right transverse muscle-spreading incision or a right upper paramedian incision.

B. The pyloric tumor is mobilized and a serosal incision is followed by division of the muscle bands until the mucosa can be inspected. Failure to completely divide the muscle on the gastric side is more common as a cause for recurrent stenosis than failure to divide the most distal duodenal muscular fibers.

C. If a perforation of the distal mucosa should occur, it is closed with 5-0 atraumatic silk and an omental patch.

D. *Postoperative Treatment*

*(1)* If no perforation has occurred, the nasogastric tube is removed within 8 hours postoperatively and feedings are started in the following manner: 20 ml. of dextrose and water every 2 hours twice, followed by 30 ml. of full-strength formula every 3 hours until the first postoperative day. On the first postoperative day, 45 ml. of full-strength formula are given every 3 hours, on the second day 60 ml. every 3 hours and on the third day 90 ml. every 3 hours. Standard demand feeding can then be initiated on the fourth postoperative day. If vomiting occurs during the feeding, the intake is stepped back to one of the preceding smaller feedings.

*(2)* If a duodenal perforation was observed during the operative procedure and the perforation was closed as described

above, nasogastric decompression is maintained for 24 hours and feedings are then started at the same intervals as outlined previously.

Intravenous fluids can usually be discontinued when the infant tolerates 60 ml. of feeding every 3 hours.

## Complications

1. *Unrecognized Duodenal Perforation.* Development of postoperative ileus or peritonitis should lead to the suspicion of an unrecognized duodenal perforation. Immediate laparotomy and repair of the perforation is indicated and postoperative feedings should only be resumed after the infant has recovered from his peritonitis.

2. *Intra-abdominal Bleeding.* Occasionally, bleeding may occur either from transected pyloric veins or the muscle mass itself. This is rare and usually self-limiting but may occasionally require blood transfusion postoperatively.

3. *Postoperative Persistent Vomiting.* Postoperative vomiting in patients, especially with long-standing pyloric stenosis, is not uncommon but usually subsides within one or two days. If continuous vomiting persists for more than one week and x-ray studies show unimproved gastric obstruction, the patient should be re-explored. In most cases an inadequate division of the hypertrophic muscle will be found, especially at the proximal gastric side of the pyloric tumor. These fibers should be completely divided and the infant should then be placed back on routine postoperative feedings.

4. *Hiatal Hernia, Peptic Ulcer or Obstructive Jaundice.* Although hiatal hernias, peptic ulcers and jaundice have been found in association with pyloric stenosis, they are rare and investigations of these conditions are only indicated if appropriate symptoms should occur.

## DUODENAL OBSTRUCTION

### Basic Principles

Duodenal atresia can be caused by webs, diaphragms or annular pancreas. Obstruction associated with malrotation is discussed subsequently.

## Criteria for Diagnosis

### Clinical

1. Persistent biliary vomiting
2. Upper abdominal distention with scaphoid lower abdomen
3. Inability to retain feedings
4. *Common Associated Anomalies:* Down's syndrome, trisomy, history of maternal hydramnios

### Laboratory

1. Isotonic or hypotonic dehydration
2. Hypovolemia
3. *Metabolic State:* normal or mild to moderate metabolic acidosis

### X-ray

1. Double bubble sign with gastric and duodenal gas bubble, usually with two fluid levels on the upright film
2. Contrast studies usually are not indicated. The presence of a microcolon usually indicates a low intestinal obstruction.

## Management

1. Nasogastric tube to gravity drainage with frequent intermittent irrigation with 1 to 2 ml. of saline
2. Venous cutdown
3. *Intravenous Fluids.* If no significant metabolic acidosis or hypovolemia exists, a solution of one-third isotonic, half bicarbonate and half saline, at 65 to 85 ml./kg. of body weight is adequate. Potassium chloride at 3 mEq./kg. of body weight per day is to be added after urinary output is adequate.
4. Maintain temperature by the use of a heated Isolet, overhead heater or a thermal mattress.
5. Type and crossmatch blood (including the mother's blood).
6. Respiratory support by use of the reverse Trendelenberg position

7. Broad-spectrum antibiotics
8. *Operative Procedure*
   A. *Diaphragmatic Web*
   *(1)* Diaphragmatic webs are notoriously difficult to diagnose since they are often pliable.
   *(2)* A duodenostomy should be performed at the most dependent portion of the duodenal dilatation.
   *(3)* If a duodenal web is found, excision of the web via the duodenostomy, followed by a transverse closure, is acceptable
   *(4)* If there is a simultaneous narrowing of the duodenum, an end-to-side duodenojejunostomy is the procedure of choice.
   B. *Duodenal Atresia or Stenosis.* A duodenojejunostomy with a short retrocolic jejunal loop should be performed.
   C. *Annular Pancreas*
   *(1)* The fusion of the dorsal and ventral anlage of the pancreas is often accompanied by anomalies of the pancreatic duct.
   *(2)* A division of the anlage of the pancreas is absolutely contraindicated.
   *(3)* The treatment of choice, as in duodenal atresia, consists of duodenojejunostomy.
9. Duodenojejunostomies should be accompanied by a gastrostomy with a small jejunal feeding tube introduced through the gastrostomy and threaded through the duodenojejunostomy into the upper jejunum.
10. In patients with marked dilatation of the obstructed duodenum, peristaltic activity often does not resume until the second or third week postoperatively.
11. To avoid the necessity of parenteral alimentation, intestinal feeding can be resumed after the third to fourth postoperative day via the jejunostomy, until duodenal peristalsis has returned to normal.

## Postoperative Management

1. *Gastrointestinal decompression* via gravity drainage through the gastrostomy tube
2. *Intravenous Fluids.* Unless there are marked electrolyte deficiencies or acid–base disturbances, a one-third isotonic solution, usually half saline and half bicarbonate with 3 mEq. of potassium per kg./ of body weight per day, is appropriate. The total fluid volume should be approximately 85 to 100 ml./kg. Gastrostomy drainage should be replaced by a two-thirds isotonic saline solution with 20 mEq. of potassium chloride per 1,000 ml. of gastric drainage.
3. *Respiratory Support.* Infants with abdominal distention tend to have an associated respiratory insufficiency due to the interference of diaphragmatic motion. Adequate gastrointestinal decompression may alleviate the pressure on the diaphragm. The positioning of the infant in a reversed Trendelenberg position can further reduce diaphragmatic interference by avoiding the pressure of abdominal organs. The increase of oxygen concentration to 40 per cent also may improve the respiratory status.
4. *Temperature.* An attempt should be made to avoid hypothermia which may further increase the patient's oxygen requirement and caloric expenditure. This can be achieved by increasing the environmental temperature as noted previously.
5. *Intake and Output.* Gastrostomy drainage, urinary output and the infant's weight should be measured at 8-hour intervals. Blood gases and electrolytes are done immediately postoperatively and at 1- to 2-day intervals.
6. *Antibiotic Treatment.* If the postoperative course is uneventful, antibiotics can be terminated one week postoperatively.
7. *Tube-Jejunostomy Feedings.* If the immediate postoperative course is uneventful, tube-jejunostomy feedings can be started on the third or fourth postoperative day as follows: 3 to 4 ml. of dextrose and water or a balanced electrolyte solution

every 2 hours, with an increase of 1 to 2 ml. per feeding over the next two days. Within 4 to 5 days, the infant usually will tolerate his ideal oral formula intake (2½ ounces of standard formula per pound of body weight in 24 hours).

8. *Gastrostomy Tube.* After the gastrostomy drainage declines to approximately 15 to 20 ml. per 8-hour period, the gastrostomy is elevated to about 15 to 20 cm. above the gastric level. It is not clamped, however, to allow overflow.

9. *Resumption of Oral Feedings.* If the infant tolerates the elevated gastrostomy without spillage, oral feedings are begun slowly, and simultaneously the jejunostomy feedings are decreased. After the infant has assumed complete oral intake, the gastrostomy tube can be removed, but not earlier than 3 weeks postoperatively, to assure adherence of the stomach to the abdominal wall.

## Postoperative Complications

1. *Functional Obstruction.* In spite of a patent anastomosis, the dilated end of the duodenum may prevent the recurrence of normal peristaltic activity for up to 2 or 3 weeks. Continuous high nasogastric output or inability to tolerate feedings should therefore not necessarily be interpreted as mechanical obstruction of the anastomosis.

2. *Anastomosis.* A leak of the anastomosis usually becomes apparent around the fourth or fifth postoperative day with signs of peritonitis or sepsis. Immediate re-exploration and reanastomosis or exteriorization are indicated.

3. *Additional Sites of Obstruction.* Unless saline is injected into the distal segment, additional areas of atresia can easily be overlooked and may not become apparent until peristalsis has recurred postoperatively. The clinical picture is then compatible with either a postoperative obstruction or jejunal or ileal atresia.

4. *Pulmonary Aspiration.* Unless a satisfactory nasogastric decompression or gastrostomy is utilized, postoperative aspiration is likely to occur in view of the incompetent esophagogastric barrier in the infant.

## MALROTATION

### Definition

Malrotation is the failure of the intestine to perform the normal 270-degree counterclockwise rotation on its return into the abdominal cavity in uterine life.

### Basic Principles

Although the type of nonrotation or malrotation can vary markedly (Grob classification 1 to 4), the essential features are usually similar in most patients.

1. A partial obstruction of the duodenum due to extrinsic bands

2. A persistent or intermittent obstruction due to volvulus of the small intestine caused by the lack of adequate mesenteric attachment of the small intestine

3. Lack of the mesenteric fixation leads to a volvulus of the small intestine around its axis: the superior mesenteric artery and vein. The volvulus leads to a strangulating obstruction with the intestine encircling the stalk of the mesentery, very often in a double or triple ring formation. Pressure exerted on the superior mesenteric vessels allows arterial inflow but prevents venous return, resulting first in congestion, followed by hemorrhagic infarction.

The volvulus usually occurs in a clockwise rotation; a counterclockwise rotation is therefore required at operation to relieve the obstruction. If infarction of the intestine occurs, it usually involves jejunum, ileum and occasionally the ascending and transverse colon, thus leading to an unacceptable loss of intestine if resection has to be performed. Although the incidence of volvulus is highest in the neonatal period, it can also occur later in childhood or even in adulthood. Associated internal hernias are occasionally present and should be looked for. The diagnosis of malrotation and volvulus can be extremely difficult, since the volvulus may be intermittent and therefore difficult to diagnose clinically. Clinical findings, as well as x-ray findings, in the early phase of a volvulus may be misleading, since the gas pattern and the small bowel distal to the volvulus may appear normal.

Clinical suspicion should be aroused in any patient with intermittent biliary vomiting in the absence of either sepsis, brain damage or typical findings of intestinal obstruction.

## Criteria for Diagnosis

### Clinical

1. Intermittent or persistent biliary vomiting
2. Absence of abdominal distention with either duodenal obstruction due to bands or early volvulus
3. Biliary vomiting and abdominal distention with volvulus and beginning congestion or infarction
4. Biliary vomiting, abdominal distention and abdominal tenderness and melena—indication of either marked congestion or infarction due to volvulus
5. Biliary vomiting, abdominal distention, melena and shock indicates a volvulus with infarction of the intestine and/or septicemic shock

### X-ray

Supine and upright films of the abdomen may show a dilated duodenum or an irregular small bowel pattern, often limited to the right side of the abdomen.

2. While abdominal x-rays may be normal in the presence of a malrotation with resulting volvulus and obstruction, contrast studies are usually diagnostic:

A. *Barium Enema.* The cecum is often found in the right hypochondrium, midabdomen or occasionally the left abdomen.

B. *Upper Intestinal Contrast Studies.* Upper gastrointestinal studies may show a dilated duodenum due to extrinsic bands and/or an anomalous position of the duodenojejunal junction, usually to the right side of the vertebra. In patients with volvulus, a duodenal obstruction can usually be found at the third or fourth portion of the duodenum on the right side of the vertebra.

## Management

In contrast to other intestinal obstructions, where the patient can usually be prepared for surgery with safety over a 24-hour period, once the diagnosis of malrotation and volvulus has been made, the patient should be explored immediately, correcting the hypovolemia if congestion or infaction has occured.

1. Nasogastric tube
2. Type and crossmatch blood.
3. Venous cutdown
4. *Intravenous Fluids.* Isotonic solutions (colloid and/or blood) are given to correct the hypovolemia, the type and amount depending on the patient's clinical appearance (signs of dehydration, hypovolemia or hemorrhagic shock).
5. Administration of whole blood if melena has occurred
6. Immediate exploration
7. *Operation*

A. The abdomen is opened through a right transverse incision just above the umbilicus.

B. The small intestine is eviscerated and, in patients with a volvulus, a double or triple twist around the superior mesenteric artery and vein is usually readily apparent. This occurs usually in a clockwise rotation and is therefore untwisted in a counterclockwise rotation.

C. After the volvulus has been untwisted and viability of the intestine appears intact, the cecum is mobilized and possible bands from the cecum crossing the duodenum are transected.

D. The duodenum is then freed and the duodenojejunal junction is placed in a straight line from the right upper to the right lower quadrant.

E. The large bowel is mobilized and

the entire large bowel, including cecum, is placed to the left side of the abdomen with the cecum in the left upper quadrant.

F. A routine appendectomy may help to create adhesions around the cecum. Fixation of either cecum or duodenum is rarely necessary.

G. If there is a questionable viability of the intestine, resection should be avoided as long as any hope for recovery exists, since the questionable area usually involves the entire small intestine and often part of the colon. In these patients the intestine should be returned into the abdominal cavity and an indwelling high jejunal catheter (Witzel-type jejunostomy) can be used to drip antibiotics into the intestinal lumen. This may help to lead to a recovery of the intestine, which should be re-examined within 24 to 48 hours following the primary exploration. In an occasional patient, part of the intestine may have recovered and the remaining devitalized portion can then be resected.

## Postoperative Management

1. Nasogastric tube to gravity drainage or low intermittent suction with frequent irrigations
2. *Intravenous Fluids.* If the dehydration and hypovolemia have been corrected pre- or intra-operatively, a one-half to one-third isotonic solution, usually with bicarbonate to counteract the frequently found metabolic acidosis, is given at approximately 2,500 ml./square meter of body surface/24 hours or at 100 to 150 ml./kg./day in infants below 1 week of age.
3. If there is any evidence of questionable viability, the patient should be kept in a 40 per cent oxygen concentration and care should be taken to avoid dehydration or hypovolemia to ensure adequate intestinal perfusion.
4. Postoperative hematocrit determinations
5. Broad-spectrum systemic antibiotics
6. Intraluminal antibiotics if there is any question of infarction
7. Careful examination for the development of peritonitis if there was questionable viability. If peritonitis should develop, re-exploration with re-evaluation of the viability of the intestines should be done immediately.
8. If major resection is necessary, an attempt should be made to preserve as much terminal ileum as possible since this is the major area of fluid absorption. When more than 6 to 8 cm. of terminal ileum can be preserved, nutrition and development should be adequate even though the immediate postoperative course may be difficult due to persistent diarrhea.

In the early postoperative period, high-protein and low-fat diet will increase intestinal absorption. Determination of the fecal pH may help in estimating the tolerance to ingested fat. (After major intestinal resection, unabsorbed fat will lead to a decrease in intestinal absorption due to the formation of fatty acids, with resulting low pH. Therefore, a decrease in fat intake often is essential.)

Elemental diet and/or parenteral hyperalimentation can assist in the early postoperative phase.

## SMALL BOWEL ATRESIA

### Definition

Small bowel atresia is complete obstruction of the small intestine by either single or *multiple* points of atresia.

### Basic Principles

The majority of small intestinal atresias are thought to be due to vascular accidents in uterine life. The atresia is often accompanied by an absence of a portion of the intestine, variable in size, in the presence of abnormal mesenteric vessels. Although most intestinal atresia are single, additional, sometimes multiple, areas of atresia do occur and should be ruled out in any patient with an intestinal atresia. The most common site of intestinal atresia other than the duodenum is the ileum, followed by the jejunum, but rarely seen in the colon. The proximal end is usually extremely dilated and therefore unable to resume immediate postoperative peristalsis after an end-to-end anastomosis has been performed. If possible, therefore, the dilated bulbous end of the atretic segment should be excised to allow earlier recurrence of intestinal activity. Associated diseases, such as mucoviscidosis, should be ruled out at the time of operation or evaluated postoperatively.

## Criteria for Diagnosis

### Clinical

1. Biliary vomiting
2. Inability to tolerate feedings
3. Abdominal distention (if obstruction is low)
4. Occasionally failure to evacuate meconium
5. Signs of dehydration

### Laboratory

1. Serum and electrolyte values usually indicate either isotonic or hypotonic dehydration and a mild metabolic acidosis.
2. The hematocrit usually is elevated due to dehydration.

### X-ray

1. Depending on the level of obstruction, a varying number of distended intestinal loops are visible with differential fluid levels in the upright position.
2. In low small bowel obstructions (most common site, ileum), a differential diagnosis between low small bowel versus large bowel atresia or obstruction may be difficult, unless gas is found in the rectum.
3. Distinction between small and large bowel or simple abdominal x-ray studies without contrast is extremely difficult in infancy.
4. In high jejunal obstruction, a triple bubble, similar to the one seen in duodenal obstruction but with a third air-fluid-filled loop, may be apparent.
5. Barium enema may show a microcolon in low small bowel obstruction.

## Management

1. Nasogastric tube to low gravity drainage
2. Venous cutdown
3. *Intravenous Fluids.* If the diagnosis has been made promptly and there is no evidence of dehydration, one-third isotonic fluid will be adequate. In the presence of dehydration, isotonic or one-half isotonic solutions may be used initially. After correction of the hypovolemic dehydration, one-third isotonic solution can be used.

Since these infants often are in a mild to moderate metabolic acidosis, proportional to the duration of obstruction, either a bicarbonate solution or a solution composed of half saline and half bicarbonate may be indicated
4. Potassium chloride is added when urinary output is stable. Replacement of nasogastric suction is accomplished with a two-thirds isotonic solution with 20 mEq. of potassium chloride per 1,000 ml. of nasogastric fluid.
5. Type and crossmatch blood.
6. *X-rays.* Abdomen and chest, supine and upright. In patients with low small intestinal obstruction, where the diagnosis may be difficult, a barium enema should be obtained. The presence of a microcolon usually indicates a low small intestinal obstruction.
7. *Operative Procedure*
    A. The abdomen is opened through a high transverse incision.
    B. The small intestine is eviscerated and the site of atresia identified.
    C. The dilated end should be resected, unless too much intestine would be lost, with a simultaneous decompression of the upper obstructed intestine.
    D. The distal intestine is opened, and saline is injected to rule out further distal obstructions.
    E. An end-to-end anastomosis can be performed in most instances. If there is a marked disparity in size, however, an end-upper-to-side-lower anastomosis may be preferable.

F. Other techniques include those of Bishop-Koop or Santulli.

## MECONIUM ILEUS

### Definition

Abnormality in exocrine secretion, involving multiple organ systems, can lead to "meconium ileus," with inspissation of meconium and secondary mechanical obstruction, usually located within the ileum. The obstruction can lead to perforation, intra-uterine meconium peritonitis, meconium cyst, intestinal atresia and intestinal volvulus.

### Basic Principles

Meconium ileus is one of the manifestations of a generalized hereditary disease involving exocrine glands. All glands appear to be involved, including the sweat, salivary, lacrimal and exocrine pancreatic glands, the intestine and respiratory system. Meconium ileus *per se* results from the abnormally inspissated meconium leading to obstruction. Associated diseases include:

1. Pulmonary involvement with repeated pneumonia
2. Hepatic involvement leading to cirrhosis
3. Malabsorption of the intestine
4. An increased incidence of peptic ulcers in patients who display little if any symptoms of cystic fibrosis has also been reported.

### Criteria for Diagnosis

#### Clinical

1. Meconium ileus presents as low small intestinal obstruction with abdominal distention and biliary vomiting.
2. The meconium, if passed at all, is usually gray in color and desiccated.
3. On abdominal examination, doughy intestinal loops can occasionally be palpated.
4. In view of the genetic trend, a familial history of cystic fibrosis may help in the clinical diagnosis.

5. The abnormality of the exocrine secretion can be substantiated by a "sweat chloride test," with a chloride content over 60 mEq. per liter diagnostic for cystic fibrosis. False negatives do occur, however, especially in the early weeks of infancy.
6. Precipitation of the meconium with 1% trichloracetic acid added to an extract of meconium is also diagnostic.
7. The absence of trypsin in the meconium, although suggestive, is not diagnostic.

#### X-ray

Flat and upright examinations of the abdomen reveal a pattern of intestinal obstruction with multiple dilated intestinal loops and a stepladder pattern of fluid levels. Variations in the size of intestinal loops and a coarse, foamy and granular-appearing intestine are suggestive of meconium ileus as well as the presence of calcified meconium cysts.

#### Differential Diagnosis

1. Other forms of low intestinal obstruction such as ileal atresia, megacolon and occasionally meconium plug
2. Intra-uterine perforation with secondary calcification or formation of a meconium cyst may occur in entities other than meconium ileus and can therefore be mistaken for mucoviscidosis.

### Management

1. Regardless of the severity of the intestinal involvement, attention should be paid to the precarious pulmonary condition. Broad-spectrum antibiotic coverage, liquefaction of the bronchial secretions and avoidance of cross-contamination, especially in the early postoperative phase, are necessary.
2. In patients in whom the inspissated meconium leads to an obstruction within the colon rather than the ileum, an enema of Gastrografin may help to dislodge the inspissated meconium due to its osmotic pull. Instillation of 4% acetylcysteine also has been recommended.

3. *Operative Procedure*

A. An attempt should be made at the time of operation to liquefy the meconium distal to the obstruction by the instillation of either acetylcysteine, saline or Gastrografin.

The use of hydrogen peroxide, although effective in removing inspissated meconium, is dangerous because of possible embolism which has been reported following intraluminal instillation of hydrogen peroxide.

B. If there is any evidence of inspissated meconium distal to the area of resection, an end-to-side Bishop-Koop anastomosis is preferable to an end-to-end anastomosis, since it will allow drainage of the upper intestine with slow, gradual liquefaction of the meconium distal to the anastomosis. The instillation of pancreatic enzymes into the distal part can assist the restoration of intestinal continuity.

C. Perforation or volvulus may require extensive resections.

## Complications

1. Anastomotic leak
2. Prolonged mechanical obstruction distal to the anastomosis due to the inspissated meconium
3. Pulmonary infection
4. Intestinal malabsorption
5. Cirrhosis

## MECONIUM PLUG

## Definition

Meconium plug is low intestinal obstruction in neonates due to inspissated meconium.

## Basic Principles

The meconium plug syndrome occurs in neonates, predominantly premature infants, who fail to evacuate meconium during the first 24 to 48 hours of life. The meconium, in contrast to patients with mucoviscidosis, is chemically normal. However, mucoviscidosis and aganglionosis have been reporated in in-fants with meconium plugs and should be ruled out.

## Criteria for Diagnosis

1. Failure to evacuate meconium
2. Abdominal distention
3. Biliary vomiting, rare if diagnosed early and treated appropriately
4. Supine and upright films are compatible with a low intestinal obstruction.
5. Barium enema usually demonstrates the obstructing meconium plug in the sigmoid colon but it can be present in the right colon and occasionally in the ileum. The barium enema is not only diagnostic but usually curative.

## Management

1. The management should be non-operative. If the diagnosis is suspected clinically, saline enemas often will suffice to expel the meconium plug and to alleviate the obstructive symptoms.

2. If the infant does not respond to saline enemas, contrast enema is usually diagnostic and therapeutic. Instead of barium, Gastrografin has been recommended, which, in view of its high osmolality, dislodges the meconium plug by attracting fluid into the bowel.

3. An occasional child with Hirschsprung's disease may present with a meconium plug; therefore, a clinical follow-up examination of all infants with meconium plug is recommended over several weeks to rule out Hirschsprung's disease.

## HIRSCHSPRUNG'S DISEASE

## Definition

Hirschsprung's disease refers to a lack of ganglion cells, usually in the lower portion of the colon, resulting in obstruction and dilatation of the proximal normally inner-vated colon.

## Basic Principles

The vast majority of patients with Hirschsprung's disease present with an aganglionosis of the rectum and sigmoid. The aganglionic segment, always involving the most distal part of the colon, can involve the entire colon, however, and in rare instances the entire intestine. Involvement of the entire intestine is incompatible with life.

Ganglion cells in the fetus develop in a cephalad-caudad fashion. Regardless of the level of the disappearance of ganglion cells, it is unlikely that ganglion cells can be found distal to this area. Although "skip areas" have been reported, their occurrence is either unlikely or extremely rare. The marked proximal dilatation can occasionally lead to perforation. The common cause of death consists of development of enterocolitis, unless treated immediately by either nonoperative or operative decompression. Breast-fed infants with Hirschsprung's disease are less likely to develop enterocolitis.

## Criteria for Diagnosis

### Clinical

1. *In Infancy*
   A. Although the lack of ganglion cells leads to obstruction, the newborn usually presents with obstipation, marked abdominal distention *and* often alternating diarrhea.
   B. On rectal examination, fecal material is often expelled with force.
   C. Although perforation of the large bowel in the ganglionic area can occur, it is rare in the absence of enterocolitis. The combination of obstructive symptoms, abdominal distention, a history of obstipation or constipation, together with signs of peritonitis or sepsis, is characteristic of enterocolitis, the most dangerous complication of Hirschsprung's disease.
2. *In the Older Child*
   A. In the older child, the primary symptoms consist of marked constipation or obstipation, with abdominal distention, reduced physical development and underweight.
   B. Encopresis (anal incontinence) is

rarely found in children with Hirschsprung's disease and is highly suggestive of a functional megacolon.

3. *Family History.* There is a genetic trend in Hirschsprung's disease and a history of other siblings having had Hirschsprung's disease should alert the physician examining a child with marked constipation or obstipation.

### X-ray

1. Supine and upright films in infancy are rarely diagnostic, but compatible with low intestinal obstruction.
2. Barium enema, while not always diagnostic in infancy, usually shows a normal-appearing aganglionic segment with a marked dilatation of the proximal normally innervated intestine. If Hirschsprung's disease is suspected, no cleansing enemas should be given prior to the barium enema. The cleansing enema produces a partial evacuation of the rectal ampulla and sigmoid, giving the appearance of a nondilated lower rectum and sigmoid, compatible with Hirschsprung's disease. Dilatation of the sigmoid and rectum to the level of the sphincter is characteristic of functional megacolon and not Hirschsprung's disease.

### Differential Diagnosis

1. Functional megacolon with ganglion cells present can be found in a variety of entities. These include endocrine deficiencies, such as hypothyroidism and mental retardation as found in Down's syndrome or in association with psychological problems. In patients with Hirschsprung's disease, symptoms usually can be traced back to infancy, whereas in patients with psychogenic megacolon, the symptoms usually develop after the first year of life.

2. Mechanical obstruction after repair of an imperforate anus also can lead to the development of megacolon. In a small percentage of patients with imperforate anus, a simultaneous low aganglionic segment has been reported.

## Associated Anomalies

The majority of infants with Hirschsprung's disease have no other major congenital anomalies. Although an increased incidence of obstructive uropathy, ranging from megabladder, megalo-ureter to hydronephrosis, has been reported in patients with Hirschsprung's disease, obstructive uropathy is also seen in patients with functional megacolon and is probably due to the pressure effect of the dilated colon rather than due to a ganglionic deficiency of the urinary tract.

## Management

1. The treatment of Hirschsprung's disease, after clinical and radiographic confirmation, is elective surgical repair.

2. Emergency colostomy is indicated only for enterocolitis not responding to conservative treatment (*see* Enterocolitis with Hirschsprung's Disease, p. 536).

3. Colostomy for obstruction should be placed in a ganglionic area. The colostomy should be decompressed immediately following the operation, either by maturation or by placing a large bore catheter into the colostomy for 24 hours. Failure to decompress the colostomy can lead to the development of a postoperative enterocolitis.

## NEONATAL PERITONITIS

### Definition

Neonatal peritonitis is chemical or bacterial peritonitis in the neonate caused by a variety of conditions listed below.

### Classification

1. Bacterial (i. e., following intestinal perforation)

2. Chemical (i. e., gastric or biliary perforation)

3. Hemorrhagic (i. e., after rupture of hepatic lesions such as hemangioma or tumor)

## Basic Principles

### Etiology

Gastric perforations are most often found in the first week of life, often following either a traumatic delivery or preceded by a history of anoxia and resuscitation. They are assumed to be related to the "diving reflex," with hypoxia, decreased cardiac output, mesenteric shunting with decreased intestinal flow, high viscosity of the infant's blood leading to local hypoxic changes with subsequent necrosis and perforation. Resuscitation of an infant born with a low Apgar score is assumed to play a contributing factor in gastric perforation due to gastric overdistention following respiratory resuscitation.

Similar factors such as the "diving reflex" may be the cause of single or multiple enteric perforations in the neonate, but perforations of small and large bowel are also seen in the presence of acute necrotizing enterocolitis. In many instances, an associated coagulopathy can either be apparent at the time of the perforation or shortly thereafter. Occasionally an intestinal perforation can be secondary to a distal obstruction such as in Hirschsprung's disease.

Peritonitis in the neonate leads to a rapid impairment of the infant's hemodynamic and respiratory system. The fluid loss into the intra-abdominal cavity results in an acute hypovolemia and decreased cardiac output, usually with an isotonic dehydration and metabolic acidosis. Diaphragmatic splinting secondary to peritonitis will result in an impairment of the respiratory function and an associated respiratory acidosis. While the degree of either metabolic or respiratory acidosis will vary with the extent of the peritonitis, both factors have to be considered in the immediate treatment of the infant.

In most infants the danger of septicemia is acute and the patient should be treated immediately with broad-spectrum antibiotics. In some infants with peritonitis, intravascular coagulopathy can occur and become evident at the height or the end of the peritonitis.

## Criteria for Diagnosis

1. The diagnosis of peritonitis, especially in the early phase, may be extremely complicated in the newborn since abdominal rigidity and guarding may be either absent or difficult to detect.

2. The patient's general appearance, pallor, tachycardia, tachypnea or inability to maintain temperature may be suggestive of peritonitis but can also be seen in infants with sepsis and secondary ileus.

3. The most characteristic abnormal findings consist of abdominal tenderness, signs of abdominal pain, including irritability, or crying when the infant's legs, which are usually flexed, are straightened out.

4. Distention of the abdomen and a shiny, stretched skin, occasionally with engorged veins, also suggest peritonitis.

5. Discoloration around the umbilicus may be a clue to the presence of intra-abdominal bleeding.

6. Leukocytosis may or may not be present.

7. With either a long-standing or marked peritonitis, signs of a combined metabolic and respiratory acidosis are present.

8. The irritation of the diaphragm may lead to a tachypnea which may be more apparent than the abdominal findings.

9. Abdominal films reveal dilated intestinal loops similar to those seen in the ileus. Thickening of the bowel wall and the presence of free fluid in the peritoneal cavity favor the diagnosis of peritonitis over gastrointestinal ileus. The fluid levels seen in the intestine are similar to those seen in ileus; the stepladder pattern found in intestinal obstruction is lacking. The presence of free air, best seen in the upright position or lateral decubitus position, indicates that an intestinal perforation has occurred.

10. Differential diagnosis includes general sepsis, adynamic ileus, brain damage, mechanical obstruction and electrolyte imbalance.

## Management

1. Restoration of the hypovolemia and isotonic dehydration with isotonic crystalloid solutions and/or colloids and blood

2. Blood may be indicated primarily in infants whose peritonitis is accompanied by massive blood loss, such as in patients with intra-abdominal bleeding or patients with infarction of the intestine.

3. The fluid therapy usually consists of an initial loading dose of 350 ml. per square meter of body surface area in 45 minutes or 10 to 20 ml. of isotonic fluid per kilogram of body weight.

4. The rate of the continuous hydration is determined by the patient's response, including pulse rate, respiratory rate and urinary output, and usually requires a fluid maintenance of approximately 2,500 ml. per square meter of body surface area/24 hrs.

5. In infants with a large amount of free air within the peritoneal cavity, tapping of the abdomen may relieve the tension in the abdomen and increase respiratory efficiency.

6. Nasogastric decompression in an attempt to prevent further increased abdominal distention should be accomplished as soon as a peritonitis is suspected.

7. Broad-spectrum antibiotics should be instituted as soon as the diagnosis of septicemia or peritonitis is suspected.

8. Maintenance of the patient's temperature to reduce the already increased caloric expenditure of the infant is important

## GASTRIC PERFORATION

### Definition

Gastric perforation refers to single or multiple perforations of the stomach.

## Basic Principles

There is a preceding history of hypoxia during delivery or a low Apgar score, often followed by resuscitation, with perforation at approximately the fifth day of life. Most perforations occur as a single linear tear of the stomach, but multiple areas of perforation and diffuse necrosis can also occur.

## Criteria for Diagnosis

### Clinical

1. Abdominal distention, tenderness, hyper- or hypothermia, ashy appearance, tachycardia and tachypnea
2. In contrast to patients with intestinal obstruction or ileus, infants with large gastric perforations are often unable to vomit, and the lack of vomiting in the presence of peritonitis may suggest gastric perforation.

### Laboratory

Findings compatible with peritonitis

### X-ray

1. Supine films show a pattern of adynamic ileus and occasionally free air outlining the falciform ligament.
2. In the upright film, the air is usually seen under the diaphragm, with fluid levels outside the intestinal lumen. Free air can also be seen on lateral decubitus film.
3. The nasogastric tube is occasionally outside the confinement of the stomach.

## Management

1. Nasogastric tube
2. Abdominal tap if a large amount of free air is present
3. Venous cutdown with isotonic rehydration. In infants without marked acidosis, normal saline can be used as the initial solution; in the presence of marked acidosis, half saline and half bicarbonate can be used. Potassium should be added after renal output has been re-established.
4. Broad-spectrum antibiotics
5. Operative repair as soon as the infant has been fully prepared for surgery

6. Operation may consist of simple closure or resection, depending on the number of ulcers and degree of associated gastric necrosis. A gastrostomy should be done following simple repair.

Central (sleeve) resection of the stomach may be done for diffuse necrosis with the addition of esophageal and duodenal catheters in the closed proximal and distal ends. Subsequent anastomosis can be made when the patient's condition has improved.

## Postoperative Management

1. Gastric decompression via a gastrostomy tube until all signs of peritonitis have disappeared
2. Intravenous fluids in accordance with the state of the peritonitis and the infant's general condition
3. Broad-spectrum antibiotics
4. Institution of gastrostomy feedings after the infant has recovered, to be followed by oral feedings once the gastrostomy feedings are being tolerated. The gastrostomy should be left in place for approximately three weeks to allow the stomach to adhere to the anterior abdominal wall.

## Complications

1. Breakdown of the gastric repair
2. Sepsis
3. Leaking gastrostomy
4. Perforation of additional hypoxic areas of the stomach, not detected at the time of the original operation
5. Aspiration pneumonia

## ENTERIC PERFORATION

### Definition

Single or multiple small bowel and/or large bowel perforation.

### Basic Principles

Single or multiple small or large bowel perforations may be caused by hypoxic episodes or distal obstructions (i.e.,

Hirschsprung's Disease). Multiple areas of either perforation or impending necrosis of either small and/or large bowel may be seen in acute necrotizing enterocolitis. Intestinal perforation and the resulting bacterial peritonitis lead to an intra-abdominal and retroperitoneal fluid loss similar to that seen in extensive burns. The resulting hypovolemia, combined with a usually isotonic dehydration leads to a markedly reduced cardiac output and decreased peripheral perfusion resulting in shock and metabolic acidosis compounded by a respiratory acidosis when the peritonitis interferes with diaphragmatic excursion. Septicemia, secondary to the bacterial peritonitis, can further intensify the state of shock.

In patients with single perforation and peritonitis, disseminated intravascular clotting (coagulopathy) can occasionally be seen at the end stage of the patient's downhill course. In contrast, patients with acute necrotizing enterocolitis not infrequently show signs of coagulopathy at an earlier stage, when even the necrotizing entrocolitis may not have been suspected clinically. Although the coagulopathy seen in necrotizing enterocolitis is probably the result rather than the cause of the enterocolitis, its association is so common that prophylactic heparinization has been considered in patients with enterocolitis before there is laboratory evidence of disseminated intravascular clotting. The actual cause of acute necrotizing enterocolitis is not known, but microscopic findings have been suggestive of a diffuse enteric Schwartzman type of reaction.

## Criteria for Diagnosis

### Clinical

1. Abdominal distension and tenderness
2. Inability to tolerate feedings
3. Biliary or fecaloid vomiting
4. Hyper- or hypothermia with signs of sepsis

5. Coagulopathy with petechial cutaneous hemorrhages and/or upper and lower gastrointestinal bleeding in patients with coagulopathy

### X-ray

1. Distended intestinal loops, presence of intraperitoneal fluid, and occasionally the presence of free air, usually less than that seen in patients with gastric perforations.
2. In patients with acute necrotizing enterocolitis, pneumatosis intestinalis or air in the portal venous system may be present.

### Differential Diagnosis

Adynamic ileus, gastroenteritis, sepsis, intestinal obstruction, electrolyte imbalance, diarrhea, enteropathies, Hirschsprung's disease.

## Management

### Preoperative

1. Nasogastric tube for decompression
2. Cutdown
3. Intravenous fluids:

A. Isotonic crystalloid solutions to restore intravascular volume as noted above. If there is either clinical or laboratory evidence of marked acidosis, sodium bicarbonate should be part of the isotonic crystalloid fluid.

B. In patients with marked peritonitis and obvious shock, part of the isotonic fluid should be given as colloid, approximately 10 ml./kg. body weight.

4. Maintenance of temperature
5. Broad-spectrum antibiotics
6. Intravenous heparinization if there is evidence of intravascular clotting
7. As soon as the patient's hemodynamic and metabolic status have been improved sufficiently, the patient should be taken to the operating room.
8. Operation, depending upon the findings, may consist of a resection of the involved area with a primary end-to-end

anastomosis or proximal and distal cutaneous enterostomies, followed by a secondary reanastomosis, or examination of the involved segments. Intraluminal antibiotic drip may be helpful.

## Postoperative

The immediate postoperative management is similar to that described in infants with gastric perforation.

## Postoperative Complications

1. Coagulopathy (disseminated intravascular clotting)
2. Persistent peritonitis or abscess formation
3. Leakage of the anastomosis
4. Dehydration, hypovolemia, and metabolic acidosis if the fluid losses from end-enterostomies are not compensated
5. Septicemic shock
6. Hypoproteinemia
7. Hypocalcemia or hypomagnesemia

## ENTEROCOLITIS WITH HIRSCHSPRUNG'S DISEASE

### Definition

Enterocolitis is severe inflammation of the bowel.

### Basic Principles

Enterocolitis is the most common cause of death in patients with untreated Hirschsprung's disease, especially in infants.

Although colitis is the common cause of death in infants with Hirschsprung's disease in the United States, it is rarely seen in some European countries where infants are breast-fed. It can therefore be assumed that the underlying etiology is related not only to the obstruction due to the aganglionosis but also to a different bacterial flora.

Development of colitis and the associated distal aganglionic obstruction leads to a rapid progression with necrosis, septicemia and shock. Treatment is therefore related to elimination of obstruction, restoration of volume and use of antibiotics.

## Criteria for Diagnosis

### Clinical

1. Abdominal distention, with or without signs of peritonitis in an infant with a history of either constipation or obstipation, occasionally alternating with diarrhea, since birth
2. In contrast to infants with acute necrotizing enterocolitis, who rarely have a history of preceding abnormal findings, symptoms relating to the aganglionosis can usually be obtained.
3. The abdominal findings vary in accordance with the extent of the colitis, which may range from abdominal distention without peritonitis to signs of peritonitis, shock, metabolic acidosis and "toxic colon."

### Laboratory

Findings are usually compatible with an isotonic dehydration, and moderate to severe metabolic acidosis.

### X-ray

Supine and upright films may be compatible with either a low intestinal obstruction or an adynamic ileus pattern.

### Differential Diagnosis

1. Low intestinal obstruction
2. Viral enteritis, secondary ileus, acute necrotizing enterocolitis, bacterial enteritis with septicemia

## Management

Experience has shown that in spite of the creation of a colostomy, the mortality rate in infants with fully developed Hirschsprung's enterocolitis is prohibitively high. In recent years aggressive nonoperative decompression has improved the survival rate if followed with a colostomy after the patient has responded to nonoperative treatment.

### Nonoperative Treatment

1. Continuous rectocolonic isotonic irrigations through a large bore tube. The

irrigating solution must be isotonic to avoid water intoxication and should contain topical antibiotics such as kanamycin.

The total amount of kanamycin should not be greater than three times the systemic dose, since the absorption rate from the colon in the presence of inflammation is unpredictable. The irrigations should be carried out at least at two-hourly intervals and care should be taken to avoid undue pressure resulting in perforation.

In patients with marked metabolic acidosis, the isotonic rectal irrigating solution can be mixed with sodium bicarbonate (for instance, half saline and half sodium bicarbonate).

2. After the patient has responded and the abdomen is flat and signs of dehydration, metabolic imbalance or sepsis have disappeared, a barium enema can be performed to demonstrate the transitional area for the prompt placement of a colostomy.

3. Patients not responding to the rectocolonic irrigation within the first 24 hours should be considered for a colostomy.

4. The supportive treatment is similar to that in bacterial peritonitis, with maintenance of adequate infusion of crystalloids.

## Operative Treatment

1. Colostomy should be placed into the dilated area of colon to avoid the danger of utilizing a transitional aganglionic area.

2. The colostomy should be matured immediately, since the obstruction resulting from an unopened colostomy may lead to an immediate flare-up or continuation of the colitis.

3. Care should be taken to secure the colostomy with multiple 4 or 5 atraumatic vascular sutures to both peritoneum and fascial layers, since colostomy herniation is not an uncommon complication.

4. The postoperative treatment is with restoration or maintenance of intravascular volume, repair of the metabolic acidosis and prevention and treatment of

septicemia and colitis with broad-spectrum antibiotics.

5. The colostomy can be left in place until a final repair at approximately the age of one year is undertaken after the diagnosis of aganglionosis has been confirmed by biopsy.

# APPENDICITIS

## Definition

Appendicitis is obstruction of the appendiceal lumen with subsequent inflammation of the appendiceal wall.

## Basic Principles

Appendicitis is caused by obstruction leading to inflammation, necrosis and subsequent, either localized or diffuse, peritonitis. Its rarity in the infant may be related to the relative scarcity of lymphoid tissue in the neonatal appendix.

## Criteria for Diagnosis

### Clinical

1. The classical history of the older child and adult, related to the obstructive nature, abdominal pain followed by nausea, fever and localization of abdominal pain, is lacking in the infant and so are the typical physical findings related to the pathology in the right lower quadrant.

2. History usually includes irritability or lethargy and a failure to feed properly, followed by abdominal distention and vomiting.

3. Neither diarrhea nor constipation is suggestive of the diagnosis.

4. On physical examination, abdominal tenderness, diffuse with abdominal distention, indicates diffuse peritonitis after the appendix has ruptured.

### Laboratory

1. The white blood cell count may be elevated with a shift to the left.

2. Electrolyte values and hematocrit may be elevated, indicating dehydration.

## X-ray

1. The findings in appendicitis in neonates are not diagnostic; they usually present a picture of a diffuse peritonitis.

2. Fecaliths are not found in the neonatal age-group.

## Management

### General

1. When the diagnosis of appendicitis has been made, the child should be prepared rapidly but adequately for operation.

2. The hypovolemia must be corrected prior to the operative procedure. A possible metabolic imbalance should be simultaneously corrected.

3. Antibiotics should be started immediately.

4. *Suggested Orders*

A. Nasogastric decompression

B. *Intravenous Fluids.* Depending on the state of dehydration, if severe, fluids up to 3,000 ml. per square meter of body surface area/24 hrs. are given, with the initial fluid given as isotonic fluid followed by half isotonic or one-third isotonic fluid. The solute depends on the child's metabolic state; if marked acidosis is present, part of the solute should be given in the form of sodium bicarbonate. If peritonitis is severe, colloid should be administered.

C. Intravenous broad-spectrum antibiotics

D. Control of temperature with hypothermia if necessary

### Operative Management

1. A right transverse incision in neonates will enable the surgeon to explore both the upper and lower quadrants and, in the case of appendicitis, will allow him to remove the appendix.

2. Since the formation of an appendiceal abscess is rarely seen in neonates, the necessity of peritoneal drainage, even after perforation, is highly debatable.

3. Generous warm saline irrigation of the abdomen, with or without antibiotics, is usually helpful to remove the purulent material and may decrease the postoperative incidence of diffuse or localized peritonitis.

### Postoperative Management

1. Nasogastric decompression

2. Intravenous fluid therapy, depending on the severity of the peritonitis found at surgery and the degree of ileus present postoperatively

3. Continuation of intravenous antibiotics

4. Careful measurement of intake and output and replacement of nasogastric drainage

5. Treatment follows in general the outline presented in the basic discussion on neonatal peritonitis.

### Complications

1. Sepsis
2. Persistent ileus
3. Abdominal abscesses
4. Wound infections
5. Fluid or electrolyte imbalance

## PERFORATED MECKEL'S DIVERTICULUM

### Definition

Meckel's diverticulum is the persistence of a segment of the omphalo-enteric (omphalomesenteric) duct attached to the ileum.

### Basic Principles

Meckel's diverticulum, which can vary in length, is usually found on the antimesenteric border and may or may not be attached to the umbilicus. In approximately one half of the diverticula, either gastric mucosa or ectopic pancreas can be found. The gastric mucosa is responsible for the common complications of hemorrhage or perforation. The ulcer found in Meckel's diverticulum may be at the base of the

Meckel's diverticulum, as usually seen in perforation, or occasionally on the opposing mesenteric side, associated with hemorrhage. Other complications are intussusception or intestinal obstruction, the latter often due to an attachment between the umbilicus and the diverticulum.

## Criteria for Diagnosis

### Clinical

Perforation of a Meckel's diverticulum usually presents with diffuse peritonitis without localization in a specific area.

### Laboratory

Laboratory findings may be suggestive of peritonitis but the correct diagnosis is usually made at laparotomy.

### X-ray

X-ray findings are consistent with diffuse peritonitis. There is rarely evidence of free intraperitoneal air.

### Differential Diagnosis

Entities listed under Neonatal Peritonitis. However, perforation of a Meckel's diverticulum usually occurs in children past the neonatal stage.

## Management

### General

The general preoperative management is outlined under Neonatal Peritonitis.

### Operative Management

1. In patients with the perforation at the base of the Meckel's diverticulum, a wedge resection with either a closed or an open end-to-end anastomosis may be satisfactory.
2. In contrast, patients with bleeding from a Meckel's diverticulum usually require a complete resection, including the mesenteric border of the ileum, opposite the diverticulum, to ensure that an ulcer at the mesenteric site has not been missed.

### Postoperative Management

As outlined under Neonatal Peritonitis and Appendicitis.

## Complications

1. Postoperative ileus
2. Localized or diffuse peritonitis or abscesses
3. Wound infection
4. Fluid and electrolyte imbalances
5. Anastomotic leak

## INTRAPERITONEAL HEMORRHAGE

### Basic Principles

Intraperitoneal hemorrhage in the newborn is most commonly seen immediately after delivery. It is usually related to trauma sustained during the delivery, and the organ most commonly involved is the liver, followed by the spleen. Pre-existing lesions, such as hemangiomas or hepatomas, may be responsible.

### Criteria for Diagnosis

### Clinical

1. Signs and symptoms of peritoneal irritation and hypovolemia
2. Low hematocrit

### Laboratory

1. Possible leukocytosis
2. Positive abdominal paracentesis

### X-ray

Abdominal flat film showing intraperitoneal fluid and a pattern of ileus

### Differential Diagnosis

1. In the presence of mild to moderate bleeding not leading to cardiovascular collapse, other causes of neonatal peritonitis as listed in the classification on page 514.
2. In patients with considerable intraperitoneal hemorrhage, intestinal volvulus, intraluminal bleeding such as seen with gastroduodenal ulceration

## Management

### General

1. All infants with suspected or proven intraperitoneal bleeding require operative exploration.

2. Preoperative stabilization is begun with the infusion of isotonic crystalloid solutions, followed by blood replacement.

### Operative Management

*Operative repair* depends on the specific etiology.

## NEONATAL GASTROINTESTINAL BLEEDING

### Definition

Neonatal gastrointestinal bleeding is bleeding originating from any level of the gastrointestinal tract or swallowed maternal or nasopharyngeal blood.

### Classification

1. *Secondary Bleeding*
   A. Swallowing of maternal blood
   B. Swallowing of blood due to nose bleeding, post-tonsillectomy, oral bleeding, etc.
2. Systemic disorders
3. Esophagus (hiatal hernias, esophagitis)
4. *Gastroduodenal Bleeding:* primary or secondary ulcers
5. *Small Intestinal Bleeding:* volvulus, Meckel's diverticulum, intestinal polyp (CR) intussusception, vascular malformation
6. *Large Bowel:* intussusception, polyps, anal fissures

### Basic Principles

Gastrointestinal bleeding in the newborn may either originate from the gastrointestinal tract or represent swallowed nasopharyngeal or maternal blood. The presence of blood in a gastric aspirate or in the meconium therefore does not necessarily indicate that the infant has a gastrointestinal bleeding problem.

Intestinal bleeding originating within the infant usually starts at the lower esophageal level and can involve parts of the entire intestinal tract down to the anus. As in the older child or the adult, the gastrointestinal bleeding may also be part of a systemic disorder such as coagulopathy or hypoprothrombinemia.

### Criteria for Diagnosis

#### Clinical

1. *History.* Family history (maternal) evidence of diffuse bleeding tendency. Upper gastrointestinal bleeding may be bright or coffee-ground colored. Rectal bleeding may be dark, bright, mixed with stool, coating the stool or occult.

2. *Physical Examination:*
   A. Oropharyngeal or nasogastric aspiration revealing blood
   B. *Clinical Signs:* changes in pulse, respiratory rate, blood pressure, urinary output, color or state of hydration compatible with decreased peripheral perfusion and hypovolemia.
   C. *Rectal Examination:* revealing blood in stool or local pathology.
   D. *Abdominal Examination:* association of peritonitis or peritoneal irritation

#### Laboratory

1. Hematocrit and white blood cell count
2. Examination of the blood for fetal or maternal hemoglobin
3. Bleeding and clotting time, prothrombin time, platelet count, partial thromboplastin time, fibrin split products, fibrinogen level.

#### X-ray

Contrast studies as indicated according to the suspected site of bleeding

### Management

1. Nasogastric decompression in upper gastrointestinal bleeders to confirm bleeding and estimate extent and continuation

2. Venous cutdown is done for administration of isotonic crystalloid solution in patients with major bleeding to restore normal vital signs, to be followed by whole blood transfusion as indicated.

## SECONDARY BLEEDING

The swallowing of maternal blood either during delivery or during nursing from a bleeding maternal nipple is usually minor in nature and can be diagnosed by differentiating the fetal hemoglobin of the infant from adult hemoglobin (Apt test).

The swallowing of blood following nosebleeds, etc., can be diagnosed by the history of preceding epistaxis or by the presence of intra-oral lesions such as hemangiomas.

## SYSTEMIC BLEEDING DISORDERS

1. Bleeding tendency of the newborn is usually limited to the first five days of life; it may include the gastrointestinal tract, the central nervous system or other sites. The disease is probably related to a deficiency in prothrombin which responds to the administration of vitamin K. Similar clinical entities may result from a plasma thromboplastin antecedent deficiency, plasma thromboplastic component deficiency or from other defects in blood coagulation. Congenital thrombocytopenic purpura occurs in infants of mothers with thrombocytopenia or those sensitized to platelet antigens by previous transfusion or pregnancy.

2. *Coagulopathy.* Usually secondary to septicemia, this is accompanied by a decrease in fibrinogen and platelets and abnormal thromboplastin and fibrin split products. Infants with gastrointestinal bleeding, in particular those who have evidence of other sites of bleeding such as skin petechiae, central nervous system bleeding, hematuria, etc., should be investigated for these factors.

## ESOPHAGEAL BLEEDING

### Definition

Esophageal bleeding refers to hematemesis or melena secondary to esophageal lesions usually originating in the lower esophagus due to hiatal hernia, esophagitis or hiatal ulcers.

### Basic Principles

The esophagogastric barrier is not fully developed in infants until approximately the age of six weeks. Simultaneously, there is an acute increase in gastric acidity and pepsinogen immediately following birth, which declines after several weeks of life. During this period, hiatal ulcerations are most commonly seen. They tend to be superficial, with the bleeding usually mild and exsanguination extremely rare.

### Criteria for Diagnosis

Clinical

1. Bleeding from hiatal hernia or hiatal ulcerations is usually mild. The hematemesis often consists of coffee-ground material.

2. Massive hematemesis of bright-red blood can occur, but it is rare.

Laboratory

Hiatal bleeding, with rare exceptions, does not lead to a rapid drop of hematocrit.

X-ray

Barium swallow may show either hiatal hernia or hiatal ulcerations.

### Management

1. Although hiatal hernias in neonates may persist, leading to continuous peptic esophagitis and ulceration with secondary esophageal stenosis, most hiatal ulcers and herniations are self-limiting and do not require operative intervention.

2. In the majority of patients, the treatment consists of conservative management.

A. The infant is placed in an upright position, feedings may have to be thickened occasionally, and antispasmodic drugs such as Donnatal may be indicated.

B. If the blood loss is significant, blood should be replaced.

C. Antacids can be added to the formula if necessary.

D. The disease is usually self-limiting and operative intervention is indicated only if there is massive hemorrhage or stenosis.

## GASTRODUODENAL BLEEDING

### Basic Principles

Primary gastric or duodenal ulcers in neonates are ulcers not associated with other diseases and without identifiable etiology.

In patients with mild to moderate gastric bleeding, the gastric aspirate can range from coffee-grounds to bright red; the rectal bleeding, depending on the severity of the gastric bleeding, ranges from dark melena to hematochezia. In the latter case, with marked bright rectal bleeding, large or small intestinal bleeding has to be ruled out. Frank blood obtained via a gastric tube indicates the source is gastroduodenal in origin.

1. *Primary Ulcer.* While the rapidly increasing gastric acidity and pepsinogen in the neonate may be related to the appearance of gastric and duodenal ulcers, the exact mechanism is not fully understood. The gross findings at operation range from single gastric or duodenal ulcers to diffuse superficial ulcers, occasionally resembling acute erosive or hemorrhagic gastritis. In some instances the bleeding ulcer may precede a gastric or duodenal perforation. If the patient responds to conservative treatment, the ulcers do not recur and differ, therefore, from peptic ulcers.

2. *Secondary Ulcer.* Secondary ulcers are similar to the primary ones in distribution, clinical signs and symptoms, and gross and histological findings, but are associated with an underlying or associated disease, such as cerebral pathology, systemic diseases or trauma, as for instance major surgical procedures. As in primary ulcers, the secondary ulcers are self-limiting and will disappear if the primary disease can be successfully treated.

### Criteria for Diagnosis

#### Clinical

1. Bleeding from gastric or duodenal ulcers in neonates can range from minimal manifestation, with hematemesis or coffee-ground material and minimally bloody stools, to massive hematemesis, usually preceding melena or frank hematochezia.

2. In occasional cases, the gastric bleeding can be so rapid in its onset that systemic signs such as shock or pallor may precede the appearance of either hematemesis or rectal bleeding.

3. The clinical signs of shock in the neonate may be extremely difficult to evaluate; the earliest sign usually consists of a tachycardia, which may be hard to assess in view of the already high normal pulse rate of the infant.

4. A significant drop of systolic blood pressure occurs late and is usually followed or preceded by bradycardia, an ominous sign indicating marked hypovolemia and shock.

#### Laboratory

1. In view of the high hematocrit in the newborn, a hematocrit in the "normal range" may be misleading and not reveal the actual extent of the hemorrhage.

2. A comparison of the prebleeding hematocrit and the subsequent drop may be an indication of the extent of the gastric bleeding.

3. The laboratory data should include bleeding and coagulation work-up to exclude systemic disorders as mentioned previously.

#### X-ray

Upper gastrointestinal studies occasionally may show gastric or duodenal ulcers. In the majority of patients, identifiable ulcers are not seen since superficial erosions and superficial ulcers are more common than deeply penetrating ones.

### Management

1. Clinical signs and symptoms, even in

the presence of massive hemorrhage, may be deceptive and the bleeding can be easily underestimated.

2. Continuous monitoring of vital signs such as pulse rate, respiration, blood pressure and urinary output is mandatory.

3. Continuous observation of the patient's clinical status, his response and signs of peripheral perfusion are more indicative of the extent of the internal bleeding.

4. Nonoperative treatment consists of:

A. Nasogastric tube

B. Intravenous cutdown for administration of whole blood

C. Restoration of blood volume with transfusion. Since upper intestinal bleeding leads to hypovolemia, transfusion with packed cells, although increasing the oxygen-carrying capacity, is inadequate and transfusion with whole blood is preferable. A sudden increase of 20 per cent of the total blood volume can be tolerated by all infants without cardiac anomalies even if the blood loss has been overestimated. Nevertheless, try to avoid overtransfusion which may reactivate bleeding.

D. Maintenance of adequate urinary output

E. Maintenance of body temperature

F. Neutralization of gastric acidity by the instillation of iced saline and milk, with or without antacids, either as a slow drip or irrigation. Careful administration is indicated when instillation of milk is used, however, to avoid aspiration and subsequent pneumonia.

G. *Intravenous Fluids.* Isotonic to half isotonic (According to blood pH, part of the solute may have to be administered as sodium bicarbonate as an isotonic push of 20 ml./kg. of body weight or 350 ml. square meter of body surface per 45 minutes.)

5. In patients with associated diseases, prompt and efficient treatment of the underlying disease is indicated to remove the cause of secondary ulcer.

6. *Operative Treatment*

A. If the estimated blood loss exceeds the infant's own blood volume within a 24-hour period, operative intervention is indicated.

B. Transfusions should be adequate so that the patient's blood volume is nearly normal at the time of operation.

C. If massive transfusions have to be used, care should be taken to warm the blood sufficiently to avoid the hypothermia associated with the transfusion of refrigerated blood. This can lead to an acute and marked deterioration of the already depleted infant.

D. *Operation*

*(1)* In either primary or secondary ulcers, the most conservative operative procedure that can control the bleeding should be utilized.

*(2)* Recurrence of the ulcer, either primary or secondary, is not seen as in peptic ulcers; therefore, the only objective of the operative procedure is the control of the gastric bleeding.

*(3)* In patients with a primary single ulcer, suturing of the site of bleeding and a gastrostomy will be all that is required.

*(4)* Since the majority of ulcers are multiple, other operative procedures such as vagotomy and pyloroplasty or hemigastrectomy and vagotomy are more commonly indicated.

*(5)* In infants with diffuse gastric ulcerations, subtotal gastrectomy with gastrojejunostomy may occasionally be indicated.

*(6)* It is advisable to add a gastrostomy to most operative gastric procedures to allow gastric decompression, avoidance of aspiration, assessment of continuous postoperative bleeding and easy access for gastric irrigation if such should be indicated.

*(7)* It should be emphasized again that the most simple operative procedure sufficient to control the bleeding should be used and that consideration pertaining to recurrent ulcers as seen in peptic ulcers are not valid in the neonatal group.

E. *Complications*

*(1)* If an adequate operative

procedure has been used in patients with primary ulcers, complications will be limited to the operative procedure itself and the extent of the preoperative hemorrhage.

*(2)* In patients with secondary ulcers, further ulcerations may occur as a result of the pre-existing associated underlying disease; therefore, the operative procedure of choice should take this into consideration and may therefore be more extensive than in patients with primary ulcers. This includes the use of vagotomy and gastric resection rather than simple oversewing of bleeding ulcer sites.

*(3)* In patients with secondary ulcers and intravascular clotting, immediate postoperative heparinization is indicated to prevent major postoperative gastric bleeding.

## VOLVULUS

*See* Malrotation, page 525.

## MECKEL'S DIVERTICULUM

### Basic Principles

Meckel's diverticulum rarely leads to massive bleeding in infancy and is described on page 538.

If bleeding does occur in infancy, the symptoms are similar to those in the older child–usually painless, sudden massive rectal bleeding, bright red in character, in contrast to the bleeding seen in patients with volvulus or upper gastrointestinal bleeding. Rectal bleeding in patients with intussusception or occasionally enteritis or enterocolitis may also be relatively bright but it is usually associated with either diarrhea as in enteritis or enterocolitis or with mucoid material rarely seen in patients with Meckel's diverticulum. The bleeding in intussusception, although fairly bright, is usually of the currant-jelly variety and not seen in patients with Meckel's diverticulum.

## SMALL INTESTINAL POLYPS

### Basic Principles

Significant bleeding from small intestinal polyps is rare in children of all ages and especially in the neonatal age, with the exception of congenital anomalies, such as ectopic pancreas or neoplasms or tumors such as leiomyomas. Small intestinal polyps are usually part of the Peutz-Jegher syndrome, a combination of diffuse intestinal hamartomas with abnormal melanin spots, found in the perioral and perianal areas and fingertips.

## INTUSSUSCEPTION

### Basic Principles

Intussusception in the neonate under the age of three months is rare. Lymphatic hyperplasia seen in older children, assumed to be one of the most common causes of intussusception, is not present in early infancy. Signs, symptoms and treatment are similar to that described on page 557.

## ENTERITIS

### Basic Principles

Severe bacterial enteritis, such as seen with Shigella, Pseudomonas, E. coli or staphylococcus, with abdominal distention and signs of peritonitis mimicking an acute surgical abdomen, also can be associated with rectal bleeding.

Intestinal bleeding due to enteritis in infants is usually accompanied by abdominal pain, fever, and signs and symptoms of generalized septicemia and diarrhea in most instances. Massive septicemia can lead to disseminated intravascular clotting. In the absence of intestinal perforation or frank peritonitis, the treatment is non-operative, consisting of gastric decompression, restoration of blood volume and the commonly found large fluid deficit and antibiotic coverage.

## COLONIC POLYPS

### Definition

Colonic polyps are juvenile or adenomatous polyps of the colon.

### Basic Principles

1. *Juvenile Polyps.* More than 90 per cent of all polyps found in children are of the juvenile type, a nonneoplastic polyp predominantly found in the large intestine, the stroma of which consists of fibrous tissue and interspersed cystically dilated glands. The surface epithelium is often eroded and missing due to inflammatory reaction. Juvenile polyps are thought to be either a reaction to inflammatory changes or redundant mucosa.

2. *Adenomatous Polyps.* These can occur in early childhood but are extremely rare. They can occur as single or multiple polyps, in either the familial or nonfamilial form such as the Gardner's syndrome. Adenomatous polyps usually do not appear in infancy but in early or mid adolescence. They may be associated with carcinoma when multiple or familial.

### Criteria for Diagnosis

1. Since most polyps are located in the large bowel, intussusception is rarely seen and the symptoms are usually limited to painless, asymptomatic bleeding which may be bright red.

2. Prolapse of polyps, located within the rectum or sigmoid, can occasionally be seen.

3. In contrast to adults, it is preferable to begin the examination with a barium enema preceding the proctoscopy, since proctoscopy, especially in young infants and children, may require general anesthesia.

### Management

1. Bleeding is rarely significant enough to require blood transfusion.

2. Patients with rectal bleeding suspected of originating from large bowel polyps can be worked-up electively.

3. The presence of either single or multiple juvenile polyps, if asymptomatic and not associated with massive bleeding, does not require operative intervention.

4. If a polyp is within reach of the sigmoidoscope, a biopsy should be performed to differentiate between juvenile and adenomatous polyps. If there is no polyp within reach of the sigmoidoscope, but small, single or multiple polyps have been visualized by barium enema studies, the treatment can be expectant in the absence of marked bleeding, with a repeat barium enema after several months' interval. In the majority of patients, the diminution in size or disappearance of the polyp indicates that they are of the self-limiting, juvenile type.

5. The treatment of adenomatous polyps, especially if multiple, and their potential for the development of malignancies are beyond the scope of this book.

## ANAL FISSURES

### Basic Principles

Anal fissures are the commonest cause of bright rectal bleeding in stool accompanied by pain and constipation. The latter may persist after the fissure heals.

### Criteria for Diagnosis

Bright rectal bleeding with coating of the stool, usually minor, accompanied by symptoms related to painful bowel movements and constipation

### Management

1. Mild laxatives
2. Stool softeners
3. Sitz baths
4. Dilation under heavy analgesia if above fails
5. Operation is rarely indicated.

## NEONATAL ABDOMINAL MASSES

### Basic Principles

Neonatal abdominal masses represent surgical emergencies. In view of their complexity, ranging from congenital anomalies with intestinal or urinary tract obstruction to various types of neoplasms, an experienced team of neonatologists, radiologists, chemotherapists, surgeons, and ancillary facilities is required. Operative intervention should not be performed unless the previously mentioned conditions exist; the neonate should be referred to an appropriate institution.

The diagnostic work-up should be completed within 24 to 48 hours. Unnecessary and repeat palpation of the abdominal tumor should be avoided. Since operative intervention is indicated in all patients, oral feedings should be discontinued and the patient placed on intravenous therapy. The use of upper extremity cutdowns is preferable if solid intra-abdominal tumors are expected. The preoperative preparation of the patient should include the entire team that may be responsible for the postoperative treatment.

## Criteria for Diagnosis

### Clinical

1. Abdominal masses, including congenital malformations and neoplasms, usually present without symptoms.

2. In accordance with their location or developmental anomaly, secondary signs such as intestinal or urinary obstruction can occur.

3. Trauma during delivery may lead to perforation with secondary hemorrhage and/or peritonitis.

4. The presence of associated anomalies such as myelomeningocele, imperforate anus or certain skeletal anomalies may suggest associated genitourinary anomalies leading to hydronephrosis.

5. The specific symptoms for the various types of intra-abdominal masses and intra-abdominal tumors in children are described subsequently.

6. Physical examination will obtain information concerning the characteristics of consistency, shape, mobility and tenderness of the neonatal abdominal mass.

7. Associated urinary or intestinal anomalies or obstruction should be ruled out. Abnormal vital signs may be related to local complications, such as perforation or obstruction, or systemic complications such as hypertension.

### Laboratory

Laboratory examinations should include hematocrit, white blood cell count, urinanalysis, liver profile, blood urea nitrogen, creatinine, vanyl mandelic acid and homo mandelic acid.

### X-ray

1. X-ray examinations should include supine and upright films of the abdomen, chest and skeletal review.

2. In view of the high percentage of renal lesions responsible for the formation of intra-abdominal masses, intravenous pyelogram, followed by cystogram if indicated, is warranted in all infants with abdominal masses.

3. Selective x-ray studies include inferior vena cavagram, angiography, radioactive scan and gastrointestinal or barium enema studies.

## NEONATAL ABDOMINAL AND CHEST WALL DEFECTS

### OMPHALOCELE

#### Definition

Omphalocele is congenital abdominal hernia into the base of the umbilical cord, covered by peritoneum and amniotic membrane unless ruptured.

#### Basic Principles

The formation of omphalocele is due to failure of the intra-abdominal organs to return into the abdomen at the third or fourth intra-uterine month. The normal return will lead to a closure of the rectus muscle with only enough space to allow the exit of the umbilical arteries and vein. If the return does not occur, the intestine, occasionally including liver and spleen, will remain in the extra-abdominal sac covered by peritoneum and amniotic membrane. The failure to return leads not only to the formation of an omphalocele, but also to an inadequate development of the abdominal cavity, a factor to be considered when an operative repair is contemplated.

Associated anomalies, including all organ systems, are common and are found in approximately 50 per cent of all patients. A nonrotation or malrotation of the intestine is common. If not repaired at the time of closure of the omphalocele, the possibility of volvulus has to be considered and the parents instructed accordingly.

In infants with unruptured omphaloceles without associated major congenital anomalies, no significant pathophysiologic disturbances occur until an attempt is made to correct the omphalocele by placing intestine and other intra-abdominal organs into an abdominal cavity that has not enlarged sufficiently to accept these organs. An attempt to reduce the omphalocele with a primary repair of either muscle and/or skin can lead to an elevation of the diaphragm and subsequent respiratory insufficiency.

## Criteria for Diagnosis

### Clinical

Defects into the umbilical cord with a part of the periumbilical abdominal wall uncovered by skin

### Differential Diagnosis

The diagnosis of an unruptured omphalocele is obvious, and the only differential diagnosis to be considered is that of a gastroschisis when the omphalocele is ruptured. In contrast to gastroschisis, an omphalocele is always consistent with a defect at the insertion of the umbilical cord. (*See* Gastroschisis, below.)

## Management

### Nonoperative

1. In large omphaloceles with an intact sac, conservative treatment has been successful. The treatment consists of careful maintenance of sterile or clean condition of the sac, with Mercurochrome or other antibacterial agents, as long as absorption by the cover of the omphalocele is insignificant.

2. This treatment is successful in many instances but leads to a prolonged hospitalization. An additional problem consists of the failure of the rectus muscle to close the defect, and the closure is usually limited to a skin coverage after an eschar has formed.

3. Conservative treatment is indicated in premature infants whose size and immaturity render them poor risks for operative repair.

### Operative Repair

1. *Unruptured Omphaloceles*

A. Small omphaloceles with a defect not larger than 3 to 4 cm. can usually be repaired without difficulty by approximating rectus muscles and skin.

B. Larger umbilical hernias, especially if intestine and/or other organs such as liver and spleen are contained within the omphalocele, require a staged repair.

(*1*) Although skin can be mobilized by the use of relaxing incisions, and a skin repair without an attempt of muscular repair may be tolerated by the majority of infants, the subsequent postoperative adhesions between skin and underlying intestine make a second or third operative procedure difficult.

(*2*) The use of synthetic material such as Silastic is preferable.

(*3*) The extent of the reduction of the intra-abdominal organs is dependent on the caval pressure and the effect on respiration. An attempt should be made to carry these infants under light anesthesia with spontaneous respiration, to observe the effect of the repair on the diaphragm intraoperatively.

(*4*) When synthetic material is used, no attempt at a skin closure is made.

(*5*) The intra-abdominal organs can then be reduced over a period of 2 to 4 weeks by either repeat excisions of parts of the synthetic material or by substituting smaller synthetic grafts.

C. *Preoperative and Operative Factors to Be Considered*

*(1)* Venous cutdown

*(2)* Vitamin K

*(3)* Appropriate intravenous fluids

*(4)* Maintenance of temperature

*(5)* Treatment of the unruptured omphalocele with continuous moisture with clean technique until the time of the operative repair.

*(6)* Insertion of a catheter into the superior vena cava will give the surgeon valuable information as to how much pressure he can exert when reducing the abdominal organs.

*(7)* In view of the high incidence of associated malformations, additional congenital anomalies should be looked for at the time of the operative procedure and corrected if possible.

D. When the omphalocele sac is removed, it should be removed with caution from the liver if the latter is present within the abdominal cavity.

*(1)* The sac, peritoneum and amniotic membrane are often densely adherent to the liver capsule and a removal will result in a damage of the liver capsule and considerable blood loss.

*(2)* The complete removal of the membrane is not necessary.

E. If the liver is found within the omphalocele, the suprahepatic portion of the inferior vena cava is usually elongated and a kink of either suprahepatic inferior vena cava or portal vein should be avoided.

2. *Operative Repair of the Ruptured Omphalocele.* The rupture of the omphalocele prior to delivery leads to the formation of a fibrinous exudate over the intestine, like the one seen in infants with gastroschisis. The operative treatment will be discussed under Gastroschisis, below.

3. *Postoperative Complications*

A. The major complications consist of the danger of pulmonary insufficiency or interference with cardiac return. Careful monitoring of respiration with repeat blood gas studies and the use of respirators may help the infant during the first few postoperative days.

B. Continuous nasogastric decompression in the early postoperative phase is indicated to prevent additional intra-abdominal expansion and interference with diaphragmatic motion.

C. In view of the high incidence of associated malformations which may not have been recognized preoperatively, associated intestinal, renal or cardiac problems should be ruled out. Although a repair of the intestinal malrotation may not be indicated at the time of the operation, the possibility of a postoperative intestinal obstruction related to the malrotation has to be considered.

# GASTROSCHISIS

## Definition

Gastroschisis is fusion failure of the abdominal wall in the midventral line, not related to the umbilicus.

## Basic Principles

Associated anomalies are common, including intestinal atresia. The failure of the intestines to return into the abdominal cavity leads to extraperitoneal development of the intestine bathed with amniotic fluid. The result is a thick fibrinous cover of the intestine, which greatly interferes with the operative reduction of the intestine and the identification of atretic segments.

## Criteria for Diagnosis

1. The appearance of extra-abdominal intestine and/or liver and spleen in an infant whose abdomen shows a defect not related to the umbilicus, with evidence of intra-uterine peritonitis, is diagnostic for gastroschisis.

2. A patient with a ruptured omphalocele may show a similar finding

but the defect is clearly within the base of the umbilical cord.

## Management

1. Immediate operative repair is indicated, as in infants with ruptured omphaloceles, to prevent bacterial peritonitis.

A. The preoperative and general operative preparations are similar to those in infants with omphaloceles, including central venous catheters to monitor caval pressure.

B. In view of the exudate covering the intestine, a reduction of the extra-abdominal intestine is more difficult than in the unruptured omphalocele, and the failure to remove the cover may prevent the surgeon from identifying associated atresias.

C. An attempt should be made to remove the coverage as far as possible to identify the continuity of the intestine.

D. Although removal of the coverage may lead to considerable bleeding, the latter can be controlled.

E. Associated obstructions should be identified and corrected.

F. The repair is similar to that of a large omphalocele.

G. In view of the intra-uterine peritonitis, intestinal activity usually resumes later than in the patient with an unruptured omphalocele, and the addition of a gastrostomy, jejunal feeding catheter or hyperalimentation should be considered.

2. *Postoperative Complications*
   A. Peritonitis
   B. Anastomotic leaks
   C. Intestinal obstruction
   D. Prolonged ileus
   E. Cardiac and respiratory distress if the reduction has been too aggressive at the first stage
   F. Associated diseases or anomalies, as mentioned before, including rare diseases such as the Beckwith syndrome with organomegaly and hypoglycemia

## UMBILICAL INFECTION

### Definition

Neonatal umbilical infection may present either as a granuloma, periumbilical inflammation or omphalitis with or without associated anomalies such as omphalo-enteric duct or urachal cyst.

### Basic Principles

Umbilical granuloma often consists of intestinal mucosa without a persistent mesenteric duct. While catheterization of umbilical vein or artery may lead to omphalitis, in the majority of infants the cause of omphalitis is noniatrogenic, due to heaped-up granulation tissue within the umbilicus.

### Criteria for Diagnosis

Omphalitis in the neonate usually appears as reddening of the umbilicus or the periumbilical area, occasionally with purulent discharge or drainage.

### Differential Diagnosis

Umbilical granuloma or polyp, omphalo-enteric duct, urachal cyst or duct

### Management

1. Umbilical granulomas usually respond to the application of silver nitrate.

2. If silver nitrate application is ineffective, excision of the granuloma or polyp is indicated, not only to remove occasionally remaining intestinal mucosa which leads to polyp formation but also to rule out the presence of a partially obliterated omphalo-enteric duct.

3. Although complications of umbilical granuloma and/or polyps are usually insignificant, omphalitis can lead to progressive thrombosis with eventual portal vein occlusion and extrahepatic portal hypertension.

## UMBILICAL HERNIA

### Definition

Umbilical hernia is failure of the rectus

fascia to close around the umbilical cord structures, leaving a fascial defect covered by skin, in contrast to the patient with an omphalocele.

## Basic Principles

The failure of the rectus fascia to completely encircle the cord structures leads to a fascial defect which is especially common in premature infants. In contrast to inguinal hernias, incarceration is rare; however, it does occur. This defect is especially common among Negroes. In contrast to inguinal hernias, the majority of umbilical hernias will close spontaneously at about the age of four to five years.

## Criteria for Diagnosis

### Clinical

Protrusion of the umbilicus, especially during straining or coughing, with a palpable underlying fascial defect

## Management

1. *General*
    A. Since the incarceration rate of umbilical hernias is considerably less than in inguinal hernias, the presence of an umbilical hernia in an infant is not an indication for surgery unless the hernia is symptomatic.
    B. The size of the skin protrusion can vary markedly but does not determine the need for operative intervention.
    C. If the fascial defect enlarges under observation, an operative repair is probably indicated.
    D. Persistence of the fascial defect after the age of four years or apparent enlargement in size is generally accepted as indication for surgery.
    E. Incarceration of either omentum or intestine is rare but necessitates that parents be instructed to watch for signs of incarceration while the infant's hernia is being followed.
    F. The strapping of the abdomen to prevent the herniation is useless and may mask incarceration or irritate the skin.

2. *Operative Repair*
    A. Repair consists of a primary closure of the defect through a semicircular incision at the inferior aspect of the umbilicus.
    B. Excision of the skin is contraindicated, regardless of how extensive the herniation may appear, in view of the elasticity of the skin in children.

## NEONATAL GENITOURINARY PROBLEMS

### MALE MEATAL STENOSIS

## Definition

Meatal stenosis is stenosis of the urethral meatus.

## Basic Principles

Meatal stenosis is usually not associated with other anomalies. The stenosis can lead to a low-grade lower urinary tract obstruction.

## Criteria for Diagnosis

### Clinical

Difficulty with micturition, pain or inadequate stream

### Differential Diagnosis

Hypospadias

## Management

Enlargement of the meatus, which can usually be accomplished by gently crushing the stenosed part of the meatus with fine clamps, followed by sharp division

### TORSION OF THE TESTIS (OR APPENDAGES)

## Definition

1. Torsion of the testis occurs along the long axis of the spermatic cord, either within or without the tunica vaginalis. Torsion can occur in both the descended and undescended testes.
2. Torsion may be of the testicular appendages, which are vestigial remnants

found in most male patients, attached to testis or epididymis, and the torsion of these appendages can lead to infarction.

## Basic Principles

The torsion of the testis is secondary to inadequate scrotal or tunica vaginalis attachments. Even though the torsion may occur on one side only, the inadequate ligamentous attachment is almost always bilateral.

The torsion of the testis leads primarily to a venous outflow obstruction with subsequent testicular engorgement, followed by infarction and necrosis.

## Criteria for Diagnosis

1. Intense and sudden pain in the involved testis. Since the torsion can occur during periods of rest as well as physical exercise, an onset of sudden pain without physical activity does not rule out a testicular torsion.

2. On physical examination, the involved testis is extremely tender on palpation and, depending on the duration, the testis may be remarkably swollen and tense.

3. Since torsion of the testis can occur with an undescended testis, the tenderness and appearance of a painful mass is not limited to the scrotum, but can be found in the inguinal area, usually distal to the external inguinal ring.

A previously descended testis which has undergone torsion may be pulled back into the inguinal area and present as an undescended testis.

4. In contrast to the torsion of the testicular appendages, the tenderness is uniform and involves the entire testis.

5. In orchitis or epididymitis the onset is less acute and the tenderness is usually less severe.

## Management

1. In view of the high incidence of testicular infarction or atrophy, there is no place for conservative treatment.

Operative treatment is invariably required.

2. *Torsion of the Testis*

A. The scrotum is opened, followed by an incision of the tunica vaginalis.

B. The torsion is untwisted and the testis is inspected.

C. If there is evidence of congestion or infarction, the tunica albuginea is incised to allow the accumulated blood to escape.

D. The testis is then anchored to the transverse scrotal septum with interrupted atraumatic sutures.

E. A contralateral repair is indicated even in the absence of physical findings.

3. *Torsion of the Testicular Appendages*

A. After the tunica vaginalis has been opened and the infarcted appendage has been identified, it is resected and the stalk is ligated.

B. No further treatment is necessary.

4. *Complications:* testicular infarction with either liquefaction necrosis or testicular atrophy

# EPIDIDYMITIS AND ORCHITIS

## Definition

Epididymitis and orchitis are bacterial or viral infections of epididymis and/or testis. Although either one may be infected individually, in most instances the infection involves both testis and epididymis.

## Basic Principles

Either viral or bacterial infections can lead to inflammation within the testis or epididymis. The most common viral infection is mumps orchitis. Bacterial infections may be secondary to staphylococcal, streptococcal or aerobacter infections. Gonorrhea is rarely seen as a cause of epididymitis in children.

## Criteria for Diagnosis

### Clinical

1. Swelling and tenderness of the testis and/or epididymis

2. The onset of pain, in contrast to tor- sion of the testis, is not acute.

3. Bilateral tenderness, especially in patients with epididymitis, is common.

4. On rectal examination, tenderness of the seminal vesicles also may be found.

### Laboratory

Urine examination may show bacteria and white cells.

### Differential Diagnosis

Torsion of the testis or testicular appen- dages, idiopathic scrotal edema, hydrocele, testicular trauma or tumor

### Management

1. Moist heat and antibiotic administra- tion is the treatment once the diagnosis has been established.

2. Since the differential diagnosis between inflammation and torsion of the testis may be difficult, in any child where the diagnosis of testicular torsion cannot be clearly ruled out, the testis should be ex- plored.

# Surgical Emergencies in the Child

## INTESTINAL OBSTRUCTION IN THE CHILD

### Classification

1. Inguinal hernia
2. Congenital bands
3. Internal hernia
4. Bezoar
5. Intussusception
6. Intra-abdominal tumors
7. Trauma

## INGUINAL HERNIA AND HYDROCELES

### Definition

This is partial or complete persistence of the processus vaginalis, with herniation of peritoneal contents into it.

### Classification

1. *Indirect Inguinal Hernia:* inguinal canal hernia, scrotal hernia
2. *Hydrocele*
   A. Communicating, noncommuni- cating
   B. Hydrocele of the cord, hydrocele of the testis
3. Inguinal hernia and hydrocele
(Although femoral and direct hernias do occur in children, they are extremely rare and are discussed in Chap. 16, Intestinal Obstruction.)

### Basic Principles

### Etiology

The processus vaginalis, which is present in both sexes during intra-uterine life, usually closes just prior to birth. The des- cent of the testis in males, usually during the eighth intra-uterine month, probably contributes to the obliteration of the neck of the processus vaginalis. For this reason the incidence of inguinal hernia is extreme- ly common in premature infants. Although there appears to be a genetic trend in males, this has not been statistically established.

Since the right testis descends later than the left, inguinal hernias are more common on the right side. Bilaterality, especially in newborn infants, has been described in up to 60 or 70 per cent of cases. Since not every "patent processus vaginalis" develops into a hernia, the clinical implication of this finding is difficult to assess. The unilateral repair of an inguinal hernia in infants un- der two years of age may be followed by the appearance of a contralateral hernia in ap- proximately 20 per cent of cases, a signifi- cant incidence of bilaterality.

## Associated Diseases or Anomalies

As mentioned previously, inguinal hernias are especially common in premature infants. While these hernias may not be apparent in early infancy, episodes of increased intra-abdominal strain, such as upper respiratory infections or constipation, may lead to their clinical appearance.

## Pathophysiology

The danger of an inguinal hernia, especially in early infancy, lies in the possibility of incarceration or strangulation. Strangulation is the result of the continuous arterial inflow with simultaneous venous occlusion, leading first to congestion and then to infarction. Not only is there vascular compromise to the intestine, more often a vascular compromise of the testis is found, even with nonstrangulated incarcerated inguinal hernia, due to the precarious blood supply of the testis.

A prompt repair of the incarcerated inguinal hernia is therefore indicated not only to prevent an intestinal strangulation, but to prevent testicular infarction or atrophy.

## Criteria for Diagnosis

### Clinical

1. *Uncomplicated Inguinal or Scrotal Hernia*
    A. A history of inguinal or scrotal swelling can often be obtained, especially after straining due to upper respiratory infections or constipation.
    B. Palpation of the spermatic cord over the pubic ramus reveals a "silk sign" when the empty peritoneal sac is rolled over the vas deferens.
    C. On strain the hernia may be visible.
    D. Examination through the scrotum and palpation of the ring, in contrast to adults, are not helpful in infants and children.
2. *Incarcerated or Strangulated Inguinal or Scrotal Hernia*

    A. The history reveals a sudden onset of inguinal swelling, frequently accompanied by pain in older children or irritability in young infants, followed by abdominal distention or vomiting if intestinal obstruction has occurred.
    B. On palpation a mass can be felt extending up to the external ring.
    C. On rectal examination a loop of intestine entering the internal ring can be felt occasionally.
3. *Strangulated Hernia*
    A. Incarceration leading to strangulation almost invariably will lead to tenderness over the strangulated hernia, sometimes with edema and redness of the overlying skin.
    B. Although signs of peritonitis may be absent, there is usually abdominal distention and signs of ir.testinal obstruction.

### Laboratory

1. Noncontributory in patients with hydrocele and incarcerated hernias
2. Leukocytosis is common with strangulation.

### X-ray

1. Flat and supine films of the abdomen may occasionally show dilated loops of intestine present in the inguinal scrotal hernia in patients with incarceration, or distended loops of intestine leading into the inguinal ring.
2. In patients with questionable uncomplicated inguinal hernias, the injection of radiopaque material into the peritoneal cavity has been used to demonstrate the inguinal hernia or the patent processus vaginalis. Physical examination alone is usually adequate, however, and these methods are rarely necessary.

### Differential Diagnosis

1. The differential diagnosis between an incarcerated hernia and hydrocele of the cord may at times be difficult, although in most cases of hydrocele of the cord the upper edge of the hydrocele can be separated

from the external inguinal ring by palpation and thus differentiated from incarcerated inguinal hernia.

2. Transillumination may be misleading, since incarcerated hernias can also transilluminate.

3. The presence of bowel sounds may also be misleading, since bowel sounds can be transmitted into a fluid-filled hydrocele extending to the external ring.

4. Tenderness which is usually present in patients with incarcerated hernias is rarely seen in patients with hydroceles.

5. In patients with hydroceles the history of swelling usually antedates the examination by a considerable period of time.

6. If there is any doubt as to whether the patient presents with an incarcerated inguinal hernia or a hydrocele of the cord, operative exploration is indicated.

## Management

### Indirect Inguinal Hernia

1. Inguinal hernias should be repaired whenever found in children regardless of age (with the exception of premature infants who can be observed in the hospital).

2. Since they tend to incarcerate and strangulate especially in infancy, inguinal hernias in premature infants should be repaired prior to their discharge, usually when the infant has reached 5 lbs. of weight.

3. Since the basic defect of a congenital indirect hernia consists of a failure of obliteration of the processus vaginalis, a herniorrhaphy with fascial repair is rarely indicated; a transection of the peritoneal sac with a high ligation is usually sufficient.

4. The recurrence rate in properly performed herniotomies is less than 1 per cent; the incidence of testicular atrophy after a herniorrhaphy with a superfluous fascial repair is significant, however.

5. With the exception of premature infants and older children with complicated inguinal hernias, postoperative hospitalization after herniotomy is usually

not necessary, and infants and children can be discharged the day of operation.

### Incarcerated Inguinal or Scrotal Hernia

1. Up to 90 per cent of incarcerated hernias in infants and children will reduce spontaneously by conservative treatment, consisting of sedation and Trendelenberg position.

2. Manual reduction, although relatively safe in the hands of an experienced surgeon, is rarely indicated in view of the ease of successful reduction with sedation, which does not include the danger of an *en bloc* reduction.

3. If a conservative reduction has been successful, operation is best performed within approximately 24 hours after most of the edema has subsided.

4. In a patient with incarceration, who has failed to respond to conservative treatment, herniotomy is indicated within several hours after admission to avoid intestinal or testicular vascular compromise.

A. A careful attempt should be made to inspect the intestine for viability within the hernial sac prior to the opening of the external ring, since an immediate reduction of the incarcerated intestine often occurs.

B. Regardless of the state of the intestine, whether it requires resection or simple reduction, care should be taken to inspect the testis.

C. If considerable vascular engorgement or infarction of the testis is found, opening of the tunica albuginea is indicated to prevent secondary atrophy.

5. If a strangulated hernia is found at operation, an attempt should be made to remove the infarcted segment before it spontaneously returns into the abdomen. Resection and anastomosis outside the inguinal canal are possible, but due to the narrow inlet at the level of the inguinal canal considerable edema and venous congestion usually occur.

6. An alternative operative procedure is more desirable. Through a secondary peritoneal incision, which can be placed

within the same skin incision, an anastomosis can be performed without interference with the vascular supply. A single-layer anastomosis is preferable, since it avoids the peritoneal contamination which occurs with open anastomoses.

## Direct Inguinal Hernia

The defect and repair of direct inguinal hernia are identical to those of adults.

## Hydrocele

1. The majority of hydroceles seen in early infancy are of the communicating type, and surgery is rarely indicated under the age of six months if no associated hernia is present.

2. A large percentage of these hydroceles in early infancy will absorb and disappear without operative treatment.

3. After the age of six months, operative removal appears to be indicated, especially if rapid enlargement and associated symptoms occur.

4. Hydroceles do not represent surgical emergencies. It should be remembered, however, that inguinal hernias are frequently associated with hydroceles and that the presence of a hydrocele, therefore, does not rule out an inguinal hernia. A complete resection of a hydrocele is rarely indicated if the communicating portion has been transected and ligated. Complete opening and eversion of the hydrocele is rarely followed by a recurrence and it obviates the difficult dissection of the hydrocele of the cord which may lead to arterial spasm and secondary testicular atrophy.

## CONGENITAL BANDS

### Basic Principles

The persistent omphalomesenteric duct is the most common congenital band leading to intestinal obstruction. Other congenital bands are occasionally encountered, such as the Jackson band, running from the terminal ileum to the right parietal gutter, or Ladd bands, associated with intestinal malrotation.

### Criteria for Diagnosis

The clinical picture is that of intestinal obstruction: cramping, intermittent pain, followed by abdominal distention, biliary vomiting and persistent abdominal pain and signs of peritonitis if vascular compromise has occurred. There are no specific findings by history, clinical examination or x-ray which will lead to the correct preoperative diagnosis.

### Management

1. Preoperative management is similar to that discussed in neonatal intestinal obstructions, with adequate preoperative hydration and correction of a coexisting metabolic imbalance, usually a mild metabolic acidosis in patients with long-standing intestinal obstruction.

2. The operative treatment consists of resection of the congenital band and intestine if a vascular compromise has occurred.

A. A closed single-layer anastomosis is preferable since it will avoid contamination of the peritoneal cavity.

B. In small infants, a transverse abdominal incision is preferable; in older children, due to the increased length of the abdominal trunk, a vertical incision may give a better exposure.

## INTERNAL HERNIA

### Definition

An internal hernia is a congenital herniation into abnormal intra-abdominal fossae without a true hernial sac.

### Classification

1. Paraduodenal hernia
2. Paracecal hernia
3. Sigmoidal hernia
4. Supravesicular hernia
5. Mesenteric defects

### Basic Principles

#### Etiology

The abnormal formation of peritoneal

folds, probably related to the rotation of the fetal intestine, is thought to be responsible for the formation of abnormal fossae, which can be found predominantly in the paraduodenal, cecal and sigmoid area and in the supravesicular space. Although internal hernias are rare in all ages, they have been found in the newborn and are therefore thought to be congenital rather than acquired. Another finding supporting their congenital nature is the presence of a "peritoneal sac."

Although mesenteric defects can occur at any part of the mesentery, they are most common in the area of the terminal ileum. The etiology is felt to be related to intrauterine vascular accidents. Operative treatment consists of reduction and closure of the defect.

## Associated Diseases or Anomalies

Paraduodenal hernias have been described in association with malrotation of the intestine.

### Pathophysiology

Indistinguishable from other types of intestinal obstructions

### Criteria for Diagnosis

The cause of intestinal obstruction in patients with intra-abdominal hernias is rarely suspected preoperatively, since the findings are identical to those seen in patients with intestinal obstruction due to adhesive or congenital bands.

### Management

## Preoperative Treatment

This is identical to that described under Intestinal Obstruction in the Neonate, with restoration of volume, rehydration and correction of metabolic imbalances.

## Operative Management

1. The proper diagnosis is rarely suspected preoperatively and has to be made at operation.
2. An incision of the peritoneal confines of the intra-abdominal hernia should be carried out with care to avoid major mesenteric vessel injury.
3. Since the entire small intestine is usually present within the abnormal fossa, reduction may be difficult if there is significant distention of the incarcerated intestine, and aseptic decompression of the intestine via an enterostomy catheter will be necessary.
4. Care should be taken to close the internal hernia, with preservation of the vascular supply to the intestine.
5. If there is vascular compromise of the intestine, it usually involves a large portion of the small intestine, and a method described under Malrotation in the Neonate, with re-exploration within 24 hours, intraluminal antibiotic drip, etc., may be indicated. Smaller portions may be resected at initial operation.

## BEZOAR

### Definitions

1. *Trichobezoar.* This is an accumulation of human hair in the intestine.
2. *Phytobezoar.* This is an accumulation consisting of vegetable fiber, seeds, squash, orange, celery, etc.
3. *Trichophytobezoar.* This is a bezoar consisting of hair and vegetable matter.

### Basic Principles

Swallowing of hair over an extended period of time will lead to the accumulation of a large hair bezoar in the stomach, which not infrequently will develop an extension through the duodenum into the jejunum which may make the extraction through a gastrotomy difficult. If a gastric trichobezoar has been identified, the distal small intestine should be examined carefully to detect additional accumulation of bezoars.

Intestinal obstruction due to foreign bodies can occur, but it is relatively rare. Foreign bodies, if symptomatic at all, are more likely to lead to perforation and intra-abdominal abscess formations.

## Criteria for Diagnosis

1. Although patients with trichobezoars are usually emotionally disturbed, a history of "hair swallowing" can be obtained. Vegetable bezoars (phytobezoars) can be encountered in all age-groups according to their dietary intake; trichobezoars are more common in older children and young teenagers.

2. Depending on the site of obstruction, the symptoms will be compatible either with gastroduodenal obstruction, especially in patients with a pure trichobezoar, or small bowel obstruction, which is more common in patients with phytobezoars.

3. Flat and upright films and especially barium studies may reveal the true cause of the obstruction, especially in patients with gastric trichobezoars. With low small intestinal obstruction, barium may be contraindicated if the obstruction is complete.

### Differential Diagnosis

Other causes of intestinal obstruction, such as congenital bands, adhesive bands, intussusception and others

## Management

### Preoperative Treatment

Identical to that described under intestinal obstruction due to other causes

### Operative Treatment

1. *Trichobezoar.* Trichobezoars should be removed through a gastrotomy. The removal can usually be accomplished without difficulty, unless there is a significant extension of a bezoar "tail" into the duodenum and occasionally into the jejunum. The sometimes tightly woven tail will not extract and an additional duodenostomy with transection and separate removal of the tail may be indicated.

2. *Intestinal Phytobezoar.* Enterostomy is usually indicated for the removal, since the phytobezoar can rarely be pushed into the large bowel. Multiple areas of accumulation may be encountered, and manual propulsion into one area may allow the removal of all bezoars through a single incision.

### Postoperative Treatment

In patients with trichobezoars, psychiatric evaluation with appropriate treatment is indicated in almost all patients.

# INTUSSUSCEPTION

## Definition

Intussusception is invagination of the small or large intestine into the contiguous distal portion.

## Basic Principles

### Etiology

Although the specific etiology of intussusceptions is not known, several predisposing factors such as viral upper respiratory infections, including adenovirus, have been identified. In spite of the increased incidence of organic problems in older children, such as polyps, in most series only up to 7 per cent of all children have documented organic lesions leading to intussusception.

### Associated Diseases or Anomalies

1. Viral infections in general, and upper respiratory infections in particular, are seen in these patients.

2. Tumors such as lymphosarcoma, leiomyoma, hamartoma, as in the Peutz-Jegher syndrome, Meckel's diverticulum and ectopic pancreas are anatomical abnormalities seen. The latter two are responsible for ileocolonic intussusception due to their proximity to the ileocecal valve.

3. Congenital anomalies such as the Jackson's band have also been incriminated as a cause of intussusception.

## Criteria for Diagnosis

### Clinical

1. Prior episodes of upper respiratory

infections are common, especially in children under the age of two years.

2. Symptoms classically are of intermittent colicky pain with sudden onset in a previously well child, followed by bloody stools (currant jelly).

3. On physical examination, an abdominal sausage-like mass can be palpated in the nonapprehensive child, occasionally combined with an absence of the cecum in the right lower quadrant (Dance's sign) in patients with ileocolic intussusception.

4. Depending on the length of the intussusception and the viability of the intussuscepted segment, signs of intestinal obstruction and/or peritoneal irritation and peritonitis can develop.

## Laboratory

An increased white cell count is not necessarily a reflection of the viability of the intestine but may be caused by an associated infection.

## X-ray

1. With the exception of small bowel intussusception, which in older children is usually due to pre-existing lesions such as lymphosarcoma, leiomyoma, etc., the x-ray pattern on flat and supine films is usually compatible with a low small intestinal obstruction.

2. The intussuscepted segment can occasionally be identified as a homogeneous mass.

3. Barium enema, performed in patients without signs of peritonitis, peritoneal irritation or long-standing obstruction, will reveal the typical "coil-spring" appearance in ileocolic intussusception.

4. The barium enema is not only diagnostic but therapeutic in the majority of acute, uncomplicated cases.

5. In upper intestinal obstruction, a barium swallow may delineate the area of pathology.

## Differential Diagnosis

Other diagnoses to be considered depend on the symptoms.

1. *Obstruction.* The obstruction of the colon may resemble low intestinal obstruction due to bands or Meckel's diverticulum. More uncommonly, small bowel obstruction is seen in which intussusception is the rule-out diagnosis.

2. *Rectal Bleeding.* Systemic causes of bleeding, such as coagulopathies, or local causes of bleeding, usually limited to the large bowel, such as polyps, are possibilities.

## Management

### General

1. Since the bleeding in intussusception rarely leads to a life-endangering exsanguination, the primary objective is to correct the deficiencies caused by the intestinal obstruction: restoration of volume, hydration and metabolic balance.

2. In the majority of children, regardless of age, there are no organic lesions, and the primary objective is a reduction of the intussusception by conservative means if possible.

3. In children with upper small bowel intussusception, reduction of the intussusception cannot be accomplished by barium and the barium swallow serves only for diagnostic purposes. Although a hydrostatic perforation is unlikely if the barium enema is performed properly, with a pressure head limited to 3 feet, the surgeon should be prepared in case such a perforation does occur. Intraperitoneally expelled barium can only be removed efficiently within a short time after the perforation. The inability to remove barium several hours after perforation leads to fecal and chemical peritonitis with a marked increase in mortality.

4. A successful reduction of an intussusception in a neonate under the age of two years does not require postoperative x-ray examination to rule out organic lesions responsible for the intussusception. In older children, a postoperative barium enema to rule out lesions such as polyps may be indicated, but it should be kept in mind that only 7 per cent of all children

have been found to have an organic cause for the intussusception.

(*See also:* Neonatal Intestinal Obstruction, Neonatal Abdominal Masses and Gastrointestinal Bleeding.)

## Operative Procedure

1. The intussusception is reduced by gentle but persistent pressure in a proximal to distal fashion.

2. An attempt to reduce the intussusception by traction of the distal segment can lead to perforation of a compromised intussusception, with peritonitis and serious complications.

3. If an operative reduction cannot be accomplished, or if there are signs of vascular compromise, resection with a simple end-to-end closed single-layer anastomosis appears to be a safe method.

4. Staged procedures, such as exteriorization or Mikulicz's procedure, are rarely indicated.

## Complications

Intestinal obstruction due to vascular compromise of the intussusception without necrosis may require reoperation. Necrosis of the intussuscepted segment will lead to acute peritonitis. The spontaneous slough of the intussusception, reported in the early 1920's, is rarely seen.

## INTRA-ABDOMINAL TUMORS

## Classification

Tumors that may cause intestinal obstruction can be classified into two groups:

1. *Intrinsic:* lymphosarcoma, leiomyoma, carcinoma, hamartoma (Peutz-Jegher)

2. *Extrinsic:* lymphosarcoma, neuroblastoma, rhabdomyosarcoma, presacral teratoma

## Criteria for Diagnosis

1. *Intrinsic*
    A. *Lymphosarcoma*
      (1) Involvement of the intestine may be preceded or associated with extra-abdominal lymphatic involvement. This may include enlargement of lymph nodes, change in white blood count or bone marrow or involvement of other organs.

      (2) In the absence of extra-abdominal involvement, the diagnosis may not be apparent until the time of laparotomy where intrinsic lymphosarcomas not infrequently present with intussusception. Close examination of the intestine involved usually shows a submucosal tumor which on cross-section has a fish-flesh-like appearance.

    B. *Hamartoma*
      (1) Peutz-Jegher hamartomas occur in the small intestine and are usually multiple and the obstruction is usually produced by intussusception.

      (2) The hamartoma resembles an intestinal polyp.

      (3) The association of this syndrome with perioral, perianal or subungual pigmentation should alert the surgeon to the correct diagnosis prior to laparotomy.

    C. *Leiomyoma*
      In contrast to the Peutz-Jegher polyps, leiomyomas are single and intramuscular lesions, and the mucosa is usually intact although occasional erosion and bleeding may occur.

    D. *Carcinoma*
      (1) While adenocarcinoma of the large intestine is rare in children, more than 300 cases have been reported. In contrast to adults, a preceding episode of bloody stools is even rarer and the carcinoma usually presents with intestinal obstruction.

      (2) Gross findings are similar to those in adults.

2. *Extrinsic*
    A. Extrinsic tumors leading to intestinal obstruction can usually be palpated on abdominal examination.

    B. While the diagnosis of an intra-abdominal tumor is apparent, the correct diagnosis may be difficult.

    C. The typical characteristics of the lesion, including VMA production by a neuroblastoma, multiple organ involvement in patients with lymphosarcoma, or the location of a rhabdomyosarcoma originating from pelvic structure, may give a clue to the diagnosis.

D. Presacral teratomas, which unlike other pelvic tumors such as ovarian tumors cannot escape into the abdominal cavity, may lead to rectal obstruction and the diagnosis can usually be confirmed by rectal examination.

E. The specific findings, including signs and symptoms, are discussed later in the section on Abdominal Tumors in the Child, page 580.

## Differential Diagnosis

Lesions other than true abdominal neoplasms leading to obstruction which may present similar findings are intestinal duplications and mesenteric cysts.

## Management

1. *Intrinsic*

A. *Lymphosarcoma.* Those limited to either intestine or mesentery adjacent to the intestine should be removed completely unless major structures are involved. The follow-up treatment is discussed under the treatment of lymphosarcoma, page 586.

B. *Hamartoma.* Since Peutz-Jegher hamartomas usually are multiple throughout the small intestine, only the lesion leading to the acute complication, usually intussusception, should be removed.

C. *Leiomyoma.* Since leiomyoma is usually solitary, a local excision by segmental resection of the intestine is all that is required.

D. *Carcinoma.* The treatment of carcinoma of the colon in children is identical to that in adults, even though the outcome is less favorable.

2. *Extrinsic Lesions.* The treatment of extrinsic sarcomas is discussed in the section on Abdominal Tumors in the Child, page 580.

# TRAUMA

## Basic Principles

Intestinal obstruction due to trauma can occur in an acute form such as duodenal hematoma or a chronic form such as fibrosis following an intramural hematoma. The blunt trauma of the midabdomen in the prevertebral area may lead to the injury of the duodenum, with intramural hematoma dissecting external to the muscularis as well as submucosally. Similar pathology can be found in the small intestine. The hematoma then can lead to either perforation or intestinal obstruction.

In acute cases associated pancreatic injury with hemorrhagic pancreatitis may be more striking and may mask an underlying duodenal obstruction.

## Criteria for Diagnosis

### Clinical

1. The most common site of intestinal obstruction following trauma is the duodenum.

2. In most cases the intestinal obstruction is acute following blunt intestinal trauma, especially following handlebar injuries in children. The blunt trauma to the abdomen usually involves the fixed portion of the duodenum overlying the vertebrae.

3. In patients without perforation or intra-abdominal bleeding leading to peritoneal irritation or peritonitis, the findings are limited to a high intestinal obstruction, with mild to moderate abdominal pain, occasionally crampy, with biliary vomiting.

4. Occasionally external injuries such as abrasions over the upper abdomen or midline may help in establishing the correct diagnosis.

### X-ray

1. Flat and upright films of the abdomen are usually noncontributory since

duodenal dilatation usually occurs only in long-standing obstructions.

2. The use of contrast material may show a mild to moderate dilatation of the duodenum, however, with obstruction in the prevertebral area.

## Management

### General

In children with duodenal hematomas leading to obstruction without perforation, the preoperative treatment is usually limited to rehydration, gastric decompression and observation for a coexisting pancreatitis.

### Operative Procedure

1. The abdomen is explored through an upper transverse or a midline incision.

2. If a duodenal hematoma is suspected, the colon should be mobilized completely, so that the entire duodenal sweep can be carefully inspected to rule out perforations.

3. In the absence of perforations, the duodenal hematoma can be incised and drained.

4. In patients with old injuries with fibrous stenosis, or in patients with perforations requiring closure which may lead to stenosis, a bypass with a duodenojejunostomy usually is indicated.

## Complications

Undetected duodenal perforations, peritonitis, pancreatitis, injury to the biliary system, leaking anastomosis or delayed rupture of the duodenal hematomas are complications to be anticipated.

## PERITONITIS IN THE CHILD

### INTESTINAL INFLAMMATORY CONDITIONS

## Classification

1. Regional enteritis
2. Ulcerative colitis
3. Appendicitis
4. *Foreign Bodies*
   A. Esophagus
   B. Stomach
   C. Intestine
5. Rectal and perianal inflammatory conditions

### *Regional Enteritis*

## Definition

Regional enteritis is granulomatous inflammation of the intestine, predominantly involving the terminal ileum, but also found in other portions of the intestine, including the stomach, duodenum and small and large bowel.

## Basic Principles

The etiology of regional enteritis is unknown, but a genetic and ethnic background is often found. It is extremely uncommon in young Negro children. The site most commonly involved is the ileum, but jejunum, duodenum, stomach or colon can also be involved, either as single or multiple areas. In keeping with the scope of this book, only acute emergencies resulting from regional enteritis will be discussed, including peritonitis, intestinal obstruction, gastrointestinal bleeding and internal and external fistulae formation.

## Criteria for Diagnosis

### Clinical

1. The extent of the disease determines the type of symptoms, including intermittent abdominal pain, diarrhea, failure to gain weight, growth failure, intermittent febrile episodes, debilitation, the development of an acute surgical abdomen, fistula formation and gastrointestinal bleeding. Careful probing of the history will usually elicit one or more of these symptoms.

2. The most common manifestation of regional enteritis in young children is the appearance of an acute intra-abdominal inflammation, compatible with acute appendicitis.

3. In patients with more severe and protracted symptoms, intestinal obstruction or intestinal bleeding can occur.

4. Although the development of internal and external fistulae represents one of the indications for operative intervention (although some of these patients can be treated effectively with hyperalimentation), fistula formation is usually not an acute emergency but follows a prolonged history of debilitating illness.

### X-ray

Although contrast studies usually are not obtained in a child presenting with findings compatible with appendicitis, in patients with a clearly established history of previous intra-abdominal manifestations, contrast studies are indicated to demonstrate the extent and the site of involvement.

## Management

### General

1. In patients not presenting an acute surgical emergency, the nonoperative treatment includes dietary regimen, sulfasuxidine, steroid, hyperalimentation and immunosuppressive agents.

2. Preoperative preparation is routine in most cases.

### Operative Procedure

1. In an acute emergency, the most common finding is the unexpected presence of an inflamed ileum with the characteristic overgrowth of mesenteric fat.

2. Unless there are significant pathologic alterations, such as fistula formation or intestinal obstruction, resection is not indicated.

3. In contrast to reports in the literature, indicating that biopsy or appendectomy will lead to fistula formation in a large percentage of cases, in our experience a carefully performed inverted appendectomy or full-thickness biopsy can be performed safely to establish the correct diagnosis.

4. In patients whose disease has progressed to a point that resection is indicated, an attempt should be made to clearly identify the areas of proximal and distal involvement by frozen section technique, to decrease the possibility of anastomotic involvement and postoperative stricture.

## Complications

Recurrence of regional enteritis, involvement of new areas, fistula formation and intestinal obstruction also are seen in the child.

### *Ulcerative Colitis*

## Definition

Ulcerative colitis in children is indistinguishable from ulcerative colitis in adults. In contrast to granulomatous colitis, the disease involves primarily the mucosa, with diffuse ulcerations.

## Basic Principles

Etiology is unknown although various causes are considered: autoimmune disease, emotional disturbance, imbalance of the autonomic nervous system, allergies and alteration of enzyme activities. A social or genetic factor has not been established. An ethnic background is apparent since ulcerative colitis is rarely seen in Negro children under ten years of age, in contrast to Caucasian children.

Associated conditions include arthralgia, pyoderma, hepatic involvement leading to cirrhosis, and failure of weight gain or growth. A significant increased incidence of adenocarcinoma in patients with ulcerative colitis has been proven, especially if the disease has been present for more than ten years.

## Criteria for Diagnosis

### Clinical

1. Intermittent abdominal pain with frequent mucoid stools, bloody diarrhea, crampy abdominal pain and failure to gain weight or grow.

2. Intermittent remissions occur frequently.

3. Although emotional problems are frequently found in adults and children alike, no definite correlation between the psychological make-up of the patient and the disease can be made.

4. Arthralgia, pyoderma and hepatic involvement are found in patients with long-standing disease.

5. On proctoscopy the rectal or sigmoid mucosa is friable. Diffuse petechiae and bleeding are found in the early stage, followed by the formation of pseudopolyps with diffuse mucosal ulceration.

6. Perianal, perineal, rectovaginal and vesicular fistulae occur as complications.

### X-ray

In the early stage, a saw-tooth appearance of the involved colonic segment, with reduced or absent peristalsis, followed by a rigid "lead pipe" formation with or without stenosis

### Differential Diagnosis

1. Nonspecific proctitis
2. Granulomatous colitis
3. Amebic colitis

## Management

### General

1. In contrast to patients with granulomatous colitis, the use of steroids has been beneficial, although the over-all rate of patients requiring operative intervention has not changed significantly.

2. While dietary regimen, such as the avoidance of milk products, has been helpful in some cases, no specific diet has been proven to be effective.

3. The use of sulfa drugs is still recommended.

4. Topical application of steroid appears to be effective only in early cases of ulcerative colitis limited to rectum and sigmoid.

### Indications for Operation

1. Prolonged disease with failure of growth or sexual development is an indication for operation in children with ulcerative colitis.

2. Other indications are identical to those in adults: intestinal obstruction, toxic megacolon, formation of fistula, development of pyoderma, joint or hepatic involvement.

### Operative Procedure

1. Bypass procedures have been almost uniformly abandoned.

2. Argument still exists whether subtotal colectomy with ileoproctostomy is justified in children to avoid a permanent terminal ileostomy. While many patients with ileoproctostomy may be symptom-free for a variable period of time, the vast majority will develop recurrent disease in the retained rectum. Not only is the recurring disease a factor to be considered, but the incidence of carcinoma in the retained rectum appears to be of such magnitude that a total colectomy with removal of the rectum and a terminal ileostomy is preferable as definitive procedure.

3. In patients with toxic megacolon with or without perforation, colectomy may not be feasible as the initial procedure. Decompressing ileostomy and secondary colectomy may be the procedure of choice.

## Complications

1. Retardation of growth, puberty and weight gain
2. Pyoderma, arthralgia, cirrhosis
3. Perineal fistula or abscess formation
4. Intestinal obstruction, internal fistula or toxic megacolon
5. Development of colonic or rectal adenocarcinoma

*Appendicitis*

## Definition

Appendicitis is inflammation of the appendix.

## Classification

1. Acute appendicitis

2. Perforated appendicitis with localized abscess formation

3. Perforated appendicitis with diffuse peritonitis

4. Chronic appendicitis

## Basic Principles

1. The etiology of appendicitis may be obstruction related to the formation of fecaliths or due to swelling of lymphatic tissues. The obstruction is followed by an increase of intraluminal pressure within the appendix, with subsequent local inflammation, necrosis and perforation which may lead to a localized, walled-off abscess or diffuse peritonitis.

2. Appendicitis is rare in children under the age of two years. Its peak incidence occurs between the seventh and tenth year in childhood. The clinical signs and symptoms follow the basic pathology: obstruction followed by inflammation, local necrosis and perforation.

## Criteria for Diagnosis

### Clinical

1. The classical symptoms consist of para-umbilical pain shifting to the right lower quadrant, followed by anorexia or nausea, signs of peritoneal irritation, right lower quadrant tenderness and rebound tenderness.

2. Signs of diffuse peritonitis develop when perforation has occurred without localization.

3. In patients with abnormal appendiceal location, such as retrocecal appendix, the classical signs and findings may be absent, and urinary findings may dominate, such as flank pain, dysuria or the presence of white cells in the urine.

4. The degree of fever may vary considerably, but high temperatures are usually only seen with purulent appendicitis and perforation.

5. Both diarrhea and constipation can occur; neither one is particularly helpful in the differential diagnosis.

6. In patients with a retrocecal appendix, either the obturator or psoas sign may indicate the presence of an inflammatory process in the retroperitoneal area, suggestive of appendicitis.

7. Local tenderness on rectal examination, while helpful when present, is often absent in children.

8. In apprehensive children, where the physical examination is difficult due to the lack of cooperation, mild sedation with Nembutal R will facilitate the examination.

### Laboratory

Leukocytosis with shift to the left

### X-ray

1. In view of the high incidence of fecaliths causing appendicitis, abdominal x-ray films should be taken in all patients with either questionable appendicitis or signs of perforation.

2. Calcification can be seen in 20 to 30 per cent of cases.

3. Although there are no other specific x-ray findings for appendicitis, the accumulation of gas around the cecal area within intestinal loops or the formation of a mass in patients with perforation and abscess formation may be suggestive of appendicitis.

### Differential Diagnosis

1. Upper respiratory infections with mesenteric adenitis

2. Gastroenteritis

3. Urinary tract infections

4. *Systemic Diseases*
   A. Sickle cell disease
   B. Rheumatic fever
   C. Porphyria
   D. Abdominal epilepsy
   E. Juvenile diabetes

5. In young girls during their menarche, an imperforate hymen with metrocolpos may be present with symptoms compatible with appendicitis.

## Management

### Acute Nonperforated Appendicitis

1. *Preoperative Management*

A. Dehydration is mild and due to the lack of oral intake, vomiting or fever, and intraperitoneal fluid losses are minimal or nonexistent.

B. Preoperative hydration can be accomplished with a one-third isotonic crystalloid solution (2500 ml. per square meter of body surface per 24 hours).

C. In view of the frequently associated increased temperature, the preoperative administration of atropine or scopolamine is contraindicated until the fever has been brought under control and the patient is on the operating table in a normothermic state.

2. *Operative Management*

A. The appendix is removed through a muscle-splitting McBurney incision.

B. Open inversion of the appendiceal stump (inversion of an untied stump) appears to be advantageous over closed inversion, since the latter can occasionally lead to secondary abscess or mucocele formation.

### Perforated Appendicitis

1. *Preoperative Management*

A. In contrast to the patient with acute nonperforated appendicitis, there usually is a significant intra-abdominal fluid loss, and adequate preoperative preparation with restoration of hydration and intravascular volume is needed.

B. The rehydration of patients with perforated appendicitis and peritonitis consists of an initial administration of isotonic fluid until vital signs have returned to normal, tachycardia is reduced and urinary output is established.

C. This is followed by a half-isotonic solution without potassium at 2500 ml. square meter of body surface per 24 hours.

D. Broad-spectrum antibiotics are indicated preoperatively.

E. Nasogastric suction is started to prevent further abdominal distention.

F. As in the patient with nonperforated appendix, the frequently associated hyperthermia should be controlled prior to the operative exploration. Normothermia can be achieved by the use of cooling mattresses or alcohol sponges, but only after the patient has been sedated to prevent shivering which increases the metabolic rate and tends to increase the patient's temperature.

2. *Operative Management*

A. In most children with perforation of the appendix with or without abscess formation, removal of the appendix and inversion of the stump are possible.

B. The presence of a calcified fecalith on x-ray should alert the surgeon to the possibility of a free intraperitoneal fecalith. Its removal may prevent postoperative abscess formation.

C. In patients with abscess, drainage via a Penrose or sump drain through the wound is advisable, not only to drain the abscess cavity but also to drain the contaminated wound.

D. Although the drainage of diffuse peritonitis is frequently performed, the benefit of the drainage in diffuse peritonitis is questionable.

E. In patients with perforation of the appendix, where dissection and removal of the appendix is either extremely difficult or might endanger other structures, a simple drainage followed by an interval appendectomy after approximately three months is preferable.

3. *Postoperative Complications*

A. Intra-abdominal abscess formation

B. Pyelephlebitis

C. Fecal fistula

D. Septicemia

E. Spontaneous rectal perforation of pelvic abscess

F. Intestinal obstruction

*Foreign Body*

## Definition

Foreign body in this section refers to material not usually found in the gastrointestinal tract at that level.

## Basic Principles

Ingestion of foreign bodies occurs predominantly between 6 months and 3 years of age. Foreign bodies passing the esophagus and entering the stomach, unless unusually long or shaped in a form interfering with their intraluminal propulsion, such as open safety pins, will usually pass through the intestinal tract over a period of time. Certain anatomical conditions will lead to a temporary or permanent arrest in the following areas: duodenum, ligament of Treitz and ileocecal valve. In the esophagus the upper third is the most likely area of retention.

Approximately 90 per cent of foreign bodies will pass through the intestinal tract without difficulties once they have reached the stomach. Symptoms are primarily due to lodgment with obstruction or perforation.

## Criteria for Diagnosis

### Clinical

1. History of ingestion
2. Choking and inability to swallow with foreign body retained in the esophagus
3. Symptoms secondary to perforation of foreign bodies, most commonly seen in the duodenal sweep, ligament of Treitz or ileocecal valve. Since the perforation usually occurs slowly, signs of diffuse peritonitis are rare, and symptoms are compatible with local abscess formation.

### X-ray

1. The majority of foreign bodies ingested are radiopaque and their progress can be followed by x-rays.
2. Round objects, such as coins, once having entered the stomach will pass through the gastrointestinal tract even though the progress may take weeks at times.
3. Interval x-rays in asymptomatic patients at approximately 1-week intervals usually suffice.

### Differential Diagnosis

With retained esophageal foreign bodies, a pre-existing lesion should be ruled out when the foreign body is either relatively small, nonrigid or a food particle normally passed in a patient of that age.

### Associated Diseases or Abnormalities

Pre-existing anatomical narrowing such as esophageal or duodenal webs.

## Management

### General

1. Gastrointestinal foreign bodies having passed the esophagus rarely require operative removal unless symptoms develop or the foreign body is retained within one area for several weeks.
2. Even foreign bodies that appear harmless because of shape or lack of symptoms should be considered for removal if absorption of toxic substances, such as lead or nickel, can lead to complications.

### Esophagus

1. Foreign bodies retained in the esophagus will require prompt removal since they invariably will lead to symptoms of choking, inability to swallow or occasional respiratory difficulty.
2. Occasionally foreign bodies with a smooth shape located in the upper esophagus can be removed by the passage of a Foley catheter distal to the foreign body with gentle inflation of the balloon and extraction of the catheter.
3. The accepted and safer method is the removal under direct vision through an esophagoscope under general anesthesia.

### Stomach

1. The propulsion of round and smooth

objects entering the stomach can be facilitated with increased undigestible roughage, such as asparagus, or by heavy, thickened barium meals.

2. If the foreign body has not moved after several weeks or if the shape or length of the foreign body makes spontaneous propulsion into the intestine unlikely, removal via a gastrotomy is then indicated. Remember, however, that the gastrointestinal tract can adapt even to rather unwieldy foreign bodies, and removal is only indicated in the absence of symptoms if the patient has been given an adequate chance for spontaneous evacuation.

## Intestinal Tract

1. Foreign bodies, with the exception of open safety pins, long pins or needles, will usually progress through the intestinal tract without difficulties once they have passed the pylorus and the duodenum.

2. If foreign bodies like pins are noted to remain in the same area for a prolonged period of time, perforation has to be considered.

3. Acute peritonitis rarely occurs, since the foreign body will perforate slowly, thereby setting up an inflammatory reaction around the serosa which leads to an abscess formation rather than free peritonitis.

4. Contrast studies are indicated to ascertain the intra- or extraluminal position of the foreign body.

## Operative Removal

1. X-rays immediately prior to celiotomy to locate the foreign body

2. In patients with a small foreign body near the ileocecal valve, removal can be performed via an appendectomy.

3. In patients in whom a perforation has occurred, the local inflammatory response will dictate the type of operation: either removal and primary closure or resection of the involved segment.

4. In patients with perforation due to nonopaque foreign bodies, such as chicken bone or toothpicks, etc., the perforating object is often not identified but the peculiar pathologic process, with abscess formation around a small area of intestine without any apparent extra- or intraluminal disease, is usually suggestive of the diagnosis.

### Rectal and Perianal Inflammatory Conditions

## Definitions

1. *Perianal Abscess.* This is located in the perianal area usually without extension into the ischiorectal area, with or without rectal communication.

2. *Perirectal Abscess.* This is an abscess in the peri- or ischiorectal area, usually communicating with the rectum.

## Basic Principles

Perianal abscess may be secondary to infected hair follicles or fissures, without rectal communication. In patients with perianal fistulae or peri- or ischiorectal abscesses, a communication with the rectum is usually present.

## Associated Diseases

1. Intra-abdominal pathology
2. Cryptitis or proctitis
3. Systemic diseases such as diabetes

## Criteria for Diagnosis

### Clinical

1. *Perianal Abscess*
   A. Perianal pain, tenderness and redness
   B. Swelling
   C. Occasionally spontaneous purulent discharge
   D. Only rarely accompanied by high temperature
2. *Perirectal Abscess*
   A. Perianal or rectal tenderness
   B. Tenderness on defecation
   C. Signs of systemic infection
   D. Occasionally purulent rectal discharge

E. Induration or swelling on rectal examination

## X-ray

1. In perirectal or ischiorectal abscess, posterior and lateral films may show a presacral mass pushing the rectum anteriorly, especially in patients with ischiorectal "horse shoe abscessess."

2. Contrast injection into a rectal or perianal fistula can demonstrate the exact outline and extension of the abscess.

## Differential Diagnosis

1. Perianal abscesses or perirectal abscesses associated with intra-abdominal pathology, such as ulcerative colitis

2. Perianal, perineal or prostatic malignancies

## Management

### Perianal Abscesses

1. Perianal abscesses undergo necrosis and require incision and drainage.

2. Conservative treatment, therefore, is only used to prepare the patient for incision and drainage.

3. Broad-spectrum antibiotics, local wet compresses and Sitz baths are continued until fluctuation has occurred, permitting incision and drainage under general anesthesia.

4. After an adequate incision, the existing cavity is loosely packed with gauze.

5. Follow-up treatment includes Sitz baths and change of the gauze until the abscess cavity has granulated in.

6. In patients with chronic perianal abscesses, especially if not responding promptly to incision and drainage, underlying malignancies, in particular rhabdomyosarcoma, have to be ruled out.

### Perirectal and Ischiorectal Abscesses

The operative drainage of these abscesses follows the same basic rules as observed in adults: adequate drainage with preservation of sphincter function. A communication with the rectum can usually be found and further treatment depends upon location and extent of the fistula.

## INTRA-ABDOMINAL INFLAMMATORY PROCESS

### Classification

1. Primary peritonitis
2. Intra-abdominal abscess
3. Perinephric abscess

### *Primary Peritonitis*

### Definition

Primary peritonitis is peritonitis without primary intra-abdominal pathology.

### Classification

1. Pneumococcal or streptococcal peritonitis, in particular in patients with nephrosis or patients under cortisone treatment

2. *E. coli* peritonitis in patients with cirrhosis

### Basic Principles

Primary streptococcal and pneumococcal peritonitis appears to be hematogenous in origin, with blood cultures usually positive for the same organism. Either form occurs in debilitated children, in particular nephrotic children or those under steroid treatment. The primary *E. coli* peritonitis is usually associated with marked cirrhosis, rare in childhood and more commonly seen in adults.

Since the infection is hematogenous without peritoneal localization, the peritonitis is diffuse and the colloid loss is far out of proportion compared with regional inflammatory changes such as appendicitis.

This loss of colloids produces subsequent hypovolemia and acute dehydration. General septicemia is usually present with positive blood cultures.

### Criteria for Diagnosis

#### Clinical

1. Rapid onset of peritonitis with ab-

dominal distention, hypoactive or absent bowel sounds

2. Rapid dehydration
3. High temperature
4. Especially seen in children between the ages of one to five years with underlying kidney disease such as nephrosis, or in children who are undergoing steroid treatment.

## Laboratory

1. Leukocytosis, shift to the left
2. Abdominal paracentesis which reveals only one strain of bacteria, either pneumococcus or streptococcus, is diagnostic of primary peritonitis.

## X-ray

A pattern of ileus is often seen, with evidence of free intraperitoneal fluid.

## Associated Diseases

Nephrosis or diseases necessitating steroid treatment

## Management

Nonoperative Treatment Directed to Two Aspects
1. The acute hypovolemia and dehydration
2. The septicemia and the causative organism
3. Operative intervention is only indicated if the diagnosis can not be clearly established. In patients in whom the diagnosis has been made only after a laparotomy has been performed, antibiotic irrigation of the abdomen is done and parenteral antibiotics started (intravenous penicillin for pneumococcus and streptococcus). Adequate replacement infusion of colloids and isotonic crystalloid solutions is started.

### *Intra-abdominal Abscesses*

## Classification

1. Loculated intra-abdominal abscess
2. Subdiaphragmatic abscess (suprahepatic or infrahepatic abscess)

3. Intra-abdominal abscess
4. Pelvic abscess
5. Retroperitoneal abscess

## Basic Principles

With the exception of appendicitis, largely responsible for the formation of abdominal abscesses in older children, postoperative abscesses are most common, followed by intestinal or gastroduodenal perforation, hepatic, perinephric, pancreatic and tubo-ovarian abscesses. Although intra-abdominal abscesses can occur in infancy, in view of the short omentum localization in infants is rare. The location of the abscess may give a clue, preoperatively or at exploration, to the underlying pathology.

## Criteria for Diagnosis

### Clinical

1. Clinical history will depend on the etiology and location of the abscess.
2. In general, intra-abdominal abscesses will present with vague abdominal signs, occasionally tenderness, diarrhea secondary to intestinal irritation, ileus or intestinal obstruction and signs of systemic infection.
3. Preceding episodes of intra-abdominal pain, suggesting appendicitis or intestinal perforation with localization, are significant.

### Laboratory

1. Leukocytosis and shift to the left
2. Occasionally positive blood cultures
3. With associated pyelephlebitis, a deranged liver profile with increased bilirubin, due either to hepatic involvement or due to septicemia

### X-ray

1. X-ray examination may be the most helpful technique for localizing the intra-abdominal or retroperitoneal abscess.
2. Depending on the suspected abscess site, in addition to plain flat and upright films, contrast studies, such as intravenous

pyelogram, upper gastrointestinal series or barium enema, can be done.

3. In patients with suspected hepatic involvement, arteriogram, umbilical venogram, scan or sonogram may be indicated.

4. Pleural effusion suggests a subdiaphragmatic collection.

### Differential Diagnosis

1. Diffuse peritonitis
2. Intra-abdominal or retroperitoneal neoplasm
3. Pancreatitis
4. Pancreatic pseudocysts
5. Chronic granulomatous disease
6. Pyelephlebitis

## Management

### General

1. An attempt should be made to localize the intra-abdominal abscess preoperatively.

2. The underlying disease responsible for the formation of the abscess should be diagnosed if possible.

3. Since numerous causes may be responsible, treatment will vary but prompt adequate operative drainage is indicated in all cases.

4. If possible, the operative approach should be limited to the area of involvement without spreading the localized infection throughout the intra-abdominal space.

5. The treatment of retroperitoneal abscesses, such as perinephric abscesses, should be done through an extraperitoneal approach.

6. In patients with associated partial or complete intestinal obstruction, release of the obstruction is indicated at the time of the abscess drainage.

7. Diffuse cellulitis, especially after operation for perforated appendicitis, is not an indication for exploration since conservative treatment with antibiotics usually suffices. Similarly, after the closure of perforated gastroduodenal ulcers,

diaphragmatic cellulitis with or without pleural effusion may occur, responding to conservative treatment without operative intervention.

### *Liver Abscess*

## Definition

Single or multiple liver abscesses may occur secondary to:

1. Nonspecific infections, pyogenic organisms
2. Specific inflammation (amebiasis)
3. Systemic disease (chronic granulomatous disease)

## Basic Principles

Pyogenic abscesses are often associated with pyelephlebitis, an infection involving mesenteric veins due to intra-abdominal inflammation such as appendicitis. Amebic abscesses are usually associated with intestinal amebiasis. Chronic granulomatous disease usually leads to diffuse hepatic abscesses but rarely as the first manifestation. Usually there has been involvement of the lymphatic or pulmonary system prior to the development of hepatic abscesses.

## Criteria for Diagnosis

### Clinical

1. Pyogenic liver abscesses usually are multiple.

2. Frequently there is a history of intra-abdominal inflammatory processes such as intra-abdominal abscesses, perforated appendicitis, etc.

3. Liver tenderness, weight loss, dehydration, chronic debilitation and jaundice with or without hepatomegaly are frequently seen.

4. Enteric manifestation of amebiasis or a history of known exposure to ameba may suggest amebic abscess which, in contrast to pyogenic abscesses, usually is large and single.

5. In patients with chronic granulomatous disease, a previous history

may disclose occurrence of multiple abscesses involving lymph nodes, lung and pleura, starting in early childhood usually under the age of one year.

## Laboratory

1. Abnormal liver profile and elevated bilirubin
2. Enteric amebiasis in patients with amebic liver abscesses
3. With chronic granulomatous disease, inability of white cells to destroy phagocytosed bacteria due to enzymatic deficiencies (NTB test)

## X-ray

Special x-ray studies such as angiograms, radioactive scan or sonograms can localize and differentiate between multiple and single abscesses. Other studies as indicated can be done to localize a primary source of infection.

## Differential Diagnosis

1. Hepatitis
2. Primary or secondary hepatic neoplasms
3. Extrahepatic and intrahepatic biliary duct anomalies associated with cholangitis
4. Intra-abdominal abscesses

## Management

1. The presence of multiple pyogenic abscesses following intra-abdominal disease necessitates the eradication of the primary inflammatory focus within the abdomen.
2. Conservative treatment with broad-spectrum antibiotics usually suffices after the primary focus has been successfully treated; only large pyogenic abscesses will require drainage.
3. Amebic abscesses, more often single than multiple, can respond to simple aspiration and proper medical treatment (chloroquine).
4. With chronic granulomatous disease, aggressive operative treatment with open drainage and appropriate antibiotic coverage is mandatory.

## *Perinephric Abscess*

## Definition

A perinephric abscess is a retroperitoneal abscess adjacent to the kidney, most often due to renal infection, obstruction or trauma.

## Basic Principles

Perinephric abscesses occur most often in patients with infected and obstructed kidneys. Trauma to the kidney, with or without pre-existing anomaly or disease, may lead to rupture and development of a perinephric abscess.

## Criteria for Diagnosis

### Clinical

1. Flank pain, often associated with the appearance of flank mass
2. Signs of local and systemic infection

### Laboratory

1. Elevated white blood count with leukocytosis
2. Presence of white cells in the urine in associated pyelonephritis or incomplete obstruction

### X-ray

Intravenous pyelogram may show evidence of renal displacement. Additionally, pyelonephritis, hydronephrosis often associated with obstruction or nonfunctioning kidney may be seen.

### Differential Diagnosis

1. Intra-abdominal abscesses
2. Pott's abscess (tuberculosis)
3. Hydronephrosis
4. Renal tumor
5. Retroperitoneal hemorrhage

## Management

### General

1. Although the immediate treatment of a perinephric abscess consists of retroperitoneal drainage, in patients with

complete destruction of the renal parenchyma nephrectomy may be indicated.

2. Unless the associated pathology has been demonstrated and the function of the contralateral kidney proven to be adequate, resection is contraindicated and the primary treatment should be limited to incision and drainage.

3. In patients in whom an unsuspected perinephric abscess is encountered during a laparotomy, the drainage should not be performed through the peritoneal space but via the extraperitoneal route, with subsequent urologic work-up.

## GASTROINTESTINAL BLEEDING IN THE CHILD

*See also* Neonatal Intestinal Bleeding.

### GASTRODUODENAL STRESS ULCERS

### Definition

Gastroduodenal stress ulcers are multiple or single ulcers of either stomach and/or duodenum, associated with stressful conditions such as trauma, operation, burn, encephalopathies or associated diseases.

### Basic Principles

In most children with secondary or stress ulcers, the underlying etiology, such as postoperative complications or burns, is apparent. Patients with cerebral lesions, however, may present with a stress ulcer before the prior disease has been recognized. In a child with sudden gastrointestinal bleeding originating from the stomach or duodenum without apparent underlying disease or trauma, an unsuspected primary disease has to be ruled out before the tentative diagnosis of peptic ulcer is made. The exact mechanism of the formation of stress ulcers is unknown; it does not appear to be related to an increase of gastric acidity, since patients with "Cushing" ulcers with cerebral pathology are often found to have low gastric acidity.

### Criteria for Diagnosis

#### Clinical

1. In contrast to adults, in children gastric or duodenal ulcers not infrequently present with bleeding prior to perforation.

2. The clinical picture of hematemesis and/or melena usually resembles that of the adult; exsanguination with minor clinical manifestations can occur more rapidly in the child.

3. Hematemesis may be coffee-ground or bright red.

4. Melena from upper gastrointestinal bleeding is usually dark in color, but with massive bleeding, "hematochezia," bright-red rectal bleeding can occur.

5. In patients with melena without hematemesis, aspiration of a nasogastric tube will usually document blood within stomach.

6. In an occasional patient, gastric blood may not be encountered either due to a cessation of bleeding or in patients with duodenal ulcers with little or no gastric reflux.

#### Laboratory

1. Low hemoglobin or hematocrit with chronic bleeding or several hours after the onset of acute bleeding

2. Normal liver profile in contrast to patients with intrahepatic block and esophageal and/or gastric varices

3. Gastric analysis for free acid is not helpful in patients with stress ulcers, since stress ulcers in children usually occur with normal or low gastric acidity.

#### X-ray

1. In chronic or subacute bleeding, a barium swallow may show deep ulcer craters or distortion of the duodenal bulb.

2. In the majority of children with stress ulcers, the ulcers are multiple and superficial and not apparent on x-ray.

3. During an acute bleeding episode, the presence of blood clots in the stomach and duodenum interferes with the correct interpretation of the x-rays.

4. Angiography may demonstrate the source of bleeding.

5. Technetium radioactive studies may differentiate gastroduodenal bleeding from a bleeding Meckel's diverticulum, with gastric mucosa within the diverticulum retaining the technetium.

## Differential Diagnosis

1. Systemic causes as listed above
2. Peptic ulcer, hemorrhagic gastritis, portal hypertension, Meckel's diverticulum

## Management

### Conservative Treatment

1. Insertion of a nasogastric tube with iced saline or milk irrigations
2. Blood transfusions as indicated to maintain adequate perfusion
3. Criteria for adequate perfusion are the patient's clinical responses, such as alertness, color and maintenance of normal vital signs, including pulse rate, blood pressure and urinary output.
4. Overtransfusion should be avoided since it may reactivate or increase gastroduodenal bleeding.
5. Sedation in patients who show signs of restlessness or anxiety without evidence of hypotension
6. Maintenance of hydration with intravenous isotonic or half-isotonic crystalloid solutions
7. Gastric antacids via a nasogastric tube or orally when the patient resumed oral intake.

### Indications for Operative Intervention

*Uncontrollable Bleeding*
1. If the gastric blood loss approximates the patient's blood volume within 24 hours, operative intervention is indicated.
2. Operative intervention is directed toward the control of the gastroduodenal bleeding.
3. Considerations determining the type of operative procedure employed in peptic ulcers to prevent recurrence do not apply

to patients with stress ulcers in view of the difference in the underlying etiology. The most limited operative procedure allowing control of bleeding should be selected.

### Operative Treatment

1. *Single Duodenal Ulcer*
   A. In patients with a punched-out single duodenal ulcer with active bleeding, closure of the ulcer crater with hemostatic suture ligation of the bleeding vessel suffices.
   B. In patients in whom continuous stress is anticipated, pyloroplasty and vagotomy should be added.

2. *Diffuse Superficial Gastroduodenal Ulcers.* In patients with diffuse superficial ulcerations, occasionally resembling corrosive gastritis in adults, vagotomy and pyloroplasty may be sufficient to control the bleeding. Vagotomy decreases the mucosal blood flow with submucosal shunting and may therefore decrease the amount of gastric bleeding.

3. *Patients With Diffuse Gastroduodenal Ulcerations*
   A. In patients with multiple deep ulcers or patients who fail to respond to vagotomy, a subtotal resection may be indicated. Resections up to 80 per cent with a gastrojejunostomy are well tolerated by children without an apparent deleterious effect on growth and development.
   B. The technique of the various operative procedures is identical to that in adults.

4. *Bleeding Ulcers Leading to Perforation*
   A. These ulcers are usually located in the duodenum. The operative treatment depends on the local anatomical findings.
   B. Suture ligation of the bleeder with a Roscoe-Graham-type of closure can be employed in most cases.
   C. If either ulcer crater or perforation is too large for a simple closure, gastrectomy and gastrojejunostomy are indicated.

## Complications

1. *Complications Related to the Operative Procedure*

A. Anastomotic leak

B. Continuous hemorrhage

2. *Other Complications*

A. Recurrent bleeding, especially if the underlying cause leading to the formation of stress ulcers has not been treated successfully

B. Development of disseminated intravascular clotting

## PEPTIC ULCERS

### Basic Principles

Although peptic ulcers are rare in early childhood, they do occur in the preteen-age years and become more common in the midteens. Etiology, pathophysiology and treatment are similar to the adult.

In addition to the various factors determining the choice of therapy, the effect of a debilitating peptic ulcer on a child's growth and development has to be considered.

## PORTAL HYPERTENSION

### Definition

Portal hypertension occurs with obstruction of the portal venous outflow leading to venous hypertension.

### Classification

The classification of portal hypertension is based on the site of the portal venous outflow obstruction.

1. Suprahepatic obstruction
2. Intrahepatic obstruction
3. Subhepatic obstruction

### Basic Principles

Etiology

1. *Suprahepatic:* cardiac failure, constrictive pericarditis

2. *Intrahepatic:* posthepatic cirrhosis, biliary cirrhosis, cirrhosis in patients with systemic diseases such as fibrocystic disease, galactosemia, Wilson's disease

3. *Subhepatic:* thrombosis of the portal vein and/or splenic and superior mesenteric vein; possibly related to ascending omphalitis

Pathophysiology

The obstruction of the portal venous blood flow leads to an increased venous pressure within the portal system and subsequent varices formation, predominantly in the esophagogastric submucosal area. Mechanical trauma, related to food intake and gastric acidity, may cause mucosal and then venous erosion with subsequent bleeding. In patients with secondary hypersplenism, the bleeding tendency can be aggravated if a thrombocytopenia has occurred.

The combination of bleeding and hepatic coma in children with intrahepatic blocks secondary to liver failure is similar to that seen in adults.

Establishment of portal venous systemic shunts can increase the rate of hepatic failure. It should be emphasized that patients with intrahepatic blocks due to cirrhosis may present with additional pathologic findings, complicating diagnosis and therapy: the presence of gastric ulcers and secondary portal venous thrombosis.

### Management

General

1. *Intrahepatic Block.* Conservative therapy is preferable, especially if advanced cirrhosis is present.

A. Blood transfusion, isotonic or half-isotonic crystalloid solutions

B. Nasogastric suction with evacuation of intragastric blood, *and*

C. Iced saline irrigations (or iced milk with antacids)

D. Platelet transfusions in patients with secondary hypersplenism

E. Esophagogastric balloon tamponade if bleeding cannot be controlled

F. Pitressin

G. Intestinal antibiotics to decrease the danger of hepatic coma

H. In patients with anticipated or actual hepatic coma, treatment of the metabolic alkalosis which is usually found by the use of sodium chloride usually is sufficient.

I. Arginine chloride is occasionally indicated, ammonium chloride is contraindicated.

J. Glutamic acid to prevent ammonia intoxication has not proven to be effective.

2. *Subhepatic Block.* Conservative treatment is identical to patients with intrahepatic blocks with the exception of measures designed to prevent hepatic failure.

## Operative Procedures

1. *Intrahepatic Block*

A. In view of the underlying etiology, cirrhosis, operative intervention is only indicated if a life-threatening hemorrhage cannot be controlled by other means.

B. In children, the central splenorenal shunt or mesocaval shunt has the lowest incidence of postoperative occlusion.

2. *Subhepatic Block*

A. *Portosystemic Shunts*

(1) *Central Splenorenal Shunt.* Although the side-to-side splenorenal shunt has been proven feasible in adults, thereby eliminating a splenectomy, in children a central splenorenal shunt with a simultaneous splenectomy is technically easier and appears to have a higher patency rate.

(2) In patients in whom a central splenorenal shunt cannot be performed, a mesocaval (Clatworthy) shunt, with ligation of the distal cava and anastomosis of the distal end of the proximal inferior vena cava to the side of the superior mesenteric vein, can be performed if the superior mesenteric vein is free of thrombosis.

B. *Patients Who Cannot Be Shunted*

(1) Transthoracic or transabdominal esophageal ligation

(2) *Tanner Procedure.* Transection of the stomach with division of the gastric varices and reanastomosis. Although the procedure temporarily reduces the blood flow into gastric and esophageal varices, the effect is only short-lived.

(3) *Colonic Interposition.* Transection of the stomach with removal of the fundus, closure of the distal end of the esophagus, cervical esophagostomy with retrosternal colonic interposition. Closure of both ends of the esophagus is well tolerated if no gastric remnant is included. Failure to transect and close the esophagus proximal to the gastric glands will lead to fluid accumulation and possible esophageal perforation.

C. *Postoperative Shunt Complications*

(1) *Patients with Intrahepatic Block:* development or enhancement of hepatic failure

(2) *Patients with Subhepatic Block*

(a) Recurrent bleeding with thrombosis of the shunt

(b) Cardiac failure if the shunt is too large

(c) Encephalopathy as a late complication

## MECKEL'S DIVERTICULUM

*See* page 544, Neonatal Gastrointestinal Bleeding.

## INTESTINAL POLYPS

*See* pages 544-545, Neonatal Gastrointestinal Bleeding.

## INTUSSUSCEPTION

*See* page 557, Neonatal Gastrointestinal Bleeding.

## VOLVULUS

*See* page 525, Neonatal Gastrointestinal Bleeding.

## COLITIS

*See* page 562, Ulcerative Colitis.

## RECTAL PROLAPSE

### Definition

Rectal prolapse is incomplete (mucosal) or complete (procidentia) prolapse of the rectum.

## Basic Principles

In the majority of infants and children, no underlying pathology is evident, and either redundancy of the rectal mucosa or the straight course of the rectum is thought to be a contributing cause. Dietary habits and occurrence of either diarrhea or constipation, aggravated by early and prolonged toilet training, are other possible etiologic factors. The prolapse of the rectum can range from a small mucosal prolapse to a complete procidentia with secondary infarction and hemorrhage.

### Associated Diseases or Anomalies

Neurogenic deficits or fibrocystic disease

## Criteria for Diagnosis

### Clinical

1. Rectal prolapse is most common in infants and children under the age of three years.
2. It is often accompanied by a history of:
   A. Malnutrition
   B. Prolonged diarrhea and/or constipation
   C. Neurologic deficits
   D. Associated diseases such as fibrocystic disease

### Laboratory

In view of the frequent occurrence of rectal prolapse in patients with fibrocystic disease, a sweat chloride test should be performed.

### X-ray

Although rectal polyps, occasionally sigmoid polyps, can lead to a rectal prolapse, they are usually clinically identifiable. A barium enema in the absence of polyps will rarely demonstrate any other pathology.

### Differential Diagnosis

Prolapse of polyps

## Management

1. In most instances the rectal prolapse is self-limiting once associated diseases or underlying causes such as malnutrition have been corrected.
2. In infants in whom the rectal prolapse recurs in the absence of other findings, the strapping of buttocks appears to be successful. Care should be taken, however, to avoid the breakdown of gluteal skin by continuous reapplication of tapes. The following method is recommended:
   A. Several vertical strips of tape are applied to each buttock; both buttock halves are then pressed together with a horizontal strip overlying the vertical strips.
   B. Once the infant or child has defecated or soiled the horizontal strip, it can be removed and a new one applied to the vertical strips without continuous skin irritation.

### Operative Management

In a very small group of patients, because of failure of conservative treatment or major anatomical or neurologic defects predisposing to rectal prolapse, the following operative procedures can be used:

1. *Modified Thiersch Procedure.* Four small subcutaneous incisions are placed in the perianal skin overlying the external sphincter. A subcutaneous sling, consisting of nonabsorbable suture material such as nylon, Teflon, or silicone, is placed through these incisions, securely tied around the operator's index finger and the incisions are closed.
2. *Lockhart-Mummery Procedure.* An incision is placed posterior to the anal opening, and the retrorectal space is bluntly dissected and packed with gauze. The gauze is removed over a period of approximately one week, leading to presacral adhesions.
3. In patients with major associated malformations and continuous complete rectal prolapse, resection of the prolapsed

segment and reanastomosis have been reported as successful.

4. More extensive, but successful in patients with complete prolapse, is the abdominoperineal resection and pull-through procedure.

## Complications

1. *Preoperative.* In patients with untreated complete rectal prolapse, spontaneous infarction can occur.

2. *Postoperative*

A. *Thiersch Procedure:* partial rectal obstruction and constipation with fecal impaction

B. *Lockhart-Mummery Procedure:* perirectal abscess

C. *Mucosal Resection and Reanastomosis:* stricture formation

D. *Perineal Pull-through Procedure:* pelvic abscess, anastomotic leak, cuff infection, intra-abdominal complications

## PANCREATIC LESIONS IN THE CHILD

### PANCREATITIS

## Definition

Pancreatic lesions refer to acute or chronic inflammation of the pancreas. Chronic recurrent pancreatitis, similar to the adult form with alcoholism or "common channel theory" due to biliary disease, is rare in children and usually only found in familial pancreatic disease such as hyperlipemia and amino-acidemia.

## Classification

1. Viral pancreatitis—mumps
2. Idiopathic—possible trauma, bacterial
3. Postoperative pancreatitis
4. Metabolic anomalies—hyperlipemia, amino-acidemia
5. Parasitic (ascaris)

## Basic Principles

The etiology of the various types of pancreatitis is as listed under Classification, above. Associated diseases are frequent and are discussed under Criteria for Diagnosis, below.

Regardless of the cause of acute pancreatitis, the degree of pancreatitis will determine the functional and hemodynamic disturbances. These disturbances can range from ductal obstruction to diffuse pancreatitis and abscess formation with intra-abdominal perforation and secondary peritonitis. If the exocrine secretion of the pancreas reaches the intra- or retroperitoneal cavity, fat necrosis and marked protein loss followed by local calcification occur. The fluid loss in diffuse hemorrhagic pancreatitis is marked, with subsequent hypovolemia, hypocalcemia and shock. The cause of associated organic manifestations, such as pulmonary problems and psychogenic alterations, is not understood.

## Criteria for Diagnosis

### Clinical

1. *Viral Pancreatitis*

A. Associated with mumps and can usually be diagnosed by the simultaneous parotid swelling

B. Amylase levels can be exceedingly high, often related to the parotitis.

C. The pancreatitis is usually self-limiting and disappears after the initial onset of mumps.

2. *Idiopathic Pancreatitis*

A. This has been described in children and infants and by definition is without known etiology. The association with biliary anomalies, such as stones, is exceedingly rare.

B. The diagnosis of acute, hemorrhagic or bacterial pancreatitis, not related to trauma, is usually made at operation in children presenting with an acute abdomen without prior known diagnosis.

C. In an occasional child, pancreatic calcifications or peripancreatic calcifications can be visualized preoperatively, indicating a subacute or chronic process.

D. Since the chronic recurrent type of pancreatitis does not occur in children with the exception of the familial type, pancreatitis is usually accompanied by an elevation of serum amylase and lipase.

E. Clinical findings are similar to those in adults, with signs of acute peritonitis, ileus and occasionally back pain.

F. Since a history of trauma may not be obtained in children, it may be assumed that some of the "idiopathic pancreatitis" found in children is not primarily bacterial but secondary to unknown trauma.

3. *Postoperative Pancreatitis*

A. The treatment of an annular pancreas by transection of the pancreas is known to lead to acute pancreatitis.

B. Other operative procedures, including gastrectomy or splenectomy, are likely to lead to pancreatitis following direct operative trauma to the pancreas.

4. *Metabolic Anomalies*

A. Various metabolic anomalies, primarily hyperlipemia and amino-acidemia, are known to lead to a recurrent form of pancreatitis.

B. In amino-acidemia, a pre-existing mental retardation can exist.

C. The actual anatomical findings are limited, and pancreatic necrosis is not seen.

5. *Parasitic Pancreatis.* The development of pancreatitis in a patient with known ascaris infestation can be assumed to be secondary to ductal invasion by the ascaris.

## Laboratory

1. Serum amylase and lipase determinations
2. Urinary amylase
3. In patients with suspected metabolic anomalies, determination of serum lipids, serum and urine amino acids, especially lysine
4. Stool examination for ova and parasites to determine the presence of ascaris

## X-ray

1. X-ray findings in acute pancreatitis are usually compatible with peritonitis and paralytic ileus.
2. "Sentinel loops" are suggestive of pancreatitis, as well as retrogastric and duodenal edematous swelling.
3. At operation a direct pancreaticogram may be helpful.

## Differential Diagnosis

1. Acute peritonitis due to unknown causes (appendicitis)
2. Intra-abdominal trauma
3. Pancreatic tumor, pseudocysts or congenital cysts

## Management

### General

With the exception of pancreatic abscess, pancreatic transection or cysts, the treatment in most cases is conservative:

1. Decrease of pancreatic activity with nasogastric suction and administration of Pro-Banthine
2. Restoration of hydration, intravascular volume, oncotic pressure and calcium replacement
3. In patients with psychological manifestations, sedation is indicated.
4. The use of hypothermia has not proved to be effective.
5. Broad-spectrum antibiotics are used to obviate secondary infection.

### Operative Management

In patients in whom the diagnosis of acute pancreatitis was unsuspected and made during operative exploration, drainage of the pancreatic bed appears indicated if abscess, necrosis or acute hemorrhagic pancreatitis is found.

### PANCREATIC CYSTS

## Classification

1. *Pseudocysts.* These are acquired intra-abdominal cysts communicating

with the pancreas without the pancreatic epithelial lining.

2. *Congenital Cysts.* These are congenital cysts with pancreatic elements within cyst's wall or lining, if preserved.

3. *Neoplastic Cysts.* These are pancreatic cysts associated with pancreatic adenoma or adenocarcinoma.

## Basic Principles

Acute or chronic pseudocysts in children follow abdominal trauma. Congenital cysts can originate anywhere along the pancreatic anlage but appear to be most common along the body and tail. Neoplastic cysts are exceedingly rare, especially in the pediatric age-group.

## Criteria for Diagnosis

### Clinical

Pancreatic cysts, regardless of origin, are rare in children. Presenting symptoms are:

1. Asymptomatic mass
2. Mass and abdominal pain
3. Growth failure and failure to gain weight with or without abdominal pain and abdominal mass
4. A history of abdominal trauma followed by vague abdominal complaints such as abdominal fullness or intermittent pain; weight and growth failure, or signs of chronic infection

### Laboratory

Serum amylase may be elevated.

### X-ray

Pancreatic cysts, regardless of etiology, have a similar pattern on x-rays if located in the head or midbody with widening of the duodenal sweep, with anterior displacement of the stomach.

### Differential Diagnosis

1. Abdominal tumor
2. Hydronephrosis
3. Intra-abdominal abscess
4. Pancreatitis

## Management

### General

1. All pancreatic cysts in childhood, regardless of etiology, should be explored.

2. Pseudocysts, the most common type, differ from congenital cysts by their adhesions to surrounding structures secondary to their inflammatory origin.

3. Congenital cysts are usually isolated structures and well defined.

### Operative Management

1. Since proximal ductal obstruction is rarely present in pseudocysts in children, internal anastomosis is rarely necessary and external drainage by catheter is preferable to marsupialization which leads to skin necrosis and inflammatory abdominal wall reaction.

2. Congenital pancreatic cysts are rarely adherent to surrounding structures, and a primary resection can usually be accomplished in contrast to pseudocysts. If resection is difficult, enterostomy drainage can be performed.

3. Treatment of neoplastic cysts depends on the underlying pathology and is identical to that in adults.

4. Occasionally intestinal duplications may be attached to the pancreas and appear as pancreatic cysts. Aspiration of the cyst content and amylase determination should suggest the diagnosis. Treatment consists of resection.

## HYPOGLYCEMIA

### Definition

Hypoglycemia in this section refers to paroxysmal or continuous hypoglycemia, leading to convulsions, mental retardation and death.

### Basic Principles

In the context of this chapter, hyperinsulinism is the primary interest. Although it occurs rarely in infancy and usually after the age of three to four years, functioning insulinomas have been reported in neonates. After the elimination of other possible causes, blood serum insulin levels can verify the diagnosis of either insulinoma or islet cell hyperplasia. In islet cell tumors or hyperplasia, the production of insulin is related to an increase in beta cells.

## Criteria for Diagnosis

### In Infancy

1. Intermittent episodes of convulsions, irritability, cyanosis, lethargy or coma in infants with blood sugar below 50 mg.% (often below 20 mg.%)
2. Only a few clinical signs may be present, such as macroglossia seen with the Beckwith syndrome.
3. The diagnosis of hypoglycemia does not imply hyperinsulinism, since the latter is the most uncommon cause of hypoglycemia in infancy.

### In Children

History of mental retardation, coma, overeating, convulsions

### Laboratory

1. Blood glucose levels below 50 mg.%
2. *Laboratory Tests for Differential Diagnosis*
    A. Insulin blood level determinations
    B. ACTH assay
    C. Adrenocortico steroid levels
    D. Epinephrine infusion tests

### Differential Diagnosis

1. Idiopathic hypoglycemia
2. Glycogen storage disease (types I and III)
3. Leucine sensitivity
4. Pituitary-adrenal-cortical insufficiency
5. Insulinoma or islet cell hyperplasia

## Management

### General

1. Idiopathic hypoglycemia requires no operation.

    A. Maintenance with hypertonic glucose infusions up to 20 per cent glucose
    B. Administration of cortisone acetate
    C. Oral administration of diazoxide
2. In patients with elevated insulin secretion, maintenance of normal blood glucose with infusion is preoperative preparation.

### Operative Management

1. The operative repair of a suspected islet cell adenoma or adenomata is not an emergency procedure and should not be carried out without appropriate study.
2. Approximately 20 per cent of the tumors are multicentric, and ectopic pancreatic insulinomas have been found in various parts of the intestinal tract.
3. Most of these tumors are benign, but islet cell carcinoma with lymph node, liver, pulmonary and osseous metastasis has been reported.
4. The extent of the pancreatic resection depends on the lesions present.

## ABDOMINAL TUMORS IN THE CHILD

### Definition

Abdominal tumors may be primary or secondary intra-abdominal and retroperitoneal neoplasms.

### Classification

Various classifications of tumors can be used, depending on the anatomical location (i.e., intra-abdominal versus retroperitoneal tumors), whether they are primary or secondary, or by their symptoms.

### Basic Principles

1. Intra-abdominal and retroperitoneal tumors rarely present as acute surgical emergencies, with the exception of patients in whom trauma has led to an acute surgical abdomen. The most common intra-abdominal and retroperitoneal tumors are included, however, because:

A. They may be encountered inadvertently during an operative exploration of the abdomen.

B. Intra-abdominal and retroperitoneal neoplasms in children are in general considered to be emergencies whose work-up should be completed within a 24- to 48-hour period with subsequent definitive therapy.

2. Since symptoms may vary considerably, from an asymptomatic mass to hypertension, intestinal obstruction, hematuria or acute abdomen, no attempt has been made to classify the following lesions in a particular order. Malignancies in children constitute the second most common cause of death in children following accidents. Approximately one half of the neoplasms will require surgical care. Wilms' tumor and neuroblastoma constitute the majority of solid intraabdominal tumors.

. 3. It should be stressed, however, that the definitive therapy does not only depend on the surgeon's ability to render proper operative care. Tumor therapy in children, probably more than in any other area, demands the presence of a completely trained and equipped team, consisting of surgeon, radiotherapist, chemotherapist, rehabilitation specialist and psychotherapist. If these facilities are not available, a patient with a suspected intraabdominal malignancy, although presenting as an emergency, should be referred to an appropriate institution.

4. Intra-abdominal masses in children occur approximately in the following sequence:

A. Hydronephrosis secondary to obstructive uropathy

B. Wilms' tumor

C. Neuroblastoma, liver tumors, ovarian tumors, lymphosarcoma

D. Sarcoma botryoides, embryonal carcinoma, pheochromocytoma

## Criteria for Diagnosis

Clinical

1. Most intra-abdominal or retroperitoneal tumors present as an asymptomatic mass, occasionally associated with symptoms according to their location or hormonal activity.

2. Tumors leading to *hypertension* include:

A. Neuroblastoma

B. Wilms' tumor

C. Pheochromocytoma

D. Occasionally lymphosarcoma invading the kidney

3. In view of the relative frequency of hypertension associated with neoplasms, the determination of the child's blood pressure is mandatory.

4. Since the majority of tumors occur in the perirenal area, renal lesions such as hydronephrosis, neuroblastoma and Wilms' tumor have to be ruled out by intravenous pyelogram in all patients with intra-abdominal neoplasms.

5. Signs and symptoms secondary to the presence of an intra-abdominal mass may include the following:

A. Complete or partial intestinal obstruction

B. Diarrhea due to hormonal activity as in neuroblastoma

C. Abdominal pain due to pressure

D. Uropathy due to bladder, ureteral or kidney involvement

E. Jaundice due to liver involvement or extrahepatic obstruction

F. Musculoskeletal pain, occasionally resembling arthritis or arthralgia, due to osseous metastasis

G. Headaches or visual disturbances secondary to hypertension

H. Failure to gain weight or growth retardation

I. Hematuria

J. Symptoms related to distant metastases

6. Physical examination of the abdomen may give information as to the:

A. Consistency of the tumor: solid or cystic

B. Contour of the tumor (Wilms' tumor usually round, neuroblastoma irregular)

C. Presence of tenderness

D. Mobility (Duplications and ovarian tumors are often mobile, whereas retroperitoneal tumors are usually fixed.)

E. Location: upper and lower quadrant lesions, indicating site of origin

7. Although in most patients a differentiation between intra-abdominal and retroperitoneal tumors can be made on physical examination, in young infants retroperitoneal tumors may present as intra-abdominal lesions. In older children retroperitoneal lesions are more likely to present as lateral flank masses.

8. A complete and thorough physical examination should rule out other secondary lesions or metastases, or the possibility of a primary lesion in an extra-abdominal area.

### Laboratory

The routine work-up in all patients with intra-abdominal masses should include:

1. Physical examination with blood pressure

2. Complete blood count with differential count

3. Urinary analysis (Intrarenal lesions, especially Wilms' tumor, may present with microscopic hematuria.)

4. Determination of urinary VMA and HMA

5. Bone marrow aspiration

### X-ray

1. Flat and upright films of the abdomen

2. Posteroanterior film of the chest

3. Complete skeletal review

4. Intravenous pyelogram, inferior vena cavagram and angiography as indicated

5. Radioactive scans and sonograms as indicated

6. Gastrointestinal contrast studies as indicated

### Differential Diagnosis

1. *Intra-abdominal Lesions Likely to Be Mobile*

A. Intestinal duplications

B. Ovarian tumors

2. *Cystic Lesions*

A. Hydronephrosis

B. Multicystic kidneys, duplications, mesenteric cysts

3. *Tumors Which May Lead to Hypertension*

Wilms' tumor, neuroblastoma, pheochromocytoma, tumors invading the kidney

### WILMS' TUMOR
(Renal Embryoma or Nephroblastoma)

### Definition

Wilms' tumor is an intrarenal neoplasm with features of both carcinoma and sarcoma. Bilaterality is seen in approximately 6 per cent of cases. Primary extrarenal Wilms' tumors have been reported but are exceedingly rare.

### Basic Principles

Wilms' tumor occurs primarily in young infants and children and is assumed to be embryologic in origin. Although familial history has been reported in several instances, there is no clear evidence of any hereditary factors. The average age is approximately two to three years. An increased incidence of Wilms' tumor has been reported in association with other abdominal congenital anomalies, such as horse-shoe kidney, hypospadias and cryptorchidism.

The most common sites of metastases consist of the lungs, possibly related to the frequency of caval involvement, followed by liver. Skeletal metastases are extremely rare.

As in patients with neuroblastoma, the cure rate is partly related to the age of the patient. Infants under the age of two years appear to have a better prognosis than older children.

### Criteria for Diagnosis

Clinical

1. Asymptomatic mass presenting in the

left or upper right quadrant, midabdomen or flank.

2. Vague abdominal pains such as fullness, anorexia, intermittent pain

3. With hypertension, symptoms such as headaches, etc.

4. Sudden appearance of an abdominal mass, usually related to hemorrhage within the tumor

## Laboratory

Gross hematuria is almost never seen; microscopic hematuria is seen in 10 to 20 per cent of cases.

## X-ray

1. On supine and upright films, a homogeneous mass is seen on the involved renal side. Calcifications, in contrast to the neuroblastoma, are rare.

2. *Intravenous Pyelogram*

A. "Moth-eaten appearance" of the caliceal system with distortion and apparent intrarenal origin

B. The long axis of the kidney may be shifted.

C. Complete nonvisualization of the kidney or calcification is rare.

3. *Inferior Vena Cavagram*

A. Injection of the contrast material for the intravenous pyelogram through either saphenous or femoral veins may demonstrate the patency of the inferior vena cava.

B. Obstruction of the inferior vena cava is more frequently seen with neuroblastoma but is rare with Wilms' tumor.

C. Renal vein invasion can occur with Wilms' tumor and a thrombosis of the renal vein extending into the inferior vena cava may be recognized on the inferior vena cavagram.

D. False positives occur; when a child cries during the injection, thereby producing a Valsalva maneuver, vertebral collaterals may fill, mimicking caval obstruction.

4. *Arteriography.* In patients in whom the intravenous pyelogram is nondiagnostic, a renal arteriogram through the femoral artery can establish the diagnosis of Wilms' tumor. It is, however, rarely necessary.

5. *Radioactive Scan and/or Sonogram*

A. In an occasional patient, a radioactive scan or sonogram may help to confirm the diagnosis.

B. On the sonogram the Wilms' tumor appears as a solid mass, in contrast to hydronephrotic or multicystic kidneys, whose echo reveals their cystic structure.

6. *Metastases Studies.* The most common site of metastases in patients with Wilms' tumor is the pulmonary parenchyma. The presence of pulmonary metastases does not contraindicate operative removal of the involved kidney.

## Differential Diagnosis

1. *Congenital Anomalies.* Hydronephrosis, multiple cystic kidney, duplication, mesenteric cyst.

2. *Neoplasms:* neuroblastoma, lymphosarcoma, other intrarenal or retroperitoneal lesions

3. Renal tumors other than Wilms' tumor can occur in children, such as hypernephroma; they are, however, exceedingly rare. Solitary renal cysts can mimic Wilms' tumor on both abdominal examinations and x-rays.

4. *Others.* In patients with left renal Wilms' tumors, the differential diagnosis between splenomegaly and Wilms' tumor may at times be difficult on physical examination. X-ray should clearly delineate the correct diagnosis, however.

## Management

### General

After the diagnostic work-up has been completed expeditiously, the child is prepared for operation:

1. Type and crossmatch blood.

2. Nasogastric tube

3. Intravenous line in the upper extremities

4. *Palpation of the abdomen is to be avoided after the diagnosis has been established.*

## Operative Procedure

1. The tumor is approached through a high transverse abdominal incision to allow inspection of the liver and the contralateral kidney, even if the intravenous pyelogram did not show any evidence of bilaterality.

2. The colon is mobilized and the renal pedicle identified, doubly ligated and transected. Local lymph nodes, adrenal gland and Gerota's fascia should be removed with the specimen.

3. Manipulation of the tumor should be avoided until the renal pedicle has been transected to avoid intracaval dissemination of tumor cells or thrombi.

4. The ureter is ligated with heavy chromic ties and transected close to its entrance into the bladder.

5. After the tumor has been removed, the area occupied by the tumor is marked with silver clips to facilitate the postoperative radiation.

6. Drainage of the retroperitoneal space is rarely necessary.

7. It has been our practice to start chemotherapy preoperatively to cover the patient during the operative procedure.

## Postoperative Treatment

1. *Intravenous Fluids.* Since the intra-abdominal fluid loss is limited, maintenance with 1500 to 2000 ml./square meter of body surface area per 24 hours of a one-third isotonic solution is usually sufficient.

2. Continuous nasogastric decompression until peristaltic activity has recurred, usually in 24 to 48 hours

3. Antibiotic coverage is usually not necessary.

4. If radiotherapy is indicated, it is usually started within 24 hours after the operative procedure.

5. Postoperative chemotherapy and radiotherapy have to be coordinated since chemotherapy may potentiate the radiation effect.

6. *Chemotherapy:* actinomycin D and vincristine or Cytoxan radiation: 700 to 4,000 r, average 2000 r

*Post-treatment Complications.* Postoperative complications are usually not related to the operation, but to chemotherapy and radiotherapy, including radiation nephritis, pneumonitis, occasionally cirrhosis of the liver, bone marrow depression, alopecia, scoliosis and gastrointestinal complaints.

## Bilateral Wilms' Tumor

1. If the exploration of the contralateral side indicates that a small area of the contralateral kidney is involved with a Wilms' tumor, a simultaneous partial resection of the contralateral kidney can be performed if no more than one third of the kidney has to be resected.

2. In tumors too extensive to allow nephrectomy on one side and partial nephrectomy on the other, a biopsy should be obtained, the extent of the tumor marked with silver clips and chemotherapy and radiotherapy initiated postoperatively.

3. In patients with renal Wilms' tumor and pulmonary metastasis, the treatment will depend on the extent of the pulmonary metastasis. Even in the presence of multiple pulmonary metastases, if the patient's general condition is satisfactory, the Wilms' tumor should be removed.

4. The treatment for multiple pulmonary metastases consists of chemotherapy and radiotherapy. In patients with a single pulmonary metastasis, either radiotherapy or segmental resection is indicated.

5. Bilateral nephrectomy in patients with bilateral Wilms' tumor and subsequent renal transplant have been reported on several occasions; this has not yet been accepted, however, as standard treatment.

## NEUROBLASTOMA

### Definition

Neuroblastoma is neurogenic neoplasm arising from the sympathetic nervous system or the adrenal medulla (other terms: sympathicoblastoma, neurocytoma).

### Classification

1. Type III undifferentiated; type III R with rosette formation
2. Types II and I beginning differentiation with ganglionic elements

### Basic Principles

The neuroblastoma is considered to be embryonic in origin. In contrast to all other tumors, a small percentage of patients with undifferentiated malignant neuroblastoma may undergo spontaneous maturation with change into a benign ganglioneuroma. Spontaneous "maturation" is exceedingly rare, however, and has no therapeutic implications.

The symptoms depend on the location of the tumor, local invasion or displacement of other organs. General symptoms are related to the high incidence of hormonally active tumors, with hypertension and diarrhea. While the hormonal activity is not directly related to the degree of maturation, the most undifferentiated neuroblastoma, type III without rosette formation, infrequently produces elevated VMA or HMA levels.

### Criteria for Diagnosis

#### Clinical

1. In view of its origin, the neuroblastoma can arise anywhere in the body where sympathetic elements are present, including neck, chest, abdomen and pelvis. The most common site is intra-abdominal, arising in the adrenal medulla.
2. Clinical findings may be related to its locations: upper or midabdominal mass, occasionally extending toward the flank and often crossing the midline.
3. With the tumor's hormonal activity, symptoms may be secondary to the hormonally induced diarrhea and hypertension.
4. More than 60 per cent of all children with intra-abdominal neuroblastomas present with metastases at the time of admission, the most common sites being in the skeletal system with symptoms resembling arthralgia or rheumatic fever.
5. In early infancy, metastases are more commonly seen in skin or liver.
6. Pulmonary metastases do occur but are rare.
7. General symptoms include loss of weight, anemia and lethargy, and occasionally bizarre head movements.

#### Laboratory

1. White blood count and hematocrit are noncontributory, although anemia is not infrequent.
2. The incidence of bone marrow metastases is very high and bone marrow aspiration is therefore mandatory in all children with abdominal tumors.
3. Twenty-four-hour urinary determination of VMA and HMA while on an appropriate diet

#### X-ray

1. Flat and upright films of the abdomen and chest
2. In contrast to Wilms' tumor, calcification is frequently seen in neuroblastoma.
3. The inferior vena cavagram may show a deviation over the midline with partial obstruction, rarely seen with Wilms' tumor.
4. The intravenous pyelogram may reveal a distortion of the caliceal system, but rarely with intrarenal invasion as seen with Wilms' tumor.
5. In view of the location of the adrenal neuroblastoma, a shift of the renal axis without invasion of the renal parenchyma is suggestive of neuroblastoma.
6. In an occasional patient, non-

visualization of the kidney may occur secondary to ureteral obstruction.

7. If the inferior vena cavagram and intravenous pyelogram fail to differentiate between a Wilms' tumor and a neuroblastoma, angiography may be indicated.

8. Radioactive scan and sonogram

9. *Skeletal Review.* In contrast to Wilms' tumor, osseous metastases, including long bones and skull, are common.

## Management

### General

The preoperative approach is similar to that in patients with Wilms' tumor.

### Operative Management

1. General

A. The presence of metastases is not a contraindication to removal of the primary intra-abdominal tumor, as long as the child's general condition permits the operative procedure. Cures have been achieved in children with diffuse osseous and other metastases after the primary tumor has been removed.

B. A complete removal of the tumor is desirable but not indicated at the expense of other important structures. Although the adjacent kidney may have to be removed in order to accomplish a complete resection, transection of aorta and vascular grafts is not indicated.

2. *Preoperative Management.* This is identical to the preoperative management for the patient with Wilms' tumor.

3. *Operative Procedure*

A. Transverse abdominal or paramedian incision over the involved side

B. Thorough abdominal exploration to evaluate the extent of tumor and metastatic involvement, especially lymph nodes and hepatic involvement

C. As mentioned before, removal of the kidney is often indicated in patients with adrenal neuroblastoma, but extensive resections, such as removal of a portion of

the aorta with subsequent grafting, are not indicated.

D. As much of the tumor and metastases to regional lymph nodes should be removed without endangering the patient.

E. The tumor areas are marked with silver clips for immediate postoperative radiation within 24 hours.

4. *Postoperative Treatment of Neuroblastoma*

A. *Radiotherapy:* 2,000 to 4,000 r, depending on the location, within 24 hours postoperatively

B. *Chemotherapy:* at present, vincristine and Cytoxan

5. *Postoperative Management.* Urinary VMA and HMA determinations are indicated at periodic intervals, since a sudden elevation of either of the two substances may indicate metastases or local recurrence before either clinical symptoms or radiological signs develop.

6. *Complications:* as described under Wilms' Tumor

## LYMPHOSARCOMA

### Classification

1. Lymphosarcoma involving the intestine and/or mesentery

2. Lymphosarcoma involving the retroperitoneal nodes

3. Lymphosarcoma limited to the abdomen

4. Lymphosarcoma with extra-abdominal spread

5. Lymphosarcoma and leukemia

### Basic Principles

In a small number of patients, the lymphosarcoma may be limited completely to the intestine, intestinal mesentery or to the intra-abdominal area, with or without invasion of adjacent organs. A "staging procedure" is used in most patients to determine the extent of tumor. In a considerable number of patients, lymphosarcoma occurs as part of a leukemia; careful peripheral blood examination and bone marrow studies are therefore indicated.

## Criteria for Diagnosis

### Clinical

1. Asymptomatic abdominal mass
2. Gastrointestinal symptoms—related to partial or complete intestinal obstruction
3. *Findings Related to Multiple Organ Involvement*
    A. In patients without intestinal obstruction, abdominal findings are limited to an asymptomatic or slightly tender irregular, hard mass.
    B. Careful examination for peripheral lymphadenopathy is indicated, since the abdominal lesion may be part of a diffuse lymphosarcoma.
    C. Bone marrow
    D. Liver profile

### X-ray

1. Upper gastrointestinal series or barium enema
2. Intravenous pyelogram is indicated in all patients, preferably in conjunction with inferior vena cavagram.

### Differential Diagnosis

1. Wilms' tumor
2. Neuroblastoma
3. Duplication
4. Mesentery cysts
5. Obstructive uropathy
6. Intestinal obstruction

## Management

### Operative

1. In patients in whom the lymphosarcoma, limited to the intestine, leads to intestinal obstruction such as intussusception, complete resection is indicated.
2. In patients with a diffuse lymphosarcoma not obstructing the intestine, complete resection is rarely possible or indicated.

3. A laparotomy is performed to establish the diagnosis and the extent of the lesion by staging: tumor biopsy, pelvic and mesenteric node biopsy, open bone marrow biopsy, liver biopsy and splenectomy.
4. A biopsy of peripheral nodes, if enlarged, should be included.

### Postoperative Treatment

Radiotherapy and chemotherapy according to the extent of the tumor, the presence of metastases and/or evidence of leukemia

## PHEOCHROMOCYTOMA

## Definition

Pheochromocytoma is a tumor arising from the medullary portion of the adrenal gland or adrenal rests, with epinephrine or norepinephrine secretion leading to hypertension.

## Basic Principles

The pheochromocytoma is not a tumor to be removed without adequate preparation and availability of an experienced team. Treatment of an unexpectedly encountered pheochromocytoma consists of deferment of the definitive treatment until adequate preparation can be accomplished.

## Criteria for Diagnosis

### Clinical

1. The predominant clinical signs consist of signs and symptoms related to sustained hypertension in children: headaches, vision disturbances, tachycardia, sweating and irritability.
2. An abdominal mass may be found in either the adrenal area of the midabdomen, if the pheochromocytoma arises from the organ of Zuckerkandl.
3. Manipulation of the tumor may lead to a rapid increase of the already existing hypertension.

## Laboratory

1. Catecholamine determinations, including norepinephrine and epinephrine

2. The histamine stimulation test is dangerous and rarely indicated.

3. Regitine, producing adrenergic blockade, is equally diagnostic and safer.

## X-ray

1. Since the pheochromocytoma rarely reaches the dimensions seen in Wilms' tumor, neuroblastoma or lymphosarcoma, the flat and upright film may be nondiagnostic.

2. If a tumor is suspected, angiography can demonstrate the tumor.

3. Increased hypertension during angiography has been reported and should be treated accordingly.

4. X-ray work-up should include investigation of distant metastases or extraabdominal location of the primary tumor.

## Management

### General

1. If an unsuspected pheochromocytoma is encountered during a laparotomy, excision is contraindicated unless the patient has been fully prepared. The risk of sudden hypertension during manipulation, followed by hypertension after its removal, is unacceptably high when the patient and operative team are unprepared.

2. Closure of the abdomen and evaluation of the patient's status, including the assessment of possible cardiac myopathy, are absolutely essential before an operative removal is contemplated.

### Preoperative Treatment

An attempt should be made to keep the patient for at least one week at normotensive levels by conservative methods, including medication such as Regitine.

### Operative Removal

1. A well-planned team approach, including anesthesiologist, endocrinologist and surgeon, is necessary to discuss and anticipate possible adverse reactions which include hyper- and hypotension, cardiac irregularities, shock and pulmonary edema.

2. After patient and team are thoroughly prepared, the abdomen is opened through an appropriate incision depending on the location of the tumor.

3. Prior to manipulation and dissection of the tumor, all veins leading from the tumor are clamped and ligated.

4. At least two large bore cutdown catheters in the upper extremities have to be available to permit sudden infusion of medication and occasionally large quantities of blood to correct a suddenly occurring hypovolemia after the resection.

### Postoperative Complications

1. In children without long-standing hypertension, the systolic pressure will return to normal within a short period postoperatively.

2. Failure to do so indicates that either multiple primary tumors exist (approximately one third of all patients) or that metastases may be present.

3. In patients with long-standing hypertension, the latter may persist for several months due to secondary renal changes.

## OVARIAN TUMORS

### Definition

An ovarian tumor is a tumor arising from the ovary or ovarian remnants.

### Classification

1. *Ovarian Tumors Which May Lead to Sexual Precocity*
    A. Granulosa cell tumor
    B. Mixed dysgerminoma
    C. Carcinoma (embryonal)
2. *Tumors Without Hormonal Activity:* ovarian teratoma—solid or cystic

## Basic Principles

Hormonally active tumors, such as granulosa cell tumor, or malignancies such as carcinoma are exceedingly rare in children. Dysgerminomas occur slightly more frequently but only a small number will lead to sexual precocity. Occasionally ovarian cysts without neoplastic changes have been reported in association with sexual precocity, disappearing after the cysts have been removed.

Bilaterality can occur with ovarian tumors regardless of origin. It appears to be most frequent in patients with teratomas.

## Criteria for Diagnosis

### Clinical

1. In patients without signs of sexual precocity, findings are usually limited to:
   A. Asymptomatic abdominal mass
   B. Sudden excruciating abdominal pain due to an ovarian torsion
   C. Symptoms related to the large size of the ovarian tumor, such as dysuria or constipation
2. In patients with hormonally active tumors, precocious development including breasts, pubic hair, external genitalia and the premature onset of menarche may be the first presenting signs.

### Laboratory

In hormonally active tumors, steroid level evaluation may be indicated.

### X-ray

1. In solid teratomas, calcification is frequently seen. The calcification is usually localized in one area and differs from the diffuse calcification seen in neuroblastoma.
2. The intravenous pyelogram shows noninvolvement of the kidney, but a mild unilateral or bilateral hydronephrosis or megalo-ureter may be present due to the pelvic pressure in patients with large ovarian tumors.

## Management

### General

1. The preoperative work-up is identical to that described in patients with Wilms' tumor and neuroblastoma.
2. Vaginal examination, under sedation or anesthesia, should be included, especially if there is a possibility the tumor may either be uterine in origin, such as a sarcoma botryoides, an early pregnancy or a hematocolpos.

### Operative Procedure

1. In patients who present with sudden excruciating abdominal pain, indicating the presence of an ovarian torsion, laparotomy should be performed as an emergency.
2. Most ovarian torsions occur in association with ovarian tumors, but in young girls torsion can occur with a normal ovary and, unless the torsion is untwisted early, infarction and necrosis occur.
   A. In patients with ovarian torsion in whom the presence of a tumor can be ruled out, the torsion should be untwisted, the ovary carefully inspected and, if infarction has occurred, the ovary should be bivalved to allow the escape of the trapped venous blood.
   B. Unless complete liquefaction necrosis has occurred, the ovary is placed back into the peritoneal cavity if there is any evidence of even marginal viability.
3. With solid or cystic ovarian teratomas, dysgerminoma or tumors without invasion of adjacent structures, a simple salpingo-oophorectomy is performed.
   A. The base of the fallopian tube is doubly ligated with heavy chromic gut ligatures; vascular structures in the ligament are ligated with interrupted silk stitch ligatures.
   B. The contralateral ovary is carefully inspected. If there is any suggestion of a possible contralateral tumor, the ovary is

bivalved and, in patients with teratoma, a partial ovarian resection can be performed on the contralateral side.

## TESTICULAR TUMORS

### Classification

1. *Primary*
   A. *Germinal*
      *(1) Benign:* teratoma
      *(2) Malignant:* orchioblastoma or adenocarcinoma, embryonal carcinoma
   B. *Nongerminal*
      *Benign:* Sertoli's cell, interstitioma, androblastoma
2. *Secondary.* The most common secondary tumor consists of the lymphosarcoma. All other tumors originating in the stroma, including connective tissue and muscle, can occur, such as rhabdomyosarcoma.

### Basic Principles

Although testicular tumors are rare in infants and children, they do occur in a considerable variety, based on their embryologic background, hormonal activity, primary or secondary origin, benign or malignant. Only the more common tumors are included in this description. In spite of the histological variety, all primary testicular tumors in infants and children show an intimate relation to the embryologic background.

### Criteria for Diagnosis

#### Clinical

1. Most testicular tumors are found as asymptomatic testicular masses. Occasionally an incidental trauma will attract the parents' attention to the pre-existing lesion.
2. In a small number of patients with hormonally active tumors, sexual precocity, including testicular enlargement, appearance of pubic hair or the development of breasts, may precede the appearance of the testicular mass.

#### Laboratory

1. Urinary ketosteroids
2. Liver function tests to rule out metastases or primary involvement
3. White blood count and differential to rule out lymphosarcoma

#### X-ray

1. Abdominal and chest films to rule out metastases or other primary tumors
2. Intravenous pyelogram

### Differential Diagnosis

1. Hydrocele
2. Testicular trauma
3. Testicular torsion
4. Primary or secondary testicular tumors
5. Epididymitis
6. Orchitis

### Management

#### General

1. Simple orchiectomy is sufficient in all patients with benign testicular tumors and patients with secondary tumors.
2. In view of the increased instances of pelvic node metastases in primary malignant testicular tumors, such as embryonal carcinoma and teratocarcinoma, complete removal of the spermatic cord with pelvic node dissection appears indicated.
3. Since there is no statistical evidence that radical pelvic node dissection improves the survival rate in patients with embryonal carcinoma and teratocarcinoma, a selective pelvic node dissection (removal of all identifiable nodes) appears to be sufficient.

#### Operative Procedure for Undiagnosed Testicular Lesions

1. After the testis has been exposed through either a scrotal or inguinal incision, the vascular pedicle should be secured and temporarily occluded until the tunica albuginea is opened to perform a biopsy and inspect the gross lesion.

2. The failure to occlude the spermatic cord may otherwise lead to an increased dissemination of tumor cells within the blood stream during the testicular manipulation.

## TUMEFACTIONS OF THE BREAST IN THE CHILD

### Classification

1. *Breast Abscess:* bacterial mastitis
2. *Tumors*
    A. *Male*
        *(1) Benign:* gynecomastia
        *(2) Malignant:* carcinoma
    B. Female
        *(1) Benign*
            *(a)* Adenofibroma
            *(b)* Giant adenofibroma
            *(c)* Cystic mastitis
            *(d)* Adenosis
            *(e)* Intraductal papillomatosis
        *(2) Malignant*
            *(a)* Cystosarcoma phylloides
            *(b)* Carcinoma

### Basic Principles

Although breast tumors do not present as surgical emergencies, the unilateral early development of the breast or the appearance of a breast abscess is occasionally mistaken for a tumor. For this reason breast abscesses, breast development and breast tumors are included here.

Normal breast development in the young girl may occur unilaterally for a considerable period of time before menarche and the development of other sex characteristics. The enlarging subareolar disk, which is often slightly tender and painful, can be mistaken for either infection or tumor and the removal of this disk will result in ablation of the entire breast tissue. Bilateral breast development and the appearance of secondary sex characteristics at an early age may be idiopathic, but underlying hormonal causes such as ovarian tumor, etc., have to be ruled out.

Breast abscesses can occur in infancy, since under the influence of maternal hormones the infantile breast secretes a whitish fluid and during this period obstruction and secondary infection, unilateral or bilateral, are common.

The etiology of breast tumors is unknown but the rapid enlargement of giant adenofibromas or the development of "virginal hypertrophy" is assumed to be a local tissue hypersensitivity rather than an abnormal hormone production.

### Criteria for Diagnosis

Clinical

1. *Breast Abscess.* This occurs most often in neonates, with a tender, red swelling of the breast and cellulitis preceding fluctuation. It may be unilateral or bilateral.

2. *Tumors*
    A. *Adenofibromas*
        *(1)* These may be single or multiple, and constitute approximately 90 per cent of all premenarchal tumors. Their appearance is similar to that in adults, (2) through (6) below.
        *(2)* Painless or slightly tender mass
        *(3)* Well delineated
        *(4)* Not attached to the skin
        *(5)* Rubbery or firm in consistency
        *(6)* Without nipple discharge
    B. *Giant Adenofibroma*
        *(1)* History compatible with the appearance of a small adenofibroma, with rapid enlargement and tenderness
        *(2)* On physical examination, the lesion is well delineated and firm, the skin is stretched and reddened with prominent venous engorgement and there is tenderness on palpation.
    C. *Cystosarcoma Phylloides*
        *(1)* May be indistinguishable by history and physical examination from the giant adenofibroma
        *(2)* Although most large fast-growing breast lesions in young children and teenagers are clinically assumed to be

cystosarcoma phylloides, the histological composition is different.

*(3)* Since the cystosarcoma phylloides originates as a small lesion, it can therefore also be mistaken for a regular adenofibroma.

*D. Adenosis or Intraductal Papillomatosis*

*(1)* Cystic mastitis, adenosis and papillomatosis are similar in clinical appearance, with vaguely delineated areas of tenderness, mild pain and occasional nipple discharge.

*(2)* In contrast to adults, where florid papillomatosis is considered premalignant, neither of these lesions is considered premalignant in the premenarchal child although a follow-up is indicated.

*E. Carcinoma.* The carcinoma in males and females is similar to that seen in adults on physical examination.

## Laboratory

Noncontributory

## X-ray

Mammography in large tumors

## Differential Diagnosis

Breast abscess, breast trauma, primary breast tumor as listed above or secondary breast tumors such as hemangioma or lymphangioma

## Management

### Breast Abscess

1. If signs of cellulitis dominate, without fluctuation, conservative treatment with antibiotics and warm, wet compresses

2. When fluctuation has occurred, incision and drainage without damage to the remaining breast tissue

### Breast Tumors

1. *Benign*

A. The removal of adenofibromas or biopsy of areas of adenosis, or cystic mastitis can usually be accomplished through a semicircular areolar incision which, while technically adequate, is cosmetically superior to other incisions.

B. In patients with giant adenofibromas, an inferior submammary incision is utilized, removing the adenofibroma while retaining the adjacent, usually subareolar, normal tissue.

C. Although the breast skin may appear markedly redundant, in view of the elasticity of skin in children excision of skin is not indicated.

D. Since cystosarcoma phylloides rarely, if ever, metastasizes in children, local removal is adequate and radical mastectomy is not indicated.

2. *Malignant.* The treatment of cancer of the breast in both male and female is identical to that in adults. The results, however, are inferior to those in adults.

## Complications

The major complication in breast surgery in infants and young children consists of the inadvertent damage or removal of the subareolar disk, which represents the anlage for future breast development.

# HEAD AND NECK LESIONS IN THE CHILD

## PAROTITIS

### Definition

Parotitis is inflammation of the parotid gland secondary to viral or bacterial infection.

### Classification

1. Viral parotitis
2. Nonobstructive bacterial parotitis
3. Obstructive bacterial parotitis

### Basic Principles

The etiology of infantile parotitis is not known, but it is frequently found in debilitated premature infants and the incidence has been markedly reduced during the last decade. In older children, obstruction, either at the level of Stensen's duct or duct stones, is felt to be responsible in a majority of cases.

## Criteria for Diagnosis

### Clinical

1. *Infantile Parotitis*

A. Parotitis in infancy, either unilateral or bilateral, is bacterial in nature and is most commonly found in debilitated premature infants.

B. The parotid area is swollen, tender and soft or cystic on palpation.

C. The tenderness and reddening of the skin differentiates the unilateral parotitis from parotid tumors such as hemangioma or hygroma.

2. *Parotitis in the Older Child*

A. Bacterial parotitis in the older child is often accompanied by dilatation of parotid ducts, with or without stone formation, or occasionally obstruction and inflammatory changes at the oral opening of Stensen's duct.

B. In contrast to infantile parotitis, it is unilateral, the physical findings are identical, and occasionally periods of previous inflammation and swelling have been present.

### Laboratory

1. Since the amylase level is elevated in all types of parotitis, it does not help in the differential diagnosis.

2. Bacterial parotitis, in contrast to viral parotitis, usually is associated with leukocytosis.

### X-ray

1. Obstructive parotitis in older children, especially recurrent parotitis, may show the presence of ductal stones in the parotid glands. Calcifications also can be seen in hemangiomas involving the parotid and must be differentiated.

2. In patients past infancy—with the exception of patients with mumps parotitis—sialogram is indicated to rule out obstruction or possible parotid tumors.

## Differential Diagnosis

1. *Parotitis*
   A. Viral
   B. Bacterial
   C. Tuberculous
2. Parotid tumor

## Management

### General

1. *Infantile Parotitis*

A. In the absence of parotid abscess formation, systemic antibiotic treatment

B. If a parotid abscess with fluctuation develops, incision and drainage or aspiration are indicated. In the absence of ductal obstruction, occurrence of parotid fistula is unlikely.

2. *Parotitis in the Older Child.* In older children with parotitis, especially recurrent parotitis, the treatment consists of:

A. Systemic antibiotics

B. Alleviation of obstruction or stones if present

## CERVICAL LYMPHADENITIS

### Definition

Cervical lymphadenitis is acute or chronic inflammation of cervical lymph nodes due to specific or nonspecific organisms.

### Basic Principles

The most common organism responsible for nonspecific lymphadenitis is a coagulase-negative or coagulase-positive staphylococcus. In patients with tuberculosis, both typical and atypical strains may be responsible. Fungal lymphadenitis is most commonly caused by Actinomyces. Lymphadenitis in cat-scratch fever is due to a virus transmitted by young kittens.

### Criteria for Diagnosis

#### Clinical

1. *Acute, Nonspecific Lymphadenitis*
   A. Painful and tender swelling in the

anterior or posterior cervical chain occasionally following an episode of an upper respiratory or ear infection

B. On palpation, one or several lymph nodes may be enlarged, tender, with surrounding cellulitis.

C. The lymph nodes are usually soft, nonfused and not attached to the skin. With necrosis, increased tenderness, reddening of the skin, attachment to the skin and beginning fluctuation occur.

D. A regional entry can occasionally be found, such as evidence of tooth disease or ear involvement.

2. *Chronic Lymphadenitis*

A. Enlarged asymptomatic lymph nodes may be present for months after an acute episode, especially when treated with antibiotics.

B. On palpation, the lymph nodes are discrete, nontender and not attached to the skin or surrounding structures.

3. *Tuberculous or Fungal Lymphadenitis*

A. Either may be indistinguishable by history or symptomatology from acute lymphadenitis.

B. On palpation, single lymph nodes are rarely palpated; lymph nodes are usually found matted together and usually less tender than during an acute nonspecific lymphadenitis.

C. A history of exposure to actinomycosis, such as visits to a farm or exposure to known tuberculous adults, should be investigated.

## Laboratory

1. *Skin Tests*

A. Regular or atypical tuberculosis

B. Fungal tests if indicated

C. Cat-scratch antigen if the child was exposed to young cats

2. White blood count and differential

## X-ray

A chest x-ray is indicated in all patients with cervical lymphadenitis to rule out pulmonary or mediastinal involvement.

## Differential Diagnosis

Acute or chronic nonspecific lymphadenitis, tuberculous or fungal lymphadenitis, lymphosarcoma (Hodgkin's disease), infected branchial cyst, infected cystic hygroma

## Management

### Acute Nonspecific Lymphadenitis

1. *If No Fluctuation Is Present*

A. Conservative treatment is instituted with antibiotics specific for staphylococcus. At present ampicillin appears to be the drug of choice.

B. Warm wet compresses

2. If fluctuation occurs, incision and drainage are done, with cultures and Grams, stains to identify the underlying organisms, followed by appropriate antibiotic therapy.

### Chronic Lymphadenitis

1. *Persistent, Chronic Lymphadenitis.* If abnormal lymph nodes persist more than 8 weeks after the initial treatment, even if asymptomatic, they should have an excisional biopsy with microscopic and bacteriological examination.

2. *Tuberculous Lymphadenitis*

A. If abscess or fistula formation has not yet occurred, appropriate antituberculous treatment will control most cervical lymphadenopathies.

B. If abscess formation has occurred, however, excision of the involved lymph nodes is done with primary closure after starting and continuing antituberculous therapy.

C. If spontaneous decompression with fistula formation has occurred, antituberculous treatment should result in spontaneous closure. If closure does not occur, subsequent excision of the fistula tract together with underlying lymph nodes should be performed.

3. *Fungal Infection*

A. Incision and drainage of an unsuspected fungal abscess, usually actinomycosis, should be followed by penicillin therapy.

B. Spontaneous closure usually occurs and secondary excision of the involved node is rarely necessary, unless the tract does not heal.

4. *Cat-Scratch Fever.* Simple incision and drainage usually suffice to cure the necrotizing lymphadenitis.

## Complications

1. Incision and drainage of a tuberculous lymphadenitis without appropriate chemotherapy may result in a persistent fistula. Proper identification of the underlying organism and systemic work-up, including skin test and chest x-ray, may prevent this complication.

2. In patients with lymphadenitis not responding to appropriate conservative therapy, excisional biopsy is indicated to rule out primary or secondary malignancies.

## BRANCHIOGENIC SINUS OR CYST

### Definition

Branchiogenic sinuses or cysts are persistent remnants of the first or second branchial cleft.

### Classification

1. *First Branchial Cleft.* The internal opening is in the auditory canal; the external opening is below the ear on the mandibular angle.

2. *Second Branchial Cleft.* The internal opening is in the peritonsillar fossa; the external opening is between the lower third of the neck to the infraclavicular area following the anterior margin of the sternocleidomastoid muscle.

### Basic Principles

Branchial sinuses or cysts are persistent remnants of the first and second branchial clefts. Most sinuses and cysts communicate with either the auditory canal or the oral cavity. Branchial "rests," as a rule, do not communicate with either opening and constitute cartilaginous remnants without the danger of infection seen in the other two types.

### Criteria for Diagnosis

#### Clinical

1. Branchial sinuses with an open communication with the external skin are more common than cysts without communication.

2. Depending on their embryology, the external opening, usually pinpoint in size, can be found along the anterior border of the sternocleidomastoid, occasionally reaching to the infraclavicular area.

3. A history of intermittent, clear discharge from the sinus opening confirms the diagnosis.

4. In complicated cases, especially in patients with branchial cysts without external communication, infection occurs and the presenting symptom is similar to that in acute lymphadenitis: a tender, fluctuant mass in the area of the anterior cervical chain.

#### Laboratory

Leukocytosis if associated with infection

#### X-ray

Noncontributory

#### Differential Diagnosis

1. Lymphadenitis
2. Infected cystic hygroma
3. Lateral thyroglossal cyst
4. Secondary tumor

### Management

#### General

1. In view of the high incidence of infection, elective removal of branchiogenous sinuses and clefts is indicated.

2. If an infection has occurred, removal is difficult. Incision and drainage may be required, followed by excision after the inflammatory changes have subsided.

## Operative Treatment

The most common type, originating from the second branchial cleft, begins in the peritonsillar fossa, passing between external and internal carotids, and terminates in the lower third of the neck. It requires a stepladder incision for its removal.

## Complications

If not removed electively, infection may occur with duct obstruction.

## THYROGLOSSAL CYST

## Definition

Thyroglossal cyst is the persistence of an epithelial lined duct ending in a midline cyst following the descent of the thyroid from the foramen caecum.

## Basic Principles

The thyroid descends from the base of the tongue into the neck, and a persistent tract from the foramen caecum may remain with lymphoid tissue and occasionally thyroid follicles in its wall. Due to its communication with the oral cavity, bacterial invasion and infection occur frequently.

## Criteria for Diagnosis

### Clinical

1. A midline cyst, occasionally deviating slightly to one side, is found between the hyoid bone and the mid neck.
2. On palpation, it is not attached to the skin and is nontender if not infected, and it moves with deglutition.
3. If infected it is tender and indistinguishable from cervical adenitis.

### Laboratory

Noncontributory

### X-ray

No tracheal compression

### Differential Diagnosis

1. Ectopic thyroid
2. Submental lymphadenitis
3. Submental dermoid
4. In a slightly lateral position, a branchiogenous cyst

## Management

1. *Noninfected Thyroglossal Cyst.* The treatment is operative as follows:
*Operative Procedure* (Systrunk's Procedure)
A. The thyroglossal cyst is dissected through a transverse incision after the underlying normal thyroid has been identified to rule out an ectopic thyroid.
B. The tract is followed to the midportion of the hyoid bone which is excised in continuity with the tract and followed to the base of the tongue.
C. The duct is then ligated and transected.
D. The failure to resect the midportion of the hyoid bone results in a high rate of recurrent infection and cyst formation
2. *Infected Thyroglossal Cyst*
A. In the anterior midline location, major complications are rare and the treatment consists of drainage, followed by resection after inflammatory changes have subsided.
B. In thyroglossal cysts with a lateral or posterior position, perforation and respiratory distress have been reported. Incision and drainage providing adequate tracheal decompression also are indicated in these patients, followed by the secondary definitive procedure.

## Complications

Infections and perforation

## DERMOID CYST

## Definition

Dermoid cysts are cysts arising from misplaced ectodermal elements.

## Basic Principles

Dermoid cysts originating from ectodermal cells are benign in contrast to solid teratomas. Most dermoid cysts occur at the lateral aspect of the orbit; they are non-tender, not attached to the skin but occasionally attached to the periosteum and therefore nonmobile. Dermoid cysts in the midline or the bridge of the nose or the scalp may be indistinguishable from encephaloceles. Occasionally a communication with the skin, a dermal sinus, may be present which leads to subsequent infection.

Sublingual dermoids may communicate with a submental dermoid and present in a dumbbell-shaped type of lesion. By increasing growth, due to sequestration of squamous cells, they may interfere with swallowing and respiration. Since they are not attached to the hyoid, the characteristic movement during deglutition seen with thyroglossal cyst is usually absent.

## Criteria for Diagnosis

### Clinical

1. Dermoid cysts or benign teratomas occur in the periorbital subglottic or submandibular area.
2. Position tends to distinguish the lesion.
3. Nontender and not attached to the skin
4. Nonmobile because frequently attached to periosteum
5. In the subglottic or submandibular region, they do not move with deglutition.

### X-ray

In all dermoid cysts of the scalp or periorbital area, especially the midline, accurate x-ray evaluation is mandatory to differentiate encephaloceles.

### Differential Diagnosis

1. *Periorbital or Scalp Dermoid Cyst*
   A. Encephalocele
   B. Epidermal cyst
   C. Sublingual or submental cyst
2. *Submental Cyst*
   A. Ranula
   B. Submental lymphadenitis
   C. Thyroglossal cysts

## Management

1. Periorbital dermoid cysts can be removed without difficulty through a linear incision in the eyebrow, which should not be shaved.
2. Sublingual or submental cysts can be removed through a single incision if no communication exists.
3. If a dumbbell-type tumor between the sublingual and submental space exists, a dissection of the submental part with ligation and subsequent sublingual removal is indicated.
4. If dermoid cysts with dermal sinuses become infected, the primary treatment consists of incision and drainage, followed by a resection after the inflammatory changes have subsided.

# RESPIRATORY EMERGENCIES IN THE CHILD

## UPPER AIRWAY CONDITIONS

### *Retropharyngeal Abscess*

## Definition

1. *A retropharyngeal abscess* is an abscess formation in retropharyngeal lymph nodes.
2. *A parapharyngeal abscess* is infection and abscess formation in the parapharyngeal area secondary to pharyngeal infection or trauma.

## Basic Principles

Although the incidence of retropharyngeal abscesses has decreased since the advent of antibiotics, they still occur due to suppuration in retropharyngeal lymph nodes, predominantly in children under the age of three years.

Associated diseases which may impair the normal immune mechanism, such as chronic granulomatous disease, should be ruled out. Direct extensions of pharyngeal inflammatory changes or perforations into the parapharyngeal compartments produce abscess in this region.

## Criteria for Diagnosis

### Clinical

1. *Retropharyngeal Abscess*

A. History usually reveals an upper respiratory infection, such as tonsillitis, with persistent temperature elevation.

B. Dysphagia followed by respiratory difficulties, occasionally with stridor

C. External examination of the neck may be completely within normal limits.

D. The retropharyngeal abscess presents as a submucosal bulge. It is easily missed during oral examination unless the pharynx is closely inspected.

2. *Parapharyngeal Abscess*

A. Parapharyngeal abscesses are in a lateral or posteriorlateral position and less likely to cause acute onset of respiratory difficulties, as compared with the retropharyngeal abscess.

B. They may be accompanied by a history of pharyngitis or pharyngeal trauma such as perforation with foreign bodies.

C. Occasionally pre-existing lesion such as an infected branchial or thyroglossal cyst may perforate and may dissect into the parapharyngeal compartments.

D. They usually are palpable on external examination.

### Laboratory

Leukocytosis

### X-ray

Anteroposterior and lateral films of the neck demonstrate an acute anterior deviation of larynx, trachea and esophagus with retropharyngeal abscesses and anterolateral deviation with parapharyngeal abscesses.

### Differential Diagnosis

Retropharyngeal tumors (juvenile fibromatosis, hemangioma, neurogenic tumors)

## Management

### General

1. Decompression of the retropharyngeal abscess represents an emergency procedure in view of the respiratory distress caused by the pharyngeal obstruction.

2. The decompression should be performed *only* in the operating room.

3. Since endotracheal intubation is complicated by the anatomical distortion of the pharynx, needle aspiration of the abscess with a large bore needle not only identifies the site of the abscess formation, but facilitates intubation by decompression of the abscess.

4. Preparations for tracheostomy should be made in all cases,

5. Although repeat aspiration may be effective, incision and drainage under anesthesia, with endotracheal intubation to prevent aspiration, appear most preferable.

6. The incision of a retropharyngeal abscess should be performed in a vertical line to avoid transection of major retropharyngeal vessels; transection of these vessels leads to bleeding which is substantial and difficult to control.

7. In patients with parapharyngeal abscesses, the incision and drainage depend on the compartment involved; this can usually be accomplished through external drainage.

8. In either case antibiotic coverage is started as indicated by the Gram's stain and bacterial cultures at the time of drainage.

### *Epiglottiditis*

## Definition

Epiglottiditis is inflammatory laryngeal obstruction.

## Basic Principles

Epiglottiditis occurring after the age of two years is due to laryngeal, glottic and rarely subglottic inflammation caused by *Haemophilus influenzae.*

## Criteria for Diagnosis

### Clinical

1. Rapid onset of respiratory distress with stridor, hoarseness and fever

2. Direct laryngoscopy is not advisable unless preparations for intubation or tracheostomy have been made, since the child's excitement and even minor trauma during laryngoscopy may lead to complete obstruction.

### Laboratory and X-ray

Noncontributory, but can rule out other causes

### Differential Diagnosis

Laryngeal obstruction due to other causes, such as aspirated foreign bodies.

## Management

1. All patients with haemophilus epiglottiditis are to be considered as possible candidates for emergency tracheostomies.

2. In patients in whom the respiratory exchange is still adequate, treatment consists of sedation, high humidity and antibiotics (tetracycline of chloramphenicol).

3. Signs of clinical deterioration or a continuous increase in $PCO_2$ are indications for tracheostomy.

4. An occasional patient can be carried with endotracheal intubation, but the latter is not advisable in patients with epiglottiditis in view of the marked laryngeal inflammatory changes.

5. Although the disease is only short-lasting, rapid onset of complete laryngeal obstruction requires tracheostomy in the majority of patients.

### *Aspirated Foreign Bodies*

## Definition

This refers to aspiration of foreign bodies with retention in the laryngotracheobronchial airway.

## Basic Principles

Foreign bodies are retained in the hypopharynx, larynx, trachea or bronchus. Foreign bodies which have been present for a prolonged period of time, especially in small bronchi or bronchioli, can perforate and remain within the pulmonary parenchyma.

## Criteria for Diagnosis

### Pharyngeal or Hypopharyngeal Foreign Bodies

1. *Clinical*

A. The majority of foreign bodies in this area are of a shape which leads to perforation of the pharyngeal wall and retention, such as toothpicks, chicken bones, fish bones and occasionally pins.

B. The history of ingestion shortly before, with sudden pain, choking or inability to swallow

C. Respiratory distress is usually absent, separating this group from patients with aspiration of foreign bodies located within larynx or trachea.

2. *Laboratory and X-ray*. These are usually noncontributory unless the foreign body is radiopaque.

### Laryngeal Foreign Bodies

1. *Clinical*

A. History of ingestion

B. Sudden onset of dyspnea and respiratory distress, usually without change of voice

2. X-ray. Radiopaque materials can be seen on x-rays in an anteroposterior position, in contrast to esophageal foreign bodies which are usually seen in a lateral position.

### Tracheobronchial Foreign Bodies

1. *Clinical*

A. History of ingestion

B. Sudden onset of respiratory difficulty with choking or coughing and continuous or intermittent respiratory distress

C. The voice is normal.

D. Inspiratory or expiratory stridor may be present.

E. Smaller foreign bodies which do

not lead to respiratory difficulties often cause a "brassy" continuous cough, which may be the only indication of the foreign body aspiration.

(1) If the foreign body is lodged in one of the smaller bronchi, the development of either pulmonary collapse and pulmonary infection or pulmonary overaeration caused by a ball-valve mechanism may result.

(2) The clinical findings with small impacted bronchial foreign bodies can therefore change from absent or diminished breath sounds to hyperresonance.

2. *X-ray*

A. The majority of aspirated foreign bodies in children, particularly between the ages of one to three years, are not radiopaque since they are mainly vegetable material such as peanuts.

B. If the foreign body is lodged within one of the lobar bronchi, pulmonary collapse or overexpansion with radiolucency may be an indication of the presence of a foreign body.

## Management

### Pharyngeal or Hypopharyngeal Foreign Bodies

Removal of the foreign body under sedation can usually be performed without difficulties. General anesthesia is rarely required.

### Laryngeal Foreign Bodies

1. Since most children with aspirated laryngeal foreign bodies are excited, thereby further increasing their respiratory difficulties, sedation is indicated.

2. Removal of the laryngeal foreign body should be performed in the operating room.

3. Direct laryngoscopy under sedation, either without anesthesia or with only mild anesthesia, is usually sufficient. The foreign body can usually be extracted without difficulties.

### Tracheobronchial Foreign Bodies

1. Bronchoscopy, especially in young children, is best performed under general anesthesia.

A. After the patient has been anesthetized, a laryngoscope is introduced and larynx and vocal cords are examined.

B. The ventilating bronchoscope is then inserted between the cords, the laryngoscope is removed and the patient is ventilated through the bronchoscope.

2. Aspirated foreign bodies which do not change their size, such as metallic or plastic foreign bodies, can usually be removed with bronchoscopy forceps without undue difficulties.

3. Vegetable matter, especially peanuts which have been present for several days, may be difficult to remove in view of the swelling of the foreign body occurring after aspiration. They may therefore be too large to be removed through the vocal cord.

A. Biopsy forceps are used to diminish the size of the foreign body, but care must be taken to avoid complete fragmentation.

B. This may lead to separation of small fragments which can be driven into smaller bronchi or bronchioli where they cannot be reached with biopsy forceps.

C. Occasionally a small fragment left behind may be responsible for a segmental collapse, requiring repeat bronchoscopy at a later date.

D. The majority of these small fragments, however, will be cleared by the patient spontaneously by coughing, unless they have been forcibly pushed into a bronchial opening.

4. Elongated metallic foreign bodies, such as needles and pins, may end up in bronchi too small for the introduction of the bronchoscope.

A. Bronchoscopy under an image intensifier may facilitate their removal, directing small biopsy forceps into even minor bronchi too small for the introduction of a bronchoscope.

B. In patients in whom needles and

pins have been present for a prolonged period of time, the removal via bronchoscopy may be impossible if perforation has occurred and the foreign body is located within the pulmonary parenchyma. In these patients a thoracotomy for the removal of the foreign body is indicated.

C. *Caution:* in patients with pulmonary foreign bodies, when a thoracotomy is considered, a repeat chest film on the operating table is indicated on *all* patients, since foreign bodies may change their location even though they may have been present in one position for a prolonged period of time. The failure to repeat the chest film on the operating table may cause the surgeon to perform either an unwarranted thoracotomy or a thoracotomy on the wrong side.

## INTRAPLEURAL AND PULMONARY PROBLEMS

### *Empyema*

### Definition

Empyema is pleural accumulation of a purulent exudate.

### Basic Principles

Empyema, especially in young infants and children, is commonly seen following staphylococcal pneumonia. In rare instances the perforation of an infected lung cyst or pulmonary abscess may also lead to the development of an empyema. The empyema may be accompanied by a pneumothorax (pyopneumothorax), with or without tension, or the formation of a bronchopleural fistula.

Uncomplicated empyema, if untreated, can lead to an "entrapment" of the lung with a peel formation.

### Criteria for Diagnosis

#### Clinical

1. The development of an empyema, especially in young infants and children, is usually preceded by a staphylococcal pneumonia with signs and symptoms of either cough, dyspnea and/or chest pain.

2. On physical examination, dullness is noted over the involved chest with diminution of breath sounds.

#### Laboratory

1. Leukocytosis
2. Bacterial cultures of nasopharyngeal and tracheal aspirate
3. Thoracocentesis

#### X-ray

Loculated or diffuse fluid accumulation with obliteration of the costophrenic angle. If the involved lung can be visualized, there is usually evidence of pneumonia.

### Management

#### General

1. In contrast to patients with pleural effusion, patients with empyema require primary tube thoracostomy after a single needle thoracocentesis has been performed to identify the site and nature of the empyema, by cultures and Gram's stains to identify the underlying causative organism.

A. The thoracocentesis is followed by local infiltration of Novacain, skin incision and placement of a thoracostomy tube.

B. This can be accomplished with a hemostat in infants or a trocar in older children.

C. In patients with a nonloculated empyema, the tube is best placed in the midaxillary line in the sixth or seventh interspace.

D. A posterior position will interfere with the patient's supine position or lead to kinking or obstruction of the tube.

2. Inadequate drainage or loculation may require the insertion of several thoracostomy tubes.

#### Treatment of Entrapped Lungs

In patients with inadequately drained empyema leading to pulmonary entrapment or the formation of a constrictive peel, decortication is indicated.

## Complications

1. Peel formation
2. Septicemia
3. Pyopneumothorax
4. Bronchopleural Fistula. In patients with persistent broncopleural fistula, in spite of adequate thoracotomy tube drainage, operative intervention is indicated.

### Lung Abscess

## Definition

Lung abscess is a formation of an abscess cavity within the pulmonary parenchyma.

## Basic Principles

The majority of pulmonary abscesses follow pneumonia. In rarer instances, fungal infections such as coccidioidomycosis or foreign bodies may be the underlying cause. Pulmonary abscesses following pneumonia are more common in the middle and lower lobe, hematogenous abscesses in the upper lobes. Pulmonary abscesses following the aspiration of a foreign body are likely to be in the right middle or lower lobe.

## Criteria for Diagnosis

### Clinical

1. A lung abscess in children is usually preceded by symptoms of pneumonia.
2. In a small number of patients, the preceding symptoms may be absent, with the presenting symptoms limited to a febrile episode, cough, weight loss and occasionally hemoptysis.

### Laboratory

Leukocytosis and occasionally anemia

### X-ray

Presence of an abscess cavity within the pulmonary parenchyma

## Differential Diagnosis

1. Tuberculosis
2. Fungal abscesses
3. Abscesses due to foreign bodies
4. Infected lung cysts

## Management

1. Endotracheal culture should be obtained since appropriate antibiotic therapy is effective in the majority of cases.
2. Bronchoscopy should be performed to rule out endobronchial involvement and foreign body obstruction, and to obtain cultures.
3. In some patients bronchoscopy will permit aspiration and drainage of the abscess cavity if it is freely communicating with the endobronchial tree.
4. Persistent lung abscesses not responding to conservative treatment require semental resection or lobectomy.

## Complications

1. Empyema
2. Perforation into the endobronchial tree
3. Endobronchial dissemination
4. Massive hemoptysis
5. Metastatic brain abscess

### Pneumatoceles

## Definition

Pneumatoceles are acquired pulmonary cysts, usually multiple.

## Basic Principles

Pneumatoceles in infancy and childhood are almost invariably secondary to a staphylococcal pneumonia. Cysts may involve several lobes but are usually found on one side only. A single pneumatocele, developing after a staphylococcal pneumonia, may be indistinguishable from a congenital cyst. Rapid expansion of the cyst or perforation may lead to a tension pneumothroax with marked mediastinal shift and interference with the function of the contralateral lung.

## Criteria for Diagnosis

### Clinical

1. History of symptoms and signs compatible with a preceding staphylococcal pneumonia

2. Patients with multiple pneumatoceles, without rapid expansion or persistent infection, may be completely asymptomatic.

3. If either single or multiple pneumatoceles expand rapidly, the findings are compatible with a tension pneumothorax: diminished breath sounds on the involved side, hyperresonance and mediastinal shift to the contralateral side.

4. Symptoms can be aggravated if spontaneous perforation with pneumothorax or tension pneumothorax occurs.

### X-ray

Chest films usually reveal the presence of multiple pulmonary cysts varying in size.

### Differential Diagnosis

Congenital lung cysts

## Management

1. In patients with pneumatoceles without evidence of respiratory distress the treatment is conservative, and in the vast majority of patients the pneumatoceles will disappear within one year. The pulmonary parenchyma then will appear normal on x-ray.

2. Rapid expansion leading to respiratory distress may require the insertion of one or several thoracostomy tubes. The treatment is far less satisfactory than in patients with pneumothorax or tension pneumothorax, since the mediastinal shift may be due to the expansion of numerous small cysts.

3. Since these cysts do not freely communicate, decompression of one cyst will not decrease the tension in another cyst. Tube thoracostomy therefore is only indicated to drain large cysts in patients with severe respiratory distress.

## Complications

1. Spontaneous perforation of pneumatoceles with pneumothorax or tension pneumothorax

2. Empyema

## MEDIASTINAL EMERGENCIES

*Acute Mediastinitis*

## Definition

Acute mediastinitis is acute inflammation of the anterior or posterior mediastinum.

## Basic Principles

Acute mediastinitis may originate within the mediastinum: esophageal perforation, breakdown of purulent mediastinal nodes and mediastinal operative complications.

Mediastinitis may also be secondary to nonmediastinal processes: dissection of cervical or retropharyngeal abscesses into the mediastinum, cervical injuries with cellulitis and abscess formation extending into the mediastinum.

## Criteria for Diagnosis

### Clinical

1. Chest pain
2. Sepsis
3. Dyspnea
4. Tachycardia
5. Occasionally a superior mediastinal syndrome with venous congestion of the head and neck area and facial edema
6. Depending on the underlying cause, the patient's history may include:
    A. Neck or chest trauma
    B. Cervical infections
    C. Preceding operative manipulations including esophagoscopy
    D. Mediastinal node biopsy
    E. Esophageal operations
    F. Other operative procedures which may lead to esophageal perforation
    G. Cervical or thoracic trauma
7. Physical examination in patients with

posterior mediastinitis rarely defines the site and cause of the mediastinitis.

8. In patients with anterior mediastinitis, swelling, tenderness or subcutaneous emphysema of the supraclavicular area may be present.

### X-ray

1. Widening of the posterior mediastinum may be visible.

2. Air may be present in the posterior or anterior mediastinum, especially after esophageal or tracheal injuries.

3. Esophageal contrast studies may show a displacement of the esophagus or an esophageal leak.

### Differential Diagnosis

Intrathoracic lesions leading to infection or obstruction

### Management

### General

In only a few instances is conservative treatment likely to be effective, primarily in the treatment of purulent mediastinal lymphadenitis. In the vast majority of patients, regardless of the underlying cause, operative drainage is required.

### Anterior and Superior Mediastinitis

1. The anterior and superior mediastinum can be drained through a low transverse neck incision, with a dissection carried down bluntly into the superior anterior mediastinum.

2. When this approach is inadequate, drainage can be accomplished through the second or third anterior rib bed.

### Posterior Mediastinum

1. Extrapleural or transpleural drainage through an appropriate posterior rib or intercostal space, depending on the cause and site of the mediastinitis

2. In patients with recent esophageal perforation, operative closure may be indicated.

3. In all patients the operative drainage

is combined with antibiotic and intravenous fluid administration, and nasoesophageal gastric decompression in patients with esophageal perforations.

### *Superior Mediastinal Syndrome*

### Definition

Superior mediastinal syndrome refers to obstruction of the superior mediastinal structures.

### Basic Principles

The most common cause for the obstruction of superior mediastinal structures in children is lymphosarcoma.

### Criteria for Diagnosis

### Clinical

1. Development of facial and cervical edema and cyanosis, occasionally involving the upper extremities

2. Respiratory impairment may occur

3. Dysphagia is usually not a prominent feature.

### Laboratory

In patients with lymphosarcoma, the presence of a leukemia may be confirmed by peripheral and bone marrow studies.

### X-ray

1. Posteroanterior and lateral films of the chest may show the presence of a mass density within the upper mediastinum.

2. Venography, either through an upper extremity or jugular vein, confirms a partial or complete venous obstruction with the formation of collateral veins.

### Differential Diagnosis

1. Mediastinitis
2. Acute traumatic superior mediastinal syndrome (acute traumatic asphyxia, blast injury)

### Management

1. In the absence of a confirmative peripheral or bone marrow study, a

mediastinal node biopsy should be performed to confirm the diagnosis of lymphosarcoma.

2. If lymphosarcoma has been diagnosed as the cause of the obstruction, operative treatment is not indicated.

3. Conservative treatment consists of radiotherapy and chemotherapy.

4. When the syndrome is due to other expanding lesions, their removal is mandatory.

## EXTREMITY LESIONS IN THE CHILD

### LYMPHADENITIS

#### Definition

Lymphadenitis is infection of regional lymph nodes.

#### Classification

1. Acute
2. Chronic
3. Viral
4. Bacterial
5. Tuberculous
6. Fungal

#### Basic Principles

Infections (including such minor infections as folliculitis which may have healed and disappeared by the time the lymphadenopathy appears) are the usual cause of lymphadenitis. In patients with persistent and repeated infection, immune deficiencies such as agammaglobulinemia should be ruled out. Peripheral lymphadenitis is most commonly seen in the femoral-inguinal area, followed by axillary and iliac nodes. Recent minor injuries such as cuts, abrasions and small abscesses should be looked for by history and physical examination. In acute lymphadenitis, one or several enlarged lymph nodes can be palpated, and the lymph nodes are well-delineated, neither fused nor matted as in tuberculosis, and not as firm as in lymphosarcoma.

#### Criteria for Diagnosis

##### Clinical

1. Tenderness, edema and reddening of the overlying skin may be present.

2. The presence of a distal lymphangitis, with a characteristic linear reddish discoloration leading toward the involved nodes, suggests a distal source of infection.

3. History should include information of previous infections, exposure to hospital infections or hospital carriers and contact with animals carrying cat-scratch fever (young cats under the age of one year).

4. Physical examination of all lymph-node-bearing areas, including head and neck, axilla and inguinal area, femoral and epitrochlear area, to rule out diffuse lymphadenopathy

##### Laboratory

1. Hematocrit
2. White blood cell and differential count

##### X-ray

Chest posteroanterior film (for mediastinal widening)

##### Differential Diagnosis

1. Diffuse lymphadenopathy
2. Lymphosarcoma and/or leukemia

#### Management

1. Treatment should include both the primary cause, if present and identifiable, and the lymphadenitis.

2. If there is no evidence of fluctuant abscess formation, only conservative treatment with antibiotics, usually broad-spectrum, local heat and rest is indicated.

3. If fluctuation is present, incision and drainage should be done with culture and Gram's stain studies.

4. Patients with persistent enlarged nodes not responding to conservative treatment, suggesting chronic lymphadenitis, should have excisional biopsy for microscopic histological fungal and bacterial examination.

## ABSCESS FORMATION

### Definition

Abscess formation refers to loculated necrosis with liquefaction.

### Basic Principles

Extremity abscesses usually follow minor trauma, foreign bodies, infections such as folliculitis, subcutaneous or intramuscular injections or underlying osteomyelitis. On physical examination, differential diagnosis between cellulitis and/or abscess formation may be difficult if the abscess is deep in the muscular tissue. It is necessary to look for associated diseases such as diabetes or immune deficiences.

### Criteria for Diagnosis

Clinical

Classical:
1. Rubor—redness
2. Dolor—pain
3. Calor—heat
4. Tumor—swelling
5. Plus fluctuation

Laboratory

1. Peripheral white blood count
2. Blood sugar
3. Urinalysis

X-ray

Views of the underlying osseous structure to rule out foreign bodies or osteomyelitis

Differential Diagnosis

1. Cellulitis
2. Osteomyelitis
3. Necrosis in primary or secondary tumors such as rhabdomyosarcoma

### Management

1. *Incision and drainage,* under general anesthesia in children, with the exception of small superficial abscesses
2. In chronic abscesses or abscesses not responding to appropriate treatment, a biopsy of the abscess wall should be obtained to rule out primary or secondary neoplasms.

## CELLULITIS

### Definition

Cellulitis is diffuse acute inflammation involving skin and subcutaneous tissue.

### Classification

1. Streptococcal (erysipelas)
2. Nonspecific

### Basic Principles

Rapidly spreading cellulitis is usually caused by streptococcal infection. Cellulitis, especially in association with minor local infections, can also be caused by a variety of bacteria.

### Criteria for Diagnosis

Clinical

1. Localized or diffuse reddening of the skin, followed by moderate swelling without localization or abscess formation
2. Streptococcal infections display rapid development of intense bright-red discoloration of the skin, which usually is accompanied by high fever and marked leukocytosis.

Differential Diagnosis

1. Contact dermatitis
2. Abscess formation

### Management

1. The treatment of cellulitis is conservative, with immobilization, warm to hot compresses and appropriate antibiotic therapy.
2. If streptococcal infection is suspected, intravenous penicillin in high doses should be effective within 24 to 48 hours.

## LYMPHEDEMA

### Definition

Lymphedema is swelling, usually affecting one or both of the lower extremities, due to congenital lymphatic malformation.

## Basic Principles

Congenital lymphedema usually becomes apparent shortly after birth and leads to the appearance of "elephantiasis," with marked enlargement of the involved extremities, without pitting and longitudinal overgrowth. The etiology of lymphedema is poorly understood. Several types have been described histologically and by lymphangiography; all appear to be related to a congenital lymphatic malformation.

Lymphedema does not represent a surgical emergency, but it is extremely susceptible to massive infections and difficult to treat in view of the lymphatic malformation. Infection without lymphatic drainage and the resulting stasis can lead to an overwhelming infection which responds poorly to conservative therapy. The extent of cellulitis or infection in a patient with lymphedema is difficult to assess, since skin changes which ordinarily occur are often absent in patients with lymphedema.

## Criteria for Diagnosis

### Clinical

1. Diffuse swelling of one or both legs
2. Skin changes vary from reddening and formation of blisters to diffuse necrosis and slough.
3. Signs of diffuse septicemia which can occur rapidly

### X-ray

Lymphangiography (only to be performed in the absence of acute inflammation) may show dilated lymphatic channels without connection or with marked delay in drainage into normal proximal lymph channels.

### Differential Diagnosis

*Lymphangioma.* In contrast to diffuse lymphedema, lymphangiomas or cystic hygromas are localized and more cystic in character, involving the skin in most patients. The cystic hygroma, like lymphedema, is also susceptible to infection.

## Management

1. The treatment of congenital lymphedema, without superimposed infection, is not an emergency procedure and therefore is not included here.
2. The treatment of the acutely infected lymphedema consists of:

    A. Immobilization

    B. Aggressive antibiotic and local treatment, including wide incision, drainage and excision, is indicated.

    C. If aggressive local therapy fails with the patient displaying signs of spreading cellulitis and skin necrosis accompanied by sepsis, amputation with secondary closure is indicated.

## HEMANGIOMA

## Classification

1. Capillary hemangioma
2. Cavernous hemangioma
3. Arteriovenous fistulae

## Basic Principles

Capillary hemangiomas, single or multiple, with a bright-red appearance, usually undergo early fibrosis indicated by the development of diffuse areas of grayish fibrosis. Patients with large cavernous hemangiomas, with or without skin involvement, may develop platelet trapping in early infancy. The resulting thrombocytopenia can lead to a systemic bleeding tendency. If local ulcerations of the hemangioma occur, massive bleeding may result.

Arteriovenous fistulae, which can be found in both upper and lower extremities, are usually multiple and lead to an excessive growth of the involved limb. If the arteriovenous shunt is large, secondary cardiac manifestations due to the high left ventricular output may occur, such as cardiac failure. The presence of an elongated extremity with a positive Branham sign (a decrease of pulse rate when the major arteries supplying the extremities are occluded) is diagnostic of peripheral arteriovenous fistulae.

## Criteria for Diagnosis

### Clinical

1. Typical "port-wine" stain on skin
2. Subcutaneous spongy tumor with bluish discoloration of the extremity
3. Hemihypertrophy of the limb associated with palpable thrills or audible bruits
4. Positive Branham-Nicoladoni sign

### Laboratory

1. Platelet count in infants to rule out platelet trapping
2. Bilateral venous and arterial oxygen determinations (increased venous $pO_2$ on the involved side)

### X-ray

Arterial angiography, including venous phase, to demonstrate the extent or multiplicity of the hemangioma, arterial feeders and the presence of arteriovenous fistulae

### Differential Diagnosis

1. *Vascular Tumors:* pericytoma
2. *Other Factors Leading to Differential Growth:* hemihypertrophy

## Management

1. *Capillary Hemangiomas*
   A. Observation
   B. Excision only if sudden enlargement should occur
2. *Cavernous Hemangiomas.* Excision is indicated if platelet trapping should occur or if there are ulcerations leading to major bleeding.
3. *Arteriovenous Fistulae*
   A. Excision or ligation of single arteriovenous fistula to prevent overgrowth of the involved extremity or cardiac failure

B. In patients with diffuse congenital arteriovenous fistulae, operative treatment is ineffective. Stapling of the epiphysis is indicated to equalize the growth of both extremities.
   C. In infants with rapidly enlarging, unresectable hemangiomas, the administration of steroid may result in the arrest of growth or diminution in size of the hemangioma.

## OSTEOMYELITIS

### Definition

Osteomyelitis is pyogenic inflammation of the bone.

### Classification

1. Hematogenous osteomyelitis
2. Local extension of an inflammatory process

### Basic Principles

Acute osteomyelitis in infants and children is usually caused by hematogenous infection with streptococcus, staphylococcus or salmonella (especially in children with sickle cell disease), and usually involves the lower extremities. Due to the capillary increase at the metaphyseal-epiphyseal junction, osteomyelitic changes are usually found here. Inflammation and necrosis are limited to the metaphysis, and the epiphyseal plate acts as a boundary. Subperiosteal extension of the inflammatory process leads to a secondary ischemia of the cortical bone and necrosis.

In chronic osteomyelitis a fenestration of the bone occurs with new bone formation from the surrounding periosteum. This leads to a cycle of bone necrosis, abscess formation, cavitation and new bone formation.

Patients with sickle cell disease with thrombosis of nutrient osseous vessels are particularly prone to salmonella osteomyelitis.

## Criteria for Diagnosis

### Clinical

1. Systemic symptoms include:
   A. High fever
   B. Signs of septicemia
   C. Irritability or lethargy
   D. Weight loss or failure to gain weight
2. On physical examination
   A. Localized tenderness over the involved area, usually over the metaphysis of the lower femur and upper tibia
   B. Limitation of motion
   C. Effusion into the adjacent joint

### Laboratory

1. Leukocytosis with a shift to the left
2. Positive blood cultures

### X-ray

1. In the early stages of osteomyelitis, x-ray findings may be absent for up to three weeks.
2. Positive x-ray findings consist of bone necrosis with rarefaction and subperiosteal bone formation or calcification or the formation of a sequestrum in chronic osteomyelitis.

### Differential Diagnosis

1. Rheumatic fever
2. Primary osseous malignancies
3. Secondary metastases (neuroblastoma)
4. Sickle cell disease

## Management

1. *Early Osteomyelitis Without Bone Necrosis*

A. If blood culture or local aspiration reveals the underlying organism, the appropriate antibiotic can be administered.
B. This is always combined with local immobilization.
C. In the absence of positive cultures, broad-spectrum antibiotics, covering gram-positive and gram-negative organisms, are indicated.
D. If the response to the treatment is satisfactory, without radiologic signs of necrosis, the treatment can be terminated several weeks after symptoms have subsided.

2. *With Radiographic Evidence of Osteomyelitis*

A. Operative intervention with incision, curettage and drainage of the involved area is indicated.
B. The incision should be adequate but limited, and periosteum should be preserved to prevent further devascularization and necrosis of the adjacent bone.
C. Inlying catheters can be used for continuous irrigation and suction.
D. Antibiotic coverage will be depending on the underlying organism.
E. Even with prompt and satisfactory response, antibiotic coverage is indicated for a period of approximately three months.
F. In patients with chronic osteomyelitis, excision and curettage of the sequestrum (the underlying necrotic bone) with irrigation and drainage should be performed.
G. Primary skin closure should be attempted to prevent the formation of sinus tracts.
H. Catheters or drains are necessary if a primary closure is performed.

# Common Emergency
# Pediatric Surgical Procedures

## NASOGASTRIC DECOMPRESSION

### Basic Principles

Nasogastric decompression is indicated in all infants and children with: (1) intestinal obstruction, (2) adynamic ileus, and (3) respiratory impairment due to abdominal distention.

## Technique

1. Prior to the insertion of a nasogastric tube, the patency of both choanal openings should be ascertained.

2. If a unilateral choanal atresia exists, intubation of the open choana may lead to respiratory distress and is therefore contraindicated. Gastric decompression can be achieved in these infants through the insertion of an orogastric tube.

3. Efficient nasogastric decompression depends on the internal diameter of the nasogastric tube, its patency and length. Nasogastric feeding tubes, with small diameter and considerable length, create an increased peripheral resistance if used as drainage tubes and are *not* designed for nasogastric decompression.

4. In infants and young children, the largest catheter that easily passes through the ala and choana should be placed into the stomach.

5. After the catheter has been introduced, injection of a small amount of air with auscultation over the stomach and aspiration of gastric material will confirm its correct position.

6. Catheters should be taped in place, *avoiding:*

A. Pressure on the ala with possible resulting necrosis of the cartilage

B. Occluding the nostrils by the securing tape to permit the infant to continue its nasal breathing

7. Gravity drainage is sufficient in most infants for adequate decompression, but even if intermittent suction is used, frequent injections of either small amounts of air or saline are indicated to either verify the patency of the tube or to restore its patency.

8. *A nonfunctioning nasogastric tube is more deleterious than no tube at all.*

9. In children over the age of one year, sump drains can be used with continuous suction. Although the continuous inflow of air through the sump drain makes a clogging of the tube more unlikely, frequent manual irrigations and aspirations are still indicated to assure patency.

## Warning

1. *Don't* use a small feeding tube for gastric decompression.

2. *Don't* occlude both nostrils or apply pressure to the ala while securing the catheter.

3. *Don't* assume that "intermittent" or "continuous" suction provides suction without manual check.

4. *Don't* clamp the tube. The irritation of a nonfunctioning nasogastric tube may lead to air swallowing and more gastric distention than if no tube is used.

5. *Don't* consider that even a functioning nasogastric tube is a guarantee preventing vomiting and aspiration.

## RECTAL TUBES

### Basic Principles

Rectal tubes for the evacuation of gaseous distention of the large bowel may be indicated in patients with rectal strictures, toxic megacolon or Hirschsprung's colitis.

### Technique

1. A multifenestrated rectal tube should be placed so that its tip lies at least in the rectosigmoid.

2. Rectal tubes have to be irrigated and aspirated at regular, frequent intervals.

3. The insertion of a rectal tube without irrigation and aspiration is as effective as the insertion of a plug. It leads to increased external sphincter contraction and, in the absence of patency, which can only be confirmed by frequent irrigation, obstructs rather than decompresses the large bowel.

### Warning

*Don't* forget to maintain rectal tube patency by irrigation.

## VENOUS CUTDOWN

### Basic Principles

In contrast to adults, where lower extremity venous cutdown may lead to thrombophlebitis and embolism, the lower saphenous vein is the preferred site for an intravenous cutdown in infants and children. This is so only if *no* operative injury or occlusion of major intra-abdominal vascular structures is anticipated, such as in major abdominal trauma or with resections of major abdominal tumors or hepatic lesions.

## Technique

1. A venous cutdown should be performed under complete sterile conditions with the surgeon gowned, gloved and masked.

2. After adequate skin sterilization and draping, an incision measuring approximately 3 mm. is made 1 cm. above the anterior third of the medial malleolus into the subcutaneous tissue.

3. The incision is gently spread in a vertical fashion and with the use of a blunt nerve hook the saphenous vein can easily be delivered into the field.

4. The distal end is ligated with a 4-0 or 5-0 silk tie; another tie is loosely placed around the proximal portion and the vein is incised between them. An intravenous catheter with a blunted tip, approximately twice the size of the collapsed vein, is then gently inserted *but no higher than midcalf.* Attempting to pass the catheter past the popliteal fossa will either result in the perforation of the saphenous vein or in obstruction of the catheter when the leg is bent.

5. The catheter is secured in place with the upper tie and the wound is closed with one single atraumatic nylon suture.

6. The wound is covered with a small dressing soaked with a bactericidal solution, such as Betadine, and the catheter is securely taped in place.

7. The adhesive tape encircling the catheter extends past the incision and is securely taped but not in circular fashion to the calf. This eliminates restraints like foot boards, which are not only uncomfortable for the child, but may mask infiltration.

8. In patients undergoing operative procedures, the junction of catheter and intravenous tubes should be securely taped

so that separation does not occur unobserved during the operative procedure.

9. The catheter is removed as soon as signs of infiltration, tenderness, pain or reddening occur.

## Warning

1. *Don't* use encircling tapes.

2. *Don't* use stiff or pointed catheters.

3. *Don't* use hypertonic infusions, especially with pumps, in peripheral veins.

4. *Don't* perform a cutdown procedure under unsterile conditions unless it is a lifesaving emergency.

5. *Don't* use lower extremity cutdowns if possible laceration or occlusion of intra-abdominal aorta or vena cava is anticipated.

6. *Don't* leave a cutdown catheter in place with signs of local infiltration, infection or sepsis possibly related to a contaminated catheter.

## JUGULAR VENOUS CUTDOWN

A venous cutdown of either the internal or external jugular veins may be preferable in children for:

1. Continuous measurement of central venous pressure

2. Anticipated intravenous hyperalimentation

3. An intravenous line when accessible peripheral veins are absent (previously used or collapsed in shock)

4. Patients with intra-abdominal vena cava compression, injury or anticipated operative caval occlusion

### Selection of Veins

Both external and internal jugular veins can be used for the insertion of intravenous cutdown catheters. Although an occlusion of all four veins can result in temporary facial cyanosis and venous congestion, collateral veins will usually prevent serious complications. While external jugular veins are usually easily identifiable in older, particularly skinny, children, the identification of the external jugular vein may be difficult in children in shock or in obese children, especially under one year of age.

Catheterization of the left jugular vein, especially the external jugular vein, may be difficult since the catheter may not advance into the superior vena cava but may go into peripheral veins. It is easier to catheterize the right jugular veins, especially the internal jugular vein, in an emergency.

## Venous Cutdown Technique

1. Maintenance of sterility as described above, in particular if intravenous hyperalimentation is anticipated
2. *External Jugular Vein*
   A. The easiest point to identify and catheterize the external jugular veins is at the junction of the lower and middle third of the anterior border of the sternocleidomastoid muscle.
   B. The distance from this point to the approximate entry into the atrium should be measured, and a catheter should be marked accordingly and inserted into the jugular vein.
   C. Regardless of which jugular vein is used, the proper location of the catheter should be checked by:
      *(1)* Fluctuation of the central venous pressure during inspiration and expiration
      *(2)* X-rays to determine the exact location of the tip of the catheter
3. *Internal Jugular Vein*
   A. Although the internal jugular vein can be ligated proximal to the insertion of the catheter, a small circumferential purse-string suture of 6-0 or 7-0 silk is preferred. This allows patency of the jugular vein and prevents the damping of the central venous pressure which can occur after ligation of the vein around the catheter.
   B. If a long-term position of the catheter is anticipated, as in patients with hyperalimentation, the ipsilateral postauricular site should be prepared for the entrance of the catheter. An area above and behind the ear should be shaved and thoroughly prepared. A small incision is carried into the subcutaneous tissue, and a groove director is advanced subcutaneously to the neck incision, immediately over the jugular vein catheterization. The catheter is brought through the postauricular opening and then inserted into the jugular vein as described before. The catheter is sutured to the scalp to prevent movement. Antibacterial and antifungal ointment is placed around the opening and the incision is occluded by a water-tight dressing.

## Warning

1. *Intravenous Pressure.* If the catheter is introduced into peripheral veins or into the intra-abdominal vena cava, erroneous intravenous pressure readings can be obtained, especially if intra-abdominal pressure is increased. Proper identification of the tip of the catheter by (1) radiologic identification and (2) evidence of negative and positive pressure within the thoracic cavity is essential.

2. *Perforation.* The use of stiff catheters, especially if used in the left jugular vein, can lead to perforation with a resultant "glucose thorax" with escape of the administered fluid into the intrapleural or retropleural space.

3. *Arrhythmias.* The dissection of the jugular vein, especially of the internal jugular vein, may lead to cardiac arrhythmias in premature infants. Careful dissection and administration of atropine may be necessary in these patients.

4. *Hyperalimentation.* Hyperalimentation should not be attempted unless all ancillary services and trained personnel are available (proper solutions, sterile preparation, adequate facilities to follow metabolic changes and laminar flow for preparation of fluids).

## BRACHIOCEPHALIC CUTDOWN

Preparation for brachiocephalic cutdown is as discussed under Venous Cutdown, above.

## Warning

If an antecubital cutdown is used, the brachial artery can easily be mistaken for a vein. For this reason a needle aspiration should be performed to properly identify the brachial artery and vein. If the brachial artery is transected by mistake, restoration of arterial flow is indicated since peripheral gangrene can occur in children with ligation of the brachial artery.

## FEMORAL CUTDOWN

A femoral vein cutdown is rarely indicated in children. Although thrombosis of the femoral vein after cutdown is tolerated by most children, the insertion of the catheter through the saphenous vein approximately one-half centimeter distal to the junction of femoral vein is preferable to a direct femoral vein catheterization.

## ENDOTRACHEAL INTUBATION

### Basic Principles

Even though endotracheal intubation may be lifesaving in many instances, improper use may be more detrimental to the patient, especially in the hands of a physician used to adults but not familiar with infants.

Emergency endotracheal intubation is only indicated:

1. If airway and assisted mask ventilation fail
2. If there is glottic or supraglottic obstruction
3. If appropriate endotracheal tubes and laryngoscopes are available

In the majority of acute respiratory emergencies, the insertion of an airway and mask or mouth-to-mouth assisted ventilation is preferable to an attempt at intubation, until endotracheal intubation can be attempted by personnel familiar with the procedure. Repeated attempts at unsuccessful intubation not only can lead to severe local trauma, preventing further successful intubation, but can lose valuable time with increase in hypoxia and further deterioration of the patient. If a satisfactory air exchange can be obtained through oral assisted ventilation, as confirmed by auscultation, clinical observation of chest expansion and maintenance of a normal heart rate, intubation can be postponed until circumstances are appropriate. The addition of a nasogastric tube to prevent gastric overdistention, vomiting, aspiration and interference with diaphragmatic motion is indicated in all patients undergoing prolonged mask or mouth-to-mouth respirations.

### Technique

Endotracheal intubation for the inexperienced physician is best accomplished in the following way:

1. Prepare various sizes of endotracheal tubes likely to fit into the glottic space without trauma (for infants, sizes 8 to 12).

2. Measure and prepare an internal stylet if the endotracheal tube is flexible and soft.

3. Select an appropriate laryngoscope blade.

4. Clear the oropharynx of secretions prior to the insertion of the laryngoscope.

5. Have an assistant to maintain hyperflexion of the head and slight pressure on the larynx if necessary.

6. Insert a nasal catheter attached to 100% oxygen.

7. Introduce the laryngoscope blade gently without pressure on pharynx or palate toward the base of the tongue, lift up the base of the tongue without touching the base of the epiglottis and have your assistant put slight pressure on the larynx. This will bring epiglottis and vocal cords into view.

8. Evaluate the existing pathology, and if intubation is possible select the appropriate endotracheal tube and insert it between the vocal cords for a distance of 3 to 4 cm.

9. Use mouth inflation of the endotracheal tube with simultaneous auscultation and examination of the chest.

10. If the attempt of intubation was unsuccessful, remove tube and laryngoscope and hyperventilate with mask or mouth-to-mouth and repeat the procedure after the condition of the patient has stabilized.

11. Although an experienced endoscopist can lift up the tip of the epiglottis and insert the tube without difficulties, manipulation of the epiglottis may lead to laryngospasm and make intubation impossible for the inexperienced. The use of the base of the tongue as fulcrum is therefore safer for the inexperienced endoscopist.

12. If the patient has been intubated successfully, confirm that both lungs are properly ventilated. Avoid deep intubation since the endotracheal tube may extend into the right main stem bronchus, occluding the left main stem bronchus.

13. Tracheostomy without intubation is rarely indicated. It is reserved for the patient in whom existing pathology or trauma prohibits both assisted mask or mouth ventilation and intubation.

### Warning

1. *Don't* attempt intubation when mask or mouth-to-mouth ventilation may be successful.

2. *Don't* waste valuable time by repeat intubations without attempting to ventilate the patient by mask or mouth-to-mouth.

3. *Don't* laryngoscope the patient without having cleared his secretions prior to laryngoscopy.

4. *Don't* attempt intubation unless your equipment is appropriate.

### Postintubation

1. Endotracheal tubes can be kept in place for several days if there is no associated trauma during introduction.

2. In patients with observed or anticipated trauma, or if prolonged respiratory support is indicated, tracheostomy is preferable to avoid the superimposed trauma created by the indwelling tube.

3. If prolonged assisted ventilation by respirators is expected, nasotracheal intubation is preferable to orotracheal intubation, since it will decrease the trauma on the vocal cords imposed by the continuous motion of the endotracheal tube during the positive-pressure phase of the respirator.

4. After the orotracheal or nasotracheal tube has been secured and the patient has stabilized, confirm the exact position of the tracheal tube by x-ray.

5. Prior to the introduction of the endotracheal tube, under elective circumstances, the length of the largest catheter capable of passing through the lumen of the endotracheal tube should be marked. This catheter is not used for aspiration, but as a guide to the personnel responsible for endotracheal suctioning. By comparing the guide catheter and the catheter used for suctioning, a beginning obstruction at the end of the endotracheal tube interfering with the passage of the endotracheal suction catheter can easily be identified.

## TRACHEOSTOMY

### Basic Principles

A tracheostomy in an infant or a child is neither a minor procedure nor with rare exceptions, should it be performed on the ward or in the emergency room.

If possible, the tracheostomy should be done under general anesthesia in the operating room following endotracheal intubation. Complications following tracheostomies are frequently related to tracheostomies performed with faulty technique or improper site. The internal diameter of the trachea in children, especially in infants, is relatively narrow at the level of the first and second ring and begins to widen at the third and fourth ring just prior to the intrathoracic entrance. Therefore, the location least likely to create a postoperative stenosis is at the fourth tracheal ring.

## Technique

1. Endotracheal intubation with general anesthesia and controlled ventilation
2. Hyperextension of the neck
3. A transverse neck incision over the midline, approximately 1 to 2 cm. cephalad to the manubrium
4. Transection of the platysma, identification and separation of the strap muscles
5. The areolar tissue anterior to the trachea is dissected bluntly and retracted until the tracheal rings can be visualized.
6. The fourth tracheal ring is identified.
7. A vertical incision is made into the fourth ring, and a nonabsorbable suture is placed on each side of the incision encircling the transected cartilaginous ring.
8. Gentle traction on these sutures will elevate the trachea into the wound, and an appropriate tracheostomy tube, preferably a Silastic tube, is selected in accordance with the internal diameter of the trachea.
9. If the incision appears inadequate, the proximal or distal ring can be incised to enlarge the opening.
10. The tracheostomy tube, after removal of the endotracheal tube, should be inserted without undue pressure on the trachea.
11. If a metal tube is used, the length of the tube has to be measured to avoid a placement into one of the main stem bronchi. If the metal tracheostomy tube appears too long, the tube should only partially be inserted with a stent between the skin and the tube until a proper tube can be obtained.
12. After the tracheostomy tube has been inserted, dental rolls are tied to the end of each traction suture and left in place (Haller procedure). If the tracheostomy tube should inadvertently dislodge, the personnel in the recovery room or the ward can simply lift the trachea into the wound by a pull on the traction suture and reinsert the tracheostomy tube.
13. A closure of the skin around the tracheostomy tube is unnecessary.

## Warning

1. *Don't* perform a tracheostomy without an endotracheal tube unless intubation is impossible.
2. *Don't* try to force a tracheostomy into an inadequate tracheal incision.
3. *Don't* use a metal tracheostomy tube if the curvature or size is inappropriate.

### Tracheostomy Extubation

1. After the respiratory emergency leading to the tracheostomy has subsided, extubation should be performed gradually.
2. In children, gradual change to smaller tracheostomy tubes will permit extubation over the period of several days.
3. The partial or complete "blocking" of tracheostomy tubes, in particular in infants, is contraindicated since the plugged indwelling tracheostomy tube leads to considerable airway obstruction.
4. Removal of a tracheostomy tube in an infant can be facilitated by the immediate insertion of a small plastic catheter which can be used for temporary ventilation if the removal of the tracheostomy tube leads to respiratory distress.

## ABDOMINAL PARACENTESIS

### Basic Principles

Indications for abdominal paracentesis in children are:
1. Evaluation of intraperitoneal trauma in the unconscious patient with multiple trauma
2. Differentiation between abdominal wall and intraperitoneal trauma following blunt injury
3. Decision not to operate on a patient with penetrating abdominal trauma
4. To establish the diagnosis of primary peritonitis

### Technique

1. Paracentesis should only be performed in the right or left lower quadrant; the introduction of a paracentesis needle in the upper quadrants may result in damage to either liver, gallbladder or spleen.

2. The supine patient is slightly rotated with a padding behind his back, so that the lower quadrant to be aspirated is in a slightly inferior position.

3. Various types of needles can be used for the aspiration or lavage; 18-gauge spinal needles with an indwelling stylet or needles with an outer Teflon sheath are both suitable.

4. In the noncomatose patient, a small intradermal injection of procaine is followed by a small incision with a pointed blade to facilitate the slow introduction of the paracentesis needle.

5. Loss of resistance indicates that the needle has perforated the peritoneum. Either the stylet or the needle within the Teflon catheter is withdrawn, and the latter is slightly advanced.

6. A syringe is attached and slowly aspirated. The presence of blood which fails to clot is indicative of defibrinated intra-abdominal blood due to trauma. In patients with suspected primary peritonitis, the presence of purulent material confirms the proper location of the needle. The material is aspirated for Gram's stain and bacteriological culture.

7. In patients with suspected intraperitoneal trauma, where neither peritoneal fluid or blood can be obtained, 100 to 250 ml. of saline are slowly infused through the needle or catheter, followed by reaspiration. The return of sanguineous fluid indicates that intra-abdominal trauma with bleeding has occurred.

8. Peritoneal lavage is a much more sensitive test than paracentesis, so that even minute amounts of intraperitoneal bleeding, not necessarily requiring operative intervention, may yield a positive lavage. One ml. of blood dispersed in 500 ml. of saline will produce a bright-red color. The finding of a positive lavage in the absence of a positive paracentesis is a matter of interpretation, and in the absence of peritoneal signs the decision to perform exploratory celiotomy is an individual one.

## Warning

1. *Don't* perform paracentesis in either upper quadrant.

2. *Don't* interpret the aspiration of fecal material as evidence of peritonitis. If the suspicion exists that the paracentesis needle inadvertently entered a loop of intestine, a repeat paracentesis and/or lavage is indicated. The perforation of intestine with a paracentesis needle rarely leads to persistent leak or complication.

3. *Don't* regard a negative paracentesis as a negative diagnostic study.

## TUBE THORACOSTOMY

### Basic Principles

Tube thoracostomy is indicated in instances of pneumothorax, tension pneumothorax, pleural effusion and empyema, or following thoracic operations.

Effective drainage of intrapleural fluid is best accomplished through a dependent portion of the chest, and the most accessible dependent portion of the chest in a patient lying in bed is a low midaxillary position which does not interfere with the patient's resting position. Evacuation of air, with or without tension, can be accomplished through any intrapleural site, but in contrast to adults, where the anterior second or third intercostal space is frequently used, the introduction of a thoracostomy tube in infants and young children is difficult in this area due to the proximity of major vascular structures. Evacuation of both fluid and air in infants and children is therefore best accomplished through a midaxillary thoracostomy tube in the sixth or seventh interspace.

### Technique

1. The child is placed in a lateral position lying down, with the involved side elevated.

2. Procaine is injected over the site of entrance, and a small incision, ap-

proximately the size of the tube to be introduced, is carried through the skin into the subcutaneous space.

3. In infants and young children, a curved hemostat is slowly advanced between the intercostal muscles until the pleura is reached.

4. The pleura is perforated with the tip of the hemostat in a position parallel to the thoracic wall, to avoid injury to the underlying lung.

5. The exchange of air or the escape of fluid indicates an open communication between the intrapleural space and the skin.

6. The hemostat is intermittently opened and advanced, thereby enlarging the entrance into the intrapleural space.

7. A thorocostomy tube, approximately the size of the intercostal space, with two or three side holes, is then advanced into the chest and secured with two nonabsorbable skin sutures tightly closing the skin around the tube to prevent an air leak.

8. Depending on the underlying pathology, the tube is then attached to either a simple water seal drainage or negative suction.

9. An air-tight dressing, preferably Furacin or Vaseline dressing, is applied and covered by tape, additionally anchoring the thorocostomy tube.

## Post-thoracostomy Management

1. When the thoracostomy tube is attached to simple water seal drainage, its patency can be checked by observation of the continuous fluctuation of the water level during inspiration and expiration.

2. Lubrication of the tube with mineral oil will facilitate the "milking" required at frequent and regular intervals to preserve patency of the tubing.

3. In patients on negative suction, the fluctuation may not be apparent and patency is therefore more difficult to evaluate. Intermittent disconnection, unless an air leak exists, is therefore required

to allow the nursing personnel to monitor the tube's patency.

4. If a chest tube has become occluded and further drainage is indicated, irrigation of the chest tube is contraindicated since it may allow retrograde contamination. A nonfunctioning chest tube should be removed and replaced by a new tube.

### Warning

1. *Don't* insert a chest tube under unsterile conditions.

2. *Don't* use a chest tube larger than the intercostal space; it will be compressed and become nonfunctional.

3. *Don't* clamp chest tubes when the patient is transported to the operating room or other facilities if an active air leak exists.

4. *Don't* irrigate chest tubes to restore patency.

## THORACOCENTESIS

### Basic Principles

Thoracocentesis is indicated in patients with pneumothorax, tension pneumothorax or empyema or for diagnostic aspiration of a pleural effusion.

### Technique

1. The patient should be in an upright sitting position or slightly tilted toward the involved side.

2. A small intradermal wheal with procaine precedes the introduction of the larger bore needle.

3. Instead of entering the chest at a right angle, a slanted angle will allow the entrance of the needle through the pleura parallel to the thoracic wall, which probably is less likely to injure the lung, especially in nonsedated apprehensive children or crying infants. The bevel of the needle should face the thoracic wall, with the shorter side toward the lung.

4. The syringe is attached to the needle prior to the introduction of the needle, and the movement of the piston is tested prior

to aspiration. If the intent of the thoracocentesis is aspiration and evacuation of pleural effusion, a three-way stopcock is placed between the syringe and the needle to allow the change of syringes without introduction of air.

5. In patients with suspected tension pneumothorax, the upright position and tangential introduction of the needle are unnecessary. Since the patient's respiratory and cardiac status may be compromised, aspiration is best done in a supine position.

6. After the diagnosis of tension pneumothorax has been made, the piston is removed from the syringe to allow the continuous escape of air until a thorocostomy tube can be introduced.

# 37. PEDIATRIC TRAUMA

*Peter K. Kottmeier,* M.D.
*Gerald W. Shaftan,* M.D.
*Donald Klotz,* M.D.

## INTRODUCTION

Substantial differences are found in the causation, type, assessment and treatment of trauma between the pediatric and adult age-groups. *Since history, initial findings and symptomatology of the traumatized child on admission may either be non-diagnostic or misleading, the detection of a change in symptoms, findings or vital signs since the time of the first examination becomes the most important parameter in evaluating the injured child.*

### History

1. The history of a child's accident and the circumstances around it often can not be obtained because of the child's age or his fears and anxieties on admission to the hospital.
2. Not infrequently parents have either been unaware of the cause of the trauma or in certain cases, such as battered children, the information obtained may be misleading.
3. Additional history, therefore, may have to be obtained from playmates, relatives or social workers.

### Physical Findings

1. Fear and apprehension, caused by both the accident and the admission to the hospital, may either mask or exaggerate findings.
   A. An attempt to alleviate the child's apprehension is therefore mandatory in all cases.
   B. In patients without impending or actual shock, mild sedation may be required to allow a thorough physical examination.
2. The differences between major and minor trauma may be exceedingly subtle.
   A. With blunt abdominal trauma, the findings with a minor abdominal wall contusion may be indistinguishable from major intra-abdominal injury.
   B. For instance, the absence of bowel sounds, considered an ominous sign in adults with possible intra-abdominal injury, is frequently seen in children with either no abdominal injury, such as with neurologic injuries, or with minor abdominal injuries.

### Blood Loss

In children with considerable blood loss the signs and symptoms of hypovolemia, especially hypotension, may occur late.
1. The actual extent of the blood loss may not be apparent at the time of admission.
2. Findings such as thirst, irritability, lethargy or change of pallor may precede a systolic hypotension due to substantial blood loss by a considerable period of time and may become important criteria in the evaluation of an injured child.

### Other Diagnostic Considerations

1. A history of a minor trauma followed by signs and symptoms indicating major injury usually points toward a pre-existing lesion, an enlarged hydronephorotic kidney, a renal neoplasm or an enlarged spleen.
2. The pliable rib cage in the child is easily compressed, and therefore not as protective, and leads to injuries such as liver lacerations, which are not as common in adults.
3. Conversely, when underlying pathology can be suspected in adults with rib fractures, children whose pliable rib cage is less susceptible to fractures may mask injuries such as splenic lacerations or pulmonary contusions which may not be apparent for over 24 hours.

4. The causes of trauma in the pediatric age-group vary depending on the child's age, sex, sociological factors and environment (urban or rural).

A. Our most common cause for major injuries is related either to:

*(1)* Vehicular accidents, either as pedestrian or occupant

*(2)* Falls out of windows or off of fire escapes, which are especially common during summertime in urban ghetto areas

B. The physical abuse of children by adults crosses all sociological lines, but it is most common in the young infant and pre-school-age child in sociologically deprived groups.

*(1)* Certain effects of the underlying assault, such as rape, are apparent.

*(2)* In the majority of battered or abused children, the cause of a single injury may not be apparent, and only repeated injuries or the multiplicity and type of injury may arouse suspicion.

*(3)* To protect the child, even on the basis of only a minor suspicion the pertinent authority should be informed to investigate the circumstances of the child's injury.

C. The injuries sustained during play, such as a single blow or a fall on a handle bar, usually cause single organ injury (duodenal hematoma, rupture of the spleen). The correct history may therefore be helpful in the interpretation of the signs and symptoms at the time of admission.

## RESUSCITATION OF THE CHILD WITH MULTIPLE MAJOR INJURIES

### Airway

1. Maxillofacial and/or oropharyngeal trauma leading to airway obstruction should be ruled out by direct examination.

2. If airway obstruction exists, place an oropharyngeal plastic airway of proper size.

3. If this is inadequate:

A. Endotracheal or naso-tracheal intubation (page 613)

B. Tracheostomy (For the technique of tracheostomy, *see* page 614.)

C. If neither of these procedures can be performed safely, a large bore needle can be introduced into the cricopharyngeal membrane, with 100%-oxygen-assisted respiration until intubation or tracheostomy can be performed.

### Respiratory and/or Cardiac Arrest

1. *Assisted Respiration*

A. Unless obvious airway blockage exists, immediate mouth-to-mouth respiration, followed by the introduction of an oral airway and mask ventilation, will be sufficient to deliver adequate oxygen to the lungs. This is more likely to be successful than the attempt of endotracheal intubation by the unexperienced.

B. Excessive overinflation, particularly with sustained peak pressures exceeding 25 to 30 cm. of water, are dangerous in infants and young children and may lead to alveolar emphysema or spontaneous simple or tension pneumothorax.

C. Auscultation and visual observation of chest expansion combined with peripheral signs of restored oxygenation can be used as parameters for assisted ventilation.

2. *Assisted Circulation.* Closed cardiac massage, especially in small children, should be performed gently with a rate of approximately 80 to 100 massages per minute.

A. The pressure is applied to the midsternum and simultaneous palpation of peripheral pulses is done to check the adequacy of the cardiac resuscitation.

B. Unnecessary force may not only lead to other organ injury such as rupture of the liver or spleen but may traumatize the heart.

3. Assisted respiration cannot by synchronous with the cardiac massage because of the rapid cardiac massage rate.

4. *Medications*

A. Intravenous epinephrine, 0.05 mg./kg. of body weight/minute, or intracardiac epinephrine, 1:10,000 dilution, 2 to 4 ml.—if body weight is less than 4 kg., 2 ml.; if 4 to 18 kg., 3 ml.; if more than 18 kg., 4 ml.

B. Intravenous sodium bicarbonate, 3 mEq./kg. of body weight

C. Calcium gluconate or chloride, 100 mg./kg. of body weight, especially if sodium bicarbonate has been used

D. Isuprel if cardiac action is unstable after resuscitation or if repeated cardiac arrests have occurred

5. *Intravenous Fluids*

A. The restoration of an adequate blood volume, which may be substantially higher than the normal blood volume, is determined by central venous pressure.

B. In patients with a prolonged period of cardiac-respiratory arrest, or with recurrent periods, the combined respiratory and metabolic acidosis which is commonly found is treated by administration of isotonic solution of Ringer's lactate or isotonic sodium bicarbonate as the initial solution.

C. Continuous determination of $pO_2$, $pCO_2$ and pH is essential for the rational administration of intravenous fluids and medication.

D. The repeated administration of 7% sodium bicarbonate at 3 mEq. per kilogram of body weight may lead to rapid increase of the intravascular volume and pulmonary edema in patients whose arrest occurred in the presence of a normovolemia. This danger is particularly present in small infants.

## Respiratory Distress Caused by Thoracic Injuries

1. Oral airway with mouth-to-mouth or mask-assisted respiration

2. Endotracheal intubation followed by tracheostomy, if indicated

3. *Warning:* an emergency tracheostomy in a child is a major and difficult procedure and should be performed without prior intubation *only in cases of dire emergency* where intubation cannot be accomplished due to technical problems.

4. All patients with respiratory distress requiring assisted ventilation should have a nasogastric tube inserted to:

A. Prevent gastric distention

B. Prevent secondary aspiration

## Shock

1. With impending or actual shock, two intravenous catheters should be placed.

A. Upper extremity cannulation is preferable, especially since intra-abdominal bleeding may require cross-clamping of the vena cava. For that reason intravenous lines are always placed in the upper extremity unless a simultaneous extremity injury, such as displaced fractures or major lacerations can interfere with the function of the utilized vein.

B. Either catheter can be used for the initial administration of isotonic crystalloid solutions, either saline or Ringer's lactate.

C. After stabilization, one central catheter can be used to monitor the intracaval pressure as a reflection of the hemodynamic state.

2. After the catheters have been inserted, an immediate blood type and crossmatch is obtained. The administration of untyped blood (O negative blood) is rarely necessary and the initial administration of isotonic salt solutions may be preferable to the administration of blood alone.

3. Although an abnormally low systolic blood pressure is compatible with hypovolemia in children, the maintenance of a normal systolic pressure is by no means related to the restoration of a normal volume.

A. Tachycardia, especially in the conscious and alert child, may be an expression of his anxiety and fear rather than of his blood volume.

B. More reliable criteria for the

restoration of adequate perfusion are:

(1) The patient's clinical appearance

(2) Mental status

(3) Signs of peripheral perfusion

(4) Adequate urinary output determined by hourly measurement of urinary volume obtained through an indwelling catheter

## Neurologic Injury

1. The initial assessment of an unconscious patient without obvious signs of major cerebral injury (open skull fracture, brain laceration, escape of blood and spinal fluid through the ears or nose) may be difficult in the absence of localizing signs.

2. The coexistence of cerebral injury and shock should be interpreted as multi-system injury with hemorrhagic blood loss in either the intra-abdominal or intra-thoracic space, since even major cerebral injury rarely leads to hypotension.

3. All children admitted with signs or history of unconsciousness should be followed closely to detect alterations in their state of consciousness or the appearance of localizing signs indicating major cerebral injury.

4. Nasogastric decompression to avoid aspiration and endotracheal intubation for respiratory assistance are indicated in all patients who are unresponsive at the time of admission (*see* p. 609 and 613).

## Extremity Injury

1. In all patients with apparent extremity injuries or in unconscious patients the following parameters should be examined:

A. Deformities

B. Abnormal mobility

C. Signs of peripheral pulses and perfusion

D. Sensation in patients who are responsive

2. The application of tourniquets in patients with major extremity injury and massive bleeding is justifiable only during their transport to the hospital.

A. Once a patient has been admitted, hemostasis usually can be obtained with relative ease and tourniquet should be removed to avoid secondary vascular injury.

B. In the majority of children even major arterial injury to the extremities will not lead to exsanguination. Reduced blood volume and the arterial spasm that occurs at the site of injury usually will lead to thrombosis and limitation of major bleeding.

## ABDOMINAL TRAUMA

Trauma to the abdomen may result in injury to:

1. The abdominal wall

2. Intraperitoneal structures

3. Retroperitoneal structures

## Basic Principles

The technique of selective conservative approach to operation for both blunt and penetrating abdominal injuries is as true for children as for adults. Fortunately, penetrating injuries are less frequently encountered than blunt trauma. The following observations are applicable for either type of injury.

## Criteria for Diagnosis

1. *Clinical Criteria*

A. *History.* The history obtained from the patient, parents or observers should concern the following:

(1) Type of Injury

(2) Time of Injury

(3) Location

(4) Nature and type of first aid rendered

(5) Patient's condition at the time of injury

(6) Subsequent changes or treatment rendered during transportation or referral

B. *Physical Findings*

(1) Neurologic

(a) State of consciousness

(b) Alertness

(c) Irritability or lethargy

*(d)* Local neurologic signs: reaction and size of pupils; inspection of eardrums to rule out retrotympanic hemorrhage; escape of aural or nasal spinal fluid

*(2) Chest*

*(a)* Observation of inspiration for even excursion of both thoracic cavities

*(b)* Auscultation

*(c)* Presence of pain or tenderness spontaneously or on palpation or motion

*(3) Abdomen*

*(a)* External signs of abdominal injury such as abrasions, hematomas, tire marks or umbilical hematoma

*(b)* Localized, diffuse or referred pain or tenderness

*(c)* Evaluation of the abdomen for gaseous or fluid distention

*(d)* Presence of localized spasm, guarding or rigidity

*(e)* Auscultation of bowel sounds

*(f)* In unconscious patients with suspected multiple system injury or in patients with vague abdominal findings suggestive of intra-abdominal injury, abdominal paracentesis and lavage should be done (*see* p. 158).

*(4) Genitourinary System*

*(a)* Patient's ability to void

*(b)* Gross appearance of the urine

2. *Laboratory Tests*

A. Typing and crossmatching of blood

B. Hemoglobin, hematocrit, white blood cell count and differential count

C. Serum and/or urinary amylase

D. Complete urine examination

3. *X-ray Studies*

A. Posteroanterior view of the chest

B. Supine view of the abdomen

C. Upright or lateral decubitus study of the abdomen

D. With hematuria, even if minimal and only microscopic, intravenous pyelogram

## Management

1. Nothing by mouth

2. Intravenous catheter either percutaneously or by cutdown, depending on the severity of the injury

3. Nasogastric tube, multifenestrated plastic with radiopaque line

4. Do not routinely catheterize the patient. Use voided urine catch unless catheterization is specifically indicated.

5. Crossmatch and type blood. Do not routinely request blood delivery.

6. One-half isotonic saline solution to run at 1500 to 2000 ml./square meter of body surface/day

7. Repeated (1½ to 2 hours) observation of abdominal physical signs until unquestionably stable

8. Abdominal paracentesis and lavage with a Teflon needle if any doubt exists

## INJURY TO THE SPLEEN

### Basic Principles

The spleen is the most commonly injured solitary intra-abdominal organ. The cause of the injury can vary from a single blow to a massive injury leading to multisystem injury.

Blunt trauma may lead to intracapsular bleeding, partial or complete laceration, avulsion, infarction or delayed bleeding.

Although major bleeding can occur from a splenic laceration or splenic avulsion, the bleeding is usually self-limiting after a moderate degree of hypotension has occurred, and exsanguination is rare. Subcapsular hemorrhage with subsequent rupture can lead to delayed bleeding ranging from several days to several weeks later.

### Criteria for Diagnosis

1. *Clinical Criteria*

A. History of abdominal or lower chest trauma, which in a patient with pre-existing splenic enlargement can be trivial

B. Localized left upper quadrant or left lower chest pain

C. Occasionally referred pain to the shoulder

D. Rib fracture is rarely present in children; if present, it is *highly* suggestive of underlying splenic injury.

E. Bowel sounds diminished or absent

F. Signs of hypovolemia may be present, but frank shock is rare in isolated splenic injury.

2. *Laboratory Tests*

Leukocytosis and normal or lowered hemoglobin and hematocrit

3. *X-ray Studies*

A. Supine and upright films may demonstrate:

(1) An enlarged splenic shadow

(2) Shift of the stomach

(3) Left upper quadrant fullness or increased gastric serrations

B. Radioactive scan can show incomplete splenic uptake, indicating fracture or laceration.

C. Angiography, while diagnostic, is rarely indicated in children and has a risk of complications.

## Differential Diagnosis

1. Unrelated rib fractures
2. Abdominal wall contusion
3. Retroperitoneal hemorrhage

Associated Injuries

While splenic injury is usually solitary, in multiorgan trauma, injuries to the pancreas, liver, kidney and lung are most frequently seen.

## Management

Operative Procedure

1. In young children with an anticipated isolated splenic injury, a left upper transverse incision provides the best exposure. If an associated pancreatic or hepatic injury has occurred, extension across the midline will provide adequate exposure.

2. In older children with a longer abdominal trunk, or with suspected multiple injury, a vertical midline incision is preferable.

3. After the peritoneal cavity has been opened and the splenic injury has been identified, control of the splenic pedicle should be achieved even if active bleeding is not encountered.

4. With splenic avulsion or diffuse hemorrhage surrounding the splenic pedicle, control of the splenic artery is best accomplished by opening the lesser sac and applying finger compression to the splenic artery running along the upper posterior third of the pancreas, followed by suture ligation of the visualized transected vessel.

5. If there is no evidence of major continuous bleeding, the spleen is mobilized by transecting the colonic, lienal and diaphragmatic attachments.

6. After complete mobilization, the spleen can be brought into the abdominal wound.

7. The splenic pedicle is identified and the artery and vein are ligated individually, followed by transection and ligation of the short gastric vessels.

8. Complete mobilization of the spleen not only allows thorough inspection of the pancreatic tail for an associated injury, but also prevents inadvertent operative trauma to this structure.

9. Complete hemostasis can usually be accomplished with ease and a drainage of the splenic bed is not indicated in children unless associated pancreatic trauma has been found.

### Postoperative Complications

1. Pancreatitis
2. Subphrenic cellulitis or abscess formation
3. In infants and young children with pre-existing splenic pathology, a risk of postoperative sepsis has been demonstrated. In patients without pre-existing pathology, statistical evidence of an increased susceptibility to septicemia is lacking.

## INJURY TO THE LIVER

### Definition

Injury to the liver is caused by direct or

indirect trauma to the liver, resulting in:
1. Small superficial liver laceration
2. Major transection of the hepatic parenchyma
3. Diffuse fracture of the liver parenchyma
4. Liver injury with associated caval or hepatic venous injury

## Basic Principles

Minor injury due to trauma may result in a superficial tear with minimal and self-limiting bleeding. Occasionally simple tears are associated with deep parenchymal infarction, leading to necrosis, biliary leak, subdiaphragmatic abscess or hematobilia. In patients with significant parenchymal damage the initial bleeding episode may be mild but subsequent erosion of major vessels can lead to delayed massive hemorrhage, intraperitoneally or within the biliary tract.

## Criteria for Diagnosis

1. *Clinical Criteria*
   *History*
   A. Minor hepatic injuries can result from direct blows.
   B. Major hepatic injuries are usually caused by extensive direct or diffuse injuries, often leading to multiple system injury.
2. *Laboratory Tests*
   Leukocytosis and normal or lowered hemoglobin and hematocrit
3. *X-ray Studies*
   A. Supine and upright films of the abdomen are usually nondiagnostic for hepatic injury but may show signs of free peritoneal fluid or peritonitis with adynamic ileus.
   B. Pleural effusion can occur in unsuspected and untreated hepatic lacerations.
   C. Traumatic diaphragmatic hernia on the right side caused by abdominal compression may be associated with hepatic injury.
   D. In patients without evidence of major intra-abdominal bleeding,

angiography or radioactive scan can demonstrate lacerations or areas of parenchymal necrosis.

## Differential Diagnosis

1. Renal or retroperitoneal injury
2. Traumatic peritonitis due to other causes

## Associated Injuries

Although multiple organ injuries are common with major hepatic injury, in children the involvement of the extrahepatic biliary tree is less common than in adults.

## Management

1. In children, laparotomy in suspected liver injury is best performed through a midline or a right paramedian incision. Either can be extended into a right thoraco-abdominal incision if necessary.
2. Specific technique of management is discussed elsewhere (p. 167).
3. Even if a major hepatic resection is performed in children, common duct or gallbladder cannulation does not appear to be necessary as long as the perihepatic area is drained sufficiently through indwelling sump drains.

## Postoperative Complications

1. Recurrent bleeding
2. Subdiaphragmatic or hepatic abscesses
3. Septicemia
4. Hematobilia
5. Biliary fistula

## INJURY TO THE PANCREAS

## Classification

Blunt trauma to the pancreas results in:
1. Hemorrhagic pancreatitis
2. Contusion of the pancreas
3. Partial or complete laceration of the pancreas

## Basic Principles

The position of the pancreas overlying the vertebrae renders it vulnerable to direct forces applied over the abdominal midline. In patients with splenic injuries, the force of trauma or operative injury is usually limited to the tail of the pancreas. Transection usually occurs at the midline. The head of the pancreas is rarely involved in pancreatic injury. The most commonly injured organs in association with pancreatic injury are the spleen and duodenum.

## Criteria for Diagnosis

1. *Clinical Criteria*
A. History of a single blow or single-object injury against the midabdomen (e.g., Bicycle handle bar)
B. *Physical Findings*
(1) Usually not specific
(2) Often overshadowed by signs and symptoms related to injuries to other organs such as splenic rupture or duodenal trauma
C. With isolated pancreatic injury, the onset of peritonitis, retroperitoneal edema and pain radiating to the back are suggestive of pancreatic injury.
D. Accumulation of fluid in the lesser sac or pseudocyst formation is a probable sign of missed injury.
2. *Laboratory Tests*
Elevated serum and urinary amylase; especially serial changes are diagnostic.
3. *X-ray Studies*
A. X-ray findings in patients with acute pancreatic injury are nondiagnostic although compatible with acute peritonitis.
B. In patients with pancreatic abscess or pseudocyst formation, retrogastric accumulations within the lesser sac pushing the stomach anteriorly are suggestive and require further study.

## Differential Diagnosis

1. Peritonitis
2. Intestinal perforation

## Management

### Acute Injury

1. In children, major injury to the tail or midportion of the pancreas with partial or complete transection usually requires a distal resection with ligation of the pancreatic duct and subsequent drainage.
2. With pancreatic contusion, especially of the pancreatic tail in association with splenic injury, only substantial drainage of the injured pancreas is indicated.

### Pancreatic Pseudocyst

1. In children with pancreatic pseudocysts without the formation of a firm, fibrous capsule, tube drainage through the abdominal wall constitutes the procedure of choice.
2. Children, in contrast to adults, even with well-formed and chronic pseudocysts appear to do favorably with drainage procedures, so that cyst enterostomy is less often indicated in children than in adults.

## Postoperative Complications

1. Peritonitis
2. Pancreatic abscess formation
3. Subdiaphragmatic abscess
4. Pseudocyst formation

## INTESTINAL TRAUMA

### Definition

Intestinal trauma is direct or indirect injury resulting in intestinal or mesenteric laceration or hematoma formation.

### Basic Principles

Most intestinal perforations and hematomas occur in the duodenum or jejunum overlying the vertebrae and are therefore caused by direct injury compressing the intestine against the unyielding bony background. The force of the injury may be minor, and not infrequently symptoms occur slowly.

### Criteria for Diagnosis

1. *Clinical Criteria*
A. History of abdominal trauma
B. Diffuse abdominal pain with rebound tenderness, followed by abdominal guarding and rigidity and intra-

abdominal distention with hypoactive or absent bowel sounds

    2. *Laboratory Tests*

      A. Leukocytosis

      B. Abdominal paracentesis may yield bloody fluid with white cells or intestinal contents. The presence of bile-colored fluid indicates a high intestinal perforation.

    3. *X-ray Studies*

      A. With minor intestinal perforations, subdiaphragmatic air may be apparent on the upright films.

      B. In the majority of patients, however, radiologic findings are limited to a pattern of peritonitis with free fluid and separation of intestinal loops.

## Differential Diagnosis

    1. Retroperitoneal hemorrhage

    2. Peritonitis

    3. Pancreatitis

## Management

### Intestinal Perforation

    1. In blunt trauma, the perforation is usually located in the jejunum on the antimesenteric border.

    2. If small, it can be closed with a two-layer repair, an inner chromic catgut and an outer interrupted atraumatic silk layer.

    3. If the perforation is extensive, or if adjacent necrosis or hematoma have occurred, resection with an end-to-end anastomosis is indicated.

### Duodenal Injury

    1. In children with a suspected duodenal injury (retroperitoneal hematoma extending to the midline, hemorrhage within the right mesocolon, injury to the midportion of the pancreas), mobilization of the right colon and complete inspection of the duodenum are indicated

    2. In duodenal hematoma without perforation, drainage of the hematoma suffices

    3. With minor perforations, a two-layer closure may be adequate

    4. With extensive perforations and/or necrosis of the duodenum, a repair of the involved side with a duodenojejunostomy cephalad to the area of trauma may be required to eliminate the possibility of duodenal obstruction and/or perforation.

## Postoperative Complications

    1. Postoperative leak

    2. Peritonitis

    3. Stricture formation

# RETROPERITONEAL HEMORRHAGE

## Definition

Retroperitoneal hemorrhage is hemorrhage in the extraperitoneal space due to bleeding from:

    1. Major kidney injury

    2. Pelvic fracture

    3. Vertebral collaterals or lumbar vessels

## Basic Principles

The source and the extent of the retroperitoneal hemorrhage can vary widely. Bleeding from renal injury, with the exception of avulsion, is usually self-limiting, and tamponade is thought to occur unless Gerota's fascia is torn or incised. With diffuse retroperitoneal hemorrhage, the bleeding may be self-limiting if no major vessels are involved, but the amount of blood sequestered in the retroperitoneal space may be tremendous, exceeding the child's own blood volume. Major vessel injury in blunt abdominal trauma is usually limited to major venous structures. Blunt transection of major arterial vessels is rare even with extensive pelvic crush injuries, whereas penetrating wounds can injure any structure.

## Criteria for Diagnosis

    1. *Clinical Criteria*

      A. History of a major crush or blow to the abdominal region

      B. *Physical Findings*

        *(1)* Signs of external injury

        *(2)* Flank, inguinal and suprapubic

swelling and/or ecchymosis occasionally extending into the femoral triangle

*(3)* Secondary abdominal signs, predominantly ileus and abdominal distention with absent bowel sounds and abdominal tenderness, may develop

*(4)* In the unconscious or relaxed child, the retroperitoneal swelling may be felt on abdominal examination, mimicking an intra-abdominal mass

*(5)* The signs of hypovolemia and/or shock vary greatly, depending on the amount of retroperitoneal hemorrhage. In patients with major vascular injury, shock may be the primary symptom and indistinguishable from major intraperitoneal bleeding

*(6)* Other findings may be related to apparent renal or urinary tract injury

2. *Laboratory Tests*

A. Hematuria is present in most patients with associated renal or bladder injury.

B. Decrease in hemoglobin and hematocrit in accordance with the blood loss

3. *X-ray Studies*

A. Loss of the psoas shadow, secondary ileus and flank distention with loss of the properitoneal fat line.

B. Intravenous pyelogram is indicated in all patients with suspected retroperitoneal hemorrhage even in the absence of hematuria. In patients with retroperitoneal hemorrhage, a non-visualized kidney on the IVP warrants an angiographic study or renal scan to rule out renal avulsion or arterial injury.

C. Angiography, both venous and arterial, may give information as to the site of hemorrhage.

## Differential Diagnosis

Intraperitoneal hemorrhage

## Management

1. Treatment is primarily conservative, although due to the small reserve blood volume in the child exploration may be required for control of bleeding

2. Preoperative evaluation through venograms and arteriograms may significantly aid in the operative procedure

3. Bleeding from a pelvic crush is usually caused by numerous collaterals, bony fragments or major venous structures. Arteries are rarely involved. If after the major venous structures have been dissected bleeding continues from bony fragments or collaterals, ligation of the internal iliac arteries may safely control it

## Complications

1. Exsanguination

2. Retroperitoneal infection and abscess formation, unrecognized

3. Renal, ureteral, bladder or urethral injury

# TRAUMA TO THE GENITOURINARY SYSTEM
## KIDNEY INJURY

## Classification

1. Contusion
2. Intrarenal extravasation
3. Laceration (shattered kidney)
4. Renal avulsion
5. Renal arterial or venous thrombosis

## Basic Principles

The most common result of blunt abdominal injury to the kidney is renal contusion with temporary hematuria. Intrarenal injuries such as laceration leading to intrarenal extravasation usually heal without operative intervention. Even mild extrarenal extravasation is unlikely to lead to major complications. The remarkable ability of the kidney to recover from injuries and the rarity of post-traumatic complications such as renal hypertension have led to an increasingly conservative approach to the treatment of renal injuries, especially in children. Only injuries leading to either marked or continued hemorrhage, marked and continuous urinary extravasation or interference with the blood supply represent entities necessitating early operative intervention.

## Criteria for Diagnosis

1. *Clinical Criteria*

A. History of trauma varing from a minor flank or abdominal injury from a simple blow or fall with pre-existing renal pathology, to a violent injury causing multisystem damage.

B. *Physical Findings*

(1) Minor renal extravasation can produce peritoneal irritation or ileus with abdominal distention

(2) Renal arterial occlusion may lead to few symptoms other than flank pain, mild ileus and/or abdominal tenderness

(3) With apparent intra-abdominal injuries, the associated renal injury may be missed on physical examination and examination of the urine in abdominal trauma is therefore essential

2. *Laboratory Tests*

A. Over 90 per cent of patients with renal injuries will present with at least microscopic hematuria

B. Hematuria may be absent in patients with arterial occlusion or renal avulsion

3. *X-ray Studies*

A. In every patient with hematuria or suspected renal injury, an intravenous pyelogram is mandatory

B. In most children, the excretory urogram using the infusion technique (*See* p. 159) will readily demonstrate the type and extent of the renal injury

C. With nonvisualization of a traumatized kidney, either a renal angiogram or renal scan is indicated. If arterial occlusion such as caused by intimal transection has occurred, the kidney will not be visualized on either angiogram or scan and early exploration is indicated

## Differential Diagnosis

1. Intraperitoneal injury
2. Retroperitoneal injury not related to the kidney
3. Lower urinary tract injury

## Management

### Renal Contusion

1. Conservative treatment with bed rest
2. Frequent and regular determinations of the extent of hematuria and repeat IVP's to check renal function

### Minor Renal Lacerations with Internal Bleeding or Extrarenal Extravasation

1. Careful observation of the patient's clinical status. Check for evidence of retroperitoneal infection, perinephric abscess, continuing hematuria and degree of secondary adynamic ileus

2. *Indications for Operation*

A. Evidence of a shattered kidney on the intravenous pyelogram or angiogram

B. Continued hemorrhage while on bed rest

3. Nephrectomy, regardless of the underlying condition, is contraindicated unless proof has been obtained that the contra-lateral kidney is functioning. Even if a preoperative intravenous pyelogram could not be obtained, it can be performed on the operating table

### Renal Avulsion

Retroperitoneal hemorrhage and nonvisualization on the intravenous pyelogram or angiogram require immediate operative exploration

### Arterial Occlusion

Nonvisualization on the intravenous pyelogram, angiogram or scan demands immediate operative repair

## Complications

1. Hemorrhage
2. Perinephric abscess
3. Renal hypertension

## BLADDER DISRUPTION

## Classification

1. Intraperitoneal
2. Extraperitoneal

## Basic Principles

### Extraperitoneal Bladder Rupture

Extraperitoneal rupture is invariably due to blunt trauma resulting in pelvic injury and usually accompanied by apparent pelvic fractures. The extraperitoneal extravasation of urine leads to perivesicular swelling, which may be prominent either in the pubic, femoral or perineal area, with periprostatic swelling in males. The ability to void is usually maintained with extraperitoneal rupture, unless complete transection of the bladder neck has occurred. If urine is obtained, microscopic or gross hematuria is present.

### Intraperitoneal Bladder Rupture

Intra-abdominal rupture of the bladder usually follows a compression injury to the abdomen in contrast to extraperitoneal bladder rupture. With intraperitoneal rupture of the bladder, free fluid is evident clinically, by tap and on prone and supine x-rays.

## Criteria for Diagnosis

*See* pages 175 and 423.

## Management

*See* pages 175 and 424.

## URETHRAL TEAR

### Definition

A urethral tear is transection of the membranous portion of the urethra.

### Basic Principles

Blunt trauma leading to a transection of the urethra is violent in nature and often accompanied by pelvic fracture. Early physical findings may consist only of a few blood drops in the urethra; hematuria is absent in view of the inability to void. The appearance of urethral blood without voiding is diagnostic of urethral transection. Perivesicular swelling, often difficult to distinguish from hemorrhage, results, with urinary extravasation in the peripubic area. In contrast to bladder urine, which is usually sterile, urethral urine often contains bacteria and can therefore set up a more acute and marked inflammatory response.

## Criteria for Diagnosis

*See* page 426.

## Management

*See* page 426.

## VAGINAL INJURY

### Classification

1. Accidental injury (perineal injury)
2. Self-induced injuries (foreign body)
3. Forced rape (medical, not considering legal terminology)
4. Continuous abuse by adults

### Basic Principles

In young girls with vaginal trauma, regardless of the underlying etiology but especially if rape is suspected, vaginal examination should be performed under heavy sedation to avoid the additional psychological trauma of a repeat vaginal manipulation in an already frightened child. In contrast to other situations, the physician if he is a male is not the one who should, or is likely to, obtain a precise history from the patient. The child for obvious reasons is more likely to verbalize her experience to a female member of the staff. In all cases of suspected rape, acute or chronic, vaginal smears to demonstrate sperm are indicated with a notification of the pertinent authorities.

Those patients suspected of having retained foreign bodies should have a gentle but thorough rectal examination, which will usually reveal the presence of the foreign body. Its absence can be ruled out by vaginoscopy which can be done according to the patient's age and the size of the vaginal introitus with a nasal speculum, a small pediatric proctoscope or an esophagoscope. If vaginoscopy is indicated, it is usually best performed under light anesthesia.

## Criteria for Diagnosis

1. *Clinical Criteria*

   A. *Accidental Injury*

   *(1)* History of an injury sustained during an accident such as on a picket fence, a sled or a bicycle

   *(2)* Straddle injuries usually involve the vagina, perineum and/or rectum, so that inspection alone should determine the likelihood of injury.

   *(3)* Vaginoscopy is diagnostic (*see* above).

   B. *Self-induced injury* usually presents with minor symptoms:

   *(1)* Vaginal discharge or minor bleeding

   *(2)* Associated with retained small foreign bodies, especially in younger children

   C. *Forced Rape*

   *(1)* In contrast to accidental injury to the vagina, which usually includes the perineum, in forced rapes the primary injury is to the vaginal introitus, vaginal wall and occasionally the cervix.

   *(2)* A perineal injury is rare unless a tear of the introitus and vagina is coexistent.

   D. *Continuous Abuse by Adults.* Continuous intercourse of adults with children (as young as two years of age) may lead to the formation of a patulous adult vagina, with minor symptoms such as discharge and minor bleeding. In children with evidence of continuous sexual abuse, ascending infection may lead to salpingitis or tubo-ovarian abscess.

2. *X-ray Studies*

   X-rays of the pelvis are indicated in all cases where the presence of vaginal foreign bodies is suspected.

## Management

### Accidental Injury

1. The vaginal or perineal repair, unless involving the rectum, is technically simple and can usually be performed with muscular and serosal interrupted chromic catgut sutures.

2. In patients seen more than 24 hours after the injury, subcutaneous drainage may be indicated.

3. In patients with involvement of the rectum, a simultaneous repair of the external sphincter should be performed.

### Foreign Bodies

1. Removal by vaginoscopy

2. Following removal, vaginal smear and bacterial culture with antibiotic therapy as indicated

### Rape or Continuous Sexual Abuse

While the repair of the anatomical defect rarely presents a problem, emphasis should be placed on psychological and sociological therapy and assistance. A thorough examination of the child's home surroundings should be done since in the majority of cases the males responsible for the rape are either family members or friends of the family.

## RECTAL INJURIES

### Classification

1. Accidental, usually involving the perineum

2. Self-induced injury due to foreign bodies

3. Continuous abuse by adults

### Basic Principles

Accidental injuries of the rectum due to accidents usually involve parts of the perineum and are therefore readily identifiable. In patients with rectal foreign bodies, mild rectal bleeding may occur; perforation rarely occurs.

### Criteria for Diagnosis

1. *Clinical Criteria*

   A. History of an accident producing perineal trauma, similar to that seen in vaginal trauma

   *(1)* Accident on a picket fence

   *(2)* Straddle injuries

   *(3)* Accident on a sled

   B. Rectal examination may demonstrate the injury.

C. Rectal bleeding necessitates proctoscopy to rule out injury.

D. With rare exceptions, rectal foreign bodies in childhood consist of broken retained thermometers.

E. Patulous anal sphincter with perianal tears suggests chronic anal intercourse.

2. *X-ray Studies*

X-rays are indicated in patients with a history of a rectal foreign body to determine the level and position of the foreign body and whether it is intra- or extraluminal.

## Management

### Accidental Rectal Injury

1. For rectal injuries accompanied by perineal lacerations, a repair of the external sphincter should be attempted.

2. Colostomy is rarely indicated even with extensive rectal trauma.

3. If primary sphincter repair was not performed or has failed, resulting in fecal incontinence, a secondary repair should be performed after an interval of at least three months. At that time the severed and scared ends of the rectal sphincter are re-anastomosed. *Do not* attempt to excise the fibrotic ends and approximate the debrided muscular ends; *this usually fails.* In patients in whom a repair of the sphincter is not possible due to extensive previous injury, the use of a Thiersch procedure or the revision of the levator sling may improve the patient's condition.

### Foreign Bodies

In children, rectal foreign bodies should be removed under general anesthesia unless the foreign body is at the sphincter level. The removal can usually be accomplished with ease in patients over the age of six months through an adult-size proctoscope.

### Acute or Chronic Sexual Abuse

Acute or chronic sexual abuse requires psychological and sociological management.

### Complications

1. Perianal or rectal abscesses
2. Fecal incontinence with destruction of the external sphincter

## THORACIC TRAUMA

### Basic Principles

The pathophysiology, etiology and clinical findings in children with penetrating wounds of the chest are similar to those in adults, although their occurrence is less frequent. The results of blunt injury of the chest in children are also similar with the exception that intrathoracic injury (pulmonary contusion) without rib fractures is more likely to occur in children than in adults.

### PULMONARY CONTUSION

### Definition

Pulmonary contusion is pulmonary parenchymal hemorrhage following blunt chest trauma.

### Basic Principles

Contusion of the pulmonary parenchyma leads to a diffuse hemorrhage with arteriovenous shunting followed by infection. Although pulmonary contusion occurs not infrequently in children with major accidents, it is rarely suspected at the time of admission since rib fractures are commonly absent and x-ray findings do not appear until approximately 24 hours after the pulmonary contusion has occurred.

### Criteria for Diagnosis

1. *Clinical Criteria*

A. The first presenting clinical signs consist of diminished breath sounds on the involved side, occasionally accompanied by a slowly developing pleural effusion.

B. Hemoptysis rarely occurs.

C. With diffuse or extensive pulmonary contusion, respiratory difficulties leading to respiratory acidosis may occur before x-ray findings are diagnostic.

2. *Laboratory Tests*

A. Laboratory studies are rarely obtained unless an extensive pulmonary contusion is suspected clinically.

B. In view of the underlying pathophysiology (i.e., arteriovenous shunting), a differential in alveolar-arterial $O_2$ concentration precedes x-ray evidence.

C. If the alveolar-arterial oxygen difference cannot be determined, the results of $pO_2$ and pH may be used to estimate the increase or decrease of arteriovenous shunting.

3. *X-ray Studies*

A. Pulmonary contusion, which usually becomes apparent within 24 to 48 hours after the trauma has occurred, usually presents with a diffuse pulmonary infiltrate which does not follow the usual anatomical boundaries seen in pneumonia.

B. Pleural effusion, usually mild, may be present, with obliteration of the costophrenic angle or outlining the interlobar fissures.

## Differential Diagnosis

1. Pulmonary hematoma (localized and well defined)
2. Pneumonia
3. Atelectasis

## Management

1. Expectant conservative therapy

A. Liquefaction and aspiration of retained secretions

B. Antibiotic coverage

2. Positive-pressure breathing or assisted ventilation for correction of respiratory acidosis

## Complications

1. Arteriovenous shunting
2. Pulmonary infection

## HEMOPNEUMOTHORAX

*See* pages 134, 515 and 616.

## ESOPHAGEAL BURNS

### Definition

Esophageal burn is the injury that occurs following the oral intake of caustic material.

### Basic Principles

In children, burns of the esophagus caused by the inadvertent swallowing of lye or acid are almost exclusively limited at the present time to the intake of lye available in most households. This ingestion leads to a burn of the esophagus, which may involve both mucosa and muscularis. The formation of eschar, adhesions and fibrosis can lead to a stricture of the esophagus, usually involving long segments in contrast to congenital esophageal stenosis.

### Criteria for Diagnosis

*Clinical Criteria*

1. A history of choking, chest pain, inability to swallow and salivation after the accidental intake of lye

2. Physical findings may include:

A. Dehydration

B. Vascular collapse

C. Acute dehydration

D. Oropharyngeal burns

3. In patients seen several days or weeks after the ingestion of lye, the symptoms may be solely related to dysphagia.

4. Esophagoscopy should be performed within 24 hours following the ingestion of lye to confirm the diagnosis and to estimate the extent of the damage.

## Differential Diagnosis

1. Acid ingestion (rare), often associated with gastric corrosion
2. Congenital intrinsic or extrinsic esophageal obstruction

### Management

General Management

Antidotes are not used since the effect of the burn is immediate and irreversible.

Treatment of Systemic Changes

1. Rehydration

2. Broad-spectrum antibiotic coverage

3. Although there is no general agreement on the use of early esophagoscopy or steroids, we use the following regimen:

A. Esophagoscopy within 24 hours under general anesthesia to confirm the diagnosis and to estimate the degree of burn

B. Steroid treatment for one week

4. Esophageal dilation as indicated

5. Esophageal barium swallow to determine stricture formation

6. In patients with stricture development either after an unsuccessful primary treatment or when first seen with already existing stenosis:

A. Gastrotomy

B. Esophageal dilation with Tucker dilators attached to a No. 5 nasogastric silk string

7. Patients with strictures not responding to repeat dilation and with marked dysphagia require retrosternal colonic interposition.

## Complications

1. Esophageal perforation
2. Stricture formation
3. Oropharyngeal complications
4. Long-term complications of increased incidence of esophageal squamous cell carcinoma

## EXTREMITY TRAUMA

### Basic Principles

1. The management of injuries of the soft tissue and osseous portions of the extremity is essentially the same in children as in adults. Major differences in diagnosis and management, however, concern:

A. The inability of children to give accurate histories so that diagnosis is primarily dependent upon the physical and x-ray findings

B. The difference in potential for growth and remodeling that exists both in the bones and in the nonosseous structures

2. Extremity injuries in children will frequently yield good results despite apparently inadequate management, thus confirming the aphorism that "God is good to fools and surgeons that treat children's injuries." Nevertheless, proper reapproximation of nerve, blood vessel and musculotendinous structures as well as proper axial, rotary and angular realignment of bone will yield results superior to those cases in which a surgeon depends upon "Mother Nature" and "Father Time" to correct his inadequacies.

## INTEGUMENT INJURY

### Basic Principles

Open extremity trauma in children, unlike the wartime management of such injuries in adults, is best treated, following meticulous debridement, by closure. Skin closure is especially important when underlying artery, nerve, tendon or bone has been injured and repaired. Split-skin grafting, the movement of flaps with grafting of the resultant defect, or coverage of exposed areas with distant pedicles or burying the denuded extremity in skin pockets, all are devices for achieving wound closure. Only in the instance of heavily contaminated or infected wounds is autogenous closure not attempted, and in this instance heterogenous (in our institution, bovine) grafts are used as a temporary biological dressing for the first 2 to 5 days until closure can safely be achieved with graft and/or flaps. The sooner the wound is repaired, the lower will be the incidence of infection, edema, extremity stiffness and subsequent atrophy.

Conversely, evidently crushed or devitalized skin should be excised and replaced with viable tissue. In the instance of a clean, sharp elevation of a flap, the flap may be completely severed, defatted and replaced in its original location as a free full-thickness graft.

Although the instance of "take" of amputated fingertips brought in by anxious parents is low, they should be replaced when possible with the caution that they might subsequently have to be removed.

The failure to initially replant the fingertip is rarely appreciated by the parents, although they readily consent to subsequent elective excision and replacement of an obviously gangrenous replant. Likewise, to the astonishment of the surgeon, some of these autografts will survive to the eternal gratitude of a family for the surgical "miracle."

Aside from this consideration, however, radical excision of questionable skin and cutaneous tissue, especially in children, except on the palms or soles of the feet, produces fewer postinjury headaches for the surgeon.

### Criteria for Diagnosis

1. Lacerations and excised wounds are obvious.

2. Less obvious is the extent of damage to avulsed or crushed skin. In general, if the flap avulsion contains no subcutaneous tissue, it must be considered a nonviable flap and should be detached. Retrograde flaps and flaps with inadequate bases also should be suspect of subsequent vascular compromise.

3. Ragged, shredded or evidently crushed skin is obvious and should be debrided. Beware of the skin that contains a characteristic crush pattern such as of a tire tread. Even the normal-appearing skin probably will not survive.

### Management

1. Debridement, the exact excision of all the dirty and devitalized tissue, but only of the dirty and devitalized tissue, is usually carried out under the constant flow of room-temperature saline. This will effectively carry away small bits of tissue as they are trimmed.

2. Debridement of larger wounds requires more extensive anesthesia, and any wound necessitating the lifting of flaps, excision of flaps or skin grafting should be debrided under regional or general anesthesia.

3. Wound edges should be approximated, closing areas of potential dead space or placing a small perforated catheter for suction under a flap that has been raised.

4. Plain catgut or 3-0 or 4-0 Dexon sutures may be used for the subcutaneous tissue, and 4-0, 5-0 or 6-0 nylon or polypropylene sutures may be used for the skin. Interrupted sutures are preferable for most lacerations because of their irregular pattern. Continuous sutures may be used for a straight incised wound and are preferable in children because of the rapidity of placement and the ease of removal.

5. If wound closure is tight (heavier suture than 4-0 is required to prevent breakage or slippage of the knots), relaxing incisions must be done to permit primary wound healing.

6. Although primary skin grafting of these relaxing incisions is not mandatory, it assists in providing for an early closed wound.

## ARTERIAL INJURY

### Basic Principles

Direct arterial injuries are evident in most instances either by the presence of pulsatile blood flowing from the wound or by massive blood loss following an injury disrupting skin and vascular continuity. Distal ischemia is difficult to evaluate in infants because systemic hypotension often will produce coldness, pallor and absent pulsation which can confuse the diagnosis. The management of arterial injuries is discussed elsewhere (*See* Chap. 18).

Volkmann's ischemic paralysis, while not peculiar to children, is seen with greater frequency in the pediatric age-group following injury. This lesion is due to occlusion of a major arterial vessel, producing infarct of muscle, nerve and even bone and skin in its area of isolated supply. It is most commonly recognized following injuries to the distal humerus or humeral epiphysis in the child, but ischemic paralysis of the lower extremity is also occasionally encountered. Osseous injury is not a necessary prerequisite for this lesion.

## Criteria for Diagnosis

1. History of injury proximal to the area of a vessel and neurologic involvement frequently accompanied by localized swelling within a comparatively closed space

2. Ischemic pain distal to the injury is a common presenting finding.

3. Pulse (main channel flow) is often diminished or absent; paralysis, however, *can* occur without loss of pulse.

4. Hypesthesia or anesthesia is the most common consistent finding in the distal extremity.

5. Loss of motor function is a late and often irreversible sign.

6. Arteriography is rarely indicated in children for diagnosis.

## Management

1. Reduction of fractures, if present, is primary. Maintenance of reduction by external fixation usually will suffice, but if the fracture reduction is unstable, percutaneous or open fixation with Kirschner wires should be done.

2. If pulse, sensation and function don't return, immediate arterial exploration is carried out.

3. Incision down to the artery frequently will suffice as a decompressive fasciotomy to restore blood flow.

4. Vessel disruption is treated as in adults by resection and anastomosis.

5. Spasm often may be overcome by hydraulic dilatation after the technique of Mustard.

    A. Atraumatic clamps are placed proximal and distal to the area of spasm.

    B. Saline with 10 mcg. of heparin/ml. is injected with a hypodermic needle intraluminally to overdistend the vessel.

    C. Release of the distal and then of the proximal clamp should result in restored flow.

6. Spasm that does not respond to dilatation should be treated by resection and end-to-end anastomosis because of the possibility of intimal tear.

7. If vessel flow is restored, only the skin is closed. The extremity should be immobilized with a heavy plaster mold, with the elbow or knee in flexion and the wrist or ankle dorsiflexed.

8. Subsequent clinical evaluation of success should suffice—arteriography is mettlesome and dangerous.

## VENOUS INJURY

### Basic Principles

Venous extremity injuries in children are most expeditiously and adequately treated by complete division of the vein continuity and ligation of the proximal and distal ends. Care must be taken to search for small side branches which may have been injured along with the major vessel and to ligate these to prevent subsequent hematoma formation. Venous vascular repair only is indicated in the instance of replantation of an extremity.

## NERVE INJURY

### Basic Principles

Of all the injuries to structures in the extremity, lacerations of nerves are the most difficult to diagnose in the child. Even gross motor deficits will not be apparent because of the inability to reliably differentiate between that function which is lost through denervation and that which results from fear of pain. Sensory evaluation similarly is extremely misleading, with both generalized anesthesia or loss of isolated areas of sensory denervation present with or without nerve damage. Examination is time-consuming and often fruitless. When there is a flesh wound, it is better in general to explore the wound under adequate anesthesia if there is even a suggestion of nerve injury. In our experience, primary nerve repair in the child's extremity produces much more gratifying results than secondary reconstruction.

## Criteria for Diagnosis

1. Gross motor or sensory deficits distal to a wound
2. A wound in the vicinity of an anatomical nerve pathway, frequently accompanied by arterial injury
3. Visualization of a nerve end on preliminary wound exploration, generally the distal end. Although nerves themselves do not retract, they tend to follow divided tendons being pulled up as a wad of tissue after severance.
4. Remember that nerve injuries can be present even though gross motor function appears intact and sensation is apparently present.

## Management

1. Cleanly divided nerves require no debridement for suture.
2. Specific techniques of repair are discussed elsewhere (*See* Chap. 33). In nerve lacerations in children, the use of magnification facilitates accurate axonal reapproximation and permits the use of sutures in the range of 8-0 to 10-0. In the absence of a surgical microscope, a loupe or hood magnifier may be substituted.
3. Following repair, especially when the nerve has had to be mobilized to permit approximation, immobilization of the extremity should be done with circular plaster, padding the areas of flexion creases with soft fluff dressing. This is continued for 3 weeks, after which time it either may be removed or replaced with progressive extension casts.
4. EMG's are painful and add little information in children to that which may be obtained clinically in the follow-up.

## MUSCLE AND TENDON INJURIES

### Basic Principles

Injuries to the motor unit of the extremities, while frequently difficult to diagnose without the active cooperation of the patient, can be evaluated by squeezing the involved muscle groups to cause passive distal flexion or extension. Repair of tendons in children should be more complete than the repair of similar injuries in adults. For example, in lacerations of the wrist, the wrist flexors and the deep and superficial tendons of the fingers all may be repaired with the expectation that they will all function subsequently as individual units and not as a single mass scar. Primary repair of tendons in children with clean lacerations in "no man's land" is feasible with the anticipation of good subsequent function. There is little excuse for deferring musculotendinous repairs in the child until a later date, except in the instance of gross infection or massive crush. The more adequate the repair initially, the more rapid and simple will be the subsequent return of function.

### Criteria for Diagnosis

1. Lacerations which are deep to the dermis and even remotely could have injured a musculotendinous structure
2. Abnormal position of the distal extremity due to unopposed antagonistic function in muscle groups (e.g., extension of a finger while the remaining fingers are in a semi-flexed position, indicative of flexor tendon injury)
3. Inability to actively move the involved distal extremity or portion thereof
4. Inability to produce passive motion of the extremity when the muscles terminating in the involved tendons are passively squeezed between the thumb and forefinger
5. Visualization of severed tendons on preliminary wound inspection

### Management

1. Under general anesthesia following satisfactory sterile preparation, draping and wound debridement, a complete assessment of the injured and uninjured structures must be carried out. This is especially true in lacerations in the wrist, in which all 17 structures on the volar aspect should be identified.

2. The proximal and distal ends of the injured structures should be tagged as they are isolated with a fine atraumatic suture.

3. If time permits, all divided structures should be repaired. If the general condition of the patient precludes this, the order of importance of repair is arteries, nerves, tendons and muscular injuries.

4. In children, tendon repair is best accomplished using 5-0 or 6-0 Tevdek placed as a far-near, near-far suture in a box-type fashion. The use of 4-0 or 5-0 monofilament nylon sutures appears to offer no advantage in the child and it is more difficult to tie securely. We have no experience with the use of polypropylene sutures at this time. The Bunnell-type suture, while providing greater tendon-holding power, is rarely justified in initial tendon repair and is reserved by us for secondary repairs in which considerable tension will be exerted on the suture line.

5. Lacerations of the muscle or the musculotendinous junction are simply repaired with interrupted sutures of 4-0 or 5-0 Tevdek placed in the fascia overlying the muscle injury. Adequate hemostasis must be obtained prior to muscle repair. When suture of the muscle fascia will result in a large muscle dead space, the dead space should be obliterated with a few interrupted sutures of 3-0 Dexon or plain catgut.

6. Since hemostasis is always meticulously controlled, drains as such are never used. If the procedure has been carried out entirely under tourniquet control and it is not feasible (primarily because of the type of anesthesia) to remove the tourniquet prior to closure, a fine multifenestrated suction catheter may be placed for wound aspiration for 48 hours, although this is rarely necessary.

7. Circular plaster casts are used to maintain immobility of the injured musculotendinous structure. In the child, it is possible and preferable to immobilize the entire extremity, including all fingers, for 3 weeks without affecting subsequent function.

8. After removal of the plaster, active but not passive motion of all joints, both involved and uninvolved, must be done. The parents must be advised to repetitively remind the child to practice his joint exercises to the point of nagging. Loss of range of motion should neither be anticipated nor complacently accepted following musculotendinous injuries in children.

## BONE INJURY

### Definitions

1. *Greenstick Fracture.* This is an incomplete fracture in which the cortex is broken on the convex side of the fracture angulation and bent on the concave side.

2. *Torus Fracture.* This is a circumferential greenstick fracture in which the cortex is buckled in a doughnut-like fashion due to axial force injury. It is completely non-displaced.

3. *Epiphyseal Fracture.* This is any fracture passing across or through an epiphyseal plate.

### Basic Principles

Fractures in children in general are handled similarly to those in adults. There are a number of striking differences, however, and in this section only those differences will be considered.

1. Closed reduction and external immobilization with traction or plaster are the *sine qua non* of good pediatric fracture management. The aphorism of Preston Wade that is often quoted, "in children's fractures never, never, never operate, but if you have to operate, never, never, never use metal, and if you have to use metal, always take it out," summarizes our approach to pediatric fracture care.

2. The ability of pediatric fractures to remold malunion has prompted an unwarranted dependence on the child's ability to develop normality from deformity. Unfortunately, Dr. Wade's facetious remark, that in children it is only necessary to have both fragments in the same ex-

tremity, has been taken literally by too many fracture surgeons. Dr. Blount has defined the factors which will assist in the remodeling after fracture. These are:

A. Youth of the patient

B. Closeness of the fracture to the epiphyseal line

C. Deformity in the plane of motion of the adjacent joint

Therefore, axial or mild angular deformity, such as dorsal displacement of a distal radial fracture within 3 cm. of the epiphysis in a 5-year-old child, almost certainly will restore itself with time to near normal anatomical configuration. The uncertainty of the degree of this remodeling and the necessity to live with the patient's parents until the remodeling has taken place so that the deformity is not clinically evident, and the possibility of legal recourse for maltreatment until the age of majority, prompts most of us to strive for the best anatomical fracture reduction possible.

3. In the lower extremities, particularly in the femur, when there has been extensive periosteal stripping, epiphyseal stimulation and bone overgrowth during the first 18 months after fracture healing is not unusual. It is for this reason that Blount emphasized the acceptability of 1 to 1.5 cm. of overriding in the reduction of femoral shaft fractures to compensate for an-

ticipated overgrowth. Again, the degree of overgrowth cannot be accurately anticipated and is even greater during the pubescent growth spurt. In axially displaced fractures, therefore, we should not strive for end-on apposition. Neither, however, should we accept 2 or more cm. of shortening because of the anticipated overgrowth. Conversely, fractures initially seen end-on should not be displaced to permit shortening. In these instances, periosteal stripping and subsequent stimulation of the epiphysis are minimal and fracture shortening will result in a shorter extremity. *It cannot be emphasized too strongly that Blount's recommendation for 1 to 1.5 cm. shortening in femoral shaft fractures (and 0.5 to 1 cm. overriding in tibial-fibular fractures) is an optimal figure, and that greater shortening should never be tolerated.*

4. Epiphyseal fractures are unique in children. A classification of types of fracture (after Salter) is shown in Figure 37-1. The possibility of epiphysiodesis increases from type I to type V. The recognition of epiphyseal fractures is of primary importance because of the subsequent disturbance in growth, and the parents must always be told (and appropriate notations made in the record of the conversation) of the possibility of failure of growth and of abnormal growth characteristics. This

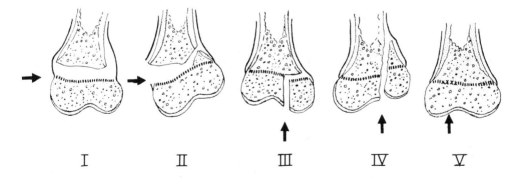

I    II    III    IV    V

Fig. 37-1. Types of epiphyseal fractures after Salter. The incidence of epiphysiodesis increases from left to right. (Salter, R. B., and Harris, W. R.: Injuries involving the epiphyseal plate. J. Bone Joint Surg., *45A*:587, 1963)

should be done even in the case of an epiphyseal fracture in which there is a small chance of growth arrest.

5. Children heal fractures rapidly, and after 10 to 21 days most fractures cannot be remanipulated to correct shortening nor can angular deformity be realigned after 14 to 21 days. Frequent check radiographs (of adequate quality and position) must be done to ensure the maintenance of reduction. Once loss of initial position is found, time should not be lost in repeating x-rays, but prompt repeat reduction under general anesthesia should be done. Slipped reductions never get better, they only get worse.

6. Children have an innate ability to break, loosen and slip out of even snug, skintight-fitting plaster. Casts must be checked frequently, especially during the first 3 weeks after reduction. Simple radiographic examination does not substitute for clinical inspection. Broken casts should be repaired, and loose casts should be replaced as soon as practical. Casts that have been bivalved or windowed should be completed prior to hospital discharge. Traction must be checked in children as frequently as every hour to be sure that they remain in proper position without the weights sitting on the floor.

## Criteria for Diagnosis

1. The signs and symptoms of fracture are essentially the same in the child as in the adult.

2. Because of the inability of the child to communicate, areas of tenderness in the extremity should be x-rayed with comparison views of the opposite extremity to differentiate fracture lines from epiphyseal areas.

## Management

1. Adequate sedation may suffice for the management of simple fractures. Nembutal, 1 mg./lb. of body weight, and Demerol, 1 mg./lb. of body weight, are given intramuscularly in children up to 50 lbs. Above 50 lbs., the per pound dose is reduced according to reaction. This dose should also be given with caution in the excessively obese child.

2. Adequate sedation should be used even before traction devices are applied to the child. This will permit manual reduction and will make the entire process of setting up the traction device less painful for both the surgeon and his young patient. Specific techniques for closed reduction and for the application of traction devices are given in Chapter 25.

3. Open fractures and epiphyseal fractures require general anesthesia with relaxation for debridement and for gentle, comparatively atraumatic reduction.

4. Open reduction, if necessary, invariably is done under general anesthesia.

5. Displaced epiphyseal fractures, as noted above, always should be reduced under general anesthesia to prevent crushing of the epiphyseal plate, which would increase the possibility of epiphysiodesis. A 70 to 80 per cent reduction of an epiphyseal fracture is preferable to repeated attempts or open reduction to achieve anatomical reposition. In some instances (epiphyseal fracture of the proximal humerus, type IV fractures of the lateral distal tibial epiphysis), open reduction is mandatory if a single attempt at closed reduction fails. Fine Kirschner wires across the epiphysis to maintain the open reduction usually do not destroy the epiphysis or provide sites of epiphysiodesis.

6. Greenstick fractures with more than 15 degrees of angular displacement, especially in the forearm, should be converted to complete fractures by breaking the cortex through entirely. In that way straight axial alignment may be obtained and retained during healing. Torus fractures merely require protection to avoid pain.

7. In the reduction of fractures in children, the order of priority is:

    A. Rotary realignment

    B. Angular correction

    C. Length

    D. Axial alignment

The use of muscle relaxants when general anesthesia is used greatly facilitates reduction. Distracting the fragments completely is necessary before reduction is carried out.

8. After reduction is obtained, plaster is applied over a single layer of stockinet or cast padding so that the subsequent cast will conform closely to the extremity contour. Casts are made heavier (in number of layers of plaster) than the adult counterparts.

9. Circular plaster is preferable to the use of plaster molds for the maintenance of reduction. However, if the primary problem relates to arterial or venous supply or to skin coverage or wound infection, appropriate anterior or posterior heavy molds may be used because of the simplicity of removal in case of supervening problems.

10. Circular plaster casts must be elevated well above heart level after application to ensure good venous return and to prevent swelling. Cyanosis, coldness of the exposed distal extremity, loss of sensation or swelling that persists after 6 hours of adequate elevation should be treated by univalving the cast and spreading it open.

11. Check radiographs must be done immediately following the application of external immobilization. This is true whether or not precasting postreduction x-rays showed good fracture position. The failure to repeat the x-rays to show maintained good fracture position following the application of plaster places the surgeon in a poor legally defensible position if subsequent x-rays show fracture slippage.

12. X-rays must also be repeated at 48 and 96 hours and whenever a cast is bivalved or changed.

13. After hospital discharge, x-rays should be repeated on a weekly basis until the first callus is visible radiographically. After that time, x-rays need only be repeated to ascertain the adequacy of healing or after removal or change of a cast.

14. After reduction of epiphyseal fractures, the immobilization is continued for the same period of time as would be carried out for a simple osseous fracture in the same region. Follow-up, however, should continue for a minimum of 3 years, with x-rays at 3-month intervals, usually with comparison views of the opposite extremity to assess epiphyseal closure.

15. Malunions or shortening should be given at least 8 to 12 months before any operative correction is considered.

16. Restoration of joint function is almost always complete in children following the removal of immobilization. The use of physiotherapy is rarely, if ever, justified. Certainly, passive range of motion exercises must be discouraged.

# APPENDIX
## SUPPLIES AND EQUIPMENT FOR THE
## EMERGENCY CARE OF THE SURGICAL PATIENT

## Common Trays for Surgical Emergency Care

1. *Minor Suture Pack*
   Large absorbent towels, 2
   4 × 4 12-ply gauze sponges, 5
   Tissue forceps, Adson, 1
   Needle holder, Baumgartner, 1
   Scissors, Metzenbaum, 1
   Sterile drape, 1
2. *Suture Removal Pack*
   Metal scissors, 1
   Metal forceps, 1
   4 × 4 gauze pads, 2
3. *Plastic Suture Set*. This is a metal tray with the following:
   Emesis basin, 1
   Prep cups, 3
   100-cc. Asepto syringe, 1
   Solution bowl, 1
   5-cc. Luer lock syringe, 1
   2-cc. syringe, 1
   Needles (22 × 1½ and 24 × ⅝), 2
   Medicine dropper, 1
   4 × 8 gauze sponges, 10
   4 × 4 gauze sponges, 10
   2 × 2 gauze sponges, 10
   Carmalt clamp, 1
   Small needle holder, Webster, 1
   Sharp scissors, 1
   Iris scissors, 1
   Mosquito clamps, 4, (2 curved, 2 straight)
   Scalpels, No. 3 handles with No. 11 and No. 15 blades, 2
   Skin hooks (large and small), 2
   Adson tissue forceps, 1
   Martin atraumatic forceps, 1
   Plain forceps, 1
   Mouse-tooth forceps, 1
   Sterile towels, 4
4. *Nasal Plastic Set*. This is a metal tray with the following:
   Large facial drape, 1
   No. 3 scalpel with a No. 11 blade, 1

10-cc. Luer lock syringe, 1
Needle, 22 × 2½, 1
Needle, 22 × 3½, 1
5-cc. syringe, 1
Needle, 22 × 1½, 1
Needle, 25 × ⅝, 1
4 × 4 compresses, 6
Nasal speculum (1 large, 1 small), 2
Scissors (iris), 1
Small curved hemostat, 1
Meede needle, 1
Large forceps, bayonet, 1
Small forceps, bayonet, 1

5. *Cutdown Tray*. This is a metal tray with the following:
   Small emesis basin, 1
   Test tube, 1
   Medicine cups, 2
   Cannulas, 3
      1 No. 18
      1 No. 16
      1 No. 14
   *Note: Mark Size on Outside Cover.*
   Needle, 24 × ⅝ or 25 × ⅝, 1
   Needle, 22 × 1½, 1
   5-cc. syringe, 1
   2-cc. syringe, 1
   No. 10 blade (no handle), 1
   Scalpel No. 3 handle with a No. 11 blade, 1
   Jansen retractor, 1
                *or*
   3-prong tracheal retractors, 2
   Needle holder, 1
   Scissors, 5-inch, 1
   Kelly clamps (2 straight, 2 curved), 4
   Mosquito clamps, 2, (1 straight, 1 curved)
   Forceps (1 anatomical, 1 plain), 2
   4 × 4 gauze pads, 2
   4 × 8 gauze pads, 2
   2 × 2 gauze pads, 2
6. *Combination Suture Pack*. This is a metal tray with the following :
   Emesis basin, 1

100-cc. Asepto syringe, 1
2-cc. syringe, 1
Needle, 24 × ⅝, 1
Needle, 22 × 1½, 1
Test tubes, 2
Solution bowls, 3
Iodine cup, 1
Medicine cup, 1
Kelly clamps, 3
Needle holder, 1
Scissors, 1
Probe, 1
Groove director, 1
Plain anatomical forceps, 1
Scalpel (No. 4 handle with a No. 20 blade), 1
4 × 4 gauze sponges, 5
2 × 2 gauze sponges, 5
Large drape, 1

7. *Tracheostomy Tray.* This is a metal tray with the following:
Scalpel, No. 3 handle with a No. 11 blade, 1
Scalpel, No. 4. handle with a No. 20 blade, 1
3-prong retractors, 2
2-prong retractors, 2
Needle holder, 1
Scissors (curved), 1
Metzenbaum scissors, 1
Kelly clamps (curved), 4
Kelly clamps (straight), 2
Allis clamps, 2
Mosquito clamps (curved), 4
Mosquito clamps (straight), 4
Forceps, anatomical plain, 1
Forceps, mouse-tooth, 1
Tracheal dilator (3-prong, Jackson-Delaborde), 1
Delaney retractors, 2
Tracheal hook (single-prong) in bag, 1
Towel clips, 4
Trach tubes (Nos. 6, 7, 8, 9), 4
Whistle-tip catheter (No. 16 or 18), 1
Emesis basis, 1
Medicine glasses, 2
2-cc. syringe, 1
5-cc. syringe, 1
Needle, 25 × ⅝, 1
Needle, 20 × 1½, 1
Towels, 4

*On Pediatric Tray:*
Doctor's gown, 1
Mask, 1
Cap, 1
Trach tubes (Nos. 0, 1, 2, 3, 4, 5,), 6
Whistle-tip catheter (No. 10), 1

8. *Thoracostomy Tray (Emergency Chest), Adult.* This is a metal tray with the following:
Plain anatomical forceps, 1
Mouse-tooth forceps, 1
Mosquito clamps, 2, (1 straight, 1 curved)
Kocher clamp, 1
Trocar and cannula No. 33 French, 1
Towel clamps, 4
Carmalt clamps 2, (1 straight, 1 curved),
Probe, 1
Groove director, 1
Kelly clamps (2 straight, 2 curved), 4
Needle holder, 1
Scissors, 1
Scalpel handles (No. 3 with No. 11 blade and No. 4 with No. 20 blade), 2
Sims suction tip, plastic, 1
Kidney basin, 1
Solution bowl, 1
Plastic connecting tubes, ⅜-inch, 2
Medicine glasses (1 metal, 2 cups), 3
Test tubes, 2
Pezzer catheters (1 No. 38 and 1 No. 40), 2
Malecot catheters (4-wing) (1 No. 38 and 1 No. 40), 2
5-cc. syringe, 1
10-cc. syringe, 1
20-cc. syringe, 1
Safety pins, 2
Needles, 5
   1 24 × ⅝
   1 22 × 1½
   1 19 × 2
   1 18 × 2
   1 15 × 3
Towel compresses, 4
*For the pediatric tray add:*
Cap, 1
Mask, 1
Gown, 1

*and substitute:*
Malecot catheters, No. 22 to No. 26f, 3
Pezzer catheters, Nos. 22 to 32f, 6

## Additional Equipment

1. Cardiac pacemaker/defibrillator
2. Max Cart which includes a:
Monitor
Pacemaker
Defibrillator/pacemaker
Monitor or defibrillator
Pacemaker synchronizer
3. ECG machines
4. Hypo/hyperthermia machine
5. The following various supplies which also are needed to function effectively may be obtained from the surgical service or the central supply department:
Anesthesia extension sets
Angiocaths (all sizes)
Asepto packs
Basins (soak, large and small)
Berman oral airways (all sizes)
Burn trays (major and minor)
Cantor tubes
Cardiac arrest tray with internal defibrillator paddles
Catheterization sets
Culture tubes
Cutdown catheters (small, medium, large, extra large x 18 inches)
    (small, medium, large, extra large x 36 inches)
Dialysis catheters and equipment
Drainage tubing
Endotracheal tubes (Nos. 6, 7, 8, 9, and 10)
Ewald tubes
Foley catheters (5-cc. and 30-cc. bags) (sizes 12, 14, 16, 18, 20, 22 and 24f)
French catheters (sizes 10, 12, 14, 16, 18, 20 and 22f)
Furacin roll and gauze
Gloves (disposable)
Infusion packs
Intracardiac needles (Nos. 20, 22, 23 × 3¼ or 6 inches)
Intracaths (all sizes)
Intravenous catheters

Kling bandage
Labor bundles
Leuken traps
Levin tubes
Medical cutdown catheters (small, medium, large and extra large)
Medicuts (sizes 14, 16, 18 and 20)
Miller-Abbott tubes
Minimeters
Morgue packs
Nasotracheal tubes (sizes 6, 7, 8, 9 and 10)
Needles (sizes 18, 19, 20, 22, 24 and 25 gauge (g))
Oxygen catheters, masks and tubing
Paracentesis sets
Pediatric feeding tubes (sizes 8 and 10f)
Pediatric scalp vein sets
Pleura-Vac sets
Prep packs
Scalpels
Sengstaken tubes
Spinal packs
Spinal needles
Sterile caps, gowns and masks
Sterile urine bottles (sizes 12, 14, 18 and 20)
Sump tubes
Syringes (sizes 2-cc. with No. 25 needles, 2-cc. with No. 22 needles, 5-cc. with No. 22 and 20 needles, 10-cc. with No. 22 and 20 needles, 20-cc., 30-cc., 50-cc., 30-cc. and 50-cc. with catheter tip)
Teflon needles (BD No. 01-0049)
Thoracocentesis sets
Tracheostomy care sets
Transfusion packs (obtained from blood bank by messenger)
Intravenous catheters
Uri-Meters
Vaseline gauze and package
Venous pressure sets
Subclavian catheter set
Solution administration set and without minidrops
Scalp vein set (all sizes)
Enema set
Clear plastic connecting tubing
Specimen bottles

# INDEX

The notation, t, indicates a table.

645